Re-Visioning Psychiatry

Re-Visioning Psychiatry explores new theories and models from cultural psychiatry and psychology, philosophy, neuroscience, and anthropology that clarify how mental health problems emerge in specific contexts and points toward future integration of these perspectives. Taken together, the contributions point to the need for fundamental shifts in psychiatric theory and practice:

- restoring phenomenology to its rightful place in research and practice;
- advancing the social and cultural neuroscience of brain–person–environment systems over time and across social contexts;
- understanding how self-awareness, interpersonal interactions, and larger social processes give rise to vicious circles that constitute mental health problems;
- locating efforts to help and heal within the local and global social, economic, and political contexts that influence how we frame problems and imagine solutions.

In advancing ecosystemic models of mental disorders, contributors challenge reductionistic models and culture-bound perspectives and highlight possibilities for a more transdisciplinary, integrated approach to research, mental health policy, and clinical practice.

LAURENCE J. KIRMAYER, MD, FRCPC, is James McGill Professor and Director, Division of Social and Transcultural Psychiatry, Department of Psychiatry, at McGill University. He is editor-in-chief of *Transcultural Psychiatry* and Director of the Culture and Mental Health Research Unit at the Institute of Community and Family Psychiatry, Jewish General Hospital in Montreal, where he conducts research on culturally responsive mental health services, global mental health, and the anthropology of psychiatry.

ROBERT LEMELSON, PhD, is currently an associate adjunct professor in the Department of Anthropology and a research anthropologist at the Semel Institute of Neuroscience, both at UCLA. He is also the president and founder of the Foundation for Psychocultural Research, a nonprofit research foundation supporting research and training in the neurosciences and social sciences.

CONSTANCE A. CUMMINGS, PhD, is project director of the Foundation for Psychocultural Research. She is coeditor of *Formative Experiences: The Interaction of Caregiving, Culture, Developmental Psychobiology* (Cambridge University Press, 2010) and a forthcoming volume on culture, mind, and brain.

Re-Visioning Psychiatry

Cultural Phenomenology, Critical Neuroscience, and Global Mental Health

Edited by

Laurence J. Kirmayer
McGill University

Robert Lemelson
The Foundation for Psychocultural Research and UCLA

Constance A. Cummings
The Foundation for Psychocultural Research

CAMBRIDGE
UNIVERSITY PRESS

CAMBRIDGE
UNIVERSITY PRESS

University Printing House, Cambridge CB2 8BS, United Kingdom

One Liberty Plaza, 20th Floor, New York, NY 10006, USA

477 Williamstown Road, Port Melbourne, VIC 3207, Australia

4843/24, 2nd Floor, Ansari Road, Daryaganj, Delhi - 110002, India

79 Anson Road, #06-04/06, Singapore 079906

Cambridge University Press is part of the University of Cambridge.

It furthers the University's mission by disseminating knowledge in the pursuit of education, learning and research at the highest international levels of excellence.

www.cambridge.org
Information on this title: www.cambridge.org/9781108431538

© Cambridge University Press 2015

First published 2015
First paperback edition 2017

A catalogue record for this publication is available from the British Library

Library of Congress Cataloging in Publication data
Re-visioning psychiatry : cultural phenomenology, critical neuroscience, and global mental health / edited by Laurence J. Kirmayer, Robert Lemelson, Constance A. Cummings.
    p. ; cm.
Re-visioning psychiatry
Includes bibliographical references and index.
ISBN 978-1-107-03220-0 (Hardback)
I. Kirmayer, Laurence J., 1952–, editor.   II. Lemelson, Robert, 1952–, editor.
III. Cummings, Constance A., editor.   IV. Title: Re-visioning psychiatry.
[DNLM: 1. Psychiatry–trends.   2. Mental Disorders–etiology.
3. Neuropsychiatry–trends.   4. Sociological Factors. WM 100]
RC454
616.89–dc23   2014050247

ISBN 978-1–107-03220-0 Hardback
ISBN 978-1-108-43153-8 Paperback

To all who struggle with "mind-forg'd manacles,"
their families, friends, and caregivers.

What is meaningful cannot in fact be isolated.... We achieve understanding within a circular movement from particular facts to the whole that includes them and back again from the whole thus reached to the particular significant facts.

– Karl Jaspers, *General Psychopathology*

Though I personally favor both alcohol and neurologizing in moderation ... psychology is intoxicating itself with a worse brand than it need use.

– D. O. Hebb, "Drives and the C.N.S. (Conceptual Nervous System)"

To make psychology into experimental epistemology is to attempt to understand the embodiment of mind.

– Warren McCulloch, *Embodiments of Mind*

We are most of us governed by epistemologies that we know to be wrong.

– Gregory Bateson, *Steps to an Ecology of Mind*

Le fait que je sois moi est hanté par l'existence de l'autre.

– Frantz Fanon, *Rencontre de la Société et de la Psychiatrie*

Contents

Section Two: Biosocial Mechanisms in Mental Health and Illness

Section Three: Cultural Contexts of Psychopathology

Figures

Color plates follow page 450.

Tables

Contributors

NEIL KRISHAN AGGARWAL, MD, MBA, MA, Assistant Professor, Department of Psychiatry, Columbia College of Physicians and Surgeons; Research Psychiatrist, NYS Center of Excellence for Cultural Competence, NY State Psychiatric Institute

KALMAN APPLBAUM, PhD, Professor, Department of Anthropology, University of Wisconsin–Milwaukee

ANNE E. BECKER, MD, PhD, SM, Maude and Lillian Presley Professor of Global Health and Social Medicine, Department of Global Health and Social Medicine, Harvard Medical School; Department of Psychiatry, Massachusetts General Hospital

GERMAN E. BERRIOS, MD, FRCPSYCH, FBPSS, FMEDSCI, Chair of Epistemology of Psychiatry, Robinson College and Department of Psychiatry, School of Clinical Medicine, University of Cambridge

ROBERT M. BILDER, PhD, Michael E. Tennenbaum Professor of Psychiatry and Biobehavioral Sciences and Psychology, UCLA Semel Institute for Neuroscience and Human Behavior

YULIA E. CHENTSOVA-DUTTON, PhD, Associate Professor, Department of Psychology, Georgetown University

THOMAS J. CSORDAS, PhD, Professor, Department of Anthropology, University of California, San Diego

CONSTANCE A. CUMMINGS, PhD, Project Director, the Foundation for Psychocultural Research

ADEL FARAH, Graduate Student, McGill Group for Suicide Studies, Douglas Mental Health University Institute, McGill University

SHAUN GALLAGHER, PhD, Lillian and Morrie Moss Professor of Excellence in Philosophy, Department of Philosophy, University of Memphis; Research Professor of Philosophy and Cognitive Science, University of Hertfordshire

IAN GOLD, PhD, Associate Professor of Philosophy and Psychiatry, McGill University

JAMES L. GRIFFITH, MD, Professor, Department of Psychiatry and Behavioral Science, George Washington University Medical Center

DEVON E. HINTON, MD, PhD, Associate Professor of Psychiatry, Massachusetts General Hospital, Harvard Medical School

NEV JONES, PhD, Postdoctoral Fellow, Department of Anthropology, Stanford University

LAURENCE J. KIRMAYER, MD, FRCPC, James McGill Professor and Director, Division of Social and Transcultural Psychiatry, Department of Psychiatry, McGill University

ARTHUR KLEINMAN, MD, MA, Esther and Sidney Rabb Professor, Department of Anthropology, Harvard University; Professor of Medical Anthropology in Global Health and Social Medicine and Professor of Psychiatry, Harvard Medical School

BRANDON A. KOHRT, MD, PhD, Assistant Professor, Global Health and Cultural Anthropology, Duke Global Health Institute; Department of Psychiatry and Behavioral Sciences, Duke University School of Medicine

BENOIT LABONTÉ, PhD, Postdoctoral Fellow, Nestler Laboratory, Fishberg Department of Neuroscience, Icahn School of Medicine at Mount Sinai

CECILE D. LADOUCEUR, PhD, Assistant Professor, Department of Psychiatry, Western Psychiatric Institute and Clinic, University of Pittsburgh School of Medicine

ROBERT LEMELSON, PhD, President, the Foundation for Psychocultural Research; Associate Adjunct Professor, Department of Anthropology, UCLA

ROBERTO LEWIS-FERNÁNDEZ, MD, Professor, Department of Psychiatry, Columbia College of Physicians and Surgeons; Director, NYS Center of Excellence for Cultural Competence, and Hispanic Treatment Program, NY State Psychiatric Institute

T. M. LUHRMANN, PhD, Watkins University Professor, Department of Anthropology, Stanford University

ETHAN MACDONALD, BS Candidate in Neuroscience; Research Assistant, Cognitive Neuroscience Laboratory, McGill University

IVANA S. MARKOVÁ, MBChB, MPhil, MD, FRCPsych, Reader in Psychiatry, Center for Health and Population Sciences, Hull York Medical School

KWAME MCKENZIE, MD, MRCPsych, Professor, Department of Psychiatry, University of Toronto; Professor, Institute of Philosophy Diversity and Mental Health, University of Lancashire

GEORG NORTHOFF, MD, PhD, FRCPC, Canada Research Chair in Mind, Brain Imaging and Neuroethics; ELJB-CIHR Michael Smith Chair in Neurosciences and Mental Health, Institute of Mental Health Research, University of Ottawa; http://www.georgnorthoff.com

JOSEF PARNAS, MD, DrMedSci, Clinical Professor of Psychiatry, Department of Clinical Medicine, Department of Neurology, Psychiatry and Sensory Sciences, University of Copenhagen

DUNCAN PEDERSEN, MD, MPH, Associate Scientific Director, International Programs, Douglas Mental Health University Institute; Associate Professor, Department of Psychiatry and Division of Social and Transcultural Psychiatry, McGill University

MARY L. PHILLIPS, MD, Professor in Psychiatry and Clinical and Translational Science; Director of the Clinical and Translational Affective Neuroscience Program, Department of Psychiatry, Western Psychiatric Institute and Clinic, University of Pittsburgh School of Medicine

EUGENE RAIKHEL, PhD, Assistant Professor, Department of Comparative Human Development, University of Chicago

AMIR RAZ, PhD, ABPH, Professor, Departments of Psychiatry, Neurology and Neurosurgery; Associate Professor, Department of Psychology; Canada Research Chair in the Cognitive Neuroscience of Attention, McGill University and SMBD Jewish General Hospital

ANDREW G. RYDER, PhD, Associate Professor, Department of Psychology and Centre for Clinical Research and Health, Concordia University and Affiliated Researcher, Culture and Mental Health Research Unit and Lady Davis Institute, Jewish General Hospital

JAI SHAH, MD, FRCPC, Assistant Professor, Department of Psychiatry, McGill University; Researcher, Douglas Hospital Research Center; Psychiatrist, Prevention and Early Intervention Program for Psychosis (PEPP-Montréal), Douglas Mental Health University Institute

NAOMI M. SIMON, MD, MS, Director, Center for Anxiety and Traumatic Stress Disorders Director, Complicated Grief Program; Associate Professor of Psychiatry, Harvard Medical School

JENNIFER J. THOMAS, PhD, Co-Director, Eating Disorders Clinical and Research Program, Massachusetts General Hospital; Assistant Professor of Psychology, Department of Psychiatry, Harvard Medical School

ANNIE TUCKER, PhD, Lecturer, Disabilities Studies Minor, UCLA; Senior Researcher, Elemental Productions

GUSTAVO TURECKI, MD, PhD, Associate Professor of Psychiatry, Human Genetics and Neuroscience; Chair, Department of Psychiatry, McGill University; Director, McGill Group for Suicide Studies; Head, Depressive Disorders Program, Douglas Mental Health University Institute

AMELIA VERSACE, MD, Instructor, Department of Psychiatry, University of Pittsburgh School of Medicine

Foreword

The trouble with psychiatry as an academic and intellectual field goes far back, as do efforts at reform and remaking. Today, psychiatry is still troubled, and efforts at reform and remaking are again under way.

Nineteenth-century alienists were often isolated, cut off from the rest of medicine and from developments in the wider society. The moral treatment movement sought to remake "dreadful asylums" with their punitive "treatments." Freudianism began as one among many types of psychological treatments aimed at making the biography of the patient, as well as a more progressive understanding of the therapeutic process, humanize care. In time, psychoanalysis swept away its psychotherapeutic rivals and became a powerful but limiting orthodoxy that not only dominated American psychiatry but also turned its back on science, while routinizing its methodology as a kind of psychic reverse engineering.

Now we are in the age of the hegemony of biological psychiatry, which seems a perfect fit with an American health care system that has replaced quality with efficiency and cost-cutting and has turned the broad competencies of psychiatrists into the narrowest framing as psychopharmacologists. Like a flood tide, it has washed away much of psychosocial and clinical research, replacing both with a romantic quest for a neuroscientific utopia as its holy grail, which has little relevance to the work of practitioners.

After a half century of serious biological research, it seems that all but the true believers are beginning to lose confidence and are feeling ashamed of the simple fact that we do not understand the pathophysiology of depression, anxiety disorders, bipolar disorder, or schizophrenia. Nor do we possess a single biological test that can be routinely applied in the clinic to diagnose these or other mental disorders – which, given the large investments in biological research, is nothing short of scandalous. Tellingly, if sadly, the Director of the National Institute of Mental Health (NIMH) at NIH – the pinnacle of science in the mental health field – has given up on the profession's controversial diagnostic system (*DSM-5*) and, seemingly, on psychiatry itself, confessing that the only hope is for a new discipline of clinical neuroscience, which will be decades in the making. The NIMH supports few academics who do other forms of research: talk about putting all your eggs in one basket!

Meanwhile, medical students are voting with their feet. They go into other fields of medicine that seem more promising. Psychologists, behavioral neurologists, primary care physicians, and geriatric specialists divide up the common mental disorders among themselves, leaving psychiatry with the psychoses, as in the days of the alienists. Add to this diminished picture the more recent outcome findings that make psychiatric medications appear barely better than placebo treatments, as well as the fact that an entire generation of psychosocial and clinical researchers has been lost due to the absence of research funding, and the need for change toward new directions seems urgent.

There are positive things to build on, of course. In spite of the irrelevance of much of academic psychiatry for clinical practice, psychiatric clinicians still have useful interventions that they can and do offer to help sufferers. Global mental health and community psychiatry are exciting fields with evidence of implementable interventions that matter. As this collection well illustrates, these fields – together with the small but enduring field of cultural psychiatry and recent efforts to connect neuroscience with social research and concerns – are all providing evidence of new directions.

My own minor contributions to this recurrent story of remaking psychiatry include a 1977 coedited volume, *Renewal in Psychiatry*, which in honoring my mentor, Leon Eisenberg, offered up distinctly different examples of psychiatric science that went against the grain of the then declining dominance of psychoanalytic approaches in psychiatry. My 1988 book, *Rethinking Psychiatry*, perhaps too precociously, advanced cultural psychiatry and psychiatric anthropology as a new paradigm for psychiatry by showing what would happen if psychiatry began with culture as an underlying principle. In 2013, together with several other physician anthropologists, I coedited *Reimagining Global Health*, which once again emphasized a new direction for mental health, calling for interventions in resource-limited societies based on comparative case studies, relevant social theories, local and global history, and implementation of proven interventions.

It is intriguing that each of those volumes, as well as *Re-Visioning Psychiatry*, begins with the prefix "re-" in the title. Almost all of the definitions listed in the *Oxford English Dictionary* (OED) for this prefix seem relevant: "going back to origins," "undoing some prior efforts," "stopping things from going forward." What the OED doesn't list that the present volume and its predecessors illustrate is a sense of strong critique combined with arguments for reform that include practical recommendations for ways forward.

Re-Visioning Psychiatry deserves a wide audience that goes well beyond the many fields canvassed by the editors and contributors. The volume offers useful demonstrations of how psychiatry is being remade anew, under the very feet of the biological hegemon, in a biosocial direction that insists on the centrality of cultural, psychosocial, and global processes in the classification and diagnosis of mental disorders, to be sure, but also in the experience of caregiving and in policies and programs. And in this refashioning there is an important place for neuroscience; a place in which social processes and neural ones are understood as interacting and interconnected.

Will such works change psychiatry? I think over the long haul they could; in fact, they must, because psychiatry truly needs to change if it is to survive as a robust and significant field. Whatever neuroscience can contribute, and I hope it is a great deal, psychiatry must engage other narratives and treatment experiences, as well as the most deeply human context of clinical relationships and caregiving. Emotions, moral life, the local worlds that patients and families inhabit, and clinicians, too, and the economic and political forces that shape those worlds and institutions – all should matter for psychiatrists, both clinically and in research. Resocializing psychiatry, and understanding that to include neuroscience, too, is the prescription to revivify the intellectual as well as the practical sides of this troubled field. "Re-Visioning" is not at all a bad metaphor for a field that has become blind both to its roots and its extensions. This is far too important and complex an intellectual and practical domain – in far too complex, uncertain, and dangerous a world – to leave psychiatry in the hands of laboratory scientists and bureaucrats. Nothing short of original, outside-the-box, interdisciplinary approaches are needed, and, as this volume attests, they are on the way.

Arthur Kleinman
Harvard University

Preface

The diagnostic language of psychiatry has come to define the ways in which we think about many human problems and predicaments. In recent years, many have hoped that brain research will give us a clearer map of the varieties of mental disorder than our descriptive categories can provide and clarify their origins, mechanisms, and effective treatment. In pursuing this vision, researchers and practitioners have often set aside the social, cultural, political, and historical contexts of suffering. Yet attention to the phenomenology of psychiatric disorders points to the importance of culture and context for understanding mental health and illness.

Re-Visioning Psychiatry explores new models from philosophy, neuroscience, and anthropology, along with cutting-edge work in social and cultural psychiatry and psychology, that clarify the ways in which mental health problems emerge in specific biological, social, and cultural contexts and that point toward the future integration of these perspectives. The book is based on the premise that psychiatric problems reflect the interactions of biological and sociocultural systems that can be described in terms of dimensions of functioning, developmental trajectories, thresholds of tolerance, and feedback loops.

Biological, psychological, social, economic, and political circumstances all may contribute to vicious circles that cause and maintain symptoms, suffering, and disability. These systems are *ecological* in the sense that they involve the individual as a biological organism embedded in and in constant transaction with the environment on multiple scales of time and space. In advancing ecosystemic models of mental disorders, the contributors challenge some of the reductionistic assumptions and culture-bound perspectives of psychiatry and highlight the possibilities of a more transdisciplinary, integrated approach to research, clinical practice, and social policy to promote mental health and well-being. This approach goes beyond the biopsychosocial approach by making explicit the causal links and mechanisms – as well as the tensions and contradictions – across levels of organization and description.

The book is based in part on presentations from the fourth interdisciplinary conference cohosted by the Foundation for Psychocultural Research (FPR; http://thefpr.org) and UCLA, which was organized by the editors in January 2010. The mission of the FPR is to support and advance interdisciplinary and integrative research and training on interactions of culture, neuroscience, psychiatry, and psychology, with an emphasis on cultural processes as central. The FPR's primary objective is to help articulate and support the creation of transformative paradigms that address issues of fundamental clinical and social concern. The 2010 conference was unique in several ways: its interdisciplinary focus; the quality of scholarship by a group of distinguished contributors from biology, neuroscience, anthropology, and psychiatry; and the emphasis on identifying key questions and research opportunities at the intersection of biology and culture. Panel discussions allowed participants to explore issues of integration across disciplines. The interdisciplinary exchanges raised some of the provocative questions that are pursued in this volume:

- What is the right conceptual vocabulary to use in thinking about mental disorders and devising effective clinical, social, and political responses?
- How can a phenomenological understanding of mental illness that explores the everyday realities for persons living with disorder inform psychiatric theory, research, and practice?
- What are the key sites for understanding brain–body–environment interactions (e.g., genome, cell, circuit, functional system, and networks)? What theoretical, computational, and experimental approaches can model the complex interactions across levels of analysis? How can concepts of dynamical systems (e.g., dimensions of functioning, developmental trajectories, thresholds of tolerance, and feedback loops) illuminate the nature of psychiatric disorders?
- How do particular adverse situations, such as those that expose individuals to early life stress, poor social support, endemic violence, forced migration, social exclusion, or discrimination, affect psychophysiological processes and neuro- and psychodevelopmental trajectories?
- How do social and cultural contexts shape psychiatric theory and practice? In particular, given that diagnostic labels have a social life beyond the confines of psychiatry, how is psychiatric nosology changing the ways in which people think about their own health and well-being or sense of self and personhood? What are the social, ethical, and political implications of these changes?

This book begins with a return to the basic phenomenology of mental disorders, with chapters from historical, philosophical, neuroscientific, anthropological, and clinical perspectives. The second part explores recent developments in biology that provide ways to understand the impact of social and cultural processes, including groundbreaking work in epigenetics, neural circuitry, and cognitive neuroscience. The third part focuses on the impact of social and cultural contexts on mental disorders, influencing underlying mechanisms and the ways in which distress is understood, expressed, and resolved. The fourth and final part explores the implications for psychiatric practice of the interactional and contextual view, moving from considerations of cross-cultural diagnosis, case formulation, and intervention, to the larger issues of the political economy of international psychiatry and the movement for global mental health. The book concludes with a chapter on future directions in the prevention, intervention, and treatment of mental illness. The aim then is to open up new ways of thinking about mental health problems, which can contribute to a revisioned and reinvigorated discipline that responds to the needs of people with interventions that are truly helpful and healing.

Moving beyond theorizing to research and treatment will be a key challenge as the complementary approaches presented in this volume evolve. The conferences organized by the FPR – *Posttraumatic Stress Disorder: Biological, Clinical and Cultural Approaches to Trauma's Effects* in 2002; *Four Dimensions of Childhood* in 2005; *Seven Dimensions of Emotion* in 2007; *Cultural and Biological Contexts of Psychiatric Disorder* in 2010; and *Culture, Mind, and Brain* in 2012 – and the volumes emerging from these conferences provide numerous examples of the ways forward. We take this opportunity to thank all of our contributing authors, as well as the speakers, panelists, and audience members of the FPR conferences, and especially the FPR board – Carole Browner, Marie-Françoise Chesselet, Douglas Hollan, Marjorie Kagawa-Singer, Marvin Karno, Steven López, and Beate Ritz – who have taken part in countless ways to shape our work; it is truly a collaborative effort.

Laurence Kirmayer thanks all the many friends and colleagues at McGill University, the Institute of Community and Family Psychiatry of the Jewish General Hospital, and the FPR who have contributed to this work. Special thanks for many stimulating conversations to Nicola Casacalenda, Suparna Choudhury, Daniel Frank, Ian Gold, Danielle Groleau, Jaswant Guzder, Eric Jarvis, Joel Paris, Duncan Pedersen, Amir Raz, Cécile Rousseau, Andrew Ryder, Robert Whitley, and Allan Young. Elizabeth Anthony was generous with her time, clinical acumen, and editorial expertise.

Robert Lemelson would like to thank the FPR board and staff. The FPR is now entering its fifteenth year with the same group of people, and he is both appreciative and proud of their deep dedication and efforts in blazing new pathways in scientific research and education.

Constance Cummings extends thanks to the following people: FPR Director Irene Sukwandi (without whom the FPR and this project could not exist); and Aleta Coursen, Dede Cummings, Alan Gesek, Erin Hartshorn, Bonnie Kaiser, Carolyn Kasper, Linda Thompson, Kathy Trang, and Mamie Wong for their close readings, expert suggestions, and skillful edits to figures and text.

Finally, the editors thank Cambridge University Press, in particular our former editor Simina Calin, and our current editor Matthew Bennett and former senior editorial assistant Elizabeth Janetschek, for their unwavering enthusiasm and patience.

Abbreviations

AA	Alcoholics Anonymous
ACC	anterior cingulate cortex
ACG	anterior cingulate gyrus
ACh	acetylcholine
aCMS	anterior cortical midline structures
ACTH	adrenocorticotropic hormone
AD(H)D	attention deficit (hyperactivity) disorder
ADRA2A	alpha-2A receptor gene
AF	arcuate fasciculus
AIDS	acquired immunodeficiency syndrome
AMY	amygdala
AN	anorexia nervosa
ANS	autonomic nervous system
APA	American Psychiatric Association
AR	androgen receptor
ASAM	American Society of Addiction Medicine
AT	attention training
AVP	arginine vasopressin
B6	stress-resilient mouse strain
BALB	stress-susceptible mouse strain
B.B.	Bahasa Bali, Balinese
BD	bipolar disorder
BDI	Beck Depression Inventory
BD-I, II	bipolar disorder type I and II
BDNF	brain-derived neurotrophic factor
BD-NOS	bipolar disorder, not otherwise specified
B.I.	Bahasa Indonesia, Indonesian
BMI	body mass index
BN	bulimia nervosa
BPQ	body perception questionnaire
BPSD	behavioral and psychological symptoms of dementia

CAG	cytosine–adenine–guanine
cAMP	cyclic adenosine monophosphate
CATIE	Clinical Antipsychotic Trials of Intervention Effectiveness (study)
CBIT	comprehensive behavioral intervention for tics
CBT	cognitive behavioral therapy
CFI	Cultural Formulation Interview
CLI	Child Led Indicators
CMA	critical medical anthropology
CMDs	common mental disorders
CMS	cortical midline structures
CNS	central nervous system
COMT	catechol-*O*-methyltransferase gene
COPSI	Community Care for People with Schizophrenia in India
CpG	cytosine–phosphate–guanine dinucleotide
CPSWs	community psychosocial workers
CRE	cAMP-response element
CRH	corticotropin-releasing hormone (also referred to as CRF; corticotropin-releasing factor)
CSF	cerebrospinal fluid
CSTC	cortico-striatal-thalamo-cortical
c/s/x	consumer/survivor/ex-patient
CST	community support team
CT	computerized tomography
DA	dopamine
DAT1	dopamine active transporter 1 gene (also known as *SLC6A3*)
DALY	disability-adjusted life year
DDNOS	dissociative disorder, not otherwise specified
DfID	Department for International Development (U.K.)
DLPFC	dorsolateral prefrontal cortex
DMN	default mode network
DMPFC	dorsomedial prefrontal cortex
DMT	dorsomedial thalamus
DNA	deoxyribonucleic acid
DNMT	DNA methyltransferase(s)
DOSMD	Determinants of Outcome of Severe Mental Disorder
DRD4	dopamine receptor D4 gene
DSM	*Diagnostic and Statistical Manual of Mental Disorders*
DTI	diffusion tensor imaging
EDE	Eating Disorder Examination
EDE-Q	Eating Disorder Examination-Questionnaire

EDNOS	eating disorder, not otherwise specified
EFNBACK	Emotional Face N-Back Task
ELA	early-life adversity
EP	epistemology of psychiatry
FA	fractional anisotropy
FDA	Food and Drug Administration (U.S.)
FIRB	fixated interests and repetitive behaviors
FKBP5	gene involved in regulating the HPA axis
FMM	factor mixture modeling
fMRI	functional magnetic resonance imaging
FSL	functional magnetic resonance imaging of the brain software library
GABA	gamma aminobutyric acid
GAD	generalized anxiety disorder
GC	glucocorticoid
GDNF	glial cell-derived neurotrophic factor
GED	General Educational Development
Glx	glutamate and glutamine
GMH	global mental health
GPPPs	global public–private partnerships
GR	glucocorticoid receptor
GWAS	genome-wide association studies
HBO	healthy bipolar offspring (8–17 years old) with at least one parent diagnosed with bipolar disorder
HC	healthy control
HIC	high-income countries
HIV	human immunodeficiency virus
HMIS	health management information systems
HPA	hypothalamic–pituitary–adrenal (axis)
HPC	hippocampus
HRT	habit reversal training
ICD	International Classification of Diseases
ICH	International Committee on Harmonization
ICPC	International Classification of Primary Care
ILF	inferior longitudinal fasciculus
IMD	institute for mental disease
IPA	International Psychogeriatric Association
IPSS	International Pilot Study of Schizophrenia
KFPEC	Kosovar Family Professional Educational Collaborative

K-SADS-PL	Kiddie Schedule for Schizophrenia and Affective Disorders Present and Lifetime
LG	licking and grooming (of rat pups)
LMIC	low- and middle-income countries
LSD	lysergic acid diethylamide
MAOA	monoamine oxidase gene
MD	maternal deprivation
MD	mean diffusivity
MDD	major depressive disorder
MdPFC	dorsomedial prefrontal cortex
MEG	magnetoencephalography
mhGAP-IG	*Mental Health Gap Action Programme Implementation Guideline*
MINI	McGill Illness Narrative Interview
MNS	mental, neurological, and substance use
mPFC	medial prefrontal cortex
MRI	magnetic resonance imaging
mRNA	messenger ribonucleic acid
MRS	magnetic resonance spectroscopy
MTR	magnetization transfer ratio
NAMI	National Alliance for the Mentally Ill
NCS-A	National Comorbidity Survey-Adolescent Supplement
NE	norepinephrine
NFP-AN	non-fat-phobic anorexia nervosa
NGF1-A	nerve growth transcription factor
NGO	nongovernmental organization
NIDA	National Institute on Drug Abuse
NIH	National Institutes of Health
NIMH	National Institute of Mental Health
NSA	National Security Agency
OCD	obsessive-compulsive disorder
OFC	orbitofrontal cortex
OSFED	other specified feeding or eating disorder
PACC	perigenual anterior cingulate cortex
PAG	periaqueductal gray
PC	primary care
PCC	posterior cingulate cortex
PCPs	primary care physicians
PD	panic disorder
PET	positron emission tomography
PFC	prefrontal cortex
PHPC	parahippocampus

PhRMA	Pharmaceutical Research and Manufacturers of America
PLOS	Public Library of Science
PMDD	premenstrual dysphoric disorder
POMC	proopiomelanocortin
PRIME	Programme for Improving Mental Health Care
PPV	public–private ventures
PTSD	posttraumatic stress disorder
PVN	paraventricular nucleus (of the hypothalamus)
rCBF	regional cerebral blood flow
RD	radial diffusivity
RDoC	Research Domain Criteria project
RMPs	rural medical practitioners
RNA	ribonucleic acid
ROI	region of interest
SACC	supragenual anterior cingulate cortex
SAD	social anxiety disorder
SCDs	social communication deficits
SLF	superior longitudinal fasciculus
SNS	sympathetic nervous system
SPL	superior parietal lobe
SRO	single-room occupancy hotel
SSDI	Social Security Disability Insurance
SSI	Supplemental Security Income
SSRI	serotonin–selective reuptake inhibitor
SWAN	strengths and weaknesses of ADHD symptoms and normal behavior
SWYEPT	Southwest Youth and the Experience of Psychiatric Treatment
T	thalamus
TBSS	tract-based spatial statistical (analysis)
TD	tardive dyskinesia
TID	task-induced deactivation
TP	temporal pole
TPJ	temporal parietal junction
TPO	Transcultural Psychocial Organization
TRIPS	Trade-Related Aspects of International Property Rights
TrkB	tyrosine receptor kinase B
TrkB.T1	astrocytic variant of TrkB
TS	Tourette syndrome

VLPFC	ventrolateral prefrontal cortex
VMPFC	ventromedial prefrontal cortex
VS	ventral striatum
WHO	World Health Organization
WHO-AIMS	World Health Organization Assessment Instrument for Mental Health Systems
WPA	World Psychiatric Association
WTO	World Trade Organization
YLD	years lived with disability

1 Introduction: Psychiatry at a Crossroads

Laurence J. Kirmayer, Robert Lemelson,
and Constance A. Cummings

Psychiatry today faces challenges on many fronts, with vigorous critiques of its theory and practice from clinicians, scholars, and people with lived experience of mental health problems. These critiques target the slow progress in understanding and treating mental illness, overreliance on medications and other biomedical treatments, and the lack of attention to patients' lifeworlds and aspirations, but extend to much broader concerns about the medicalization of everyday life, and even wholesale condemnation of psychiatry as a source of heavy-handed social control, stigma, and harmful interventions that actually undermine recovery. In recent years, many of the concerns of the antipsychiatry movement of the 1960s have been reasserted by a new critical psychiatry literature that builds on these earlier critiques but includes attention to contemporary questions of epistemology, political economy, and globalization (Bracken et al., 2012 Cohen & Timimi, 2008; Fernando, 2014; Mills, 2014; Moodley & Ocampo, 2014; Whitley, 2012). This renewed critique emphasizes the dehumanization of care that has come from a narrow, reductionistic medical model and advocates for the central place of the voice and agency of people with lived experience and the key role of community-based interventions aimed at recovery.

To some extent, this criticism reflects frustration with the limitations of existing treatments for many of the serious afflictions that psychiatry aims to help. Since the "Decade of the Brain" was inaugurated in 1990, we have witnessed twenty-five years of intensive neuroscience research aimed at finding effective therapies, yet relatively little has changed in terms of treatment options and approaches. Meanwhile, the rise of biological psychiatry has displaced psychosocial and psychotherapeutic approaches in psychiatric training and practice, resulting in what some observers have perceived as less humane and patient-centered care. From a critical and political economic perspective, the involvement of the pharmaceutical industry and managed care corporations has created conflicts of interest that threaten the credibility and accountability of psychiatry as a helping profession.

1

Mental health problems can profoundly affect social identity and relationships. Like other illnesses, they challenge our resources and coping capacities, but unlike other illnesses, they can directly affect basic cognitive and emotional processes in ways that undermine our social functioning, sense of self, and identity. The distinctive character of mental health problems often leads to stigmatization, and the more severe forms of mental illness are recognized everywhere as serious afflictions. Psychiatry has tried to provide more humane and effective care for people who have sometimes received harsh treatment, including physical confinement and social ostracism. Unfortunately, psychiatric care also has contributed its own forms of coercion and marginalization. Hence, there are enduring concerns about the negative effects of psychiatric labeling and interventions. The recovery movement aims to address the tendency of psychiatry to view outcomes narrowly in terms of symptom management by recognizing the agency and values of people living with mental health problems as central to ethical and effective care (Rudnick, 2012).

There is also growing concern with the ways that the focus on mental health has invaded the lives of people in wealthy, urbanized countries, as seen in the proliferation of psychiatric diagnoses, overuse of medications, and the medicalization of everyday problems in living (Horwitz & Wakefield, 2007; Greenberg, 2010; Whitaker, 2010). Claims that more than 50 percent of the general population suffer from a psychiatric disorder have led prominent psychiatrists and psychologists to worry that we are losing the very notion of "normal" (Frances, 2013). Although medicalization can have real benefits in terms of problem recognition, stigma reduction, and mobilizing an effective response, it can also result in diagnostic labeling that causes demoralization and disability and that leads to inappropriate treatments with harmful effects. In psychiatry, medicalizing problems tends to locate them within the individual, shifting attention away from the social determinants of health (Marmot & Wilkinson, 2006; Pickett & Wilkinson, 2010). Social scientists have pointed to the subtler ways in which psychiatric thinking has changed our self-understanding, showing up in public discourse and private soliloquy. Psychiatry is increasingly shaping the ways in which we think about ourselves in health and illness. Everyday challenges and conflicts are framed in the metaphors of neuroscience and psychology, and the new technologies of neuroscience, including genomics and brain imaging, are contributing to new forms of identity. Critical perspectives on the "psy" disciplines and on neuroscience aim to analyze this ongoing transformation of personhood, which has potential benefits, but which may also inadvertently undermine individual agency and social advocacy (Choudhury & Slaby, 2011; Rose, 1998; Rose & Abi-Rached, 2013).

To be sure, psychiatry and allied mental health professions have improved the lot of many people living with mental illness, but services and effective treatments are not equitably distributed. Although estimates suggest that mental, neurological, and substance use disorders account for 14 percent of the global burden of disease, according to the World Health Organization "most of the people affected – 75% in many low-income countries – do not have access to the treatment they need" (www.who.int/mental_health/mhgap/en/). The global mental health movement aims to ensure that people around the world have access to the same treatment resources available in wealthy countries (Patel & Prince, 2010). The effort to promote global mental health is framed as a matter of basic equity and human rights (Kleinman, 2009). The vehicle for correcting these injustices, however, is often assumed to be the same psychiatric interventions currently facing critique in wealthy, well-resourced countries. The exportation of Western mental health practices is viewed by critics as a kind of cultural imperialism (Fernando, 2014; Mills, 2014; Watters, 2010).

How can we understand these dilemmas, respond to the critiques, and chart a way forward? As a profession, psychiatry is a young discipline, and there is little reason to think that it will maintain its current modes of practice over the next decades. Will it disappear, supplanted on one front by behavioral neurology, based on understanding neural mechanisms of brain dysfunction, and on another front by psychology and social work, professions better equipped to address the personal and social contexts of suffering? Or, is there still a place for a reimagined psychiatry that aims to integrate biological, social, and cultural perspectives in a person-centered medicine that responds to the full range of mental health problems?

This volume builds on recent work in philosophy, cognitive and social neuroscience, medical anthropology, psychology, and psychiatry to answer in the affirmative and to suggest promising directions for a renewed and reinvigorated psychiatry. The contributors explore some of the innovative lines of research and critical thinking that are leading to an integrative view of the origins and nature of mental health problems, which can inform more effective clinical, public health, and social responses to the human predicament.

In this introductory chapter, we provide a brief overview of some key issues in the current crisis of psychiatry and some recent responses. We then outline the contributions to this volume. The concluding chapter considers the implications for the future of psychiatry of an ecosocial, systemic view that can integrate the diverse perspectives of the contributors. Our aim is to point toward a vision of the future, mapping some of the obstacles and promising directions to a more inclusive, humane, and effective response to the many forms of human suffering that concern psychiatry.

The Ambit of Psychiatry: What Is a Mental Disorder?

As a helping profession, psychiatry seeks to interpret and respond to the needs of people with "mental disorders." This leads immediately to problems of defining what counts as a mental disorder (McNally, 2011). Here, we briefly address three levels of definition, which are reflected in the taxonomic structure of current psychiatric nosology.

The first and most general level concerns the overall definition of mental disorder as distinct from a state of health or well-being. Despite efforts to devise a unitary and inclusive definition of mental disorders, no single definition works for the very diverse problems that are collected together in current psychiatric diagnostic systems or nosologies, such as the *Diagnostic and Statistical Manual of Mental Disorders* (5th ed.; *DSM-5*; American Psychiatric Association [APA], 2013).[1] As we discuss later in this chapter, much effort has been given to trying to refine the notion of "disorder," but it is worth noting that what counts as a specifically "mental" disorder is also not straightforward. The concept of the "mental" has a cultural history that is related to notions of personhood, agency, and morality, with important consequences for how we respond to people with psychiatric problems (Kirmayer, 1988; Miresco & Kirmayer, 2006). Every kind of affliction – from injuries and infections to everyday misfortunes – affects our thoughts and feelings, and, if sufficiently intense, can interfere with cognitive and emotional functioning. In psychiatric disorders, these disturbances of mental functioning, experience, and behavior are viewed as primary rather than secondary characteristics of the illness, but a secondary response can become a problem in its own right, as reflected in notions of "reactive" conditions or "adjustment disorders."

---

[1] *DSM-5*, the official nosology of the American Psychiatric Association (APA), offers the following definition:

> A mental disorder is a syndrome characterized by clinically significant disturbance in an individual's cognition, emotion regulation, or behavior that reflects a dysfunction in the psychological, biological, or developmental processes underlying mental functioning. Mental disorders are usually associated with significant distress or disability in social, occupational, or other important activities. An expectable or culturally approved response to a common stressor or loss, such as the death of a loved one, is not a mental disorder. Socially deviant behavior (e.g., political, religious, or sexual) and conflicts that are primarily between the individual and society are not mental disorders unless the deviance or conflict results from a dysfunction in the individual, as described above. (APA, 2013, p. 20)

The second level of definition concerns the ways that broad categories of disorders are grouped together as related (e.g., depressive disorders, anxiety disorders, and feeding and eating disorders). These superordinate groups reflect judgments of similarity based on symptomatology and behavioral manifestations (Borsboom, Cramer, Schmittmann, Epskamp, & Waldorp, 2011); assumptions about similar causality and underlying mechanisms; or comparable responses to treatment (Kendler & Campbell, 2009). However, in the absence of reliable measures of these underlying mechanisms or a fixed set of symptoms that are deemed necessary and sufficient for inclusion in a particular diagnostic group, these groupings remain contentious. Indeed, the decision to group certain disorders in one category or another often reflects the historical choice of prototypes or exemplars around which each category was built by family resemblance (Young, 1995). Although this fits well with styles of clinical reasoning (Westen, 2012), it builds a high level of cultural specificity and contingency into the categories.

The third level of definition concerns specific types of mental health problems. Here, categorization leads to the recurrent dilemma of determining the right level of detail or specification to characterize a symptom and the level of severity that makes it a clinical problem. Each individual's symptoms and modes of expressing suffering are unique in some respects, and in deciding which features on which to focus and which to ignore in defining a disorder, we must either rely on their salience for the individual or fall back on a preexisting prototype or model. Panic attacks, hallucinations, and feelings of dysphoria all come in many varieties and gradations of severity that may lie on a continuum with everyday experiences of no pathological significance. Even psychotic disorders exist on a continuum with more common milder and transient symptoms (van Os, Linscott, Myin-Germeys, Delespaul, & Krabbendam, 2009).[2] Characterizing mental health problems therefore depends on finding the right level of abstraction and threshold of severity. The great heterogeneity of individual experience results in many cases being viewed as atypical and assigned to residual categories (e.g., "unspecified" in *DSM-5*).

A pragmatic answer to the first question, about the outer boundaries of what counts as a mental disorder, could simply point to the types of problems that have been historically assigned to psychiatry. As a medical specialty, psychiatry emerged in the 1800s from the custodial

---

[2] A 2014 report by the British Psychological Society also supports a continuum model for psychotic experiences, such as hearing voices, arguing that they don't fall into neat categories (see www.bps.org.uk/networks-and-communities/member-microsite/division-clinical-psychology/understanding-psychosis-and-schizophrenia).

care of people with severe, chronic conditions that affected their ability to think clearly and function socially and emotionally in an appropriate manner (Grob, 2008; Pressman, 1997). Some of these conditions were found to reflect congenital, infectious, or traumatic injuries to the brain. Early success in identifying such underlying pathology in a few cases (e.g., syphilis) gave impetus to the disease model in psychiatry (Bolton, 2012).

Although psychiatry began with only the most severe mental illnesses as its "object," the discipline's domain expanded throughout the past century to include common mental disorders that shade into the kinds of worries, fears, and demoralization that are part of everyday challenges, adversities, life transitions, and losses. The embrace of psychoanalysis as a theory of psychopathology and treatment method encouraged this wide compass (Luhrmann, 2000; Zaretsky, 2004). With this expansion, however, came growing difficulty in distinguishing the legitimate objects of psychiatric concern from the "merely" troubling or troublesome. Efforts have been made to define the boundaries of what counts as a mental disorder, both to clarify the domain of psychiatry and to forestall pathologizing normal behavior (Wakefield, 1999, 2007). But attempts to define psychiatric disorders in biological terms – whether in relation to the machinery of the brain or human evolutionary history – founder on the essentially normative nature of diagnosis (Kirmayer & Young, 1999). Mental disorders are problems that affect our social roles and functioning, and what is expected of us in these roles depends on our culturally constructed institutions and forms of life. This dependence on culture and context is explicitly recognized in the *DSM-5* definition, which distinguishes a "culturally approved response" to a stressor or loss from a mental disorder, but this context-dependence of function and dysfunction is not always given the attention that it deserves in psychiatric research and everyday clinical practice.

The Crisis of Psychiatry: Cracks in the Scientific Foundation

The current crisis of psychiatry has deep historical roots in its ambiguous position as a medical specialty, institution of social control, and secular arena for dealing with moral, spiritual, and existential problems. In the 1960s, a common critique concerned the imprecision and unreliability of clinical diagnosis. Epidemiological studies used general measures of distress that did not correspond to the discrete diagnoses used by clinicians (March & Oppenheimer, 2014). In clinical settings, there was wide variation in the use of diagnostic categories and criteria. In courtroom or forensic settings, psychiatrists could be found to affirm contradictory or opposing clinical assessments. These troubles were an embarrassment to a profession that claimed a scientific basis to its practice and led to concerted efforts to develop a more reliable diagnostic system. The U.S.–U.K. comparative study showing great discrepancies in patterns of diagnosis of schizophrenia and bipolar disorder (BD) between psychiatrists in New York and London (Cooper et al., 1972; Wing, 1971), coupled with the availability of lithium as a relatively specific treatment for mania, added further urgency to efforts to improve the reliability and accuracy of psychiatric diagnosis.

The introduction of *DSM-III,* the third edition of the official diagnostic nosology of the APA (1980), marked an important advance in the clarity and reliability of psychiatric diagnosis (Wilson, 1993). Earlier versions of the manual had relied on descriptions of clinical entities that required a high level of inference about internal mechanisms, psychodynamic processes, or hypothetical etiology. *DSM-III* aimed for an "atheoretical" nosology based on observable clinical data through the use of specific diagnostic criteria "operationalized" in terms of symptoms and signs. This approach enabled professionals and trained lay interviewers to consistently identify major diagnostic categories. Large-scale epidemiological studies could then determine the prevalence of specific problems in the population, an important guide to developing appropriate mental health services and an essential tool for studying the course and outcome of mental health problems.

The 1980s saw a dramatic sea change in American psychiatry, in which psychoanalysis was dethroned and replaced with increasingly biological approaches in psychiatry and cognitive-behavioral approaches in psychology (Luhrmann, 2000; Paris, 2005; Shorter, 1997). Biological psychiatry assumes that mental health problems result from "broken brains" or "chemical imbalances" and focuses on drug treatments (Baldessarini, 2014; Vázquez, 2014). Cognitive-behavioral psychology views mental health problems as the result of maladaptive patterns of thought and action that can be modified through psychotherapy (Hofmann, Asmundson, & Beck, 2013).

At the same time, an ever-expanding array of human problems have been reframed as mental disorders. Whereas *DSM-I* (1952) listed 106 diagnostic categories, *DSM-II* (1968) had 182, *DSM-III* (1980) had 265, and *DSM-IV* (1994) included 297 – the precise numbers vary with how one counts subtypes and variants. *DSM-5* (2013) eliminated some conditions but added new disorders, renewing concerns about the proliferation of categories and "bracket creep" (McNally, 2011) – the lowering of thresholds and liberalization of criteria through constructing "spectra" – resulting in a very high proportion of the population meeting criteria for one or more psychiatric disorders (Whitaker, 2010). Is this an accurate picture of the human condition – at least in the urban, industrialized, wealthy countries where most epidemiological surveys take place – or is it an example of the aggressive expansion of professional turf and corresponding markets for medications and other treatments? A critical literature documents many recent examples of diagnostic inflation, including: labeling prolonged grief and sadness as depression (Greenberg, 2010; Horwitz & Wakefield, 2007); extending BD to cover a broad spectrum of mood variations and applying the diagnosis to adolescents, children, and even infants (Moncrieff, 2014; Paris, 2012); viewing difficulties in classroom adjustment as evidence of attention deficit disorder (ADD; Koerth-Baker, 2013; Thomas, Mitchell, & Batstra, 2013; Singh, 2008); treating shyness and other variations in social behavior or gregariousness as anxiety disorders (Horwitz & Wakefield, 2012); and broadening the use of the term "autism" to cover a very wide spectrum of traits (Basu & Parry, 2013).

Along with the rise in numbers of diagnostic categories and rates of diagnoses has come a dramatic increase in prescriptions for and consumption of psychiatric medications (Angell, 2011). Psychopharmacology is big business, and creating new kinds of problems and new indications for existing medications (repackaged and relabeled) is one way to keep the market growing (Angell, 2011; Collin, 2014; Healey, 2004; Horwitz, 2011). For example, in recent years there has been an enormous growth in the use of stimulants for ADD in both children and adults, as well as atypical neuroleptics for an extraordinarily wide range of symptoms and conditions (Olfson, Blanco, Liu, Wang & Correll. 2012).

Unfortunately, in this embrace of better living through chemistry, little serious attention has been given to the possibility of subtle behavioral side effects or to habituation and withdrawal symptoms that might exacerbate the course of illness or lead to increased rates of relapse and more severe episodes, refractory to treatment. For example, the new selective serotonin reuptake inhibitor (SSRI) antidepressants, marketed as more effective than older tricyclic antidepressants, not only turned out to be no more effective (Anderson, 2000) but also caused subtle signs of neurocognitive disinhibition as well as sexual dysfunction (including loss of sexual desire), with potentially serious effects on relationships, especially when the effects were misattributed to the relationship rather than to the medication (Fisher & Thomson, 2007). Still more disturbingly, meta-analyses of clinical trials revealed that in general antidepressants were little more effective than placebos for mild to moderate depression

(Kirsch, 2009; Kirsch et al., 2008). The atypical neuroleptics, heralded as more effective for schizophrenia, with fewer uncomfortable side effects, also were found to be no more effective than older antipsychotic medications (Leucht et al., 2009) and to lead to serious side effects, including diabetes and metabolic syndrome, with increased mortality (Haddad & Sharma, 2007). Despite this evidence, both SSRI antidepressants and atypical neuroleptics have largely supplanted earlier medications in routine practice in wealthy countries and are used with increasing frequency for an ever-wider range of symptoms and disorders in both adults and children, including mild conditions.

Leading figures in psychiatry have recognized the problem of over-diagnosis. Allen Frances (2012), the editor of *DSM-IV,* has become a vocal critic of this expansionism. He identifies multiple sources that contribute to diagnostic inflation, including: the *DSM* system itself, which provides a loose set of criteria; drug company marketing, which engages in "disease mongering"; and insurance companies which require diagnosis for reimbursement (Frances, 2013). In the United States, the FDA, the main regulatory body responsible for protecting public health, is largely funded by pharmaceutical company user fees, an obvious and profound conflict of interest (Light, Lexchin, & Darrow, 2013). Many consumer groups are substantially financed by drug companies and, although their explicit goal may be education and stigma reduction, the link implies tacit promotion of medications (Read & Cain, 2013). As a reflection of consumer culture, popular media regularly present tentative new research findings as "breakthroughs," contributing to fads in diagnosis and treatment.

Of course, there are real problems and suffering behind this psychia-trization of everyday life. The issue is whether the characterization of these problems as discrete psychiatric disorders leads to an appropriate and helpful response. In the case of children with behavioral or learning difficulties in the classroom, for example, psychiatric diagnoses are used to manage the uncertainty about complex issues that may involve parents, teachers, and the school setting itself, and to suggest a clear course of action that is usually focused on the child. But the labels attached to children at one point in their school career may follow them for life, changing both their own self-concept and the ways in which others treat them. Indeed, because psychiatric labels become self-reinforcing and have so many social consequences, Frances (2012) suggests that "new diagnoses in psychiatry can be far more dangerous than new drugs."

Ironically, efforts at mental health promotion and prevention have also contributed to diagnostic inflation through efforts to detect and treat common conditions and to identify early prodromes of serious mental illness. Screening for mental disorders with imprecise instruments can lead to widespread labeling and inappropriate treatment for mild, self-limited conditions (Thombs et al., 2012). The desire to promote early treatment and prevention of chronicity in schizophrenia led to efforts to define a prodromal syndrome in *DSM-5* (Carpenter & van Os, 2011). The proposal led to much controversy because the potential consequences of universal screening of children and adolescents (the usual time of onset for schizophrenia) and of early intervention are almost completely unknown. As a result, the suggestion was abandoned as premature.

Many of the psychiatric medications in use today were discovered by happenstance and, as we have noted, the newer generations of medications are not notably more effective than their forebears. Experts in psychopharmacology have decried the lack of substantial progress in developing new drugs, a lack that is sometimes attributed to not looking closely enough at biological mechanisms. Whereas many hope that neuroscience eventually will provide a coherent and complete account of the origins, mechanisms, and effective treatment of major psychiatric disorders, despite enormous advances to date there has been strikingly little clinical yield from research. Some of the most promising and widely used methodologies – for example, genome-wide analyses and functional brain imaging – present serious technical challenges, including managing the "growing torrent of results" (McCarroll, Feng, & Hyman, 2014, p. 759), as well as statistical and conceptual issues in interpreting data (Stelzer, Lohmann, Mueller, Buschmann, & Turner, 2014). Genomic-, cellular-, or network-level variations found in experimental paradigms, or in clinical studies comparing people with particular types of symptoms or pathology to those who are healthy, generally identify differences that cannot be attributed to a specific gene or single locus of pathology; instead, they are part of larger, systemic changes in functioning that manifest their effects through gene–environment interactions over developmental trajectories, in interaction with other individual systems, and in response to particular contexts of learning and performance (Kendler, Jaffey, & Romer, 2011; Kirmayer & Crafa, 2014; Kirmayer & Gold, 2012; McCaroroll et al., 2014). Despite the large scale and methodological sophistication of these studies, the focus on genetic risk factors or neural differences based on imaging research is far from the complex realities of illness faced by patients and clinicians.

The revision of nosology for *DSM-5* began with high hopes that it would reflect advances in neuroscience, and some of the early research conferences focused on ways of framing psychiatric disorders in terms of current neuroscience on, for example, fear circuitry, pair bonding, or maternal behaviors in animal models (Andrews, 2009; Beach et al., 2007). There was a sense that this engagement with neuroscience would require radical revisions: for example, shifting to a dimensional approach and identifying disorders in terms of biomarkers or endophenotypes, which can be measured at the level of underlying neurobiology and genetics, rather than overt behaviors, or symptom clusters (Kendler & Neale, 2010). In the end, however, it became clear that current neuroscience is not sufficiently developed to provide much guidance for clinical diagnosis, and the revision of *DSM-5* was very conservative (Paris & Phillips, 2013).

Nevertheless, mainstream psychiatry continues to expect biological explanations for major mental disorders, and the main U.S. funding agency for mental health research, the National Institute of Mental Health (NIMH), recently launched a new research program, the Research Domain Criteria (RDoC; www.nimh.nih.gov/research-prior ities/rdoc/), to focus on the search for neuroscience models (Cuthbert, 2014; Insel et al., 2010). The announcement by NIMH director Thomas Insel that the research establishment was parting ways with *DSM* clinical nosology two weeks before the manual's May 2013 release was timed for maximum rhetorical effect – the RDoC program had been announced much earlier and its development proceeded in parallel with that of *DSM-5,* albeit with input from a smaller number of advisors. The NIMH's approach is interesting in terms of supporting neuroscience research based on specific circuits and systems rather than discrete clinical entities, but many trenchant critiques of the RDoC have been voiced, ranging from the lack of attention to phenomenology and the patient's perspective to the kinds of experimental paradigms and levels of explanation favored.[3] A major concern is that the levels of interpersonal, social structural, and cultural processes are relatively undeveloped in the framework and therefore risk being further marginalized (Kirmayer & Crafa, 2014).

The Importance of Culture and Context

Decades of research in cultural psychiatry as well as medical and psychological anthropology have explored the social construction and context of psychopathology. Doctors and administrators working during the colonialist era, although mired in racist notions of the primitive nature

---

[3] The February 2014 issue of *World Psychiatry* presents some of these critiques from leading figures in psychiatry (see http://onlinelibrary.wiley.com/doi/10.1002/wps.v13.1/issuetoc).

of the "native mind," laid some of the foundations of a descriptive or comparative study of mental illness (Bains, 2005; Littlewood & Dein, 2000). Building in part on this problematic foundation, psychological anthropologists trained in or experimenting with psychoanalytic approaches such as Ruth Benedict, Margaret Mead, Gregory Bateson, Cora Dubois, and Edward Sapir, along with like-minded psychiatrists such as Henry Stack Sullivan and Abram Kardiner, continued the exploration of the relationships of culture and social context to mental illness (Jenkins, 2007).

By the 1950s and 1960s, anthropologists were developing ethnographic methodologies to specifically address the role of local values, beliefs, social structures, and communities in the course and outcome of mental illness. By the 1980s, the convergence of these two domains led to the maturation of the field of cultural psychiatry, which has documented substantial variations in the symptoms, course, and outcome of mental health problems (Kirmayer, 1989; Kleinman, 1980, 1988; López & Guarnaccia, 2012). This work shows how culturally varied developmental experiences, explanatory models, and social contexts shape the ways people experience and express suffering as well as the ways they cope with illness (Kirmayer & Bhugra, 2009). Psychiatric practice has integrated some of this work through efforts to implement standards of cultural competence in training and practice (Kirmayer, 2012). Building on *DSM-IV*'s engagement of how to relate cultural context to diagnosis (Mezzich et al., 1999), *DSM-5* expanded the discussion of culture by including a cultural formulation interview designed to help clinicians collect information about patients' background and current context to complement and inform psychiatric assessment, diagnosis, and treatment planning (Lewis-Fernández et al., 2014).

Although these are important steps in moving toward a contextual view of mental health problems in official nosology, there are reasons to think that attention to culture and context should play a much larger role in psychiatric research, theory, and practice (Jenkins, 2015; Kirmayer & Gold, 2012; Whitley, Rousseau, Carpenter-Song, & Kirmayer, 2011). This call for renewed attention to culture and context is not only an issue of responding to the social and political realities of human diversity but also is consistent with recent advances in our understanding of the brain's plasticity, adaptability, and attunement to social interaction (Roepstorff, 2013; Rule, Freeman, & Ambady, 2013; Wexler, 2006). Cultural variations in development and in everyday social contexts, roles, and practices appear to exert stable, long-lasting changes in brain structure and function that affect our very concepts of self and the ways in which we think about others (J. T. Cacioppo, Cacioppo, Dulawa, &

Palmer, 2014; Chiao, 2009; Han et al., 2013; Kim & Sasaki, 2014; Rule et al., 2013). The brain bears the traces of the individual's development and social experiences, all of which are culturally mediated.

Moreover, cultures frame the ways we look at the world so that existing arrangements, including inequalities, come to seem inevitable or unquestioned. Critical anthropological and social science approaches are needed to explore these tacit dimensions of social life; such approaches can also help uncover the assumptions built into psychiatric theory and practice. This is especially challenging, given how cultural practices tend to vindicate the categories we use to perceive and act on the world, through what Kleinman (1988) has called the "category fallacy" – imposing our conventional categories on the ways that others view the world – and what Hacking (1995, 1999) refers to as the "looping effect," in which socially constructed categories shape institutions, practices, and experiences that perpetuate the categories. In the case of neuroscience, there is a tendency to view neurobiological knowledge as value-free and independent of these social processes of knowledge construction, but an emerging body of work in *critical neuroscience* seeks to reveal the interests and assumptions at play in the production and application of neuroscientific research (Choudhury & Slaby, 2011).

This Volume

In this volume, we bring together contributors to address some of the challenges facing psychiatry on four main fronts: (1) through studies of the epistemology and phenomenology of mental health and illness; (2) by developing models for mind–brain–environment interactions that can capture the ways in which developmental histories and social contexts interact to cause illness and recovery; (3) by tracing the ways in which our own understandings of our selves and of mental illness shape illness experience, psychological adaptation, and the social course of affliction; and (4) by examining the interaction between local and global forces in articulating kinds of psychiatric theory and practice that can meet the needs of diverse populations. In organizing this volume, we asked contributors to consider how systems thinking at different levels (neural, developmental, psychological, family, social, and environmental) can advance psychiatric research and practice. We emphasized a dynamic perspective of mind as emergent from biological processes that are embodied and socially and culturally embedded. We advocated for an *ecosocial* approach that understands these levels as "intertwine[d] at every scale, micro to macro" (Krieger, 2001), citing Gregory Bateson's (1972) "ecology of mind" as an inspiration. Finally, we encouraged the authors to explore the relevance to their particular domain of concepts rooted in systems thinking, including *trajectories, dimensions, dynamics, complexity,* and *looping effects*. What follows is a brief "guided tour" through the book's four parts.

Restoring Phenomenology to Psychiatry

Part One focuses on restoring phenomenology to its rightful place in psychiatry. The chapters in this section take the reader from basic epistemological questions about the objects of psychiatry, through the role of phenomenological methods in research and clinical practice, to articulating a vision of neurophenomenology and understanding the cultural embedding of illness experience and healing. The contributors show how close attention to psychiatry's conceptual structure and descriptive psychopathology, on one hand, and the structures and organization of consciousness and lived experience, on the other hand, can revitalize psychiatric theory, research, and practice.[4]

The operationalized criteria of *DSM-III* reduced the phenomenology of psychopathology and illness experience to a simple checklist of symptoms and signs. Without close attention to patients' experience, however, clinicians cannot establish the trust and rapport needed to negotiate and deliver effective treatment. Moreover, much of the suffering associated with mental disorders is directly tied to the particularities of experience: from the physical distress associated with anxiety or the sense of being unable to act that is intrinsic to severe depression to the varieties of complex hallucinations and delusions central to psychotic disorders. Even neuropsychiatric conditions such as Tourette syndrome or other movement disorders have particular phenomenology that is not simply dictated by neurobiology but emerges from active processes of perception, action, and interpretation, so that the agency and meaning-making processes of the person must be included in our models of mental disorders.

The section opens with a chapter by historians German Berrios and Ivana Marková, who argue that psychiatry is a "hybrid" discipline and its subject matter – mental symptoms and disorders – hybrid objects

---

[4] For an introduction to phenomenology, see Gallagher and Zahavi (2012), and for basic readings on phenomenology in psychiatry, see Broome, Harland, and Owen (2013). Ratcliffe (2014) provides an exemplary study of depression combining empirical data on experience with phenomenological analysis. The influence of Karl Jaspers' work is explored in Stanghellini and Fuchs (2013).

with both neurobiological and meaning-based aspects. They distinguish "primary brain inscriptions," which they suggest are more directly brain-based or hard-wired, from "secondary inscriptions," which are more dependent on interpretative processes and, hence, more historically contingent and language-bound. Crucially, both forms of inscription are subject to institutional and cultural configuration and, at the same time, both forms reenter and reshape dynamic networks of neural activity. The clinical and epistemological challenges are to identify and explain the patterns of interaction between primary and secondary inscriptions (Marková & Berrios, 2012).

In the next chapter, psychiatrist Josef Parnas and philosopher Shaun Gallagher propose a phenomenological approach to clinical psychiatry that is specifically tailored to understanding "anomalies of experience." Rather than posing structured sets of yes/no questions in the clinical encounter to ascertain the presence or absence of symptoms (a method that has dominated diagnostic interviews used in research but that has proved to have serious problems of reliability and validity), the authors argue that a semistructured phenomenological interview by an experienced clinician attuned to a more hermeneutical or dialogical approach can reveal a more complete picture of how delusions, for example, have made "a patient's *life* different." The framework that they propose is based on the notion that psychiatric symptoms and syndromes cannot be understood in isolation but must be interpreted in context as part of a gestalt. Diagnosis emerges as the clinician assesses and attempts to typify another person's experiences (i.e., by searching for resemblances to certain prototypes), while also bearing in mind "the full scope of the subject's embodied engagements in ... various physical and social environments." Hence, context is central to the meaning and implications of symptoms and psychopathology. This approach not only provides a basis for person-centered clinical work but also can guide more integrative research attuned to the fine-grained structure of psychopathological experience (Nordgaard, Sass, & Parnas, 2013) as well as contributing to neuroscientific investigations into self, subjectivity, and consciousness (Cromby, Newton, & Williams, 2011).

In his contribution, psychiatric neuroscientist Georg Northoff illustrates one clinically relevant direction for engagement between neuroscience and phenomenology. His "neurophenomenal" approach explores possible linkages between basic aspects of the experience of psychopathology and differences in the brain's intrinsic or resting-state activity. Regarding depression, Northoff correlates increased self-focus seen at the phenomenal level with elevated resting-state activity in regions of the brain involved in self-specific processing (the default-mode network). In addition, functional imaging studies show abnormal resting-state and stimulus-induced activity in persons with schizophrenia, which may be related to a wider range of deficits. Northoff and others also argue that schizophrenia may involve disruptions in the brain's intrinsic activity outside the default-mode network, at more basic sensory processing levels in the cortex (Northoff, 2014). Abnormal encoding of environmental stimuli could in turn disrupt self-specific resting-state activity and ultimately alter what phenomenologists have characterized as the sense of self or "mineness" with which we experience the world.

Work like Northoff's may ultimately help us understand how symptoms are configured by neuropathology, but the patterns in the brain also represent the sedimented history of individual experience (learning, life events, biography) and culture (collective history, knowledge, and practices, social roles and contexts). The chapter by psychological anthropologist Thomas Csordas reviews the history and critical importance of cultural phenomenology in understanding first-person experience of psychiatric illness. Csordas begins by acknowledging the work of Edward Sapir, who argued that the locus of psychiatry cannot be "the human organism at all in any fruitful sense of the word but the more intangible, and yet more intelligible, world of human relationships and ideas that such relationships bring forth" (Sapir, 1932, p. 232). Csordas takes this crucial idea forward with the tools of ethnography, presenting some of his own and Janis Jenkins's work on the experience of depression among adolescent psychiatric inpatients in the American Southwest and then summarizing some key contributions to two landmark edited volumes in psychiatric anthropology by Kleinman and Good (on depression) and Jenkins and Barrett (on schizophrenia). The breadth of work represented by these edited volumes – and much other recent work in phenomenological anthropology (Desjarlais & Throop, 2011) – is an important counter to the concern that theory and research in psychology and psychiatry do not adequately represent the great cultural diversity of human experience (Henrich, Heine, & Norenzayan, 2010).

Finally, Laurence Kirmayer brings critical attention to the dynamics of empathy. Clinical understanding relies on processes of affective attunement and close listening. Understanding the strange or unfamiliar aspects of patients' experience requires not only technical models that can explain psychopathology but also knowledge of local social worlds that are conveyed through stories. Empathy can be cultivated by learning more about these lifeworlds and predicaments. Of course, empathy has its limits and clinical work must continue even in its absence by adopting an ethic of hospitality and care, as articulated in the work of philosopher

Emmanuel Lévinas. Acknowledging the limits of empathy can allow the clinician to recognize and respect radical alterity or otherness and so see the patient more clearly.

In her commentary on these chapters, anthropologist Nev Jones notes the wide gap between clinical and research studies of the phenomenology of psychopathology and the lived experience of people with mental health problems in their local worlds. As Jones points out, people living with a serious mental illness in North America interact less with psychiatrists than with front-line providers and para-professionals, as well as – all too frequently – the criminal justice and welfare systems. The contexts of clinical or research settings seem far removed from the everyday struggles with homelessness and the grinding institutional routines that preoccupy many people with severe mental illness. Among its many insights, this commentary underscores the need for psychiatry to engage more fully with the lifeworlds of those whom it hopes to understand and help.

Taken together, the chapters in this section suggest that psychiatry needs a *cultural neurophenomenology* that fully integrates neurobiological and social-cultural processes in illness experience. This kind of phenomenology depends on close listening and systematic exploration of the other's experience, as well as respect for the limits of empathy, intuition, and explanation. But it also requires a willingness to look beyond the clinical context, situating persons in their local worlds, and considering the embedding of those worlds in larger structures of power, violence, and indifference (Biehl, Good, & Kleinman, 2007).

Biosocial Mechanisms in Health and Illness

Part Two explores some examples of the kind of neuroscience that can contribute to clinical understanding of mental health problems. The rapidly developing fields of cognitive, social, and cultural neuroscience move up the hierarchy from cells and circuits to functional systems that depend on a person's learning history and social contexts. New technologies that allow us to dynamically trace pathways in the brain also show how they are modified through epigenetic processes to effectively rewire the brain by altering specific circuits and systems. Systems neuroscience emphasizes that multiple networks throughout the brain contribute to many functions (Moghaddam & Wood, 2014). The human nervous system is the substrate of behavior and experience, but its functioning depends on the body, the individual's history of development and learning, and the socially constructed environments in which we live and interact with others. Hence, we cannot fully characterize the ways in which neural processing can go wrong in mental illness without reference to personal history, psychology, and social context.[5]

Much of the discussion leading up to the publication of *DSM-5* concerned the problem of classification in psychiatry, in particular whether psychiatric disorders form discrete categories or are best described as dimensional in nature (Helzer et al., 2008). In the first chapter of this section, neuropsychologist Robert Bilder argues that researchers should adopt the stance that diagnostic boundaries *do not* exist (unless proven otherwise) because the commitment to categorical systems like the *DSM*, along with our various implicit biases, may be an "an active impediment to progress." According to Bilder, most symptoms of mental disorder (e.g., anxiety) vary quantitatively, not qualitatively, and may be best thought of as ranged along a continuum from normal to pathological. Taxometric research (using statistical procedures developed by Paul Meehl [1995] and colleagues to determine if psychological data can be divided into distinct categories) seems to bear this out (Haslam, 2007). Bilder holds out the hope that current large-scale research programs that aim to aggregate data at multiple levels – gene, cell, circuit, and so on – will lead to a new taxonomy built on dimensions that can guide both research and clinical practice.

The human genome project made it clear that much of the genome is devoted to regulating its own activity during development and in response to environmental influences throughout life (Davidson, 2010). Over the past decade, there has been an explosion of interest in epigenetics, the regulation of gene expression during development and across the lifespan in response to various environmental contexts or events (Zhang & Meaney, 2010). Epigenetics involves a particular set of regulatory mechanisms – chemical and physical modifications to the DNA base pairs or to the histone proteins around which DNA is wrapped – that turn gene transcription on and off and that are highly responsive to the environment via cell signaling pathways. Labonté, Farah, and Turecki focus on certain long-lasting epigenetic modifications, as well as on alterations in the expression of growth factors associated with brain development and plasticity, induced by early life adversity in the brains of adult suicide victims who experienced severe abuse as children. The work by Turecki's group exemplifies recent advances in our understanding of the mechanisms through which social experiences

---

[5] For a basic introduction to neuroscience applied to clinical psychiatry see: Zorumski and Rubin (2011) or Higgins and George (2013). The textbooks by Kandel and colleagues (2012) and Charney and colleagues (2013) provide more comprehensive and indepth coverage.

(adversity, social defeat, perceptions of other-ness, etc.) may influence the stress system, alter brain development and behavior, and increase risk for suicide.

The chapter by psychiatric neuroscientists Ladouceur, Versace, and Phillips discusses the search for neuroimaging biomarkers specific to (BD), a highly heritable condition that is difficult to diagnose in children and adolescents because of developmental variability in emotion regulation. Adolescents in particular are much more emotionally reactive than are younger children or adults, which may reflect increased neural plasticity in white and gray matter in regions associated with emotion processing and regulation. The authors' research focuses on interactions between brain regions implicated in automatic and voluntary emotion control networks (BD also affects reward processing). In adolescents at risk for BD, they and others have identified as possible "vulnerability markers" anatomical (white matter) abnormalities in the corpus callosum (suggesting reduced interhemispheric structural connectivity) and in the inferior longitudinal fasciculus, which connects the temporal and occipital lobes and plays a role in visual processing of emotionally salient information, such as facial expressions. In terms of the brain's dynamic or functional connectivity, the authors discuss BD-specific abnormalities in several different neural circuits related to emotion processing and emotion regulation, as well as prospects for clinically relevant biomarkers.

In their contribution to this volume, cognitive neuroscientist Amir Raz and Ethan Macdonald introduce the notion of "functional organ systems" as way to explicitly move beyond the dichotomy of functional and organic. The functional systems of attention comprise three distinct but orchestrated networks (alerting, orienting, and executive) – each with its own pattern of physiological activity, neuroanatomical structures, and neuromodulators (Posner & Fan, 2008). The orienting system can be further decomposed into two distinct (dorsal and ventral) networks related to sustaining and shifting attention, respectively. By conceptualizing attention in terms of network connectivity, the authors are able to incorporate behavioral, imaging, and genetic data and also consider the role of early experience, upbringing, and environment in individual variation. Raz and Macdonald's chapter provides support for the usefulness of nonpharmaceutical interventions that may exploit the plasticity of the brain's attentional networks, such as attention training and other cognitive-behavioral therapies.

In her commentary on these chapters, anthropologist Tanya Luhrmann suggests that the NIMH RDoC framework represents a positive step in psychiatric neuroscience, because the focus on cross-cutting intermediate phenotypes rather than nosological categories opens the door to collaboration with ethnographers studying illness experience. She discusses examples from fieldwork on voice hearing in schizophrenia that illustrate the ways in which social context interacts with psychobiological processes to shape symptoms. Her work shows how "experience-near" ethnographic research can be put into dialogue with contemporary cognitive neuroscience to yield new insights.

The chapters in this section present some of the major strategies for understanding neurobiological processes that contribute to mental functioning and psychopathology. Of course, many other new research methods, such as optogenetics (Deisseroth, 2012; Steinberg, Christoffel, Deisseroth, & Malenka, 2015), are not represented here. These hold the promise of identifying neural circuitry and larger network processes that subserve complex behavioral phenomena. Recent work in *connectomics*, for example, which attempts to map the brain's structural wiring and its real-time neural interactions, conceives of the brain in terms of dynamical systems or networks that are socially and environmentally embedded (Sporns, 2012). These extended brain–body–behavior networks shape and constrain one another across multiple temporal and spatial scales, so that researchers increasingly view them "as part of larger systems of dynamically interwoven processes that extend from the brain through the body into the world" (Byrge, Sporns, & Smith, 2014, p. 395).

Far from leading to a brain-centric view of mental disorders, therefore, the work presented in these chapters illustrates how brain and behavior are influenced by a host of internal (e.g., genetic, hormonal) and external environmental factors (e.g., early adversity and stress), requiring complementary approaches at the genetic, cellular, systems, and sociocultural levels (Kendler, 2014). As Byrge and colleagues note:

None of this can be fully understood by studying the brain in isolation. Brain networks do not arise autonomously but instead emerge in a constant dialog between intrinsic and evoked dynamics, local and global neural processing, and, perhaps most importantly, constant interaction between brain, body, and environment [...] a fuller understanding of how brain networks relate to cognition across an individual's lifespan requires extending these networks out into the world. (Byrge, Sporns, & Smith, 2014, p. 396)

The "world" here is not just the physical environment but, especially, the social world. Local social worlds or contexts contribute to patterns of interaction that not only shape symptoms but also influence the course and outcome of disorders and the response to interventions. Exploring these social worlds and understanding their embedding in larger systems is the focus of social science.

Social and Cultural Contexts of Psychopathology

Part Three applies the insights of medical and psychological anthropology and cultural psychology and psychiatry to identify the social and cultural contexts and the feedback or "looping" effects that shape illness experience and that may give rise to many forms of mental health problems. Attention to these contexts is at the center of research on social determinants of health as well as the everyday practice of clinical assessment and intervention.[6]

Addressing the interaction of social determinants of health and individual risk and protective factors, psychiatrists Kwame MacKenzie and Jai Shah propose a heuristic, four-dimensional approach to understanding psychosis based on the vulnerability-stress model, which considers *individual-level* (e.g., genetic risk factors, early adversity, and cannabis use) and *ecological* (e.g., migration, urban upbringing, and perception of social isolation) social factors and their *interactions* over *time*. Although psychosis involves "a complex and interconnected web of causation," the authors focus on migration and urban upbringing as causal influences due to the striking findings of higher incidence of psychotic disorders among migrants from the Caribbean and Africa to cities in the United Kingdom and other northern countries. They suggest these elevated rates of psychosis may reflect the effects of chronic, low-level stressors like social fragmentation or limited social networks, lack of green space, and racism and discrimination, as well as major stressors like childhood trauma, parental loss or separation, and more severe forms of social deprivation. These migration effects also have an important temporal dimension, with second-generation immigrants at an even higher risk of psychosis than their parents. This points to the importance both of multiple biological pathways and of social factors that challenge purely brain-based theories of psychosis.

In their chapter, cultural psychiatrists Devon Hinton and Naomi Simon discuss panic- and anxiety-related disorders among Cambodian refugees to show how a history of trauma and cultural conceptualizations of the body alter the psychological experience of somatic symptoms. The authors describe an approach to these disorders in terms of an integrative, "multiplex" model, according to which certain symptoms that evoke prior trauma trigger catastrophic cognitions and a positive feedback effect (bioattentional looping). Hinton and Simon describe the process in detail, using *kaeut khyâl* (wind attack), as an example.

[6] For introductions to thinking about context in psychiatry (and psychiatry in context), see Kleinman (1980, 1988) and Thomas (2014).

The multiplex model incorporates putatively universal biological processes but accommodates cross-cultural variation in terms of symptoms and causal explanations. Bioattentional looping effects, which amplify the physiological effects of the symptoms and create vicious circles, provide a way to link universal neurobiological and psychological processes of responding to threat or danger with culture-specific interpretative schemas and coping strategies. Culturally tailored intervention strategies can be built on this type of model.

One of the social interventions associated with psychiatry in the past century has been the reframing of addictions as brain diseases rather than moral problems. An increasing number of compulsive behaviors or habit problems have also been labeled addictions, including gambling, computer gaming, and Internet pornography, and even such basic bodily functions as eating and sexual behavior. An emerging consensus sees addictions as a disorder involving biological mechanisms ("hijacking" of the brain's reward circuitry), as well as material and social environments (Dackis & O'Brien, 2005). To understand these biosocial "entanglements," anthropologist Eugene Raikhel draws from Bateson's (1972) seminal essay on alcoholism, "The Cybernetics of Self," to reflect on the ways that assumptions about "mind," "self," and "volition" shape addiction and recovery. The brain-disease model is one such epistemic object, and Raikhel traces its history and influence. He identifies four promising conceptual frameworks to foster more integrative biological and social science research on addiction disorders: embodied sensations, which are shaped by context and meaning; will and habit; social and material environment; and temporal trajectories linking individual biologies with experience, events, and environments.

Psychologists Andrew Ryder and Yulia Chentsova-Dutton argue that clinical psychological "needs its own re-visioning parallel to, and in exchange with, psychiatry," which will entail a thoroughgoing engagement with cross-cultural variation. The authors propose a *cultural-clinical psychology* based on a view of culture, mind, and brain as a single multilevel system. Like many other contributors to this volume, they propose that multiple explanatory frameworks are needed to make sense of patients' difficulties. In particular, they argue that the mental processes and phenomena that psychology focuses on are emergent from the interaction of biological and social processes and must remain objects of study in their own right. In clinical practice, they suggest that broad descriptors or symptom labels, like "dysphoria" and "anxiety," are frequently a better fit than discrete *DSM* categories. Clinicians must also attend closely to the detailed quality and context of specific symptoms to better understand their patients' experiences and devise appropriate interventions. Cultural-clinical psychologists may focus on variations in the cognitive schemas or mental structures used to evaluate symptoms and the cultural scripts enacted expressions of identity and coping strategies. In a model similar to that described by Hinton and Simon, the authors suggest that cognitive and emotional responses can become part of loops or vicious circles that are the causes of persistent symptoms or disability and that can be targeted in interventions.

In the final chapter of this section, cultural psychiatrists Roberto Lewis-Fernández and Neil Aggarwal point out that although genetic or circuit-level disturbances may predispose an individual to risk, clinical syndromes arise through interactions with multiple factors, including sociocultural "patterns of distress." The authors propose a heuristic model triangulating neurobiological, sociocultural, and psychological dimensions of the illness, based on the conviction that purely descriptive or phenomenological approaches that locate pathology exclusively inside the person do not suffice, because all mental illnesses are both inscribed in the brain and locally contingent. They illustrate their approach with *ataque de nervios,* a cultural idiom of distress commonly seen in Latino Caribbean populations, characterized by a sudden attack of intense emotionality, often after a stressful or traumatic event. The final section of their chapter describes the Cultural Formulation Interview introduced in *DSM-5,* which focuses on individual experience and social context to assess cultural factors relevant to diagnosis and treatment planning using a person-centered approach (Lewis-Fernández, Aggarwal, D. E. Hinton, Hinton, & Kirmayer, 2015).

In his commentary on the chapters in this section, philosopher Ian Gold discusses how evolutionary theory and neurobiology can be incorporated into a nonreductive approach to psychiatric disorders. Understanding the nature of the specific stresses experienced in migration and adaptation to urban environments can help explain the variable prevalence of psychoses. Gold draws from his work on delusions to show both the broad similarity of psychotic processes across diverse cultures and their social, historical, and personal specificities.

The chapters in this section illustrate how social and cultural contexts affect vulnerability to illness through their effects on underlying physiological and psychological processes, as well as influence the course of illness by shaping the modes of coping, adaptation, and response to interventions. The detailed discussions of psychosis, depression, anxiety, and addictive disorders also make it clear that vicious circles or looping effects at cognitive-emotional and social-behavioral levels may be important not only in shaping symptoms and intensifying distress but also in the global spread of particular types of disorder. Mental health problems then might be characterized both by the contexts in which they occur and by the systemic processes that maintain them. This has implications for the structure of psychiatric nosology and for the ways in which we design effective interventions.

Psychiatric Practice in Global Context

Part Four considers psychiatry as clinical and public health practice, situated in wider social contexts. The aim is to show how diverse disciplinary perspectives can be integrated into a broader perspective on psychiatry that is relevant to global mental health. Psychiatric knowledge and institutions have global reach and the ways they are deployed internationally may influence their local impact. The contributors in this section build on the models presented throughout the book to consider what a culturally responsive, systemic approach to psychiatric theory and practice would look like.[7]

Responding to mental health problems across diverse settings around the globe is generally based on the assumption that people express their suffering in similar ways. A large body of ethnographic research, however, documents substantial variations in the experience, expression, and perception of mental disorders. Anthropologists Robert Lemelson and Annie Tucker discuss the embedding of psychopathology and illness experience in local and global context. Using the rich materials collected through Lemelson's longitudinal, person-centered ethnographic research and documentary film projects in Indonesia, they illustrate how both local and global are intertwined in illness experience in ways that influence the expression of distress and possibilities for coping and recovery.

Although eating disorders have the highest mortality of any psychiatric disorder, they may be difficult to detect in clinical settings due to the subtlety or nonspecificity of their symptoms. Anne Becker and Jennifer Thomas address the possibility that the prevalence of eating disorders in Fiji among *iTaukei* girls has been underestimated and, in doing so, challenge the cross-cultural applicability of Western diagnostic criteria (e.g., "intense fear of becoming fat," according to *DSM-IV*). Certain characteristics of *iTaukei* Fijian society may work to inhibit disordered eating, including robust body-type preference, discouragement of solitary or secretive eating, and close family and community scrutiny of eating habits. Although globalization, especially exposure to Western television, has had an effect on perception of body ideals, the symptoms

---

[7] For introductions to global mental health, see Patel, Minas, Cohen, and Prince (2013) and Okpaku (2014). For critiques, see Fernando (2014) and Mills (2014).

and dynamics of eating disorders may vary across cultures. To illustrate this, the authors focus on fear of fatness among four low-weight adolescent girls with possible anorexia nervosa. They find the girls' expression of such fears is ambiguous and intertwined with desire to control weight *loss* (through the use of traditional herbs) and simultaneously meet local social norms about not becoming too fat, suggesting their vulnerability to "conflicting expectations imposed by their social networks."

In recent years, the WHO and other transnational organizations, researchers, and scholars have portrayed mental illness as an escalating, global problem causing enormous suffering, particularly among residents of low- and middle-income countries (LMIC). Taking a wider lens, anthropologist Kalman Applbaum's chapter offers a critical look at the public health approach to global mental health. Like "global warming," "global mental health" poses problems on a vast scale, which the WHO describes as a crisis of epidemic proportions. This leads to a moral call to arms, "to do something." The challenge is how to scale-up interventions to have global reach. According to Applbaum, the main "solution" on offer is market-driven, with psychopharmaceuticals at its nucleus, justified with a semblance of science as "evidence-based treatment" delivered through the practice of "task shifting" by engaging community workers and others to provide care. The proper response to the global disparities in mental health deeply divides those concerned with global mental health. For some researchers, poverty and social abandonment are among the most important causes of emotional suffering and cannot be addressed by pharmaceutical interventions (Han, 2013). In addition to deleterious side effects, drug treatment for a mental illness can carry substantial stigma. Applbaum ends the chapter with a call for research that includes: close ethnographic examination of the West's own failures in delivering adequate care; a focus on collective rather than individual-based mental health models; and better understanding the embeddedness of psychiatry in "the intrigues of commercial biopower."

In the final chapter in this section, cultural psychiatrists Brandon Kohrt and James Griffith explore the various ways in which psychiatric care is delivered in LMIC from a critical medical anthropological, clinical, and ethical perspectives. The authors summarize the different players involved in critiques of the global mental health movement, with particular emphasis on the role of cultural psychiatry. Their aim is to develop a framework "for understanding and advancing global mental health *praxis*," which is ultimately based on a robust, dialogically constructed therapeutic alliance at every level of engagement, from local (healer/therapist–sufferer/client or community health worker–mental health specialist) to transnational (LMIC–IIIC mental health specialists), "within and across ecological levels" (i.e., an ecosystemic approach), with careful consideration of specific context and acknowledgment of the "unintended consequences and tradeoffs" that attend a public health approach to global mental health. Kohrt and Griffith discuss their own experiences implementing these practices on behalf of families dealing with severe mental illness and former child soldiers in Kosovo and Nepal, respectively. They argue that, whatever their merits, the global mental health critiques do not justify inaction but point to the need for more research on healer–patient interactions and other dialogical practices that can help address power differentials and stigma.

In his commentary on this section, Duncan Pedersen considers the rationale and implications of current efforts to address global inequities in mental health. To the extent that these inequities reflect structural problems in global economic systems and governance, they demand solutions at the same level. There is a risk that reframing the issues in clinical or even public health terms will miss essential dimensions of the problem and end up deflecting efforts to make real change.

There is a growing commitment to address global disparities in mental health through prevention, intervention, and effective treatment for mental illness. But in the process of sharing knowledge and redistributing resources, we risk exporting problems as well as solutions. Promoting global mental health through an ecosystemic and politically aware engagement can allow us to work toward equity while respecting diversity, and avoid a new psychiatric colonialism or imperialism.

In the concluding chapter to the volume, Laurence Kirmayer returns to the conceptual critique of reductionist models in psychiatry. He draws together several strands from the work of the contributors and other recent efforts to sketch a vision of psychiatry that integrates phenomenology, neuroscience, and social sciences in an ecosystemic approach to guide a comprehensive research program as well as multilevel clinical assessment and interventions.

Conclusion

To address the cogent critiques of psychiatry's failures and limitations, we need to rethink its conceptual foundations as well as the moral and ethical dimensions of policy and clinical practice. This rethinking depends not only on scientific advances but also on understanding the ways in which values are woven into the normative language of sickness and health, including our definitions of mental disorders, notions of good outcome, and choice of interventions.

The biological turn in psychiatry has led to reductive approaches to mental disorders. The problem lies not with the undeniable fact that the brain is the substrate of thinking, feeling, and behavior, but with the kind of neuroscience that dominates the field. Human evolutionary history makes it clear that our cognitive and emotional machinery is organized to manage the complex social worlds in which we dwell. Hence, we need a refined social and cultural neuroscience to understand the ways the brain can go wrong. This will require not only good brain theory and psychology but also good social theory.

On this view, psychiatric disorders arise from dynamic interactions within and between complex systems that operate from the molecular and cellular level all the way up to the level of society and culture (Kirmayer & Crafa, 2014). In this context, a "system" is defined as a coherent organization of elements (including other systems), the effect of which is greater than the sum of its parts. Applying systems thinking to psychiatric theory and practice requires a broad understanding of multiple disciplines, including: neuroscience (the anatomical structures and processes that comprise neural systems, their development, plasticity, and perturbation); psychology (how functional systems develop through learning, active engagement with the environment, and cognitive-interpretative processes); and the social sciences (the social interactions, including cooperation and conflict with others, that produce and sustain shared knowledge, institutions, and practices). Each of these disciplines addresses particular levels of analysis of the biopsychosocial systems that constitute human experience and behavior in health and illness. Because it is evident that psychiatry involves processes at many levels, the central conceptual problem in psychiatry is how to bring these levels together in a meaningful way.

What the contributions to this volume make clear is that moving beyond the critique of reductionistic neuroscience and decontextualized models of illness that hobble current psychiatric theory requires a broader view based on a more open-ended, socioecological, dynamical systems perspective (Kirmayer & Crafa, 2014) The biopsychosocial approach articulated by George Engel (1980) provided a schematic way to understand the multiple levels that contribute to mental health problems. Although criticized for failing to give specific guidelines for clinical practice (Ghaemi, 2010), Engel's hierarchical systems view is consistent with contemporary biology and social science. A complex systems perspective, wedded to detailed understanding of the biological, psychological, and social processes that contribute to illness and well-being, can provide an integrative framework for psychiatry.

One way to incorporate systems thinking in clinical practice is to consider the process of illness experience in terms of the constructs of *dimensions, trajectories, thresholds,* and *contexts* or *predicaments. Dimensions* are the different variables that we use to describe phenomena; in this sense, dimensions are a "systemic" concept: they are the parameters needed to describe the space within which behaviors or events occur. Within this multidimensional space, behavior can follow various *trajectories:* moving toward attractors, loops, or limit cycles, and exhibiting bifurcations or discontinuities when they cross particular thresholds (Gros, 2013). These dynamics may emerge from interactional processes within the nervous system, between the person and the environment, as well as among people and in larger social systems (Gottman, Murray, Swanson, Tyson, & Swanson, 2002).

In fact, most of the problems that people bring to the clinic are deeply rooted in the social *contexts* of local worlds and personal predicaments. Psychiatric nosology attempts to describe problems abstracted out of context in terms of certain kinds of general characteristics or processes. But in clinical practice, problems must be understood and addressed in relation to their local history, contexts, and contingencies. Here is where anthropology and other social sciences can make a crucial contribution to psychiatry by situating suffering and healing in local and global worlds of knowledge, meaning, and values. The recognition that these situations constitute *predicaments* for individuals, families, and communities highlights the questions of agency and value central to psychiatric practice. Ultimately, the problems of mental health and illness are too complex and too important to be left to any one discipline. We need the methods and perspectives of many disciplines not only to understand the underlying mechanisms of health and illness but also to understand the impact of our practices on our concepts of self and on wider social processes.

Taken together, the contributions to this volume support the call for programmatic shifts in psychiatric theory, research, and practice. Ultimately, we envision a psychiatry that approaches mind as embedded in – and co-constitutive of – the social world and mental disorders as inextricably linked to those same social realities. Of course, the social world is undergoing constant change through the forces of globalization, the Internet and telecommunications, migration, new identities and configurations of families, political conflict, and climate change. Addressing the mental health impact of these changes will require a wide-ranging program of research and theory building in psychiatry. However, as the concluding chapter tries to show, there is already a good theoretical and empirical basis for an integrative, context-sensitive psychiatry that responds more humanely and effectively to the concerns of patients, families, and practitioners.

REFERENCES

American Psychiatric Association. (1952). *Mental disorders: Diagnostic and statistical manual.* Washington, DC: Author.

American Psychiatric Association. (1968). *Diagnostic and statistical manual of mental disorders* (2nd ed.). Washington, DC: Author.

American Psychiatric Association. (1980). *Diagnostic and statistical manual of mental disorders* (3rd ed.). Washington, DC: Author.

American Psychiatric Association. (1994). *Diagnostic and statistical manual of mental disorders* (4th ed.). Washington, DC: Author.

American Psychiatric Association. (2013). *Diagnostic and statistical manual of mental disorders* (5th ed.). Washington, DC: Author.

Anderson, I. M. (2000). Selective serotonin reuptake inhibitors versus tricyclic antidepressants: A meta-analysis of efficacy and tolerability. *Journal of Affective Disorders, 58*(1), 19–36. http://dx.doi.org/10.1016/S0165-0327(99)00092-0

Andrews, G. (Ed.). (2009). *Stress-induced and fear circuitry disorders: Advancing the research agenda for "DSM-V."* Arlington, VA: American Psychiatric Association.

Angell, M. (2011). The epidemic of mental illness: Why? *The New York Review of Books, 58*(11), 20–2. Retrieved from www.nybooks.com/articles/archives/2011/jun/23/epidemic-mental-illness-why/

Bains, J. (2005). Race, culture and psychiatry: A history of transcultural psychiatry. *History of Psychiatry, 16*(2), 139–54. http://dx.doi.org/10.1177/0957154X05046167

Baldessarini, R. J. (2014). The impact of psychopharmacology on contemporary psychiatry. *Canadian Journal of Psychiatry, 59*(8), 401–5.

Basu, S., & Parry, P. (2013). The autism spectrum disorder "epidemic": Need for biopsychosocial formulation. *Australian and New Zealand Journal of Psychiatry, 47*(12), 1116–18. http://dx.doi.org/10.1177/0004867413509694

Bateson, G. (1972). The cybernetics of self: A theory of alcoholism. In *Steps to an ecology of mind* (pp. 225–43). Northvale, NJ: Jason Aronson.

Bateson, G. (1972). *Steps to an ecology of mind.* New York, NY: Ballantine Books.

Beach, S. R. H., Wamboldt, M. Z., Kaslow, N. J., Heyman, R. E., First, M. B., Underwood, L. G., & Reiss, D. (Eds.). (2007). *Relational processes and "DSM-V": Neuroscience, assessment, prevention, and treatment.* Washington, DC: American Psychiatric Press.

Biehl, J., Good, B., & Kleinman, A. (Eds.). (2007). *Subjectivity: Ethnographic investigations.* Berkeley: University of California Press. http://dx.doi.org/10.1525/california/9780520247925.001.0001

Bolton, D. (2012). Classification and causal mechanisms: A deflationary approach to the classification problem. In K. S. Kendler & J. Parnas (Eds.), *Philosophical issues in psychiatry II: Nosology* (pp. 6–11). Oxford, England: Oxford University Press. http://dx.doi.org/10.1093/med/9780199642205.003.0002

Borsboom, D., Cramer, A. O., Schmittmann, V. D., Epskamp, S., & Waldorp, L. J. (2011). The small world of psychopathology. *PLOS one, 6*(11), e27407. http://dx.doi.org/10.1371/journal.pone.0027407

British Psychological Society. (2014, November 27). *Understanding psychosis and schizophrenia* [Anne Cooke, Ed.]. Retrieved from www.bps.org.uk/networks-and-communities/member-microsite/division-clinical-psychology/understanding-psychosis-and-schizophrenia

Bracken, P., Thomas, P., Timimi, S., Asen, E., Behr, G., Beuster, C., . . . Yeomans, D. (2012). Psychiatry beyond the current paradigm. *British Journal of Psychiatry, 201*(6), 430–4. http://dx.doi.org/10.1192/bjp .bp.112.109447

Broome, M. R., Harland, R., & Owen, G. S. (Eds.). (2013). *The Maudsley reader in phenomenological psychiatry.* Cambridge, England: Cambridge University Press.

Buckholtz, J. W., & Meyer-Lindenberg, A. (2012). Psychopathology and the human connectome: Toward a transdiagnostic model of risk for mental illness. *Neuron, 74*(6), 990–1004. http://dx.doi.org/10.1016/j. neuron.2012.06.002

Byrge, L., Sporns, O., & Smith, L. B. (2014). Developmental process emerges from extended brain–body–behavior networks. *Trends in Cognitive Sciences, 18*(8), 395–40. http://dx.doi.org/10.1016/j.tics.2014.04.010

Cacioppo, J. T., Cacioppo, S., Dulawa, S., & Palmer, A. A. (2014). Social neuroscience and its potential contribution to psychiatry. *World Psychiatry, 13*, 131–9. http://dx.doi.org/10.1002/wps.20118

Carpenter, W. T., & van Os, J. (2011). Should attenuated psychosis syndrome be a *DSM-5* diagnosis? *American Journal of Psychiatry, 168*(5), 460–3. http://dx .doi.org/10.1176/appi.ajp.2011.10121816

Charney, D. S., Nestler, E. J., Sklar, P., & Buxbaum, J. D. (Eds.). (2013). *Neurobiology of mental illness.* New York, NY: Oxford University Press. http://dx.doi.org/10.1093/med/9780199934959.001.0001

Chiao, J. Y. (2009). Cultural neuroscience: A once and future discipline. *Progress in Brain Research, 178*, 287–304. http://dx.doi.org/10.1016/S0079-61 23(09)17821-4

Choudhury, S., & Slaby, J. (Eds.). (2011). *Critical neuroscience: A handbook of the social and cultural contexts of neuroscience.* Chichester, England: Wiley-Blackwell. http://dx.doi.org/10.1016/S0079-6123(09)17821-4

Cohen, C. I., & Timimi, S. (2008). *Liberatory psychiatry: Philosophy, politics, and mental health.* Cambridge, England: Cambridge University Press.

Collin, J. (2015). Universal cures for idiosyncratic illnesses: A genealogy of therapeutic reasoning in the mental health field. *Health, 19*(3), 245–62. http://dx.doi.org/10.1177/1363459314545695

Cooper, J. E., Kendell, R. E., Gurland, B. J., Sharpe, L., Copeland, J. R. M., & Simon, R. J. (1972). *Psychiatric diagnosis in New York and London: A comparative study of mental hospital admissions.* London, England: Oxford University Press.

Cromby, H., Newton, T., & Williams, S. J. (2011). Neuroscience and subjectivity. *Subjectivity, 4*, 215–26. http://dx.doi.org/10.1057/sub.2011.13

Cuthbert, B. N. (2014). The RDoC framework: Facilitating transition from *ICD/DSM* to dimensional approaches that integrate neuroscience and psychopathology. *World Psychiatry, 13*(1), 28–35. http://dx.doi.org/10.1002/wps.20087

Dackis, C., & C. O'Brien. (2005). Neurobiology of addiction: Treatment and public policy ramifications. *Nature Neuroscience, 8,* 143–6. http://dx.doi.org/10.1038/nn1105-1431

Davidson, E. H. (2010). *The regulatory genome: Gene regulatory networks in development and evolution.* New York, NY: Academic Press.

Deisseroth, K. (2012). Optogenetics and psychiatry: Applications, challenges, and opportunities. *Biological Psychiatry, 71*(12), 1030–2. http://dx.doi.org/10.1016/j.biopsych.2011.12.021

Desjarlais, R., & Throop, J.C. (2011). Phenomenological approaches in anthropology. *Annual Review of Anthropology, 40,* 87–102. http://dx.doi.org/10.1146/annurev-anthro-092010-153345

Engel, G.L. (1980). The clinical application of the biopsychosocial model. *American Journal of Psychiatry, 137,* 535–44.

Fernando, S. (2014). *Mental health worldwide: Culture, globalization and development.* New York, NY: Palgrave Macmillan. http://dx.doi.org/10.1057/9781137329608

Fisher, H. E., & Thomson, J. A., Jr. (2007). Lust, romance, attachment: Do the side effects of serotonin-enhancing antidepressants jeopardize romantic love, marriage, and fertility? In S. M. Platek, J. P Keenan, & T. K. Shackelford (Eds.), *Evolutionary cognitive neuroscience,* (pp. 245–83). Cambridge, MA: MIT Press.

Fornito, A., & Bullmore, E. T. (2015). Connectomics: A new paradigm for understanding brain disease *European Neuropsychopharmacology, 25*(5), 733–48. http://dx.doi.org/10.1016/j.euroneuro.2014.02.011

Frances, A. (2012, May 11). Diagnosing the *DSM. New York Times.* Retrieved from www.nytimes.com/2012/05/12/opinion/break-up-the-psychiatric-monopoly.html

Frances, A. (2013). *Saving normal: An insider's look at what caused the epidemic of mental illness and how to cure it.* New York, NY: William Morrow.

Frank, E. Nimgaonkar, V. L., Phillips, M. L., & Kupfer, D. J. (2015). All the world's a (clinical) stage: Rethinking bipolar disorder from a longitudinal perspective. *Molecular Psychiatry, 20,* 23–31. http://dx.doi.org/10.1038/mp.2014.71

Gallagher, S., & Zahavi, D. (2012). *The phenomenological mind.* New York, NY: Routledge.

Ghaemi, S. N. (2010). *The rise and fall of the biopsychosocial model: Reconciling art and science in psychiatry.* Baltimore, MD: Johns Hopkins University Press.

Gottman, J. M., Murray, J. D., Swanson, C. C., Tyson, R., & Swanson, K. R. (2002). *The mathematics of marriage: Dynamic nonlinear models.* Cambridge, MA: MIT Press.

Greenberg, G. (2010). *Manufacturing depression: The secret history of a modern disease.* New York, NY: Simon & Schuster.

Grob, G.N. (2008). The transformation of psychiatry from institution to community, 1800–2000. In E. R. Wallace & J. Gach (Eds.), *History of psychiatry and medical psychology* (pp. 533–50). New York, NY: Springer. http://dx.doi.org/10.1007/978-0-387-34708-0_18

Gros, C. (2013). *Complex and adaptive dynamical systems: A primer.* New York, NY: Springer. http://dx.doi.org/10.1007/978-3-642-36586-7

Hacking, I. (1995). The looping effect of human kinds. In D. Sperber, D. Premack, & A. J. Premack (Eds.), *Causal cognition: A multidisciplinary debate* (pp. 351–83). Oxford, England: Oxford University Press.

Hacking, I. (1999). *The social construction of what?* Cambridge, MA: Harvard University Press.

Haddad, P. M., & Sharma, S. G. (2007). Adverse effects of atypical antipsychotics. *CNS Drugs, 21*(11), 911–36. http://dx.doi.org/10.2165/00023210-200721110-00004

Han, C. (2014). Labor instability and community mental health. In J. Biehl & A. Petryna (Eds.), *When people come first: Critical studies in global mental health* (pp. 276–301). Princeton, NJ: Princeton University Press.

Han, S., Northoff, G., Vogeley, K., Wexler, B. E., Kitayama, S., & Varnum, M. E. (2013). A cultural neuroscience approach to the biosocial nature of the human brain. *Annual Review of Psychology, 64,* 335–59. http://dx.doi.org/10.1146/annurev-psych-071112-054629

Haslam, N. (2007). The latent structure of mental disorders: A taxometric update on the categorical vs. dimensional debate. *Current Psychiatry Reviews, 3*(3), 172–7. http://dx.doi.org/10.2174/157340007781369685

Healy, D. (2004). *The creation of psychopharmacology.* Cambridge, MA: Harvard University Press.

Helzer, J. E., Kraemer, H. C., Krueger, R. F., Wittchen, R. F., Sirovatka, P. J., & Regier, D. A. (Eds.). (2008). *Dimensional approaches in diagnostic classification: Refining the research agenda for "DSM-V."* Arlington, VA: American Psychiatric Association.

Henrich, J., Heine, S., & Norenzayan, A. (2010). The weirdest people in the world? *Behavioral and Brain Sciences, 33*(2–3), 61–83. http://dx.doi.org/10.1017/S0140525X0999152X

Higgins, E. S., & George, M. S. (2013). *Neuroscience of clinical psychiatry: The pathophysiology of behavior and mental illness.* New York, NY: Lippincott Williams & Wilkins.

Hofmann, S. G., Asmundson, G. J., & Beck, A. T. (2013). The science of cognitive therapy. *Behavior Therapy, 44*(2), 199–212. http://dx.doi.org/10.1016/j.beth.2009.01.007

Horwitz, A. V. (2011). Naming the problem that has no name: Creating targets for standardized drugs. *Studies in History and Philosophy of Science Part C: Biological and Biomedical Sciences, 42*(4), 427–33. http://dx.doi.org/10.1016/j.shpsc.2011.05.002

Horwitz, A. V., & Wakefield, J. C. (2007). *The loss of sadness: How psychiatry transformed normal sorrow into depressive disorder.* New York, NY: Oxford University Press.

Horwitz, A. V., & Wakefield, J. C. (2012). *All we have to fear: Psychiatry's transformation of natural anxieties into mental disorders.* New York, NY: Oxford University Press.

Insel, T., Cuthbert, B., Garvey, M., Heinssen, R., Pine, D. S., Quinn, K., …
Wang, P. (2010). Research domain criteria (RDoC): Toward a new
classification framework for research on mental disorders. *American
Journal of Psychiatry, 167*(7), 748–51. http://dx.doi.org/10.1176/appi
.ajp.2010.09091379

Jenkins, J. H. (2015). *Extraordinary conditions: Culture and experience in mental
illness.* Berkeley: University of California Press.

Jenkins, J. H., & Barrett, R. J. (2004). *Schizophrenia, culture, and subjectivity:
The edge of experience.* Cambridge, England: Cambridge University Press.

Kandel, E. R., Schwartz, J. H., Jessell, T. M. , Siegelbaum , S. A. & Hudspeth,
J. A. (Eds.). (2012). *Principles of neural science.* New York, NY: McGraw-
Hill.

Kendler, K. S. (2011). Levels of explanation in psychiatric and substance use
disorders: Implications for the development of an etiologically based
nosology. *Molecular Psychiatry, 17*(1), 11–21. http://dx.doi.org/10.1038/
mp.2011.70

Kendler, K. S. (2014). The structure of psychiatric science. *Molecular
Psychiatry, 171*(9), 931–8. http://dx.doi.org/10.1176/appi.
ajp.2014.13111539

Kendler, K. S., & Campbell, J. (2009). Interventionist causal models in
psychiatry: Repositioning the mind–body problem. *Psychological Medicine,
39*(06), 881–7. http://dx.doi.org/10.1017/S0033291708004467

Kendler, K. S., Jaffee, S. R., & Romer, D. (2011). *The dynamic genome and mental
health: The role of genes and environments in youth development.* New York, NY:
Oxford University Press.

Kendler, K. S., & Neale, M. C. (2010). Endophenotype: A conceptual analysis.
Molecular Psychiatry, 15(8), 789–97. http://dx.doi.org/10.1038/mp.2010.8

Kim, H. S., & Sasaki, J. Y. (2014). Cultural neuroscience: Biology of the mind in
cultural contexts. *Annual Review of Psychology, 65*, 487–514. http://dx.doi
.org/10.1146/annurev-psych-010213-115040

Kirmayer, L. J. (1988). Mind and body as metaphors: Hidden values in
biomedicine. In M. Lock & D. Gordon (Eds.), *Biomedicine examined*
(pp. 57–92). Dordrecht, The Netherlands: Kluwer. http://dx.doi.org/
10.1007/978-94-009-2725-4_4

Kirmayer, L. J. (1989). Cultural variations in the response to psychiatric
disorders and emotional distress. *Social Science and Medicine, 29*(3), 327–39.
http://dx.doi.org/10.1016/0277-9536(89)90281-5

Kirmayer, L. J. (2012). Rethinking cultural competence. *Transcultural Psychiatry,
49*(2), 149–64. http://dx.doi.org/10.1177/1363461512444673

Kirmayer, L. J., & Bhugra, D. (2009). Culture and mental illness: Social context
and explanatory models. In I. M. Salloum & J. E. Mezzich (Eds.), *Psychiatric
diagnosis: Patterns and prospects* (pp. 29–37). New York, NY: John Wiley &
Sons. http://dx.doi.org/10.1002/9780470743485.ch3

Kirmayer, L. J., & Crafa, D. (2014). What kind of science for psychiatry?
Frontiers in Human Neuroscience, 8, 435. http://dx.doi.org/10.3389/
fnhum.2014.00435

Kirmayer, L. J., & Gold, I. (2012). Re-socializing psychiatry: Critical
neuroscience and the limits of reductionism. In S. Choudhury & J. Slaby

(Eds.), *Critical neuroscience: A handbook of the social and cultural contexts of neuroscience* (pp. 307–30). Oxford, England: Blackwell.

Kirmayer, L. J., & Young, A. (1999). Culture and context in the evolutionary concept of mental disorder. *Journal of Abnormal Psychology, 108*(3), 446–52. http://dx.doi.org/10.1037/0021-843X.108.3.446

Kirsch, I. (2009). *The emperor's new drugs: Exploding the antidepressant myth.* London, England: Bodley Head.

Kirsch, I., Deacon, B. J., Huedo-Medina, T. B., Scoboria, A., Moore, T. J., & Johnson, B. T. (2008). Initial severity and antidepressant benefits: A meta-analysis of data submitted to the Food and Drug Administration. *PLOS Medicine, 5*, e45. http://dx.doi.org/10.1371/journal.pmed.0050045

Kleinman, A. M. (1980). *Patients and healers in the context of culture.* Berkeley: University of California Press.

Kleinman, A. (1988). *Rethinking psychiatry.* New York, NY: Free Press.

Kleinman, A. (2009). Global mental health: A failure of humanity. *The Lancet, 374*(9690), 603–4. http://dx.doi.org/10.1016/S0140-6736(09)61510-5

Koerth-Baker, M. (2013, October 15). The not-so-hidden cause behind the A.D.H.D. epidemic. *New York Times Magazine.* Retrieved from www.nytimes.com/2013/10/20/magazine/the-not-so-hidden-cause-behind-the-adhd-epidemic.html?pagewanted=all&_r=0

Krieger, N. (2001). Theories for social epidemiology in the 21st century: An ecosocial perspective. *International Journal of Epidemiology, 30*(4), 668–77. http://dx.doi.org/10.1093/ije/30.4.668

Leucht, S., Corves, C., Arbter, D., Engel, R. R., Li, C., & Davis, J. M. (2009). Second-generation versus first-generation antipsychotic drugs for schizophrenia: A meta-analysis. *The Lancet, 373*(9657), 31–41. http://dx.doi.org/10.1016/S0140-6736(08)61764-X

Lewis-Fernández, R., Aggarwal, N. K., Bäärnhielm, S., Rohlof, H., Kirmayer, L. J., Weiss, M. G., ... Lu, F. (2014). Culture and psychiatric evaluation: Operationalizing cultural formulation for *DSM-5. Psychiatry, 77*(2), 130–54. http://dx.doi.org/10.1521/psyc.2014.77.2.130

Lewis-Fernández, R., Aggarwal, N. K., Hinton, D. E., Hinton, L., & Kirmayer, L. J. (Eds.). (2015). *"DSM-5" handbook on the cultural formulation interview.* Washington, DC: American Psychiatric Press.

Light, D. W., Lexchin, J., & Darrow, J. J. (2013). Institutional corruption of pharmaceuticals and the myth of safe and effective drugs. *Journal of Law, Medicine & Ethics, 41*(3), 590–600.

Littlewood, R., & Dein, S. (Eds.). (2000). *Cultural psychiatry and medical anthropology: An introduction and reader.* London, England: Bloomsbury Publishing.

López, S. R., & Guarnaccia, P. J. (2012). Cultural dimensions of psychopathology. In J. E. Maddux & B. A. Winstead (Eds.), *Psychopathology: Foundations for a contemporary understanding,* (pp. 45–68). New York, NY: Routledge.

Luhrmann, T. M. (2000). *Of two minds: The growing disorder in American psychiatry.* New York, NY: Knopf.

March, D., & Oppenheimer, G. M. (2014). Social disorder and diagnostic order: The US Mental Hygiene Movement, the Midtown Manhattan study and the development of psychiatric epidemiology in the 20th century. *International Journal of Epidemiology, 43*(Suppl. 1), i29–i42. http://dx.doi.org/10.1093/ije/dyu117

Marková, I. S., & Berrios, G. E. (2012). Epistemology of psychiatry. *Psychopathology, 45*(4), 220–7. http://dx.doi.org/10.1159/000331599

Marmot, M. G., & Wilkinson, R. G. (2006). *Social determinants of health* (2nd ed.). Oxford, England: Oxford University Press.

McCarroll, S. A., Feng, G., & Hyman, S. E. (2014). Genome-scale neurogenetics: Methodology and meaning. *Nature Neuroscience, 17*(6), 756–63. http://dx.doi.org/10.1038/nn.3716

McNally, R. J. (2011). *What is mental illness?* Cambridge, MA: Belknap Press.

Meehl, P. E. (1995). Bootstraps taxometrics: Solving the classification problem in psychopathology. *American Psychologist, 50*(4), 266–75. http://dx.doi.org/10.1037/0003-066X.50.4.266

Mezzich, J., Kirmayer, L. J., Kleinman, A., Fabrega, H., Jr., Parron, D. L., Good, B. J., . . . Manson, S. M. (1999). The place of culture in *DSM-IV*. *Journal of Nervous and Mental Disease, 187*(8), 457–64. http://dx.doi.org/10.1097/00005053-199908000-00001

Mills, C. (2014). *Decolonizing global mental health: The psychiatrization of the majority world.* New York, NY: Routledge.

Miresco, M. J., & Kirmayer, L. J. (2006). The persistence of mind-brain dualism in psychiatric reasoning about clinical scenarios. *American Journal of Psychiatry, 163*(5), 913–18. http://dx.doi.org/10.1176/appi.ajp.163.5.913

Moghaddam, B., & Wood, J. (2014). Teamwork matters: Coordinated neuronal activity in brain systems relevant to psychiatric disorders. *JAMA Psychiatry, 71*(2), 197–9. http://dx.doi.org/10.1001/jamapsychiatry.2013.2080

Moncrieff, J. (2014). The medicalization of "ups and downs": The marketing of the new bipolar disorder. *Transcultural Psychiatry, 51*(4), 581–98. http://dx.doi.org/10.1177/1363461514530024

Moodley, R., & Ocampo, M. (Eds.). (2014). *Critical psychiatry and mental health: Exploring the work of Suman Fernando in clinical practice.* New York, NY: Routledge/Taylor & Francis.

Nordgaard, J., Sass, L. A., & Parnas, J. (2013). The psychiatric interview: Validity, structure, and subjectivity. *European Archives of Psychiatry and Clinical Neuroscience, 263*(4), 353–64. http://dx.doi.org/10.1007/s00406-012-0366-z

Northoff, G. (2014). Are auditory hallucinations related to the brain's resting state activity? A 'neurophenomenal resting state hypothesis'. *Clinical Psychopharmacology and Neuroscience, 12*(3), 189–95. http://dx.doi.org/10.9758/cpn.2014.12.3.189

Okpaku, S. (Ed.). (2014). *Essentials of global mental health.* New York, NY: Cambridge University Press. http://dx.doi.org/10.1017/CBO9781139136341

Olfson, M., Blanco, C., Liu, S. M., Wang, S., & Correll, C. U. (2012). National trends in the office-based treatment of children, adolescents, and adults with antipsychotics. *Archives of General Psychiatry, 69*(12), 1247–56. http://dx.doi.org/10.1001/archgenpsychiatry.2012.647

Paris, J. (2005). *Fall of an icon: Psychoanalysis and academic psychiatry.* Toronto, Canada: University of Toronto Press.

Paris, J. (2012). *The bipolar spectrum: Diagnosis or fad?* New York, NY: Routledge/ Taylor & Francis.

Paris, J. & Phillips, J. (Eds.). (2013). *Making the "DSM-5": Concepts and controversies.* New York, NY: Springer. http://dx.doi.org/10.1007/978-1 -4614-6504-1

Patel, V., Minas, H., Cohen, A., & Prince, M.J. (Eds.). (2013). *Global mental health: Principles and practice.* Oxford, England: Oxford University Press. http://dx.doi.org/10.1093/med/9780199920181.001.0001

Patel, V., & Prince, M. (2010). Global mental health: A new global health field comes of age. *JAMA, 303*(19), 1976–7. http://dx.doi.org/10.1001/ jama.2010.616

Pickett, K. E., & Wilkinson, R. G. (2010). Inequality: An underacknowledged source of mental illness and distress. *British Journal of Psychiatry, 197*(6), 426–8. http://dx.doi.org/10.1192/bjp.bp.109.072066

Posner, M., & Fan, J. (2008). Attention as an organ system. In J. R. Pomerantz (Ed.), *Topics in integrative neuroscience* (pp. 31–61). New York, NY: Cambridge University Press. http://dx.doi.org/10.1017/ CBO9780511541681.005

Pressman, J. D. (1997). Psychiatry and its origins. *Bulletin of the History of Medicine, 71*(1), 129–39. http://dx.doi.org/10.1353/bhm.1997.0044

Ratcliffe, M. (2014). *Experiences of depression: A study in phenomenology.* Oxford: Oxford University Press.

Read, J., & Cain, A. (2013). A literature review and meta-analysis of drug company-funded mental health websites. *Acta Psychiatrica Scandinavica, 128*(6), 422–33. http://dx.doi.org/10.1111/acps.12146

Roepstorff, A. (2013). Interactively human: Sharing time, constructing materiality *Behavioral and Brain Sciences, 36*(3), 224–5. http://dx.doi.org/ 10.1017/S0140525X12002427

Rose, N. (1998). *Inventing our selves: Psychology, power, and personhood.* Cambridge, England: Cambridge University Press.

Rose, N. S., & Abi-Rached, J. M. (2013). *Neuro: The new brain sciences and the management of the mind.* Princeton, NJ: Princeton University Press.

Rudnick, A. (Ed.). (2012). *Recovery of people with mental illness: Philosophical and related perspectives.* Oxford, England: Oxford University Press. http://dx.doi. org/10.1093/med/9780199691319.001.0001

Rule, N. O., Freeman, J. B., & Ambady, N. (2013). Culture in social neuroscience: A review. *Social Neuroscience, 8*(1), 3–10. http://dx.doi.org/ 10.1080/17470919.2012.695293

Sapir, E. (1932). Cultural anthropology and psychiatry. *Journal of Abnormal and Social Psychology, 27*(3), 229–42. http://dx.doi.org/10.1037/ h0076025

Shorter, E. (1997). *A history of psychiatry: From the era of the asylum to the age of Prozac.* New York, NY: John Wiley & Sons.

Singh, I. (2008). Beyond polemics: Science and ethics of ADHD. *Nature Reviews Neuroscience, 9*(12), 957–64. http://dx.doi.org/10.1038/nrn2514

Sporns, O. (2012). *Discovering the human connectome.* Cambridge, MA: MIT Press.

Stanghellini, G., & Fuchs, T. (Eds.). (2013). *One century of Karl Jaspers' General Psychopathology.* Oxford, UK: Oxford University Press.

Steinberg, E. E., Christoffel, D. J., Deisseroth, K., & Malenka, R. C. (2015). Illuminating circuitry relevant to psychiatric disorders with optogenetics. *Current Opinion in Neurobiology, 30*(9), 9–16. http://dx.doi.org/10.1016/j.conb.2014.08.004

Stelzer, J., Lohmann, G., Mueller, K., Buschmann, T., & Turner, R. (2014). Deficient approaches to human neuroimaging. *Frontiers in Human Neuroscience, 8*, 462. http://dx.doi.org/10.3389/fnhum.2014.00462

Thomas, P. (2104). *Psychiatry in context: Experience, meaning and communities.* Monmouth, England: PCCS.

Thomas, R., Mitchell, G. K., & Batstra, L. (2013). Attention-deficit/hyperactivity disorder: Are we helping or harming? *BMJ, 347*, f6172. http://dx.doi.org/10.1136/bmj.f6172

Thombs, B. D., Coyne, J. C., Cuijpers, P., de Jonge, P., Gilbody, S., Ioannidis, J. P., … Ziegelstein, R. C. (2012). Rethinking recommendations for screening for depression in primary care. *Canadian Medical Association Journal, 184*(4), 413–18. http://dx.doi.org/10.1503/cmaj.111035

van Os, J., Linscott, R. J., Myin-Germeys, I., Delespaul, P., & Krabbendam, L. (2009). A systematic review and meta-analysis of the psychosis continuum: Evidence for a psychosis proneness–persistence–impairment model of psychotic disorder. *Psychological Medicine, 39*(02), 179–95. http://dx.doi.org/10.1017/S0033291708003814

Vázquez, G. H. (2014). The impact of psychopharmacology on contemporary clinical psychiatry. *Canadian Journal of Psychiatry, 59*(8), 412–16.

Wakefield, J. C. (1999). Evolutionary versus prototype analyses of the concept of disorder. *Journal of Abnormal Psychology, 108*(3), 374–99. http://dx.doi.org/10.1037/0021-843X.108.3.374

Wakefield, J. C. (2007). The concept of mental disorder: Diagnostic implications of the harmful dysfunction analysis. *World Psychiatry, 6*(3), 149–56.

Watters, E. (2010). *Crazy like us: The globalization of the American psyche.* New York, NY: Free Press.

Westen, D. (2012). Prototype diagnosis of psychiatric syndromes. *World Psychiatry, 11*(1), 16–21. http://dx.doi.org/10.1016/j.wpsyc.2012.01.004

Wexler, B. E. (2006). *Brain and culture: Neurobiology, ideology, and social change.* Cambridge, MA: MIT Press.

Whitaker, R. (2010). *Anatomy of an epidemic: Magic bullets, psychiatric drugs, and the astonishing rise of mental illness in America.* New York, NY: Crown.

Whitley, R. (2012). The antipsychiatry movement: Dead, diminishing, or developing? *Psychiatric Services, 63*(10), 1039–41. http://dx.doi.org/10.1176/appi.ps.201100484

Whitley, R., Rousseau, C., Carpenter-Song, E., & Kirmayer, L. J. (2011). Evidence-based medicine: Opportunities and challenges in a diverse society. *Canadian Journal of Psychiatry, 56*(9), 514–22.

Wilson, M. (1993). *DSM-III* and the transformation of American psychiatry: A history. *American Journal of Psychiatry, 150*, 399–410. http://dx.doi.org/10.1176/ajp.150.3.399

Wing, J. K. (1971). International comparisons in the study of the functional psychoses. *British Medical Bulletin, 27*(1), 77–81.

Young, A. (1995). *The harmony of illusions: Inventing posttraumatic stress disorder.* Princeton, NJ: Princeton University Press.

Zaretsky, E. (2004). *Secrets of the soul: A social and cultural history of psychoanalysis.* New York, NY: Knopf.

Zhang, T. Y., & Meaney, M. J. (2010). Epigenetics and the environmental regulation of the genome and its function. *Annual Review of Psychology, 61*, 439–66, C431–3. http://dx.doi.org/10.1146/annurev.psych.60.110707.16362

Zorumski, C., & Rubin, E. (2011). *Psychiatry and clinical neuroscience.* New York, NY: Oxford University Press. http://dx.doi.org/10.1093/med/9780199768769.001.1

Section One

Restoring Phenomenology to Psychiatry

2   Toward a New Epistemology of Psychiatry

German E. Berrios and Ivana S. Marková

After a two-centuries-long alliance with medicine, psychiatry (its structure, objects, language, and praxis) remains as opaque as ever. Explaining why this is the case should be the task of the epistemology of psychiatry (EP). Surprisingly enough, until recently psychiatry lacked an epistemology to explore the nature and legitimacy of psychiatric knowledge. Instead, its problems have been addressed in part by the general epistemology of medicine (Berrios, 2006; Wulff, Pedersen, & Rosenberg, 1986) and in part by work in the philosophy of psychiatry, which began to appear after World War II (see, e.g., Blanc, 1998; Griffiths, 1994; Kehrer, 1951; Lanteri-Laura, 1963; Lewis, 1967; Natanson, 1969; Palem, 2010; Palmer, 1952; Reznek, 1991; Siegler & Osmond, 1974; Spiegelberg, 1972; Spitzer & Maher, 1990; Strauss, 1958; and others). In the hands of Anglo-American writers (such as Fulford, Thornton, & Graham, 2006; Radden, 2004) the philosophy of psychiatry has now become a voluminous industry. Given its bias in the direction of analytical philosophy, a great deal of this work has been openly justificatory of the neurosciences in general and of biological psychiatry in particular (Bolton & Hill, 2003; Kendler & Parnas, 2008; Murphy, 2006; more on this later).[1]

This predictable state of affairs throws into relief the urgent need for a dedicated epistemology that may act as an independent auditor of all psychiatric narratives, past and present, and that conceives of psychiatry as a *sui generis* discipline, broader than the conventional sciences, language-bound, and closely dependent on its historical period. This chapter will present a sketch of a new EP along these lines.

We are using the concept of "EP" to refer to the discipline of examining the various sources of knowledge underlying psychiatry and its objects in order to further develop understanding concerning their nature and stability. Because we feel that philosophy of psychiatry, while

---

[1] There are, of course, voices raised against the power of the neurosciences to define and explain psychiatric objects (e.g., Bennett & Hacker, 2003; Choudhury & Slaby, 2012), but it cannot be denied that the general trend has been to follow the official line.

pursuing a similar aim, is too constraining in its methods and sources of knowledge, we have adopted the broader term of "epistemology" to widen the field. Within EP, there will naturally be many approaches and ways of tackling the questions, but as far as the discipline is concerned we are talking about a single general epistemology rather than many epistemologies of psychiatry.

From the beginning of history, societies have put together many narratives destined to account for and manage the pervasive phenomena of mental afflictions (biological psychiatry is one of these narratives). Such narratives can be conceived of as (1) complete, independent, and "fit for purpose" narratives, carrying meanings specific to their historical context and their own predictive, therapeutic, and social value or (2) stages of a unitary, ongoing narrative of a cumulative process pointing toward the final "truth" of mental afflictions. This linear and progress-related view is favored by current biological psychiatrists. However, the success or failure of these narratives has not depended on their intrinsic "truth" (for this would be impossible to ascertain[2]), but on their social and economic usefulness (Sendrail, 1980). In general terms, narratives fail because (1) their subject-matter is elusive, opaque, or badly outlined; (2) the conceptual frames and methodologies they sponsor are inappropriate to the subject matter; (3) they do not come up to economic or social expectations; and (4) empirical research into them does not receive the support (financial, human, ideological) that their sponsors believe they deserve.

Given that presentism and "scientificism" (Budd, 2009; Butterfield, 1965; Iggers & Wang 2008) are important features of globalist societies, it is not surprising that the official view at the moment is that the biological narrative about mental afflictions is the "truthful" one, and hence what many perceive as its indifferent progress should be solely explained in terms of underresourcing (World Health Organization, 2003). In the course of this chapter, we will propose that a better explanation for this lack of success rests on a combination of poorly defined subject matter and inappropriate conceptualizations or methodologies.

Key Concepts and Chapter Overview

In order to examine questions around the nature, origin, legitimacy, and stability of psychiatric knowledge, the new EP we propose makes use of a

---

[2] This is because the required *experimentum crucis* (Laugier, 1999) is not possible to design (or undertake), and hence choosing between narratives cannot be done on a conventional "scientific" basis.

combination of tools borrowed from historiography, hermeneutics, and empirical research. At all times, the choice (and crafting) of tools is dictated by the internal needs and problems affecting the narratives under exploration. In this important sense EP differs from much of current philosophy of psychiatry in that it does not follow an "off-the-shelf" approach – be the chosen philosophies analytical (Glock, 2008); phenomenological (Spiegelberg, 1982; Strasser, 1963; Toombs, 2001); deconstructionist (Culler, 1982); or pluralist (Kellert, Longino, & Waters, 2006). Thus, EP is a centrifugal rather than a centripetal philosophical exercise (Berrios, 2006). It should also be considered as a "second-order" praxis, that is, as one whose job is to uncover and evaluate the assumptions underlying first-order research (i.e., work carried out at the coalface, such as neuroimaging and genetics research).

By "epistemological structure of psychiatry," we mean the informational vector constituted by assumptions, methodologies, institutions, venues, interventions, and views of clients and consumers that allows psychiatry (a first-order activity), to garner "data." We will propose in this chapter that both the "structure" (the discipline of psychiatry) and the "objects of psychiatry" (the mental symptoms and mental disorders) have a hybrid nature, that is, are configured by forms and practices that have been borrowed from the natural and human sciences (Berrios, 2011; Marková & Berrios, 2012). The epistemological study of hybrid structures is relatively new and complex (more on this later).

Given this hybrid nature, psychiatry needed a special language of description to capture and construct its objects. Descriptive psychopathology was constructed during the nineteenth century to fulfil this role (Berrios, 1996). The current "objects" or units of analysis of psychiatry are no longer the direct "mental afflictions" but their conceptual "transforms" (i.e., symptoms, syndromes, and diseases). ("Disorder" is a late-nineteenth-century euphemism coined to refer to conditions caused by "functional" as opposed to anatomical disturbances [Power & Sedgwick, 1882].) To illustrate some aspects of EP as well as its potential to stimulate novel research directions, this chapter will include brief accounts of: (1) the need for a new EP; (2) the epistemological structure of psychiatry; and (3) one of its "objects," namely, mental symptoms (and their brain representations).

Why a New Epistemology of Psychiatry?

Epistemology has been defined as "the theory or science of the method or grounds of knowledge" (Epistemology, 1989). Although the term was only coined in 1854 (Ferrier, 1856), the concepts and activities involved can already be found in Classical Greece when efforts started to be made to ascertain the legitimacy of human "knowledge" (Tiles & Tiles, 1993; Woleński, 2004). Depending on their tenets on truth, logic, knowledge, reality, science, and methodology, epistemological approaches range from those intent on identifying the legitimate method for reaching the truth (prescriptive epistemologies) to those that see knowledge as socially and historically determined and accept that there are many (complementary) ways of capturing reality (Soler, 2000).[3]

Falling into this second category, EP can be defined as a discipline dealing with the origin, structure, and usefulness of all narratives developed to capture what is called "mental afflictions." "Dealing" in this context means exploring the history, assumptions, and epistemo-logical structure of each narrative and then ascertaining its stability and predictive capacity by means of empirical testing. Hence the new EP does not limit itself to "philosophical analysis" but is based on a methodo-logical tripod constituted by historical, conceptual, and empirical research (Henderson & Horgan, 2011).

As mentioned earlier, since the early nineteenth century both the philosophical and empirical research carried out by alienists has closely followed the guidelines established by general medicine. This underpins the widely held belief that madness and congeners are "natural kinds," that is, "objects" that exist in space and time and hence can be said to "reside" in the brain in the same way that pneumonia might reside in the lungs. Nineteenth-century classical positivism had no difficulty in pro-viding philosophical justification for this belief (Braunstein, 2009). During the early 20th century, neopositivism fulfilled the same function; via the Vienna Circle and logical empiricism, it was succeeded by what is now called "analytical philosophy" (Dummet, 1993). This is why at present the findings of neuroscience and of biological psychiatry find easy justification in the hands of analytical philosophers (Churchland, 1986; Murphy, 2006).

Two features of analytical philosophy make it apposite to this justificatory task: First, it is wedded to the hard "truth-making" category of epistemol-ogy; and second, it has little interest in historical and hermeneutical explan-ations (Sáez-Rueda, 2002; Sorell & Rogers, 2005). Since the times of the Vienna Circle and the unified view of science (Neurath, Carnap, & Morris,

---

[3] This is the position taken in this chapter as it is not possible to determine a priori which particular narrative should be privileged over others. Conceptual analysis may help to suggest that some may be more useful, but this can only be decided after each has been tried out.

1938), analytical philosophy has been interested in developing a unitary model of knowledge acquisition. Such a model was found in the "success" of the natural sciences (particularly physics and chemistry) and duly prescribed for all sciences and knowledge-seeking activities.

This chapter claims that components such as its logical empiricism, naïve realism, unified view of science, and anti-historicism make analytical philosophy inappropriate to the study and understanding of "hybrid" disciplines such as psychiatry. The latter demands a new epistemological approach, one that is less concerned with truth, universality, and invariance and more with meaning and singularity (Marková & Berrios, 2012). The new EP should be able to handle the essential historicity, regionality, language-boundedness, and subjectivity of psychiatry and its objects.

The Epistemological Structure of Psychiatry

At the beginning of the nineteenth century, the discipline called "alienism" (called thus because *mental alienation* had until then been a popular conceptualization of mental afflictions) came under the aegis of medicine. Such "medicalization" of mental afflictions was not based on any logical or empirical findings but was the direct result of the philanthropic, social, and economic needs of the early-nineteenth-century Industrial Revolution (Foucault, 1961; Scull, 1993). This new alliance (1) imposed on alienism a new way of talking about mental afflictions; (2) professionalized alienists into medical doctors (now called psychiatrists); and (3) molded the thinking, praxis, and venues of psychiatry. Started as a philanthropic enterprise, this alliance was reconceptualized by the philosophers of the day as being an expression of progress, as a decisive step toward a new "scientific" and "objective" approach to its subject matter (Scull, 1993).

Psychiatry was thus born as a new discipline putatively dedicated to the understanding and management of "mental afflictions," reconceptualized as "mental symptoms and disorders." "Understanding" in this context should have meant a form of intellectual, emotional, and aesthetic apprehension (Martin, 2000); and "intellectual understanding," should have meant, in turn, an integrative grasping of the history, semantics, biology, contexts, and venues of mental afflictions. In practice, however, "understanding" was from the start narrowly interpreted by biological psychiatry and limited to mapping biological mechanisms.

On account of this constricted interpretation of "understanding," the medicalization of alienism never met the needs of the sufferers. The importation of a concept as complex as "disease" (Taylor, 1979) into psychiatry required major epistemological readjustments. These were not undertaken during the nineteenth century, and there is no evidence that they are being currently undertaken. For the language of psycho-pathology to work, assumptions have to be made as to where to draw the boundaries of normal behavior (Canguilhem, 1966) and an appropriate model of man, a theory of language, and a functional map of the mind must be put in place. None of these elements were available to early-nineteenth-century medicine; in consequence, alienists had to borrow them from what at the time were the nascent "human sciences" (Fox, Porter, &Wokler, 1995; Manicas 1987).

Thus, from the start, the biological narrative of psychiatry has been based on a medley of (1) Cartesian mechanicism (semantically empty[4]); (2) an Enlightenment model of man as a "rational" being; (3) a theory of signs and language (taken from the work of Rousseau, Herder, and Humboldt); and (4) a form of mosaic (or modular) neuropsycho-logy, as proposed by the Scottish philosophy of common sense and implemented by phrenology, a forerunner of current cognitive neuro-psychology; Berrios, 1988). Historical analysis shows that this hybrid epistemology has changed little ever since.

This hybrid structure did, in turn, govern the manner in which the objects of psychiatry were to be constructed. Mental afflictions became symptoms, signs, syndromes, and diseases (the latter being no more than "clusters of symptoms and signs" that for a time were provided with an independent ontology). The important point to notice is that such reconceptualization was *not* guided by "empirical" brain research (as demanded by nineteenth-century positivist prescriptions for the nat-ural sciences) but resulted from decisions molded by social and eco-nomic factors – which, at the time, were beginning to be the objects of study by the human sciences (Scull, 1993).

The medicalization of mental afflictions and the development of a biological narrative in psychiatry included, therefore, two stages. In a first stage, certain behaviors and mental afflictions were declared "abnor-mal" or "pathological" (according to social and economic canons of the time). In a second stage, the natural sciences moved in seeking to justify the "abnormality" of (socially) determined pathological objects (mental symptoms and diseases) with parts of the body (by the 1830s, the brain had become the favored body part). Alienists conflated these two inde-pendent stages, thereby gaining the impression that the natural sciences

---

[4] By definition, meaning becomes irrelevant in mechanicism, as on this view animals and human beings are machines and everything is explained on the basis of the mechanistic principle, that is, by the interaction and combination of material particles (Bunnin & Yu, 2004).

were also involved in the choice of the "abnormal objects" themselves. Indeed, some current psychiatrists may still believe that this is the case.

Historical research has confirmed that the original objects of psychiatric inquiry were exclusively configured by nineteenth-century social decisions, prescriptions, and value judgments (Conrad & Schneider, 1992; Scull, 1993). Some of these objects can still be found in current diagnostic lists; others, such as homosexuality, drapetomania (a "disease" causing slaves to run away; Savitt, 2002) or haematoma auris ("cauliflower ear"; Berrios, 1999) have shown less stability. Thus, during the second half of the nineteenth century, homosexuality was considered a serious mental disorder (Krafft-Ebing and Kraepelin were strong defenders of this view). The impact of Freud and others blurred this perspective for a while, but the renaissance of biological psychiatry after World War II resuscitated the disease view, and homosexuality was listed in earlier versions of the *DSM* series (Bayer, 1987). Although it may be claimed that these decisions were taken on the basis of putative biological markers, it is clear that the real criteria were still "social" in nature. Indeed, it would be hard to see how the available markers could by themselves have inclined the balance one way or the other. The same can be said of other forms of "mental disorder," except that in some cases, social decisions have been far less obvious and public. The point remains that the "abnormal" nature of mental states and behaviors is determined on grounds specifically studied by the human sciences, that is, by disciplines seeking to understand the ways in which at any one time individuals and cultures make sense of their world (Marková & Berrios, 2009).

The mental states and behaviors that societies demarcate as abnormal are, of course, heterogeneous. Some are highly likely to result from brain disease, and these uncontroversially should become medical conditions. Others may not, but the fact that phenomenologically they may superficially look the same as "organic" ones may lead to their misclassification. Given that differentiating these two groups should have important ethical and therapeutic implications, efforts have been made since the nineteenth century to develop criteria for such a task. Indeed, as in the case of Charcot and others, neurologists have been more willing than alienists to accept such a distinction for reasons pertaining to the sociology of medicine. Be that as it may, at an epistemological level, the role played by "brain changes" in the understanding and management of mental afflictions is complex and obscure, for the either/or (organic versus nonorganic) choice does not do justice to the way in which mental symptoms are constituted. For example, even in cases of clear organic diseases such as Alzheimer's or Huntington's or Parkinson's disease, it is highly likely that not all accompanying mental symptoms have to be "organic." A failure to recognize this simple fact has rigidified current biological psychiatry and neuropsychiatry. For example, it may be far more useful to sufferers to recognize that the memory impairment of patients with dementia may be a composite of forgetting related to brain structural changes and forgetting of emotional or dissociative origin (Berrios & Marková, 2001). Such recognition would, for example, change the manner in which the results of drug trials in dementia are interpreted and memory disorder in general is managed in these patients.

In summary, EP is necessary to understand the formation, structure, and meaning of all psychiatric objects. To achieve this understanding, a variety of tools and methods has to be borrowed from a range of disciplines (history, social psychology, anthropology, linguistics, pragmatics, and hermeneutics). For example, the history of psychiatry helps to provide knowledge about the social processes within which the objects of inquiry have been constructed; the philosophy of psychiatry can help to clarify the descriptive and definitional power of the language of psychiatry; and the hermeneutic disciplines can show how the interlocutor (clinician) contributes to the construction and interpretation of the psychiatric object. It is only after the structure of the psychiatric objects has been mapped and its components duly listed that useful empirical research can be planned and executed. Without this knowledge, empirical research in psychiatry is blind, blunderbussed, and consists of mere correlations.

The "Objects" of Psychiatry: Mental Symptoms as One Example

Much current research effort is focused on correlating mental "disorders" with brain structure and/or function. Given that "disorders" may not be more than (historical) clusters of mental symptoms, it is important to explore first mental symptoms, which remain the building bricks of psychopathology. A typical piece of research consists in correlating proxy variables representing mental symptoms or clusters thereof (usually expressed in scores obtained from questionnaires or from criterial diagnostic instruments) with proxy variables representing brain structure or function (obtained from some investigative technique). Questions concerning the validity of the correlational paradigm have been explored elsewhere (Berrios & Marková, 2002).

The underlying assumption is that some dysfunction related to a receptor population, a specific region (parcel) of the brain, or one of the large-scale networks integrating information between parcellated brain regions (together comprising the human "connectome") is associated with a given mental symptom. Since the nineteenth century, the terminology has changed without major changes in the basic correlational paradigm. From the start, the relationship is interpreted as a causal one, that is, the mental symptom in question is perceived as "arising directly" from a "pathological" alteration in an underlying brain structure. Whether this relationship is redefined as "explanatory" and the explanation is seen as exhaustive or without residuum will, of course, depend on how the mental symptom is defined. If it is considered a natural kind (Laporte, 2004), an object existing in time and space (e.g., gold, an orchid, or a dog), then the paradigm in question has exercised all of its epistemological power and the object in question can be considered "fully explained and/or understood." However, if the mental symptom is considered a hybrid object rather than a natural kind, the paradigm under analysis will be found wanting. Any real or putative relationship between "mental" symptoms and brain pathology needs to be reinterpreted and certainly can no longer be considered as a full explanation. In order to address this issue, one needs to know far more than we do know about the nature of mental symptoms.

As hybrid objects, mental symptoms are constituted by different sorts of materials or rather from elements originating from diverse types of backgrounds, from admixtures of organic/biological and sociocultural components. How can these different sorts of elements interrelate and their relationship be understood? What are the implications of reconceiving the inner structure of mental symptoms? One way of doing this is to explore the various ways in which mental symptoms might arise. At this point, it would make sense to consider separately mental symptoms that present as subjective complaints, whether volunteered or elicited (e.g., depressed mood, anxiety, hearing voices, feeling tired, and so on), and symptoms that are determined by the clinician as objective signs/behaviors (e.g., flight of ideas, psychomotor retardation, disinhibition, and the like).

Subjective Mental Symptoms

Current listings of subjective mental symptoms comprise a range of phenomena such as complaints of anxiety, fatigue, despondency, irritability, hearing voices, fear of being followed, feelings of unreality/strangeness, difficulties in thinking, believing others can hear one's thoughts, feelings of elation, believing in complicated plots against one, feeling thoughts being pulled out of one's head, incessant worrying, compulsions to do certain things, seeing things that others don't, unfamiliar bodily sensations, and many more. Even on superficial consideration, it is apparent that they are heterogeneous phenomena. Some refer to mental states that most people can relate to (e.g., worries, anxiety, or low mood), and others refer to unusual or alien experiences. Some involve everyday events and others incorporate fantastical contents; some seem to be feelings, others perceptions or beliefs, and some mixtures of all; some are volunteered freely and some are elicited with difficulty; some are uttered easily and others with hesitation and uncertainty; and so on. The question is why all these phenomena are considered *simpliciter* as exemplars of the one class, "mental symptom"? What do they have in common? Do they perchance originate in the same way, that is, by the same mechanism?

There is a clear tendency in current psychiatry to explain the difference in mental symptoms in terms of the differences shown by their putative organic substratum. This trend, which is an expression of the old Müllerian principle of the "specific energy of the nerve" (Berrios 2005), was incorporated into psychiatry during the nineteenth century and has remained unchanged ever since. Indeed, there is no a priori reason to believe that it applies to mental symptoms at all, unless, of course, it is also believed that mental symptoms are structurally just a variety of physical symptoms. As we shall see later, part of the problem is that psychopathology has not yet developed a good theory of mental symptom-formation; hence, there is little knowledge about how these complaints come to be in the first place (except that they are expressions of a disordered putative function closely linked to an altered organic structure). Let us first examine mental symptoms from a phenomenological perspective.

By definition, subjective mental states (whether considered "symptoms" or healthy mental phenomena) must refer to states about which people are aware. In other words when people complain of, for example, low mood or feelings of strangeness, then this is something that they are saying on the basis of their interpretation of internal states. Similarly, if on questioning in a clinical situation, an individual admits to hearing voices, then this is an interpretation of an internal state. The point is that all subjective phenomena are based on an awareness of something. Thus, when subjective symptoms arise, they have to develop in the context of a change in awareness. Something changes in the "normal" stream of a conscious state such that interpretative processes are triggered to make sense of the change.

The next question is, what causes the change in the conscious state or awareness? Before speculating on various possibilities, it is worth mentioning, in the light of the issues to be discussed around mental symptoms and brain representation, the relationship between the brain state and the conscious state. It seems obvious that conscious states or mental states must be dependent on brain function. Without brain function, there would be no mental state; hence, every mental state is accompanied by a neurobiological state. The issue, however, concerns the relationship between formed mental symptoms and the underlying neurobiological states, that is, to what extent does the specific neurobiological state constitute the specific mental symptom?

Returning to the change in awareness that is necessary for the production of any subjective mental state or symptom, then whatever the underlying cause of this is – for example, whether there is a primary brain "disease" process or a secondary process triggered by factors outside the individual, such as symbols or conflicts – the issue is that there must be a "perceived" change in the conscious state of the individual so that the symptom-formation mechanisms may be triggered. In this regard, at least two issues arise: What controls the content of the experienced change? And how does the change in question become a mental symptom? Various pathways have been described to account for this change (here we will only discuss one pathway, referred to as (a); see Figure 2.1).

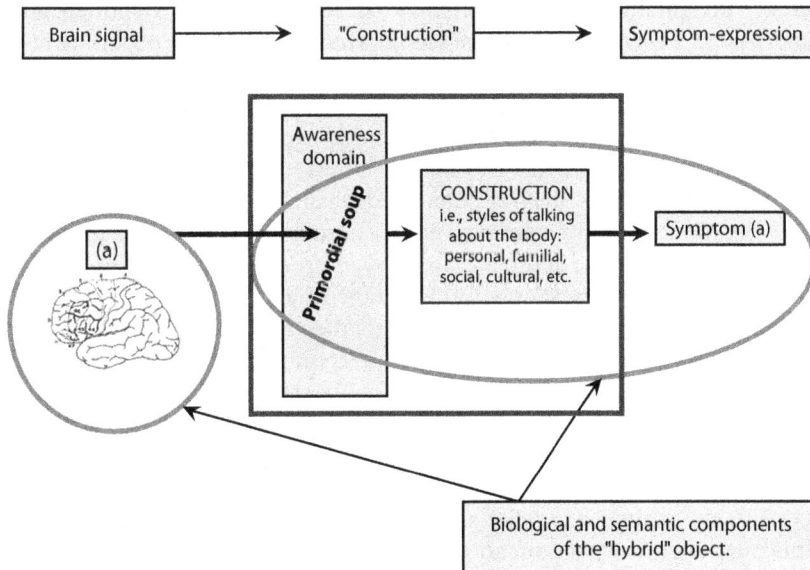

Figure 2.1. Cambridge model for symptom-formation: Pathway (a).

In pathway (a) a brain signal (say, of a perturbed network) penetrates into consciousness, causing an inchoate experience named, for lack of a better term, "primordial soup" to emphasize its prelinguistic, preconceptual nature (Berrios & Marková, 2006). To be understood by the subject or be communicated to others, the inchoate experience must be transformed/configured into "something" that fits a template familiar to the subject and into an experience that can be articulated into words and conveyed in a speech act. How might this happen? To make sense of this experience, the subject has to compare/interpret it with available templates (cognitive and emotional forms already experienced and shared with the culture). If there is no match because the experience is utterly novel, the subject must resort to the bank of forms that the local culture makes available. The cultural forms participating in the construction of the "symptom-to-be" can be conceived of as acting along different parts of the process that, for the sake of clarity, we can examine from three main perspectives (see Figure 2.1).

First, at the stage of initial appraisal of the *primordial soup* (the awareness of change experienced by the individual) we can speculate that the forms or templates made use of will relate primarily to the immediate qualities of the change itself. For example, the *rate* at which the change is happening is likely to be important. Something that builds up slowly may involve many more forms (e.g., different templates for memory, knowledge, imagination, or emotion may be accessed) than a sudden and short-lived experience. The *context* in which the change occurs is also likely to determine how and which templates will be involved. For example, some outside events may make change more "understandable" or easier to interpret. The *quality* of the experienced change is also appraised in terms of its familiarity. Thus, ordinary experiences are rapidly dismissed as they are matched against well-known templates. Novel experiences, by contrast, remain unmatched and hence force the individual to call on templates borrowed from perhaps more diverse aspects of the culture. Thus, if the change in awareness relates to some sort of alien, unfathomable internal state, then it is likely that more effort will be needed to make sense of it, to interpret it, and this in turn would involve accessing a variety of sources (see later).

Second, the interpretation of anything (in this case a change in conscious state) will depend on numerous internal and external factors (templates). Factors relating to the individual include, for example, personality traits, educational level, intelligence, past experiences, imagination, introspection, and so on. Level of education may determine the range of vocabulary an individual possesses to describe the experience. A history of past similar experiences or knowing of others with what seem like similar experiences may facilitate interpretation of particular states (e.g., depression, anxiety). A tendency to introspection might generate more detailed and colorful descriptions of experiences, and so on. In the same way that different individuals will report an external scene in different ways, individuals may likewise interpret changes in their conscious state according to their personality and background.

External factors will also interact with internal ones to influence the sort of sense that the individual makes of experience. The family, society, and culture in which the individual is brought up will structure and color (configure) their interpretation of a change in conscious state. In a society where it is frowned on to express feelings explicitly, it might be more likely that an emotional experience is described in cognitive terms. Or, in a culture lacking in obvious ways of articulating emotional distress, particular experiences might be simply described as a pain, and so on. External influences are also likely to be important in affecting the way in which experiences are interpreted and described or articulated.

Third, the other group of factors affecting the way a change in awareness will be described and named is derived from the interaction of the individual with someone else, be that a clinician or another person. Communication is not simply an exchange of independent bits of information, but involves a deep blending of meaning and thus is itself likely to contribute to the formulation or crystallisation of the experience for the individual. For example, where the individual is having difficulty in putting into words a nebulous feeling or experience, then it may be that through the exchange with the clinician, some of the descriptions offered by the clinician – in the latter's effort to try to understand the patient – may resonate with the patient or provide a reasonable "fit" for the experience. In this way, factors relating to the clinician (or other interlocutor) and their interaction may well shape the final "symptom" that is expressed.

It is important also to note at this point that tracing a path for the formation of a single subjective mental symptom, although useful for the sake of clarity, is nevertheless an artificial endeavor. Symptoms are unlikely to arise in isolation, and changes in conscious states are more likely to trigger experiences that give rise to many symptoms, parts of symptoms, and conglomerates of symptoms. The relationship between these symptoms and aspects of symptoms and clusters is an important area that remains to be explored. What is it that makes some symptoms hang together? Is there another way of understanding symptoms and their relationship to one another? To what extent and how might one symptom influence the way another is formed or experienced?

Implications

What is apparent when thinking about these sorts of ways in which subjective mental symptoms become formed is that the "final symptom" is likely to have developed through the action of many interacting factors and the use of a variety of templates and configurators. It thus represents the action of various stages of construction whose mechanisms and material are separate from the quality of the experience itself and from whatever specific content might be carried by the original biological signal. This carries major implications for the structure of the subjective symptom and consequently for its relationship with neurobiology. To make sense of this, we need to consider the general structure under-lying subjective mental symptoms. Figure 2.2 depicts such a possible structure in light of the pathway described earlier.

At the core, as with all mental states (healthy or otherwise), there has to be, as mentioned earlier, some form of neurobiological signaling for the rule that all mental states are realized in the brain to be respected. This neurobiological signaling will thus correspond to a particular state of awareness. To give it meaning, however, this state of awareness must first be subject to the layers of interpretative processes that were briefly discussed earlier. Such processes will in turn depend on and reach out to diverse aspects of each individual and their sociocultural background. Thus these multifarious factors (forms, templates relating to the

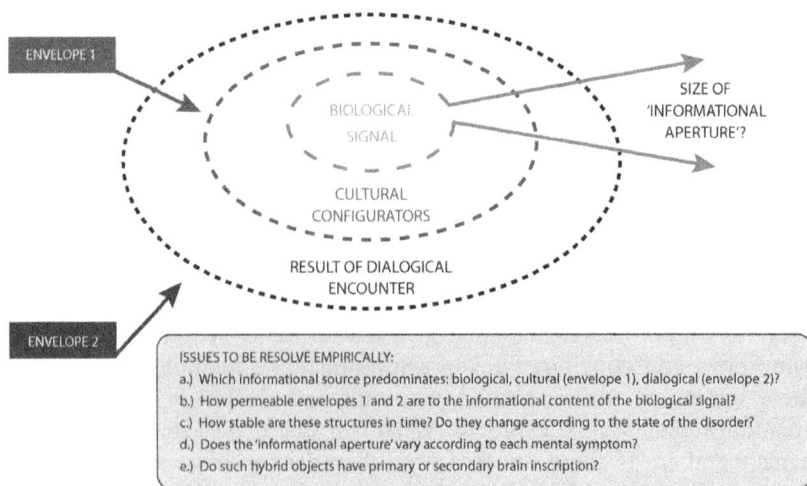

Figure 2.2. Putative structure of mental symptoms as "hybrid" objects.

individual and their background) become the wider configurators of meaning, enveloping to greater or lesser extent the original change in awareness. The symptom structure can therefore be envisaged as a core of neurobiology conferring a particular awareness state, which in turn, through the forces of the "cultural configurators," becomes a wider complex of disparate judgments. In addition, further configuration of meaning can be provided by the dialogical encounter, thereby adding another envelope of judgments (see Figure 2.2).

If, in broad terms, the structure of the subjective mental symptom is understood as the result of a layered process of configurations and interacting judgments, then the structure of the relationship between concomitant brain changes and the symptom itself becomes complicated. In the first place, it cannot be a simple cause-effect relationship between "symptom" and brain signal, as demanded by most neuroimaging research. What has been described earlier suggests that a great deal of transformation exists between the brain signal and the uttered "symptom." This transformation is likely to vary between individuals, situations/contexts, and over time to the extent that the original neurobiological signal may not govern either the form or content of the symptom as expressed.

Even if a strong "biological" stance were taken regarding the origin of mental symptoms, it is clear that each of the symptom-configurators involved would be associated with different networks; hence, the total process would have as a substratum disparate neurobiological circuitry (since it is not disputed that mental states are accompanied by neurobiological states). The point is that the *functional specificity* of the signal would be lost. One consequence would be that such functional specificity might ultimately be associated with a variety of mental symptoms, none of which necessarily preserves the original biological specificity (perceptual, emotional, and so on). The converse could also be the case: namely that a mental symptom, whose content may seem to suggest a particular functional specificity (e.g., perception), may be related to a variety of core neurobiological signals. In other words, it could not be assumed that all patients complaining of, say, depersonalization or derealization would have the same neurobiological accompaniment (or the same aspect of brain function light up in neuroimaging). (For an analysis of a specific symptom using this methodology, see Berrios & Marková, 2012.) In the same vein, it could be possible that a similar neurobiological accompaniment might be obtained in different patients complaining of low mood, fatigue, pain, anxiety, or depersonalization, respectively. The combination of these components or factors determines the hybrid nature of mental symptoms.

Objective Mental Symptoms

The other group of mental symptoms comprises those that are observed/ determined/named as such by the clinician, for example, disinhibition, psychomotor retardation, poverty of thought, flight of ideas, lability of mood, agitation, incongruence of affect, and so on. (The current, apparently "clear" distinction between symptoms and signs was constructed only during the early nineteenth century.) Again, this second category of mental symptoms forms a heterogeneous group in relation to which clinicians must make additional judgments about patients' appearances and behaviors, as well as inferences concerning changes and problems with speech/thought processes, and so on.

In contrast to subjective mental symptoms, these types of clinical phenomena are named/constructed/shaped by factors operating via the clinician's interpretation. Whatever neurobiological state is associated with a particular mental/behavioral manifestation, external factors will also contribute to the final shape of the symptom. For example, whether a particular speech pattern and content is called "poverty of thought," may depend not only on what is happening inside the patient, but also on the skill, experience, and knowledge of the clinician; thus when clinicians differ in their views on the concept of ADHD, this will influence their propensity to call a particular behavior "hyperactive." Likewise, the clinician's past experience, education, personal outlook, and so on, as well as background sociocultural factors, will determine to some extent the nature of the symptom or indeed whether or not a patient has a specific symptom. Developing "operational criteria" is never sufficient in these cases as the factors listed earlier operate at a much deeper level. This is because operational criteria are surface descriptors. How they are applied will depend on factors relevant to the individual, who may be unaware of them. Apart from the clinician's sociocultural background, their clinical experience, the context in which the interview takes place, and so forth, there will be personal experiences and biases (e.g., past traumas or emotional connections), all of which will be contributing to the way in which a clinician will identify, interpret, and name a particular "behavior" or "sign."

Like subjective mental symptoms, *objective mental symptoms* also have a hybrid structure. Including a core neurobiological state, they are wrapped up in cultural configurators that proceed both from the individual and the clinician doing the identifying ("the diagnosis"). The configuration in question also precludes a simple and direct (cause-effect) relationship between the brain signal and the symptom. It could be argued (and has been) that in the case of "signs," the relationship between the mental symptom and its neurobiological association might be more direct. (Indeed, the "higher" epistemological value attributed to signs since the early nineteenth century was based on this claim.) As with other "objects" in common (public) social space, for objective mental symptoms, "interpretative factors" may have less force because of the available external validation. Nevertheless, objective mental symptoms are also complex constructs and involve judgments and, hence, interpretative factors (Marková & Berrios, 2009).

Brain Representation and Mental Symptoms

This account of the hybrid structure of symptoms highlights the biasing effects of considering mental symptoms as "objects," *simpliciter*. Exploring brain representations (inscriptions, localizations, and so on) in relation to mental symptoms thus becomes a complicated endeavor. Unlike "blood pressure," "concentration of metabolites," "density of bone," or "levels of calcium," "mental symptoms" are structures whose defining core is "meaning" – whether from the patient's or clinician's perspective – rather than ontological stability in time and space. Now, "meaning" (used as signification, sense, intention to communicate) cannot be located in time and space, unlike the exemplar of a natural kind. In this sense, the localization of mental symptoms in the brain or their relationship to neurobiological substrata (or however this relationship may be phrased) gains a different order of complexity. Mental symptoms are not *"things"* that happen to have a content and also a "meaning" to the sufferer (where "content" and "meaning" are secondary and can be made an abstraction of the underlying entity or eliminated from the equation). This separation is not possible: an experience is called a "mental symptom" *only* when it means something to the sufferer. Mental symptoms have a wider, deeper, personal, and cultural sense and a fluidity that may not be amenable to the sort of techniques of capture that are used in relation to organic or biological dimensions of disorder or disease. The question then is whether there is a meaningful way of exploring the relationship between mental symptoms and brain representation. Are some symptoms perhaps more directly related to their neurobiology? Can other approaches be developed to understand and ultimately to manage psychopathological phenomena?

Given that two principles are worth saving – that all mental activity must have brain representation and that meaning to the sufferer is what defines and confers stability and sense to mental symptoms – a simple twofold classification of mental symptoms will be proposed to explore the complexities of brain representation. On the one hand, there are

Table 2.1 *Types of Brain "Representation."*

	Primary	Secondary
High replication rate?	Yes	No
Can it be triggered anew?	Yes	No
Proxyhood requirements	Low	High
Is it more susceptible to biological therapy?	Yes	No
Is it more susceptible to psychological therapy?	No	Yes
Functional complexity	Mono-modal	Multimodal
Structure	Process	Token
Hardwiring	Yes	No
Origin	Evolutionary, traumatic	Semantic, cultural
Alternative nomenclature	Localization	Inscription
Examples	Language functions	Delusion; brain changes post CBT

mental symptoms that, both in time and space, follow the brain activity that gives rise to them; and then there are mental symptoms that are concomitant to their neurobiological substratum. The former will be called *primary brain inscriptions*, the latter *secondary brain inscriptions* (Table 2.1).

In the case of primary brain inscriptions, the relationship between brain activity and mental symptoms is relatively direct: the brain activity precedes the mental symptoms and for its existence does not require the symptom. Functional networks in the brain may go on doing their job without ever producing a mental symptom. Alterations in their functionality or structure may on occasion generate a signal, which, on entering into awareness, triggers the process of configuration described earlier. It could be said that the primary lesion or malfunction gives rise to, or "causes," or "triggers" the process that ends up being a mental symptom. Hence, treatments that interfere with such organic substrates may well stop the mental symptom. This might be the case, for example, where organic hallucinations are triggered by an ictal focus or by the specific location of a brain tumor. Similarly, primary brain inscriptions might be more readily envisaged in relation to those symptoms captured as objective signs or behaviors (e.g., flight of ideas or disinhibition) where, as described earlier, their interpretation and naming as symptoms comes primarily from the clinician. In such situations, the brain inscriptions would have a relatively direct relationship with the mental symptoms.

Thus, they could be considered as valid proxy variables and would be etiologically informative; a number of the mental symptoms (although certainly not all) seen in the context of organic brain disease may be of this type.

In contrast, some mental symptoms are likely to have *secondary brain inscriptions*. In this case, the central and definitory core of the symptom would be its meaning or symbolism born in the intersubjective space of language. Because all mental activity must have brain representation, at some point the meaning in question is represented in the brain, but this presentation will follow, rather than precede, in time or space the construction of that meaning. No alteration of brain activity is necessary or sufficient for this type of mental symptom formation because it can only occur in an intersubjective space (Frie, 1997; Gillespie & Cornish, 2009; Stein, 1917). In such a case, no cause-effect relationship can be predicated, and physical interference with the brain representation would not affect the mental symptom at all. The latter could be affected only by unknotting the clash of meanings that generated the mental symptom in the first place. This is likely to be the case with many subjective mental symptoms that occur in the context of psychiatry. For example, stress-induced hallucinations would be inscribed differently from hallucinations in the context of a psychotic depression or indeed from those arising as a result of an organic lesion. Likewise, in the case of *folie à deux* (Berrios, 1998), the symptoms in the "inducer" and those in the "inducee" are unlikely to have the same sort of brain inscriptions. Rather, the symptoms in the latter are more likely to be secondarily inscribed.

Distinguishing between primary and secondary brain inscriptions in relation to mental symptoms has important consequences for both research and treatment. It follows from this discussion that mental symptoms associated with primary brain inscriptions will have specific brain representation; hence, it may make sense to explore correlations using neuroimaging or other localizing techniques. In the case of mental symptoms associated with secondary brain inscriptions, neuroimaging will likewise capture brain representations, but these inscriptions will have little relevance for localization of symptoms. Research focused on exploring the nature of such mental symptoms will need to take a different approach. Given the fact that these symptoms would be born in the intersubjective space of language and interaction, new ways of examining them will have to be found in hermeneutical approaches and the like. In other words, focus would need to be directed at developing methods that can help translate the symbolic representations of distress as manifested in different forms of communication and as acted out within the dialogical encounter. Similarly, from a treatment perspective, mental symptoms with primary inscriptions may be more likely to be amenable to biological therapies while those associated with secondary inscriptions may require approaches addressed at unpacking the semantic codes constituting them, using, for example, the hermeneutical-dialogical methods mentioned earlier.

Conclusion: The Hybrid Objects of Psychiatry

As opposed to conventional philosophy or epistemology, the new EP we have sketched addresses the historical and philosophical origin, meaning, predictive value, and social usefulness of all the narratives of psychiatry, both past and present. In this task, we make use of three integrated methodological approaches: history, philosophy, and empirical research. This new epistemology is of particular use in the case of disciplines like psychiatry, whose structure is hybrid, in the sense that it combines questions and methods pertaining to both the human and natural sciences.

Historiographical research shows how the current narratives of psychiatry were put together at the beginning of the nineteenth century in response to the newly forged alliance between mental afflictions and medicine. Medicine was unable to provide answers to some of the important questions posed by alienists in regard to the meaning and demarcation of their objects of inquiry. Answers had to be sought out with the epistemology of medicine and were found in the new language of the nascent human sciences. This created a hybrid structure for alienism (now psychiatry), which has endured to this day.

The objects of psychiatry resulting from the constructionist activity of the new psychopathology of alienism also acquired a hybrid structure in that their boundaries from the start were determined by social decisions and their biological anchorage provided by the natural sciences. This *sui generis* nature imposed and still imposes special demands on psychiatrists. The objects of psychiatry need to be understood, classified, and managed in specific and diverse ways, and to achieve this end, models of symptom-formation are urgently needed. Given the differential management, objects that are primarily localized in the brain need to be differentiated from those that are only secondarily localized in the brain. The overemphasis on the former is impeding the development of a psychiatry that is flexible and conceptually sophisticated. This work is required, not just for furthering our understanding of psychiatry as a discipline, but for the direct benefit of patients.

REFERENCES

Bayer, R. (1987). *Homosexuality and American psychiatry: The politics of diagnosis.* Princeton, NJ: Princeton University Press.

Bennett, M. R., & Hacker, P. M. S. (2003). *Philosophical foundations of neuroscience.* Oxford, England: Blackwell.

Berrios, G. E., & Marková, I. S. (2012). The construction of hallucinations. In J. D. Bloom & I. E. C. Sommer (Eds.), *Hallucinations: Research and practice* (pp. 55–75). New York, NY: Springer. http://dx.doi.org/10.1007/978-1-4614-0959-5_5

Berrios, G. E. (1988). Historical background to abnormal psychology. In E. Miller & P. Cooper (Eds.), *Adult abnormal psychology* (pp. 26–51). London, England: Churchill Livingstone.

Berrios, G. E. (1996). *The history of mental symptoms.* Cambridge, England: Cambridge University Press. http://dx.doi.org/10.1017/CBO9780511526725

Berrios, G. E. (1998). *Folie à deux* – A mad family by W. W. Ireland. *History of Psychiatry, 9,* 383–95. http://dx.doi.org/10.1177/0957154X9800903506

Berrios G. E. (1999). Pieterson's Haematoma Auris. *History of Psychiatry, 10,* 371–83. http://dx.doi.org/10.1177/0957154X9901003906

Berrios, G. E. (2000). The history of psychiatric concepts. In F. Henn, N. Sartorius, H. Helmchen, & H. Lauter (Eds.), *Contemporary psychiatry: Vol. 1. Foundations of psychiatry* (pp. 1–30). Heidelberg, Germany: Springer.

Berrios, G. E. (2005). On the fantastic apparitions of vision by Johannes Müller. *History of Psychiatry, 16,* 229–46. http://dx.doi.org/10.1177/0957154X05055179

Berrios, G. E. (2006). 'Mind in general' by Sir Alexander Crichton. *History of Psychiatry, 17,* 469–97. http://dx.doi.org/10.1177/0957154X06071679

Berrios, G. E. (2011). Psychiatry and its objects. *Revista de Psiquiatría y Salud Mental, 4,* 179–82. http://dx.doi.org/10.1016/j.rpsmen.2011.09.001

Berrios, G. E., & Marková, I. S. (2001). Psychiatric disorders mimicking dementia. In J. R. Hodges (Ed.), *Early-onset dementia. A multidisciplinary approach* (pp. 104–23). Oxford, England: Oxford University Press.

Berrios, G. E., & Marková, I. S. (2002). Conceptual issues. In H. D'haenen, J. A. den Boer, & P. Willner (Eds.), *Biological psychiatry* (pp. 9–39). Chichester, England: John Wiley & Sons. http://dx.doi.org/10.1002/0470854871.chi

Berrios, G. E., & Marková, I. S. (2006). Symptoms – historical perspectives and effect on diagnosis. In M. Blumenfiels & J. J. Strain (Eds.), *Psychosomatic medicine* (pp. 27–38). Philadelphia, PA: Lippincott Williams & Wilkins.

Blanc, C.-J. (1998). *Psychiatrie et pensée philosophique.* Paris, France: L'Harmattan.

Bolton, D., & Hill, J. (2003). *Mind, meaning & mental disorder* (2nd ed.). Cambridge, England: Cambridge University Press.

Braunstein, J.-F. (2009). *La philosophie de la médicine d'Auguste Comte.* Paris, France: PUF.

Budd, A. (2009). *The modern historiography reader.* London, England: Routledge.

Bunnin, N., & Yu, J. (Eds.). (2004). *The Blackwell dictionary of Western philosophy.* Oxford, England: Blackwell.

Butterfield, H. (1965). *The Whig interpretation of history.* New York, NY: Norton.

Canguilhem, G. (1996). *Le normal et le pathologique.* Paris, France: PUF

Choudhury, S., & Slaby, J. (Eds.). (2012). *Critical neuroscience.* Oxford, England: Wiley-Blackwell.

Churchland, P. S. (1986). *Neurophilosophy.* Cambridge, MA: MIT Press.

Conrad, P., & Schneider, J. W. (1992). *Deviancy and medicalization* (2nd ed.). Philadelphia, PA: Temple University Press.

Culler, J. (1982). *On deconstruction.* Ithaca, NY: Cornell University Press.

Dummet, M. (1993). *The origins of analytical philosophy.* Cambridge, MA: Harvard University Press.

Epistemology. (1989). *Oxford English dictionary* (2nd ed.). Oxford, England: Oxford University Press.

Ferrier, D. (1856). *Institutes of metaphysic* (2nd ed.). Edinburgh, Scotland: Blackwood and Sons.

Foucault, M. (1961). *Histoire de la folie à l'âge classique: Folie et déraison.* Paris, France: Plon.

Fox, C., Porter, R., & Wokler, R. (Eds.). (1995). *Inventing human science: Eighteenth century domains.* Berkeley: University of California Press. http://dx.doi.org/10.1525/california/9780520200104.001.0001

Frie, R. (1997). *Subjectivity and intersubjectivity in modern philosophy and psychoanalysis.* London, England: Rowman.

Fulford, K. W. K., Thornton, T., & Graham, G. (2006). *Oxford textbook of philosophy and psychiatry.* Oxford, England: Oxford University Press.

Gillespie, A., & Cornish, F. (2009). Intersubjectivity: Towards a dialogical analysis. *Journal for the Theory of Social Behaviour, 40,* 19–46. http://dx.doi.org/10.1111/j.1468-5914.2009.00419.x

Glock, H.-J. (2008). *What is analytical philosophy?* Cambridge, England: Cambridge University Press. http://dx.doi.org/10.1017/CBO9780511841125

Griffiths, A. P. (Ed.). (1994). *Philosophy, psychology and psychiatry.* Cambridge, England: Cambridge University Press.

Henderson, D. K., & Horgan, T. (2011). *The epistemological spectrum.* Oxford, England: Oxford University Press. http://dx.doi.org/10.1093/acprof:oso/9780199608546.001.0001

Iggers, G. G., & Wang, Q. E. (2008). *A global history of modern historiography.* Edinburgh, Scotland: Pearson.

Kehrer, F. A. (1951). *Das Verstehen und Begreifen in der Psychiatrie.* Stuttgart, Germany: Thieme.

Kellert, S. H., Longino, H. E., & Waters, C. K. (Eds.). (2006). Scientific pluralism. *Minnesota Studies in the Philosophy of Science XIX.* Minneapolis: University of Minnesota Press.

Kendler, K. S., & Parnas, J. (Eds.). (2008). *Philosophical issues in psychiatry*. Baltimore, MD: Johns Hopkins University Press.

Lanteri-Laura, G. (1963). *La psychiatrie phénoménologique*. Paris, France: PUF.

Laporte, J. (2004). *Natural kinds and conceptual change*. Cambridge, England: Cambridge University Press.

Laugier, S. (1999). Expérience cruciale. In D. Lecourt (Ed.), *Dictionnaire d'histoire et philosophie des sciences* (pp. 404–6). Paris, France: PUF.

Lewis, A. A. (1967). Empirical or rational? The nature and basis of psychiatry. *Lancet, 2*(7505), 1–9. http://dx.doi.org/10.1016/S0140-6736(67)90055-4

Manicas, P. T. (1987). *A history and philosophy of the social sciences*. Oxford, England: Blackwell.

Marková, I. S., & Berrios, G. E. (2009). Epistemology of mental symptoms. *Psychopathology, 42*, 343–9. http://dx.doi.org/10.1159/000236905

Marková, I. S., & Berrios, G. E. (2012). Epistemology of psychiatry. *Psychopathology, 45*, 220–7. http://dx.doi.org/10.1159/000331599

Martin, M. (2000). *Verstehen: The uses of understanding in social science*. London, England: Transaction Publishers.

Murphy, D. (2006). *Psychiatry in the scientific image*. Cambridge, MA: MIT.

Natanson, M. (Ed.). (1969). *Psychiatry and philosophy*. Berlin, Germany: Springer-Verlag.

Neurath, O., Carnap, R., & Morris, C. F. W. (Eds). (1971). *Foundations of the unity of science* (Vols. 1 & 2). Chicago, IL: University of Chicago Press.

Palem, R.-M. (Ed.). (2010). Psychiatrie et philosophie. *Les Cahiers Henri Ey, 25–26*.

Palmer, H. (1952). *The philosophy of psychiatry*. New York, NY: Philosophical Library.

Power, H., & Sedgwick, L. W. (1882). *The New Sydenham Society's lexicon of medicine and the allied sciences* (Vol. 2). London, England: The New Sydenham Society.

Radden, J. (Ed.). *The philosophy of psychiatry: A companion*. Oxford, England: Oxford University Press.

Reznek, L. (1991). *The philosophical defence of psychiatry*. London, England: Routledge.

Sáez-Rueda, L. (2002). *El conflicto entre continentales y analíticos: Dos tradiciones filosóficas*. Barcelona, Spain: Crítica.

Savitt, T. L. (2002). *Medicine and slavery: The diseases and health care of Blacks in antebellum Virginia*. Urbana: University of Illinois Press.

Sendrail, M. (1880). *Histoire culturelle de la maladie*. Toulouse, France: Privat.

Scull, A. (1993). *The most solitary of afflictions: Madness and society in Britain 1700–1900*. New Haven, CT: Yale University Press.

Siegler, M., & Osmond, H. (1974). *Models of madness, models of medicine*. New York, NY: Macmillan.

Soler, L. (2000). *Introduction à l'épistémologie*. Paris, France: Ellipses.

Spiegelberg, H. (1972). *Phenomenology in psychology and psychiatry*. Evanston, IL: Northwestern University Press.

Spiegelberg, H. (1982). *The phenomenological movement.* The Hague, Netherlands: Nijhoff. http://dx.doi.org/10.1007/978-94-009-7491-3

Spitzer, M., & Maher, B. A. (Eds.). (1990). *Philosophy and psychopathology.* Berlin, Germany: Springer-Verlag. http://dx.doi.org/10.1007/978-1-4613-9028-2

Stein E. (1917). *Zum Problem der Einfühlung.* München, Germany: Kaffke.

Strasser, S. (1963). *Phenomenology and the human sciences.* Pittsburgh, PA: Duquesne University Press.

Strauss, E. B. (1958). *Psychiatry in the modern world.* London, England: Michael Joseph.

Taylor, F. K. (1979). *The concepts of illness, disease and morbus.* Cambridge, England: Cambridge University Press.

Tiles, M., & Tiles, J. (1993). *An introduction to historical epistemology.* Oxford, England: Blackwell.

Toombs, S. K. (Ed.). (2001). *Handbook of phenomenology and medicine.* Dordrecht, Germany: Kluwer. http://dx.doi.org/10.1007/978-94-010-0536-4

Woleński, J. (2004). The history of epistemology. In I. Niiniluoto, M. Sintonen, & J. Woleński (Eds.), *Handbook of epistemology* (pp. 3–54). Dordrecht, Germany: Kluwer. http://dx.doi.org/10.1007/978-1-4020-1986-9_1

World Health Organization. (2003). The gap between the burden of mental disorders and resources. In *Investing in mental health* (p. 36). Retrieved from www.who.int/mental_health/publications/investing_mental_health/en/

Wulff, H. R., Pedersen, S. R., & Rosenberg, R. (1986). *Philosophy of medicine.* Oxford, England: Blackwell.

3   Phenomenology and the Interpretation
of Psychopathological Experience

Josef Parnas and Shaun Gallagher

What do psychiatrists encounter when they encounter psychopathological experience in their patients? How should we interpret such
experiences? In this chapter, we contrast a checklist approach to diagnosis, which is standard today and which treats psychiatric symptoms
and signs (i.e., "the psychiatric object"; Marková & Berrios, 2009; see
also Chapter 2, *this volume*) as readily operationalizable object-like
entities, with a nonstandard phenomenological approach that emphasizes the importance of a specific kind of interpretive interview. The
descriptive methods of today's psychiatry perpetuate what has been
called psychiatry's "problem of description" (Spitzer, 1988) because
these methods are not adequately tailored to the ontological nature of
the "psychiatric object." The psychiatric object is typically portrayed as
an objective, thinglike entity, unproblematically graspable as it exists
"in itself" through a behaviorist third-person perspective and as being
indicative of a specific and modular physiological dysfunction. We will
propose a different epistemological approach, considering the nature of
mental disorders to be primarily constituted by the patient's anomalies
of experience, expression, and existence that typically involve suffering
and dysfunction (Parnas, Sass, & Zahavi, 2013).

Introduction: Is There a Problem
in Contemporary Psychiatry?

More than thirty years ago, psychiatry, attempting to match somatic
medicine in its scientific-biological foundations, underwent an "operational revolution," introducing criteria-based diagnoses and
"operational definitions" of such criteria (American Psychiatric Association [APA], 1980). The operational project radically abridged,
simplified, and condensed the then existing corpus of clinical knowledge into diagnostic manuals accessible to the *grand publique* because
they are written in lay language and stripped of theoretical and psychopathological reflection. These manuals have long been the main

source of clinical knowledge for psychiatrists in training (Andreasen, 2007). Moreover, it is assumed that a structured interview, that is, an interview in which a psychiatrist asks the patient a series of preformulated questions in a fixed sequence, is an adequate methodology for obtaining psychodiagnostic information. We will argue that this is a mistaken assumption.

Unfortunately, the operational revolution failed to deliver on its motivating promise of a breakthrough to actionable etiological knowledge. "A gaping disconnect" is today widely recognized between the impressive progress in genetics and neuroscience and "its almost complete failure" to elucidate the causes and guide the diagnosis and treatment of psychiatric disorders (Frances & Widiger, 2012; Hyman, 2012). Moreover, it has also become clear that the reliability of psychiatric assessments in daily practice has not improved markedly since the introduction of the operational criteria of *DSM-III* (APA, 1980). On the contrary, recent "epidemics" of mental disorders (e.g., depression, ADHD, childhood bipolar disorder, PTSD, etc.) call into question the very foundations of contemporary classification (Frances & Widiger, 2012; Hyman, 2012). These obvious signs of a crisis have stimulated a variety of responses. The pharmaceutical industry has been gradually withdrawing its money from CNS research. The scientific community voices proposals to suspend research into traditional diagnostic categories, symptoms, and signs and to focus elsewhere, on domains of psychopathology (e.g., syndromes of depression, reality distortion; Carpenter, 2007), or on behavioral constructs with known neural bases (e.g., in the NIMH Research Domain Criteria [RDoC]; Cuthbert & Insel, 2010).

The phenomenological approach to psychopathology offers a different assessment of and a different remedy for psychiatry's current malaise. A key problem, in our view, is that the "psychiatric object" has been grossly oversimplified, and that this ontological oversimplification has resulted in an epistemological naïveté with reliance on methodologies (e.g., the structured interview, checklists) that are unsuited and therefore unable to capture valid phenomenal ("phenotypic") distinctions concerning the patient's experience, expression, and existence (Nordgaard, Revsbech, Sæbye, & Parnas, 2012). However, such distinctions will not go away just because we decide to ignore them. They remain crucially necessary for diagnosis, treatment, and as the *explananda* of empirical research. In short, phenomenological distinctions cannot be disregarded or marginalized, short of giving up on the very project of psychiatry itself (Parnas et al., 2013).

Operational Criteria in Psychiatry

Before presenting our critique, we need to understand what the term "operational" actually amounts to in contemporary psychiatry. Today this term is often used with a certain sense of professional pride and self-confidence. The adjective "operational" seems to transmit and guarantee a promise of scientific rigor and exactness, and therefore encourages people to dispense with any need for a critical reflection.

The origin of the term can be found in the history of logical empiricism. The issue at stake was how theories and concepts, expressed in language, might correspond to extralinguistic reality. In the early phases of logical empiricism, it was assumed that reality might be faithfully described by means of very simple, atomistic, theory-free "observational-" or "protocol-statements" (*Beobachtung- und Protokollsätze*). Critics, however, made it clear that language is never theory-free (e.g., Putnam, 1999). Moreover, what words signify is typically framed by their local context, which (by its very nature) cannot be specified in advance. An important response to these objections came from physics (Bridgman, 1927), proposing the notion of "operational definition." Operational definition was supposed to provide an objective link between a concept and its referent or counterpart in nature. This idea was presented in an influential address that neopositivist philosopher Carl Hempel (1965) delivered to the American Psychopathological Association: "An operational definition of a term is conceived as a rule to the effect that the term is to apply to a particular case if the performance of a specified operation in that case yields a certain characteristic result" (p. 123).

The operational definition specifies an *action rule* or *operation*, intended to objectively link the psychiatric concept with its counterpart in reality, as in the following example: X is *harder* than Y because X *can make a scratch* on Y, but not vice versa. It was hoped that such definitions would compensate for the unfeasibility of defining psychiatric concepts through a set of sufficient or necessary descriptive criteria. This latter solution does not work because it always requires additional specifications through the *criteria of criteria*, leading to an infinite regress.

However, psychiatry does not have, and probably cannot have, concepts that are operationalizable in the earlier sense. Consider, for instance, the recognition of "identity disturbance ... with unstable self-image or sense of self," being in a depressive state, expressing "inappropriate affect," or a "paranoid style" (*DSM-IV*). Defining such symptoms or signs cannot be performed with reference to easily observable atomic facts, or be expressed in any easily applicable action-algorithm.

This situation is very well illustrated by two diagnostically contradictory, forensic-psychiatric assessments of a Norwegian mass killer, Anders Behring Breivik. (The first assessment diagnosed schizophrenia; the subsequent assessment arrived at personality disorder diagnosis.) The main divisive psychopathological issue, that is, whether Breivik harbored delusions, was not resolved or disambiguated by an appeal to "operational criteria" (Melle, 2013; Parnas, 2013).

Thus, if viewed in a critical perspective, what operationalism in psychiatry finally amounts to is no more than simple, lay-language descriptions of symptoms and signs, deprived of any theoretical discussion and phenomenological context (Parnas & Bovet, 2014). Moreover, the clinician is able to use such descriptions correctly only on the condition of having prior conceptual grasp of, and context-sensitive and experience-based familiarity with, diagnostic symptoms and signs.

Consequences: Ontological Simplicity of the Psychiatric Object and the Structured Diagnostic Interview

Nancy Andreasen, a prominent American academic psychiatrist and scientist and influential early advocate of operationalism and biological reductionism, describes – in hindsight – the unfortunate results of the *DSM-III* operational project in the following way:

> Because *DSM* is often used as a primary textbook or the major diagnostic resource in many clinical and research settings, students typically do not know about other potentially important or interesting signs and symptoms that are not included in *DSM*. Second, *DSM* has had a dehumanizing impact on the practice of psychiatry. History taking – the central evaluation tool in psychiatry – has frequently been reduced to the use of *DSM* checklists. *DSM* discourages clinicians from getting to know the patient as an individual person. … Third, validity has been sacrificed to achieve reliability. *DSM* diagnoses have given researchers a common nomenclature – but probably *the wrong one*. (Andreasen, 2007)

In Andreasen's bleak assessment of the consequences of the *DSM* for training, person-centered care, and diagnostic validity, there is an important omission of the fact that the consequences of the *DSM* project are not independent of the adopted epistemology and metaphysics. The operational revolution in psychiatry adopted two assumptions: the first epistemological assumption was an explicit neopositivist form of behaviorism-operationalism that saw the only relevant clinical information as observable behaviors; the second assumption, involved an implicit metaphysical position, namely, physicalism. Physicalism, in the common version of neurobiological reductionism, pictures reality as graspable in a certain substantive mechanical sense, akin to the movements of objects in Newtonian mechanics (in other words, not in accord with the most contemporary models of reality provided by quantum mechanics).

According to these assumptions, psychiatric "symptoms and signs" should be considered from the third-person perspective, namely as reified (with thinglike ontological nature), mutually independent (atomic) entities that are *devoid of meaning*, and open to context-independent definitions, unproblematic objectifications, and useful quantifications. Preference is given to "external behavior," while subjective experience is for the most part dismissed, mainly because the latter is not accessible to third-person observation and description. The ensuing neurobiological (so-called neo-Kraepelinian) research program aimed, unsuccessfully, at reducing those reified psychopathological entities to modular defects in the neural substrate in order to "carve nature at its joints."

On this model, the symptom/sign and its hypothetical causal substrate are both considered to be of *the same ontological nature*: both are spatio-temporally delimited objects, that is, things. In this paradigm – which originates from the medical model – the symptoms and signs have *no* intrinsic *sense or meaning*. They are indicators or *referents* that point to the abnormalities of an anatomic-physiological substrate. This background framework or scheme of "symptoms-as-causal-referents" is automatically activated in the awareness of any physician dealing with a medical condition (e.g., jaundice → liver/gallbladder disease; coughing → lung disease).

These assumptions concerning the status of symptoms and signs are clearly reflected in the prevailing culture of obtaining psychodiagnostic information (Nordgaard et al., 2012; Nordgaard, Sass, L.A., & Parnas, 2013). The diagnosis or class membership of the contemporary classifications is determined by a positive answer to a number of predetermined questions, reflective of the "operational" criteria of a particular diagnostic class. In structured diagnostic instruments for epidemiological research, like the Composite International Diagnostic Interview (CIDI; Kessler et al., 2007), the very phrasing of the individual interview questions is usually almost identical to the phrasing of the diagnostic criteria. This isomorphism attempts to minimize the potential unreliability in the process of matching or converting the patient's response to the diagnostic criterion inquired about. Inference, reflection, or interpretation on the part of the clinician is thereby reduced almost to zero, obviating the necessity of experience, skill, and knowledge on the part of the clinician. This simplification allows for the use of inexpensive lay-interviewers in psychiatric research. In sum, the structured interview aspires to a quasi-experimental, stimulus-response purity of the behaviorist paradigm. The structured conduct of the interview is widely regarded as an adequate method of obtaining valid and reliable information by circumventing or shortcutting the complexities of subjectivity, discourse, and communication involved in the patient-clinician exchange. The symptom is thus considered to be a sort of sharply delimited, thinglike object or event, with a persistent existence in the patient's access consciousness, waiting for a standardized, prompting question in order to come into full view.

We can illustrate these crucial epistemological issues by examining two real and concrete examples of responses to questions in a structured interview, pertaining to "depression" and "thought insertion" (Nordgaard et al., 2012).

Example 1:   Depressed Mood.

If a patient says "I feel depressed, sad, or down," in response to a question concerning depression, such statements may, if further explored, be found to indicate a bewildering variety of experiences with varying affinities to the concept of depression, including not only depressed mood but also, for instance, irritation, anger, loss of meaning, varieties of fatigue, ambivalence, hyperreflectivity, thought pressure, psychic anxiety, and even hallucinatory voices with negative content. A further complication is created by the fact that mood is not an isolated mental object, easily dissociated from its experiential context, identified in an act of introspection, and eventually converted to a reportable symptom. Rather, mood is a prereflective manner of our experiencing something that, to the one who lives it, is almost too immediate and encompassing to be recognized as such. It therefore requires a skillful interviewing effort to specify the salient profile of the presented distress. Taking a confirmatory or disconfirmatory answer at face value endangers the validity of the response.

Example 2:   Thought Insertion.

A patient who answers "no" to a question from a structured interview (e.g., "Have you ever had experiences that certain thoughts that were not your own were put into your head?") may well, in fact, have experienced episodes of thought insertion. Here, a negative answer may be due to a variety of factors: for instance, a simple lack of understanding of the question, not recognizing one's experience in the formulation of the question, or anticipating that a confirmatory "yes" would be a confession of frank madness. It may also be that formulating an answer beyond "yes"

Example 2:   (*cont.*)

would be difficult. The passivity experience does not exist as a readily accessible or articulated mental object but, rather, manifests itself as a thematic accentuation of a certain habitual and prereflective manner of experiencing one's thinking processes. Perhaps, an affirmative answer might have emerged if the interviewer started his conversation with the patient by addressing, first, potential problems of concentration, followed by an inquiry about thought chaos or pressure, and finally asking about a sense of strangeness or alienation of certain thoughts, and so on. Thus, in contrast to a structured interview, a skillful, context-adapted interview sequence may eventually elicit a self-description that certain thoughts are not the patient's own but are transmitted from some external agency (Nordgaard et al., 2012).

It is important to emphasize in this critical context that a semi-structured phenomenological psychiatric interview performed by an experienced and trained psychiatrist (i.e., an interview conducted in a conversational, context-sensitive, phenomenologically adequate manner, yet with an obligation on the clinician's part to address all items of the interview schedule to assure systematicity and comprehensiveness) results in good-to-excellent interrater reliabilities, even if the targets of the interview are subtle anomalies of subjective experience or disorders of expression (Møller, Haug, Raballo, Parnas, & Melle, 2011; Nordgaard et al., 2013; Vollmer-Larsen, Handest, & Parnas, 2007). Hence, it is possible to obtain a much richer and more accurate sense of patients' symptom experience without sacrificing reliability.

Phenomenology

It is doubtful whether the "operational revolution" in diagnostic assessment is adequate even for the domain of somatic medicine. Indeed, the view that medical diagnosis can be made by attending to narrowly circumscribed symptoms and signs has long been questioned. For example, in 1937 John Dewey addressed the College of Physicians in St. Louis, advising them not to treat just the body: "we must observe and understand internal processes and their interactions from the standpoint of their interactions with what is going on outside the skin ..." (p. 326). That is, we cannot understand processes inside the body in isolation from the environment – an environment that is both physical and social. Rather, in the practice of medicine:

[W]e need to recover from the impression, now widespread, that the essential problem is solved when chemical, immunological, physiological, and anatomical knowledge is sufficiently obtained. We cannot understand and employ this knowledge until it is placed integrally in the context of what human beings do to one another in the vast variety of their contacts and associations. ... A sound human being is a sound human environment. (Dewey, 1937, p. 54)

Whatever its limitations in understanding somatic disease, however, the scheme of symptom-as-causal-referent is clearly insufficient in psychiatry. The psychiatrist, who confronts a "psychiatric object," finds himself in a situation without analogue in somatic medicine (Jaspers, 1913/1963). First, he confronts a *person*, and not a leg, an abdomen, or a skin surface; *not a thing*, or a mere organism, but broadly speaking, another phenomenally conscious person in all its dimensions.

If the human form of existence is embodied, and environmentally embedded – and if illness is experientially *a complete form of existence*, as Merleau-Ponty (1963, p. 107) suggests, that is, a specific way of being-in-the-world – then we cannot think of illness simply as something that happens to an objective body, a purely physiological condition that is explainable entirely in causal or mechanistic terms (Gallagher, 2005). It is not that the patient is simply missing something that should exist, or that there is a one-to-one correlation between isolated physiological disturbance and behavioral and psychological manifestation. The same physiological disturbance may have different outcomes in different contexts.

Psychiatry needs a framework that will help characterize the more complete picture (the positives as well as the negatives) of how illness has made the patient's *life* different. This would provide what we might call a *rich diagnosis*. The kind of practice needed to get this diagnosis, the attempt to gain a deeper understanding of the complete form of existence, is one that looks at the human as an extended *system* – an embodied and embedded living system dynamically and enactively related to its surroundings – and that takes this system as the unit of analysis.

Theoretically speaking, a psychiatric symptom/sign is not a well-demarcated thinglike object, but rather a certain configuration of consciousness that involves the phenomenal flow with its intentional content and form (structures). What the patient manifests are not isolated *symptom-referents* but rather certain wholes of interpenetrating experiences, feelings, beliefs, expressions, and actions, all of them permeated by the patient's dispositions and by biographical (and not just biological) detail. The symptom individuates itself along all these dimensions, which combine into specific meaning-wholes out of which our psychiatric diagnostic typifications start. These typifications are not constituted by *a referential function* of the symptom (which is not to say that they are totally deprived of referential function). Moreover, in psychiatry, we usually have no knowledge of potential referents in any pragmatically useful sense.

The phenomenological interview involves a second-person approach guided by phenomenological distinctions. Phenomenologists, in their analysis of experience, extract and individuate certain *repeatable invariants*, which, for reasons of tradition, are called "symptoms." A psychiatric symptom or sign emerges as an individuated entity with a certain meaning only in a synchronic and diachronic context of simultaneous, preceding, and succeeding experiences and expressions. In short, a symptom or sign is not an entity "in itself" that can be easily isolated from the ongoing flow of consciousness and objectified, defined, and described independently of its context.

Typification, Prototype, and Gestalt

If a symptom is not a referring object, what is it? We suggest that it may be best to consider the symptom in terms of a prototypical *gestalt*. This concept is equally fit for the description of single features (symptoms and signs) and larger wholes, such as syndromes or diagnostic categories.

A recent review of psychological-empirical and theoretical research on mechanisms of concept formation and concept understanding suggests that concepts are not constituted by a list of criteria but, rather, are organized around *exemplars* or *prototypes* (Machery, 2009; also see Rosch, 1973). A prototype is a central example of the category in question (a sparrow is more characteristic of the category "bird" than is a penguin or an ostrich), with a graded dilution of typicality toward the borders of the category, where it eventually overlaps exemplars from neighboring categories. A prototypical approach to psychiatric description often has been advocated (Jaspers, 1913/1963; Parnas & Bovet, 1995). During the preparations for *DSM-III*, it was originally planned to anchor psychiatric categories in prototypical descriptions, supplanted by the lists of criteria (Parnas & Bovet, 2014). Unfortunately, this approach was abandoned in favor of purely criteria-base diagnosis. However, a prototype approach has had some revival more recently in the process of preparing the eleventh edition of the *International Classification of Diseases* (Westen, 2012). Both philosophical and cognitive-scientific analyses of categorization, together with empirical studies of the diagnostic method itself (Kendell, 1975) offer a convergent picture of the actual, real-world process of coming up with a psychiatric diagnosis. This suggests that the information provided by the patient, coupled with the patient's behavior, experience, and psychosocial history, leads, in a natural conversational clinical situation, to the first *typifications*, that is, to the interviewer seeing the patient as resembling a certain prototype (Schwartz & Wiggins, 1987a, 1987b).

The concept of typification refers to a very basic human cognitive feature, especially pertinent in perception, namely, that perception of an object is always *apperceptively organized* (i.e., structured) in a semi-conceptual fashion, as a salient unity or specific gestalt. In a diagnostic encounter, the psychiatrist quickly senses a patient as being *a certain way*, for example, withdrawn, hostile, sympathetic, guarded, eccentric, and so on. In this sense, one might say that seeing is always "seeing as" (Hanson, 1965); it is always perspectival or aspectual and includes a preunderstanding of what it is that we are perceiving. Clinical diagnosis involves pattern recognition and pattern completion, thereby allowing apprehension of objects and situations as meaningful under conditions of limited or incomplete information. In typification, an interpretation is not superimposed on a perceptual act; it imbues the perception itself.

Obviously, there are potential dangers in psychiatric typifications: first, that a psychiatrist can be blinded by existing expectations and therefore may fail to recognize the data for what they really mean. Second, the repertoire of typifications that any psychiatrist has acquired through experience could always contain misperceptions and misconstruals. Third, typifications may be misused as stereotypes. Typification pervades all of our experiences and occurs outside explicit awareness. The scientific use of typifications requires a more reflective and conceptual attitude, in which psychiatrists doubt and reflect on their typifications, and repeatedly test their own interpretations by looking for additional components to support a typification or call it into question.

In the context of psychiatric diagnosis, we can think of the concept of prototype-gestalt in a narrow sense and in a wide sense, neither of which is limited to perception but can also involve more complex cognitions. In a narrow sense, a gestalt is a *unity* or organization of phenomenal aspects, a unity that emerges from the relations among the features of experience (framed in terms of part-whole relations). The whole cannot be reduced to the simple aggregate of parts ("the whole is more than a sum of its parts"). In a wider sense, the gestalt in question goes beyond phenomenal aspects of experience. It involves a dynamic interplay of factors that extend throughout and beyond the organism (Weizsäcker, 1986). In a very real sense, one has to consider not just a set of subjective experiences, or a set of mental states, but the full scope of the subject's embodied engagements in the various physical and social environments that he inhabits. To make sense of this experience and narrative reports, one needs to understand the subject's pragmatic engagements with the world and interactions with others.

The notion of a gestalt in this wide sense goes beyond the traditional dichotomies of "inner and outer," "form and content," "universal and particular" (Merleau-Ponty, 1963). The salience of an interpersonal encounter, for example, does not normally emerge or articulate itself as piecemeal or disconnected allusions to the patient's inner life plus some other, independently salient fragments of the patient's visible expressions and behavior. Rather, persons articulate themselves holistically, *jointly constituted* not simply by their experience, beliefs, and expressions, but by their actions and interactions in an environment that is both physical and social. Furthermore, this wider gestalt is reflected, and gets iterated, in the narrow gestalt of experience, in ways that can be phenomenologically characterized. There is a circle rather than a line connecting what is traditionally defined as inner and outer: "*What*" the patient reports (content) is always molded by the "*how*" (form) of cognitive processes and the experience of self, others, and the world.

A gestalt instantiates a certain *generality of type*. Yet, this type-generality is always deformed, because it inheres in a particular, concrete and situated individual. The particular token always attenuates the ideal clarity and pregnancy of type. Furthermore, the gestalt's aspects are *not independent self-sufficient symptoms*. They are interdependent in a mutually constitutive and implicative[1] manner (Sass & Parnas, 2007) and the whole of the gestalt codetermines the nature *and specificity* of its particular aspects, while, at the same time, it draws from the single features in its concrete clinical rootedness (Parnas, 2012).

Imagine a case of "social phobia," motivated by a disgust and fear of physical or tactile contact with other people, a situation that is experienced as engulfing, fusing, and annihilating. One would not consider such "phobia" as an isolated behavioral dysfunction but rather as indicative of insecure identity and porous self-demarcation, with avoidant coping behavior ensuing by implication. Another example is mumbling: *per se* it is perhaps something that 5 percent of a random sample of people do; yet in the context of other features of schizophrenia, it acquires a diagnosis-relevant role.

More detailed conceptual determinations of the gestalt proceed through the steps of phenomenological-psychiatric typifications described earlier and explicated by Schwartz and Wiggins in two seminal papers (1987a, 1987b). The clinical task is to allow the gestalt to manifest itself in more detail, to let its latent or unexpected profiles become apparent, and to conceptualize and flesh out these aspects, originally only dimly apprehended or not apprehended at all.

---

[1] This is, of course, of paramount epistemological importance and makes the operationalist project of counting the number of symptoms for a diagnostic purpose highly problematic

All of these processes should be constantly subjected to critical reflection. This necessitates training, teaching of concepts, and acquisition of skill and expertise. Such processes are open to intersubjective judgment, may be shared with other psychiatrists (Nordgaard et al., 2013; Parnas, 2011; Parnas & Zahavi, 2002; Schwartz & Wiggins, 1987a, 1987b), and are assessed with respect to interrater reliability. Moreover, a psychopathological emphasis on the gestalt-like nature of "mental objects" does not preclude that the final formal diagnosis follows a list of prespecified (e.g., polythetic) criteria.

Structured Versus Phenomenological Interviews

In a structured interview, the clinical situation is represented as a transaction between equals and the patient is portrayed as a rational consumer and a motivated informant. The theoretical framework behind the development of highly structured, preformed psychiatric interviews for use by nonclinicians is consistent with the behaviorist methodology of administering opinion polls. This form of interviewing presupposes (as its theoretical foundation) that the answers, which the patient emits, are to be considered a set of third person ("objective") *propositional signals* that can be spatiotemporally delimited in the same way as physical objects. The entire issue of *information* and *information variance* (i.e., the variability of the quantity and quality of information obtained from the patient) is seen only as a matter of reliability, a driving force behind the increasing standardization of questions (as stimuli) and permissible responses.

Thus, the very issue of the *individuation of a symptom* (e.g., whether a statement is identified as a "delusion" rather than an indicator of "social phobia") is entirely left to the patient (indeed, many now "diagnose" themselves by consulting sites listing *DSM* criteria on the Internet), and the symptoms are supposed to exist in the patient's reflective awareness each time the patient is addressed by a preformed question. The symptom is a delimited mental-behavioral object. The preformed question acts as a stimulus, evoking the presence or absence of a symptom. Not only is the symptom considered a self-delimited, naturally existing object (thing), with a referent function; it is also taken for granted that the patient has no motivation to respond negatively, if he indeed harbors the symptom.

In contrast, from the phenomenological perspective, the notions of prototype and gestalt provide psychiatrists with conceptual tools necessary for the clinical encounter with the "other mind." As already emphasized, this approach can be taught with high levels of reliability (Parnas & Zahavi, 2002). The cardinal epistemological point is that clinicians *always* perceive their patients in terms of gestalts, because a prototype lens is built into the nature of human cognition (Rosch, 1973). Omitting prototypes from the teaching and training of psychiatry disarms the clinician, placing him or her in a chaotic situation of having to confront a myriad of unconnected data, where each individual signal is *a priori* worthy of equal attention, as a potential fulcrum for a nascent diagnostic class.

If not taught the prototypes systematically, clinicians acquire their own *private* prototypes in a way that is not subjected to disciplined, critical, and peer-shared reflection. Such "private" prototypes cannot resist becoming anchored in single, contingently towering, clinical features that happen to fit an available diagnostic category. Here, the patient's first verbalizations of the complaint may play a decisive role. Someone who says, "I feel depressed" will likely be diagnosed with "depression"; someone who says, "I have a habit of cutting myself" will be diagnosed as "borderline." If a thirty-year-old habitually dysfunctional bachelor says that he has been suffering from OCD since the age of seventeen, when he was so diagnosed, the likelihood of a thorough assessment of his inner life is small (e.g., What does the word "obsession" mean to him? Is this particular obsession given as a thought, fantasy, urge, image, or picture? Is his obsession experienced from a mental distance?).

Subjective experience cannot be faithfully assessed by structured interrogation that allows only affirmative or negative responses, that is, in the manner of a preformed structured interview.[2] The assessment of the patient's experience can only be psychiatrically assessed with sufficient validity in the course of a *conversation*, which conveys a friendly-neutral, nonjudgmental atmosphere, is supportive of the patient's spontaneity, and provides a space for narrative (Gallagher & Hutto, 2008), or even poetic (Kirmayer, 2007) verbalizations of experiential examples and their contexts. It requires an active *informed attention* in order to *hear/see* and assess/typify experiences/symptoms. Such listening and seeing is apperceptively supported, as Jaspers pointed out, by the psychiatrist's basic conceptual distinctions (Parnas & Bovet, 2014). To explicitly and faithfully assess and to typify another person's anomalies of experience, belief, expression, and behavior from a second-person perspective, requires specific demands on our interpersonal, empathic, and perceptual skills – a set of "embodied and narrative practices" for the clinic (Gallagher & Hutto, 2012) – as

---

[2] Even Western police forces have abandoned such techniques of witness interrogation in favor of eliciting a more open, spontaneous narrative from the witness, yielding better and more valid results (Fisher, Geiselman, & Raymond, 1987).

well as on our analytic-conceptual (reflective) skills and knowledge. These skills and knowledge are constitutive of psychiatry as a clinical-academic discipline and are indispensable for the science of psychopathology.

It is likely that nosological and therapeutic progress cannot happen unless these epistemological root problems in psychopathology are addressed, discussed, and redressed. Improving the practice of talking with and listening to psychiatric patients is a first step toward rehumanizing the *métier* of clinical psychiatry, as well as an indispensable methodological prerequisite of scientific development.

REFERENCES

Andreasen, N. C. (2007). *DSM* and the death of phenomenology in America: an example of unintended consequences. *Schizophrenia Bulletin, 33*(1), 108–12. http://dx.doi.org/10.1093/schbul/sbl054

Berrios, G. E., & Marková, I. S. (2015). Toward a new epistemology of psychiatry. In L. J. Kirmayer, R. Lemelson, & C. A. Cummings (Eds.), *Re-visioning psychiatry: Cultural phenomenology, critical neuroscience, and global mental health* (pp. 41–64). New York, NY: Cambridge University Press.

Bridgman, P. W. (1927). *The logic of modern physics.* New York, NY: Macmillan.

Carpenter, W. (2007). Deconstructing and reconstructing illness syndromes associated with psychosis. *World Psychiatry, 6,* 92–3.

Cuthbert, B. N., & Insel, T. R. (2010). Toward new approaches to psychotic disorders: The NIMH Research Domain Criteria project. *Schizophrenia Bulletin, 36,* 1061–2. http://dx.doi.org/10.1093/schbul/sbq108

Dewey, J. (2008). The unity of the human being. In J. Boydston (Ed.), *The later works of John Dewey, Volume 13, 1925–1953: 1938–1939, Experience and education, freedom and culture, theory of valuation, and essays* (pp. 323–37). Carbondale, IL: Southern Illinois University Press.

Fisher, R. P., Geiselman, R. E., & Raymond, D. S. (1987). Critical analysis of police interview techniques. *Journal of Police Science and Administration, 15*(3), 177–85.

Frances, A. J., & Widiger, T. (2012). The psychiatric diagnosis: Lessons from *DSM-IV* past and cautions for the *DSM-5* future. *Annual Review of Clinical Psychology, 8,* 109–30. http://dx.doi.org/10.1146/annurev-clinpsy-032511-143102

Gallagher, S. (2005). *How the body shapes the mind.* Oxford, England: Oxford University Press. http://dx.doi.org/10.1093/0199271941.001.0001

Gallagher, S., & Hutto, D. (2008). Understanding others through primary interaction and narrative practice. In J. Zlatev, T. Racine, C. Sinha, & E. Itkonen (Eds.), *The shared mind: Perspectives on intersubjectivity* (pp. 17–38). Amsterdam, The Netherlands: John Benjamins. http://dx.doi.org/10.1075/celcr.12.04gal

Gallagher, S., & Hutto, D. (2012, September 10). *Embodied and narrative practices in the clinical context* [Working paper]. Roundtable on Embodied-Narrative Practices, University of Hertfordshire, Hertfordshire, England.

Hanson, N. R. (1965). *Patterns of discovery: An inquiry into the conceptual foundations of science.* Cambridge, England: Cambridge University Press.

Hempel, C. G. (1965). *Explanation and other essays in the philosophy of science.* New York, NY: Free Press.

Hyman, S. E. (2012). Psychiatric drug discovery: Revolution stalled. *Science Translational Medicine, 4*(155), 1–5. http://dx.doi.org/10.1126/scitranslmed.3003142

Jansson, L., Handest, P., Nielsen, J., Sæbye, D., & Parnas, J. (2002). Exploring boundaries of schizophrenia: A comparison of *ICD-10* with other diagnostic systems in first-admitted patients. *World Psychiatry, 1*(2), 109–14.

Jaspers, K. (1963). *General psychopathology* (J. Hoenig & M. W. Hamilton, Trans.). Chicago, IL: University of Chicago Press, 1963. (Original work published 1913)

Kendell, R. E. (1975). *The role of diagnosis in psychiatry.* Oxford, England: Blackwell.

Kessler, R. C., Angermeyer, M., Anthony, J. C., de Graaf, R., Demyttenaere, K., Gasquet I., ... Üstün T. B. (2007). Lifetime prevalence and age-of-onset distributions of mental disorders in the World Health Organization's World Mental Health Survey Initiative. *World Psychiatry, 6*(3), 168–76.

Kirmayer, L. J. (2007). Celan's poetics of alterity. *Monash Bioethics Review, 26* (4), 21–35. http://dx.doi.org/10.1007/BF03351290

Machery, E. (2009). *Doing without concepts.* New York, NY: Oxford University Press. http://dx.doi.org/10.1093/acprof:oso/9780195306880.001.0001

Marková, I. S., & Berrios, G. E. (2009). Epistemology of mental symptoms. *Psychopathology, 42*, 343–9. http://dx.doi.org/10.1159/000236905

Melle, I. (2013). The Breivik case and what psychiatrists can learn from it. *World Psychiatry, 12*(1), 16–21. http://dx.doi.org/10.1002/wps.20002

Merleau-Ponty, M. (1963). *The structure of behavior* (A. L. Fisher, Trans.). Boston, MA: Beacon Press. (Original work published 1942)

Møller, P., Haug, E., Raballo, A., Parnas, J., & Melle, I. (2011). Examination of anomalous self-experience in first-episode psychosis: Interrater reliability. *Psychopathology, 44*, 386–90. http://dx.doi.org/10.1159/000325173

Nordgaard, J., Revsbech, R., Sæbye, D., & Parnas, J. (2012). Assessing the diagnostic validity of a structured psychiatric interview in a first-admission hospital sample. *World Psychiatry, 11*, 181–5.

Nordgaard, J., Sass, L.A., & Parnas, J. (2013). The psychiatric interview: Validity, structure and subjectivity. *European Archives of Psychiatry and Clinical Neuroscience, 263*(4), 353–64. http://dx.doi.org/10.1007/s00406-012-0366-z

Parnas, J. (2011). A disappearing heritage: The clinical core of schizophrenia. *Schizophrenia Bulletin, 37*(6), 1121–30. http://dx.doi.org/10.1093/schbul/sbr081

Parnas, J. (2012). The core Gestalt of schizophrenia. *World Psychiatry, 11*(2), 67–9. http://dx.doi.org/10.1016/j.wpsyc.2012.05.002

Parnas, J. (2013). The Breivik case and "conditio psychiatrica." *World Psychiatry, 12*(1), 22–3. http://dx.doi.org/10.1002/wps.20003

Parnas, J., & Bovet, P. (1995). Research in psychopathology: Epistemologic issues. *Comprehensive Psychiatry, 36*, 167–81. http://dx.doi.org/10.1016/0010-440X(95)90078-A

Parnas, J., & Bovet, P. (2014). Psychiatry made easy: Operation(al)ism and some of its consequences. In K. S. Kendler & J. Parnas (Eds.), *Philosophical issues in psychiatry III: The nature and sources of historical change* (pp. 190–213). Oxford, England: Oxford University Press.

Parnas, J., & Zahavi, D. (2002). The role of phenomenology in psychiatric diagnosis and classification. In M. Maj, W. Gaebel, J. J. López-Ibor, & N. Sartorius (Eds.), *Psychiatric diagnosis and classification* (pp. 137–62). Chichester, England: Wiley. http://dx.doi.org/10.1002/047084647X.ch6

Parnas, J., Sass, L. A., & Zahavi, D. (2013). Rediscovering psychopathology: The epistemology and phenomenology of the psychiatric object. *Schizophrenia Bulletin, 39*(2), 270–7. http://dx.doi.org/10.1093/schbul/sbs153

Putnam, H. (1999). Problems with the observational/theoretical distinction. In R. Klee (Ed.), *Scientific inquiry* (pp. 25–9). New York, NY: Oxford University Press.

Rosch, E. H. (1973). Natural categories. *Cognitive Psychology, 4*, 328–50. http://dx.doi.org/10.1016/0010-0285(73)90017-0

Sass, L., & Parnas, J. (2007). Explaining schizophrenia: The relevance of phenomenology. In M. C. Chung, K. W. M. Fulford, & G. Graham (Eds.), *Reconceiving schizophrenia* (pp. 63–96). New York, NY: Oxford University Press.

Schwartz, M. A., & Wiggins, O. P. (1987a). Typifications: The first step for clinical diagnosis in psychiatry. *Journal of Nervous and Mental Diseases, 175*(2), 65–77. http://dx.doi.org/10.1097/00005053-198702000-00001

Schwartz, M. A., & Wiggins, O. P. (1987b). Diagnosis and ideal types: A contribution to psychiatric classification. *Comprehensive Psychiatry, 28*, 277–91. http://dx.doi.org/10.1016/0010-440X(87)90064-2

Spitzer, M. (1988). Psychiatry, philosophy, and the problem of description. In M. Spitzer, F. A. Uehlein, & G. Oepen (Eds.), *Psychopathology and philosophy* (pp. 3–18). Berlin, Germany: Springer. http://dx.doi.org/10.1007/978-3-642-74133-3_1

Vollmer-Larsen, A., Handest, P., & Parnas, J. (2007). Reliability of measuring anomalous experience: The Bonn Scale for the assessment of basic symptoms. *Psychopathology, 40*, 345–8. http://dx.doi.org/10.1159/000106311

Weizsäcker, V. von (1986). *Der Gestaltkreis. Theorie der Einheit von Wahrnehmen und Bewegen* (5th ed.). Stuttgart, Germany: Thieme.

Westen, D. (2012). Prototype diagnosis of psychiatric syndromes. *World Psychiatry, 11*, 16–21. http://dx.doi.org/10.1016/j.wpsyc.2012.01.004

4   How the Self Is Altered in Psychiatric Disorders

A Neurophenomenal Approach

Georg Northoff

Introduction

You watch a movie. You find it boring, or rather, the experience is marked by a sense of boredom. Who experiences this boredom? You. Not only are you the subject of the experience, without a "you" there is no experience. More formally, an experiencing subject (the "self") is a prerequisite not only for the possible constitution of experience, but for consciousness itself.

Clearly, much is at stake when it comes to characterizing or defining the concept of self, as well as understanding its alterations for persons living with psychiatric disorders. In order to elucidate the experience of psychiatric symptoms, I will focus on how to directly link subjective experience to neuronal mechanisms underlying the brain's resting-state activity. Methodologically, this amounts to what I describe as a *neurophenomenal* approach, as distinguished from other approaches that also seek to explore the links between neurophysiology and experience, including neurophenomenological and neurocognitive research. In the first section of this chapter, I describe some alterations of self-experience in major depression and schizophrenia. I then outline the main features of the neurophenomenal approach. Rather than going into much conceptual detail about the self (Northoff, 2011, 2013a, 2013b), I next summarize recent neuroscientific findings that suggest an overlap between the neural activity involved in what has been called "the resting state" and self-specific experience, especially in the anterior cortical midline regions. In the final section of the chapter, I relate the phenomenological features of alterations of the self to findings on resting activity in depression and schizophrenia. Space constraints prevent me from providing a more general overview on the psychopathology of the self in other psychiatric disorders like addiction (see, for example, de Greck et al., 2010; de Greck et al., 2009) and personality disorders (see, for example, Doering et al., 2013). But this same approach can be applied to a wide variety of psychiatric conditions, allowing us to link neural processing to complex behavioral and experiential manifestations of psychopathology.

The Self in Depression

Major depressive disorder (MDD) is a psychiatric disorder characterized by extremely negative emotions, suicidal thoughts, hopelessness, diffuse bodily symptoms, lack of pleasure (or anhedonia), ruminations, and enhanced stress sensitivity (see Hasler & Northoff, 2011; Kuhn & Gallinat, 2013; Northoff, 2011; Northoff, Wiebking, Feinberg, & Panksepp, 2011).

How do depressed persons experience their symptoms? This question is addressed by phenomenology, which can be loosely (and rather broadly) defined as the study of subjective experience from a first-person perspective (Northoff, 2004). A phenomenological approach differs from a psychopathological approach, which involves the observation of depressive symptoms from a third-person perspective.

A quote from a recent paper nicely describes the alterations of the self in depression:

> She sat by the window, looking inward rather than looking out. Her thoughts were consumed with her sadness. She viewed her life as a broken one, and yet she could not place her finger on the exact moment it fell apart. "How did I get to feel this way?" she repeatedly asked herself. By asking, she hoped to transcend her depressed state; through understanding, she hoped to repair it. Instead, her questions led her deeper and deeper inside herself – further away from the path that would lead to her recovery. (Treynor, Gonzalez, & Nolen-Hoeksema, 2003, p. 251)

This passage illustrates three crucial self-related characteristics of depression, which can be conceptualized as increased self-focus, association of the self with negative emotions, and increased cognitive processing of one's own self (Northoff, 2007).

Almost all depressed patients look inward more than outward; that is, they focus attention on themselves and have difficulty shifting attention to others (Figure 4.1). A variety of studies assessing self-focused attention with diverse measures and methodologies all converge on the finding of an increased and perhaps prolonged level of self-focused attention in depression (Ingram, 1990). It remains unclear, however, whether increased self-focus is purely explicit, and thus conscious, or is present on an implicit and unconscious level.

Social-psychological theory views self-focused attention as focus on internal perceptual events, that is, information sensory processes that signal changes in bodily activity (Ingram, 1990). Self-focus may also concern enhanced awareness of one's present or past physical behavior,

Increased Self-Focus   Decreased Environmental-Focus

Association with
negative emotions

Cognition of the
own self

SELF ·······▶ Other/Environment

BODY

KEY

········▶ Reduced awareness to other and environment

——▶ Feedback look with abnormal reinforcement

——▶ Shift of awareness from the other/environment to the own self

Increased Body-Focus

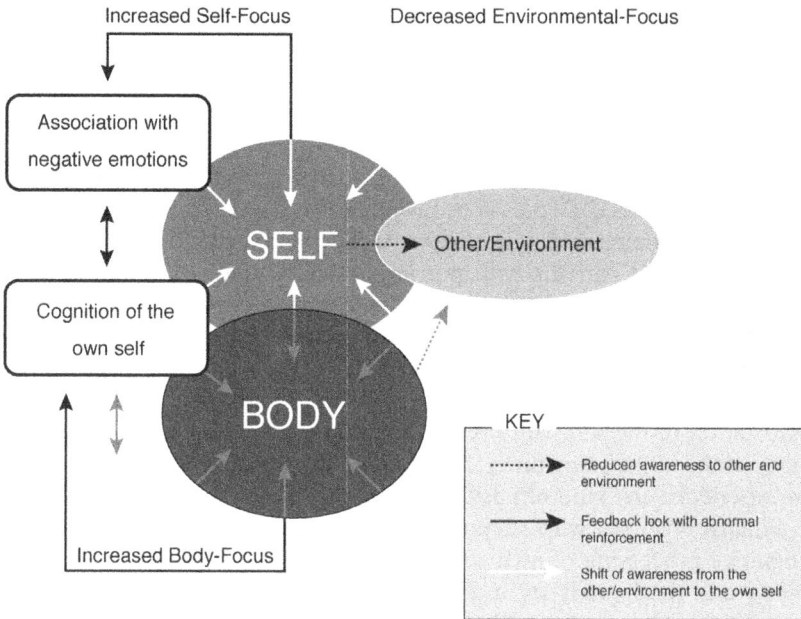

Figure 4.1. Self, body, and environment in depression. The figure
shows the relationship between the different directions of phenomenal
consciousness (here denoted as awareness) in depression.
Phenomenal consciousness can be directed either externally toward the
environment or internally toward either the own self or the body. In
depression, there is increased directedness toward the own self and the
body ("increased self- and body-focus"), while the directedness
toward the environment is decreased ("decreased environment-focus").
The increased self- and body-focus are symbolized by larger circles
and inward arrows; the decreased relationship of both self and body to
the environment is illustrated by dotted arrows. The consequences of
the increased self-focus for subsequent psychological functions are
indicated on the very left leading to increased association with negative
emotions and increased cognitions of the own self. From *Unlocking
the Brain: Volume II – Consciousness* (p. 405), by G. Northoff, 2014,
New York, NY: Oxford University Press. By permission from Oxford
University Press, USA.

including what one is doing. In addition to increased self-focus,
depressed persons show heightened awareness of their own body or
"body-focus," which results in the perception of diffuse bodily symptoms
(Wiebking et al., 2010). The increased self- and body-focus mean that
the depressed person's attention is no longer focused on their relation to
the social environment and environmental events, as in healthy people

but, rather, on themselves. Increased self-focus seems to correlate with decreased environment-focus (Figure 4.1).

Another characteristic of depression is the tendency to attribute negative emotions to one's self. The self is associated with sadness, guilt, mistakes, inabilities, death, illness, and so on, which may ultimately result in paranoid delusions. A recent study investigating symptom clusters with the Beck Depression Inventory (BDI) observed three BDI factors, including a self-blame factor (Grunebaum et al., 2005). Interestingly, depressed patients with previous suicide attempts scored significantly higher on the BDI self-blame factor than those without suicide attempts. Moreover, the self-blame factor significantly correlated with total number of suicide attempts and with known risk factors for suicidal behavior (Northoff, 2007). Such self-blame possibly results from the association of the self with predominantly negative emotions in depression, while, at the same time, these individuals apparently remain unable to experience any kind of positive emotions related to self.

Finally, people with depression typically suffer from increased cognitive processing of own self; they think about themselves and their mood and desperately try to discover the reasons for their depression, but, in the process, they only fall deeper and deeper into the depressed mood (see arrows from negative cognitions to the self in Figure 4.1). Cognitive processing of own self, or rumination, is often considered a method of coping with negative mood that involves increased self-focused attention and self-reflection (Ingram, 1990).

Based on factor analysis of a rumination scale, Treynor and colleagues (2003) suggest a two-factor model of rumination. They call the first factor "reflection," which involves a purposeful turning inward to engage in cognitive problem solving to alleviate one's depressive problems. They refer to the second factor as "brooding," which involves passive comparison of one's current situation with some unachieved standard based on others' views or what psychodynamically can be called the "ideal-self" (Boker et al., 2000). Corresponding to the reflection factor, Rimes and Watkins (2005) suggest an increase in "analytical self-focus" in depression, which they define as thinking analytically about oneself and one's symptoms; such increased self-focus is related to increased ratings of the self as worthless and incompetent and to depressed mood.

Rimes and Watkins distinguish increased "analytical self-focus" in depression from an "experiential self-focus," which refers to focus on the direct experience of one's thoughts, feelings, and sensations in the present moment. In contrast to increased analytical self-focus, experiential self-focus tends to be decreased in depression because these individuals have difficulty experiencing themselves and their self as such;

they have access to their self mainly through analytical, self-focused cognition, while experiential self-focus is decreased. Phenomenologically, this means that they remain unable to associate phenomenal features to those internal mental contents related to their self, which ultimately results in what may be described as decreased "experiential self-focus."

There is thus an imbalance between "analytical and experiential self-focus" in depression. Whether this imbalance corresponds to the increased self-focus and decreased environment-focus described earlier requires future conceptual and empirical investigation.

The Self in Schizophrenia

Based on clinical observation, early psychiatrists such as Kraepelin and Bleuler assumed abnormality of the self to be basic in schizophrenia. More specifically, Kraepelin (1913) characterized schizophrenia as "the peculiar destruction of the inner coherence of the personality" with a "disunity of consciousness" ("orchestra without conductor"). Bleuler (1911/2010) also described schizophrenia as a "disorder of the personality by splitting, dissociation" where the "I is never completely intact." Berze, a contemporary of Bleuler and Kraepelin, even referred to schizophrenia as "basic alteration of self-consciousness." Karl Jaspers (1964) also considered "incoherence, dissociation, fragmenting of consciousness, intrapsychic ataxia, weakness of apperception, insufficiency of psychic activity and disturbance of association, etc." (p. 124) to be basic or unifying "central factors" in schizophrenia.

These early descriptions of a disrupted self are complemented by recent phenomenological accounts that focus predominantly on the experience of own self in relation to the world. Josef Parnas (2003; Parnas et al., 2001) describes what he calls "presence" as being altered in schizophrenia. The experience of the world and its objects is no longer accompanied by a prereflective self-awareness. The self that experiences the world is no longer included in that very experience; that is, the self no longer experiences itself as being the subject of its own experiences:

The prominent feature of altered presence in the pre-onset stages of schizophrenia is disturbed ipseity, a disturbance in which the sense of self no longer saturates the experience. For instance, the sense of mineness of experience may become subtly affected: one of our patients reported that this feeling of his experience as his own experience only "appeared a split-second delayed." (Parnas, 2003, p. 223)

Some persons with schizophrenia thus may have difficulty referring to themselves in their experience of the world, which no longer feels like their own. Instead, they may feel that their experience belongs to or is even experienced by someone else. Due to the absence of an own self in their experience of the world, such persons with schizophrenia appear detached, alienated, estranged from their own experiences, resulting in what Sass (2003) describes as a "disorder of self-affectivity": The self is no longer experienced as one's own self, and most importantly, is no longer experienced as the vital center and source of one's experiences, actions, perceptions, thoughts, and so on. This reflects what Sass and Parnas (2003) call "diminished self-affection," meaning that the self is no longer affected by its own experiences. As a result, the self stands apart from objects and events in the world, which are experienced across a gulf or phenomenological distance that opens up between world and self (Parnas, 2003). The objects and events of the world no longer make intuitive sense and thus are no longer meaningful to the experiencing subject. The own self becomes thus almost objective and mechanical in its experience and perception of the world. The person's own self is no longer experienced as subjective, and therefore as specific to the person as distinguished from all other persons. Instead, it is viewed as one object among others.

Let us recap the situation in the case of the healthy subject. We stated earlier that ipseity is a central phenomenal feature of experience. Due to ipseity, the subject experiences "relation of mineness" and "sense of belongingness" of the contents in relation to itself as subject. And it is because of these phenomenal features, for example, ipseity, that the subject can attribute meaning and significance to the contents it experiences. Meaning of contents for the subject on the semantic level entails prior relationship between subject and content on the phenomenal level; this phenomenal relation between subject and content is realized by ipseity and its relation of mineness and sense of belongingness.

If this phenomenal relation between subject and content is disrupted, ipseity and thus its relation of mineness and sense of belongingness disappear. There is no longer a relation of mineness and sense of belongingness between subject and content. There may still be content in consciousness, but that very same content is no longer related to the subject on the phenomenal level. On the semantic level, this entails the impossibility of attributing meaning to the content in question. In summary, for a person living with schizophrenia, the contents of experience may become devoid of meaning and hence processed in a purely mechanical way.

The Neurophenomenal Approach

The neurophenomenal approach aims to link the phenomenology of psychopathology with underlying neural processes. The term "phenomenal" roughly refers to various features of consciousness, the contents of which we experience in a subjective (rather than an objective) way. For example, you experience the various contents involved in the process of reading this page not separately, but related to each other as if there were an underlying unity. This unity is considered a "hallmark feature" of the phenomenology of consciousness (see Northoff, 2014b).

Another central phenomenal feature of consciousness is its directedness toward mental contents. Consciousness is always directed toward something outside itself, whether it be an internally generated thought or a mental image of external origin. In either case, the subject experiencing consciousness stands in relation to a particular content that thereby becomes conscious. There is no consciousness without a relation between the experiencing subject and the experienced content – this is called intentionality.

Finally, the contents themselves are experienced in a subjective way. They are experienced as if they belong to me, the subject of the experience, that is, there is a certain "relation of mineness" or ipseity (Metzinger, 2003; Northoff, 2014b).

Ipseity is to be distinguished from an objective mode in which the very same contents are observed in third-person perspective, without relation to the observer. This chapter focuses on the experiencing subject, the subject in the subjective mode of experience or consciousness. How do psychiatric patients experience their own selves, and how is the subjective self altered in their experience of contents originating either in themselves (as thoughts) or in the environment (as mental imagery and perceptions)?

A neurophenomenal approach aims to directly link those phenomenal features of our consciousness and its experiencing self to the neural mechanisms of our brain. Thereby, we focus on particular neural mechanisms, namely those involved in the brain's resting-state activity or its intrinsic activity. Resting-state activity is defined in a purely operational way by the absence of the processing of any specific stimuli or tasks as, for instance, during sleep. The term "intrinsic activity" refers more to the origin of the brain's neural activity, reflecting an internal origin within the brain itself, as distinguished from the external origin of neural activity in response to extrinsic stimuli or tasks. Thus, the resting-state activity represents ongoing processing in the brain that is, to some degree, independent of specific content and that reflects the person's culture, history, and biographical trajectory as it has been sedimented in background patterns of neural processing (Northoff, 2014a, 2014b). Resting-state activity can be distinguished from the brain's extrinsic activity, its stimulus-induced and task-evoked activity, which is related to particular functions of the brain in response to cognitive, affective, motor, sensory, and social stimuli.

Distinguishing Neurophenomenal from Neurocognitive and Neurophenomenological Approaches

The focus on the brain's intrinsic activity distinguishes the neurophenomenal approach from neurocognitive approaches to the self in psychiatric disorders (see, for example, Nelson, Whitford, Lavoie, Sass, 2014a, 2014b). Neurocognitive research focuses on specific psychological (e.g., cognitive) functions and their underlying neural mechanisms. For example, disorder of the self in schizophrenia has recently been associated with cognitive functions like source memory, attention, and working memory and their respective neural correlates (Nelson et al., 2014a, 2014b). Such approaches presuppose that a certain processing of contents on the basis of particular psychological functions yields phenomenal features. But the link between neural and phenomenal features is mediated by the contents and their related psychological functions and neural correlates (see Figure 4.2a). In contrast to a neurocognitive approach (which can be extended to other functions resulting in neuroaffective, neurosocial, and neurosensorimotor approaches), the neurophenomenal approach posits a direct link between neural and phenomenal features, unmediated by contents.

The neurophenomenal approach focuses on the brain's intrinsic activity, such that the phenomenal alterations of the self in psychiatric disorders are directly related to abnormal intrinsic activity patterns, rather than being mediated by the brain's extrinsic activity as related to sensorimotor, cognitive, affective, and social functions. In the case of the self, this means that the resting-state activity, the brain's intrinsic activity, must contain some features related to self-specific organization, which make possible and predispose the constitution of an experiencing self, a subjective rather than merely objective self. These predisposing features must be encoded in the resting state itself and, as we will see later, there is indeed empirical support for this theory (see Figure 4.2b).

The neurophenomenal approach also can be distinguished from neurophenomenological approaches. As indicated in its name, neurophenomenology emphasizes a particular method developed in phenomenological philosophy, which aims to use information derived from the first-person perspective to reveal the features of consciousness (Lutz & Thompson, 2003). The neurophenomenal approach is not committed to any particular method, but focuses on the phenomenal features of consciousness, irrespective and independent of the method or means by which they are acquired (see Appendix 1 in Northoff, 2014b, for details).

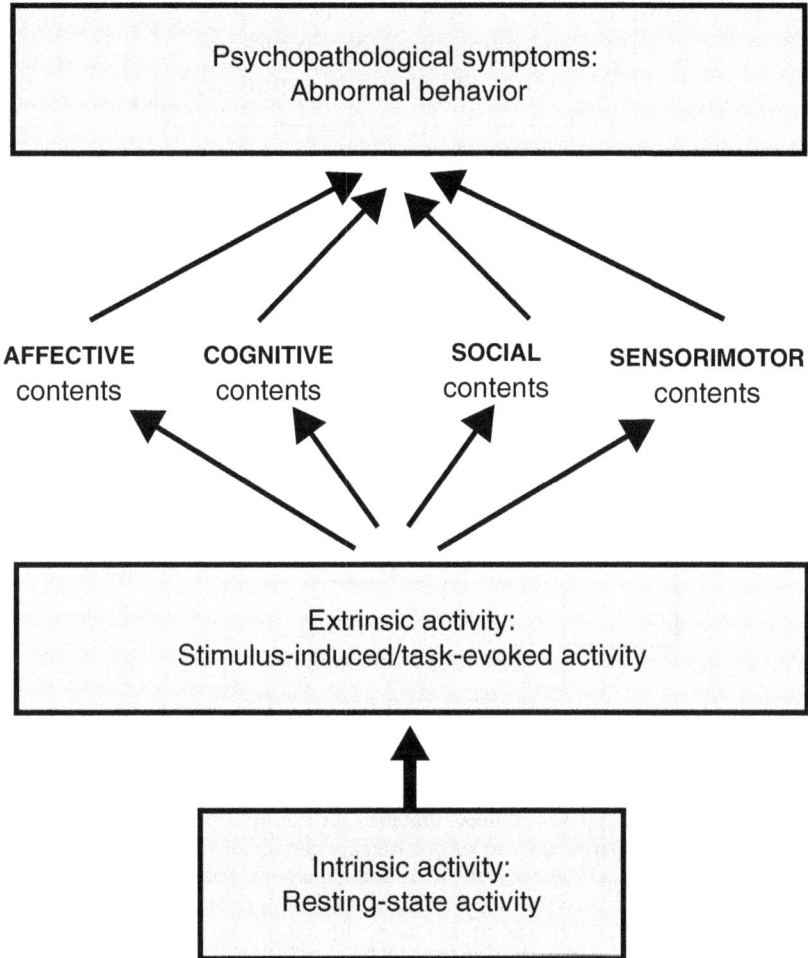

Figure 4.2a. Neurocognitive approach to psychopathology. The neurocognitive approach considers the content of the various functions (affective, cognitive, social, and sensorimotor) to be related to the various psychopathological symptoms (upper part). This attributes a central role to extrinsic activity, task-evoked or stimulus-induced activity. In contrast, the brain's intrinsic activity (lower part) bears no direct relationship to the psychopathological symptoms albeit a yet unclear indirect one. Although this approach can explain the psychopathological symptoms in terms of the functions and their extrinsic activity, the neural mechanisms underlying the abnormal sense of self in particular and subjective experience, for example, consciousness of the environment in general remain unclear in the neurocognitive approach.

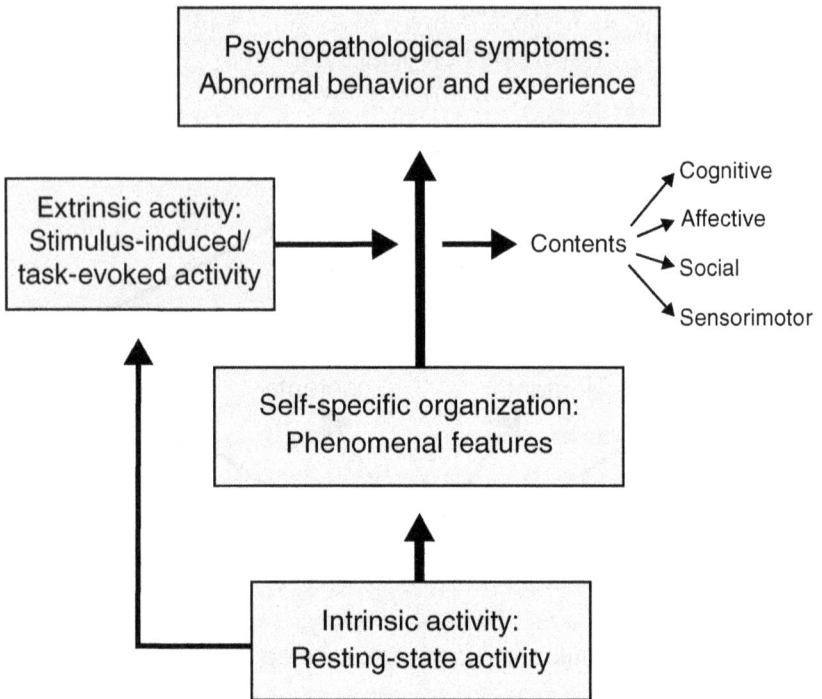

Figure 4.2b. Neurophenomenal approach to psychopathology. The neurophenomenal approach attributes a central role to the brain's intrinsic activity in that it characterizes it by self-specific organization which is supposed to make possible, for example, predispose, the sense of self in particular and subjective experience, for example, consciousness in general. Alterations in resting state activity in psychiatric disorders consequently entail abnormal sense of self (lower part). That, in conjunction with abnormal extrinsic activity, as based on abnormal resting activity (left arrow), and the consecutively abnormal functions (cognitive, social, affective, sensorimotor) (middle part) leads the various psychopathological symptoms including abnormal experience, for example, consciousness of the environment (upper part).

Neural Substrates of the Self and Resting-State Activity

The self has been the formal subject of neuroscientific investigation over the past decade, primarily through the use of functional brain imaging studies. These have detected differences in neural activity between self-specific and nonself-specific stimuli or tasks. In one type of experiment, for example, subjects view and judge words (or other stimuli-like pictures or sounds) that are closely related to themselves – for instance, the word "piano" for a concert pianist. Responses to these self-specific words are then compared to responses to other words that are unrelated or non-self-specific to the person (Gillihan & Farah, 2005; Legrand & Ruby, 2009; Northoff et al., 2006; Qin & Northoff, 2011; van der Meer, Costafreda, Aleman, & David, 2010). Interestingly, most of these studies find strong activity in specific areas of the brain including: anterior and posterior cortical midline regions like the pregenual anterior cingulate cortex (PACC); the supragenual anterior cingulate cortex (SACC); the ventro- and dorsomedial prefrontal cortex (VMPFC, DMPFC); the posterior cingulate cortex (PCC); the precuneus; and the retrosplenium (Christoff, Cosmelli, Legrand, & Thompson, 2011; Northoff et al., 2006; Qin & Northoff, 2011; van der Meer et al., 2010). These findings have led to the suggestion that cortical midline structures specifically process the stimuli's degree of self-specificity, and can thus be considered a network specific to the self.

The assumption that a cortical network underlies self-specificity has been challenged, however, because tasks and stimuli other than those focusing on the self recruit the same brain regions (Christoff et al., 2011; Gillihan & Farah, 2005; Legrand & Ruby, 2009). Such tasks include various cognitive functions like mindreading (guessing the intentions of other people) and decision making, as well as social functions like empathy, reward, and emotional-affective functions. Moreover, another line of research suggests that self-specificity not only recruits cortical midline structures. If self-specific stimuli are presented independent of any associated cognitive tasks (like judgment), they also elicit neural activity changes in subcortical midline regions like the dorsomedial thalamus, the ventral striatum, the tectum, the periaqueductal gray, and the colliculi (Northoff & Panksepp, 2008; Northoff et al., 2009; Panksepp & Northoff, 2009; Schneider et al., 2008).

Thus, while there is some neuroanatomical evidence supporting the notion of a subcortical-cortical midline system mediating the self, other researchers consider the midline regions to be too unspecific; they presuppose a different and more cognitive notion of the self than the one developed here (Christoff et al., 2011; Gillihan & Farah, 2005; Legrand & Ruby, 2009).

This distinction between a cognitive self (characterized by self-reflexivity) and a more basic phenomenal self is reflected in the well-documented structural organization of the brain in terms of three concentric inner, middle, and outer rings that span subcortical to cortical regions (Northoff, 2013a, 2013b; Northoff, Wiebking, Feinberg, & Panksepp, 2011). As shown in Figure 4.3 and also summarized in

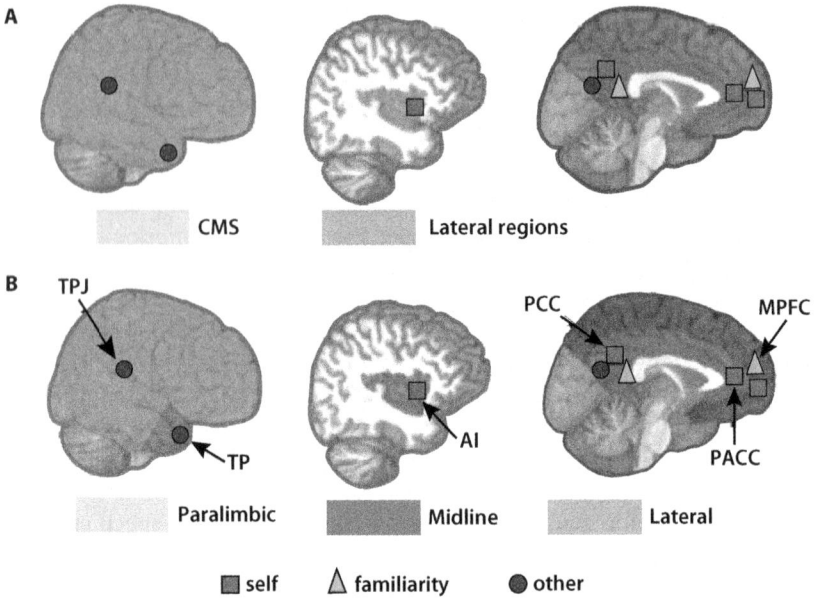

Figure 4.3. Self-specificity and anterior cortical midline regions. (A) The traditional medial-lateral twofold anatomical dichotomy: cortical midline structures (pink); lateral regions (cyan). (B) Threefold anatomical distinction: paralimbic (pink); midline (purple); lateral (cyan). Red squares represent the regions activated under *self* condition in meta-analysis; green triangles represent the regions activated under *nonself* familiarity condition in meta-analysis; Blue circles represent the regions activated under *other* condition in meta-analysis. See also Table 4.1. TPJ = temporal parietal junction; TP = temporal pole; AI = anterior insula; PCC = posterior cingulate cortex; MPFC = medial prefrontal cortex; PACC = pregenual anterior cingulate cortex; CMS = cortical midline structures. Reprinted from *Consciousness and Cognition, 20*(1), G. Northoff, P. Qin, & T. E. Feinberg, "Brain Imaging of the Self: Conceptual, Anatomical and Methodological Issues," p. 57, Copyright 2011, with permission from Elsevier. (See Color Plate.)

Table 4.1, the inner ring lies immediately adjacent to the third ventricle and extends from the subcortical to the cortical level, where it includes the cingulate cortex. The middle ring includes the paramedian and lateral core, which is sandwiched between inner and outer rings. On the cortical level, the middle ring includes regions like the VMPFC and the DMPFC. Finally, the outer ring contains regions on both subcortical and cortical level that mark the outer boundary of the brain, the visible surface in the case of the cortex.

Table 4.1 *Comparison Between the Two- and Threefold Anatomical Characterizations with Regard to Meta-Analytic Results from Self, Familiarity, and Other*

	Self	Familiarity	Other
Paralimbic			
Anterior	PACC, Insula	–	–
Posterior	PCC	PCC	PCC, TP
Midline			
Anterior	MPFC	MPFC	–
Posterior	–	–	–
Lateral	–	–	TPJ
CMS			
Anterior	PACC, MPFC	MPFC	–
Posterior	PCC	PCC	PCC
Lateral regions			
Anterior	Insula	–	–
Posterior	–	–	TPJ, TP

The table represents the results from the meta-analysis of studies on the self when compared to nonself (familiar and nonfamiliar). Most important, it represents the results in a way ordered along the threefold anatomical distinction into paralimbic regions (upper), midline regions (upper middle), cortical midline structures (CMS; lower middle), and lateral regions (lower). We can see that for instance the insula which seems to show self-specific activity is once ordered in the paralimbic regions as part of the inner ring when one presupposes the threefold anatomy with inner, middle, and outer ring. If, in contrast, one presupposes the traditional medial-lateral anatomy, the insula is listed as lateral region. This though makes it hard to understand why it shows self-specific activity because only paralimbic but not lateral regions show such activity pattern. PACC = perigenual anterior cingulate cortex; PCC = posterior cingulate cortex; MPFC = medial prefrontal cortex; TP = temporal pole; TPJ = temporoparietal junction. Reprinted from G. Northoff, P. Qin, & T. E. Feinberg, "Brain Imaging of the Self: Conceptual, Anatomical and Methodological Issues." *Consciousness and Cognition, 20*(1), 59. Copyright 2011, with permission from Elsevier.

This threefold subcortical-cortical anatomical distinction shows how subcortical and cortical regions are directly related to each other and form one unified system. The relationship between subcortical and cortical regions is important for understanding the links between aspects of the self that are associated with specifically higher-order cognitive functions and those that are associated with noncognitive functions (like affective processes) that involve subcortical regions (Panksepp, 1998).

Importantly, this threefold anatomical organization is also found in resting-state activity, where it mirrors the continuous inputs from body (inner ring) and environment (outer ring) that the brain receives even in the resting state. Hence, this anatomical organization can be related to how the self is constituted on the basis of different functional organization in the brain's resting-state activity.

Anatomical Rings and Self-Specificity

How is this threefold subcortical-cortical neuroanatomical distinction related to the self? Does it map self-specificity better than the neuro-cognitive approach, which associates the self with cognitive functions like source memory, attention, and/or working memory, linked especially to activity in the lateral prefrontal cortex (Nelson et al., 2014a, 2014b)?

Neurologist Todd Feinberg, who has undertaken careful study of patients with lesions in particular regions of the brain that are associated with changes in their phenomenal consciousness, has attempted to explain his patients' unusual experience of the self in terms of this threefold anatomical organization (Feinberg, 2009; Feinberg, 2011; Feinberg, Venneri, Simone, Fan, & Northoff, 2010). Feinberg (2009, 2010) suggests that the inner ring reflects the bodily or "intero-self," whereas the outer ring may be related to the environmental or "extero-self." The middle ring may reflect integration between inner and outer rings, that is, the self proper, or the "integrative self," which spans intero- and exteroceptive stimuli and thus body and environment.

Pengmin Qin from my group (Northoff, Qin, & Nakao, 2010; Qin & Northoff, 2011) conducted a meta-analysis of all imaging studies on the self, using self-specific, familiar, and nonfamiliar stimuli (e.g., the city in which one lives, the prime minister of one's own country, and nonfamiliar names). The self-specific condition yielded activity changes in the inner ring regions (the PACC, the insula, and the PCC), as well as in the middle ring (the VMPFC and the DMPFC). The familiarity condition, in contrast, did not yield any signal changes in the inner ring and its anterior regions (the insula and the PACC). The familiarity condition did induce signal changes in the middle ring (the VMPFC and the DMPFC), as well as in the posterior regions of the inner ring (the PCC). Finally, the posterior regions of the inner ring, including the PCC, were also recruited during the nonfamiliar condition. Unlike familiarity, the nonfamiliar condition did not recruit any other midline regions in the anterior parts but, rather, the temporoparietal junction and the temporal pole.

Taken together, these findings suggest an inner-to-outer gradient coupled with an anterior-to-posterior gradient in the brain with regard to self-specificity. The more inner and anterior regions like the PACC and insula allow for the neural processing of high degrees of self-specificity, while the converse holds for the more outer (lateral) regions and posterior regions (the PCC and precuneus), which are more closely associated with low degrees of self-specificity. Simply put, one's own self is associated with activity in anterior and inner parts in the brain, whereas others' selves are more related to activity in posterior and outer parts.

We have to be careful, however. The aforementioned description primarily relies on findings at the cortical level; there are much less data on the subcortical regions. Hence, further investigation is needed to reveal whether, for instance, the inner-to-outer gradient also applies at the subcortical level. One step in this direction has been taken by Hans Lou and colleagues at Aarhus University. Their research focuses on the neural causality of consciousness (Lou, Gross, Biermann-Ruben, Kjaer, & Schnitzler, 2010; Lou et al., 2011; Lou et al., 1999; Lou et al., 2004; Lou, Luber, Stanford, & Lisanby, 2010; Lou, Nowak, & Kjaer, 2005). Lou and colleagues suggest that a subcortical-cortical paralimbic network is central in mediating self and consciousness. This network includes the thalamus (pulvinar), the subgenual and pregenual anterior cingulate cortex, the medial prefrontal cortex (VMPFC, DMPFC), the striatum, and the posterior cingulate cortex/precuneus. The network can be characterized as a self-reference system that interacts with other networks associated with reward, emotion, and executive-cognitive functions (see Raz & Macdonald, Chapter 10, *this volume*). Lou considers this network central for consciousness.

In advancing this model, we have to distinguish between the self-specificity of internal and external contents and their recruitment of midline regions. Internal contents concern one's own thoughts and own body, whereas external contents are related to objects and events in the environment. Further studies are needed to show that both internal and external contents with high degrees of self-specificity are processed in the subcortical-cortical midline regions.

Activity of Midline Brain Regions in the Resting State and Self-Specific Thought

The cortical midline structures are core regions of the default-mode network, a midline network that shows particularly high levels of neural activity in the resting state – for example, in the absence of particular or specific stimuli or tasks demands (Buckner, Andrews-Hanna, &

Schacter, 2008; Raichle et al., 2001). Because the midline regions have been shown to be implicated in mediating self-specificity, neural activity during self-specificity may strongly overlap with high resting-state activity in the very same regions. This is indeed the case, as several studies show.

D'Argembeau and colleagues (2005) conducted a positron emission tomography (PET) study in which subjects underwent four conditions: (1) thinking/reflection about one's own personality traits, (2) thinking/ reflection about another person's personality traits, (3) thinking/reflection about social issues, and (4) a pure rest condition in which subjects could relax. This allowed the investigators to compare self- and nonself conditions as well as to explore the relation between self-conditions and resting state. The VMPFC showed significant increases in regional cerebral blood flow (rCBF) during the self condition when compared to (2) and (3) earlier. In addition, when all three task-related conditions were compared to (4) the rest condition, they showed increased rCBF in the DMPFC and the temporal regions, while no differences were observed in the VMPFC. Conversely, the rest condition showed rCBF increases in a large medial frontoparietal and posterior medial network with, again, no differences in the VMPFC.

Differentiating self and rest conditions allowed the authors to directly compare the two conditions. Comparison showed a strong overlap in the VMPFC, where rest and self-specificity had similar rCBF increases. In contrast, (2) other and (3) social conditions induced rCBF decreases in the same region. Postscanning reports of experience indicated that self-referential thoughts were most abundant in the self condition while being diminished in the other three conditions. The authors therefore correlated the post-scanning measures of self-referential thinking with the rCBF changes. This yielded a positive relationship in the VMPFC. The higher the rCBF in the VMPFC, the higher the degree of self-referentiality in subjects' self-reported thoughts across all four conditions.

The strong association between self-related thoughts and resting-state activity, especially in the regions of the inner ring, was further confirmed by a recent meta-analyses by Pengmin Qin (Qin & Northoff, 2011; Whitfield-Gabrieli et al., 2009). Qin analyzed human imaging studies on the self when compared to nonself. Most importantly, he also included studies on the resting state to compare their neural activity pattern to the one during self- and nonself-specific stimuli. This approach allowed him to directly compare resting state in the default-mode network with the regions recruited during self- and nonself-specific stimuli. Results confirmed the regional overlap between self-related thought and resting-state activity. More specifically, the regional activities during self-specific stimuli and the ones during resting state overlapped in the PACC, extending to the VMPFC, while no such regional overlap with the resting state was observed in the other conditions (that is, familiarity and nonfamiliarity) in either the PACC or any other region. Taken together, these results suggest neural overlap between self-specificity and resting-state activity in the anterior midline regions including the VMPFC.

The high degree of anatomical overlap between resting-state activity and regions recruited during self-specific thought was further confirmed in a study by Whitfield-Gabrieli and colleagues (2009). They directly tested for the neural overlap between self-related activity and resting-state activity. As expected, participants showed recruitment of stronger neural activity in anterior and posterior midline regions (VMPFC, DMPFC, PACC, PCC, precuneus) during the self-task, which did not differ from the level of resting-state activity in the same regions. The authors also conducted analyses that suggest a close relationship between the neural activities underlying rest and self, especially in the regions of the inner ring, the PACC and the PCC, while in the middle ring (precuneus, DMPFC), neural activities during self and rest seem to be distinct from each other.

The overlap between rest and self is further supported by a recent magnetoenceophalographic (MEG) study by Lou and colleagues (2010). They investigated judgment of self-related words and focused on three main regions, precuneus, thalamus/pulvinar, and anterior midline regions (including VMPFC, DMPFC, and PACC). Using Granger causality analysis (which allows testing of the direction of functional connectivity), they observed that the three regions were bidirectionally connected to each other (i.e., showed high degrees of statistical covariance in their signal changes). Most interestingly, the increase in functional connectivity occurred 900 ms *before* stimulus onset, while it was further enhanced by the stimulus itself for the first 900 ms. This suggests that self-related processing occurs on top of the resting state's already existing functional connectivity and just accentuates it even further; this further supports the suggested overlap between neural resting state and self-related activity. This is accompanied by accentuation of activity fluctuations in especially the gamma range between 30 and 45 Hz before and after stimulus onset during the self-condition. Accordingly, the resting state seems to provide both spatial (functional connectivity) and temporal (gamma fluctuations) predispositions for the processing of self-related stimuli.

Taken together, these studies show strong overlap between high resting-state activity and stimulus-induced activity, as elicited by high self-specific stimuli in anterior and posterior midline regions, including both cortical and subcortical (albeit with limited evidence) regions. Hence, the resting-state activity in the anterior regions of the inner ring seems to be closely related to self-specificity in as yet unclear ways. What does this overlap between resting-state activity and self-specificity imply for the kind of psychopathological symptoms we observe in schizophrenia and depression? This will be the focus in subsequent sections.

The Neural Basis of Self-Experience in Depression

There are distinctive alterations of resting-state activity in MDD. There are several excellent reviews of the structural and functional brain changes in MDD (Alcaro, Panksepp, Witczak, Hayes, & Northoff, 2010; Mayberg, 2002, 2003, 2009; Phillips, Drevets, Rauch, & Lane, 2003; Price & Drevets, 2010). Here, I will briefly highlight only the main findings and conclusions and then relate them to functional networks as delineated in normal-healthy brains (see Hasler & Northoff, 2011; Northoff, 2011).

Alcaro and colleagues (2010) conducted a meta-analysis of all imaging studies in human MDD that focused on resting-state activity. This yielded hyperactive regions in the PACC, the VMPFC, thalamic regions like the dorsomedial thalamus (DMT) and the pulvinar, pallidum/putamen and midbrain regions such as the ventral tegmental area, the substantia nigra, the tectum, and the periaqueductal gray (PAG). In contrast, resting-state activity was reduced in the dorsolateral prefrontal cortex (DLPFC), the PCC, and adjacent precuneus/cuneus (Alcaro et al., 2010).

These results are in accord with other meta-analyses (Fitzgerald et al., 2006; Price & Drevets, 2010; Savitz & Drevets, 2009a, 2009b), which have emphasized the role of the hippocampus, the parahippocampus, and the amygdala. Interestingly, the same regions, as well as the PACC, also show structural abnormalities in depressed patients, with reduced gray matter volume in imaging studies and reduced cell-count markers of cellular function in postmortem studies (Price & Drevets, 2010; Savitz & Drevets, 2009a, 2009b).

Involvement of these regions in MDD is further corroborated by the investigation of resting-state activity in animal models of MDD. Reviewing evidence for resting-state hyperactivity in various animal models yielded diverse participating brain regions – the anterior cingulate cortex, the central and basolateral nuclei of the amygdala, the bed nucleus of the stria terminalis, the dorsal raphe, the habenula, the hippocampus, the hypothalamus, the nucleus accumbens, the PAG, the DMT, the nucleus of the solitary tract, and the piriform and prelimbic cortex (Alcaro et al., 2010). In contrast, evidence of hypoactive resting-state activity in animal models remains sparse with no clear results (Alcaro et al., 2010).

Taken together, these findings indicate abnormally high resting-state activity in extended subcortical and cortical medial regions of the brain. This has led authors like Phillips (2003; Ladouceur et al., Chapter 9, *this volume*), Mayberg (2002, 2003, 2009), and Drevets (Price & Drevets, 2010; Savitz & Drevets, 2009a, 2009b) to assume that there is dysfunction in the limbic system in depression or, more specifically, in the "limbic-cortico-striato-pallido-thalamic circuit," with reciprocal interactions between medial prefrontal and limbic regions being crucial (Price & Drevets, 2010).

How do these findings fit into the anatomical characterization of the brain as characterized by inner, middle, and outer rings? What was conceptualized as inner and middle rings at the cortical level, the paralimbic areas, and the cortical midline structures, generally show hyperactivity during resting state in MDD. The outer ring covers the lateral regions on the cortical level, such as the DLPFC and the sensory and motor regions; resting-state hypoactivity has been consistently observed in MDD in the DLPFC, and also in part in the motor cortex (Alcaro et al., 2010).

Considering these findings together, resting-state activity in MDD may be characterized by a subcortical-cortical imbalance between inner/middle and lateral rings. More specifically, the inner and middle rings' regions seem to be hyperactive in the resting state. In contrast, subcortical and especially cortical regions of the lateral-cognitive ring, such as the lateral prefrontal cortex and the sensory-motor cortices, seem to show hypoactivity in the resting state (Northoff et al., 2011).

Resting-State Hyperactivity and Increased Self-Focus in Depression

The aforementioned findings indicate imbalance in the resting-state activity between inner/middle and outer rings. More specifically, they show that resting-state activity in the anterior portions of the inner ring (and also to some degree in the middle ring) is abnormally elevated, while the outer ring's resting-state activity is decreased. This means that there is an imbalance in the resting-state activity in depression along the inner-to-outer and anterior-to-posterior gradients.

The balance between the three anatomical rings and their corresponding functional connectivity may be central in constituting the balance between self- and nonself-specific organization in the resting state. The neural balance between midline and lateral networks appears to be central in designating contents as internal or external as well as in constituting the directedness toward contents. Since the neuronal balance between the three anatomical rings is altered in depression, one would expect a shift toward increased internal contents and decreased external contents. This indeed is the case and surfaces on the phenomenal level.

Phenomenally, a core symptom in MDD is the extremely intense focus of thought and feelings on the own self (Northoff, 2007, 2011). This increased self-focus goes along with detachment from the environment, that is, from the persons, objects, and events from which patients feel disconnected. The question becomes how the shift in focus from environment to self is generated.

One would consequently expect elevated resting-state activity in the midline regions to lead to increased self-specificity and hence to abnormally increased personal concerns in patients with MDD during both resting-state and stimulus-induced activity. Although it remains to be demonstrated for the resting-state activity, it holds true indeed for stimulus-induced activity. Grimm and colleagues (2011, 2009) from our group, as well as Lemogne and colleagues (Lemogne, Bergouignan, et al., 2009; Lemogne et al., 2012; Lemogne, le Bastard, et al., 2009; Lemogne et al., 2010), have observed significantly increased scores for self-specificity with regard to especially negative emotional pictures. Neuronally, this finding went along with decreased signal changes during self-specific stimuli in anterior cortical midline regions. This could reflect the abnormally high resting-state activity, which increases the assignment of self-specificity to stimuli.

The assumption of increased self-specificity on the phenomenal level is further supported by the observation of a correlation between the increased behavioral scores of self-specificity and the decreased stimulus-induced activity in especially the anterior midline structures. The increased self-specificity observed behaviorally in depression might therefore stem from the abnormally increased resting-state activity in the midline regions and their apparently increased self-specific processing (Grimm et al., 2011; Grimm et al., 2009).

What do these findings imply neurophenomenologically? We observed decreased stimulus-induced activity in the anterior midline regions, while at the same time, the stimuli were assigned increased degrees of self-specificity. Decreased stimulus-induced activity may go along with increased self-specificity due to the carryover and transfer of the increased resting-state activity and its abnormal self-specific organization onto subsequent stimulus-induced activity. The increased resting-state activity makes it difficult for the stimulus to induce major activity changes. The associated carryover and transfer of the resting state's abnormal self-specific organization lead to the assignment of abnormally high degrees of self-specificity to stimuli; hence the conjunction of neuronal decreases in stimulus-induced activity and behavioral increases in self-specificity.

Abnormal Exteroceptive Processing in Depression

Patients with MDD often suffer from bodily symptoms like heart pounding or palpitations, increased breathing rate (with yawning, sighing, and hyperventilation), and multiple, diffuse bodily aches and pains. These symptoms seem to go along with abnormally increased awareness of their own bodily processes (body perception), including sensitivity to stress and autonomic-vegetative changes, as demonstrated in a recent work (Wiebking et al., 2010).

The same study also investigated the neuronal activity during exteroceptive and interoceptive awareness (using tone and heartbeat counting, respectively) in relation to the brain's resting-state activity. Interoceptive stimuli by themselves (e.g., the heartbeat) induced a "normal" degree of brain signal changes (activation) in the bilateral anterior insula in depressed patients when considered relative to the preceding resting-state activity levels. This suggests that in depression, there is no abnormality in interoceptive stimulus processing.

In contrast, we observed abnormally reduced activity during exteroceptive stimuli. More specifically, we observed that exteroceptive stimuli induced decreased stimulus-induced activity in the insula in depressed patients when compared to healthy subjects. This reduced activity was related to the abnormal resting-state activity levels, as we observed increased resting-state activity in the insula part of the inner ring core-paralimbic system.

To test for independent changes in exteroceptively related stimulus-induced activity, we then calculated this activity relative to the preceding resting-state activity levels. Interestingly, when we statistically controlled for the resting-state activity level, there was no difference between healthy and depressed subjects in signal changes during exteroceptive processing; this suggests that the abnormalities in the exteroceptive condition were not related to changes in exteroceptive processing itself, but rather to abnormalities in the underlying resting-state activity level.

This suggests that the exteroceptive processing itself is preserved, but that the resting state and its interaction with exteroceptive stimuli are abnormal.

In contrast to the exteroceptive stimuli, no differences between healthy and depressed subjects were evident in interoceptive stimuli in both relative and absolute signal changes. This difference between interoceptive and exteroceptive stimuli with regard to relative and absolute signal changes suggests differential interaction of both kinds of stimuli with resting-state activity. Either rest–stimulus interaction is reduced during exteroceptive stimuli or rest–stimulus interaction is increased during interoceptive stimuli – which activity is occurring cannot be differentiated on the basis of our findings. What is clear is that there is an imbalance in activity between intero- and exteroceptive stimulus processing, including their respective interactions with the resting-state activity level. Because of the paucity of work in this area, additional imaging studies are needed to clarify changes in interoceptive processing in depression.

The study by Wiebking and colleagues (2010) also investigated psychological measures of body perception, employing the body perception questionnaire (BPQ). We found that BPQ scores were significantly increased in depressed patients, indicating increased bodily awareness. Most interestingly, unlike in healthy subjects, the increased BPQ scores no longer correlated with the signal changes during the resting-state and the exteroceptive condition. This suggests that in depressed patients, neuronal activity is not properly modulated in response to changes in the body or the environment. This finding may correspond to the difficulty that people have in shifting attention from the body to the environment and could help explain the many somatic complaints that characterize MDD. Although tentative, such lack of correlations with abnormally increased neuronal activity has also been seen for other psychological measures in depression, such as excessive negative affect, self-specificity, and negativistic temporal projections to future possibilities (Grimm et al., 2009; Lemogne et al., 2012; Lemogne et al., 2010; Wiebking et al., 2010).

Self-Perspectival–Intentional Imbalance in Depression

These findings are indicative of an imbalance in neural processing between interoceptive and exteroceptive stimuli, with only the latter inducing decreased neural activity. This may lead to relatively increased neural processing of interoceptive processing and rest–interoceptive interaction, when compared to the apparently absolutely reduced exteroceptive processing and rest–exteroceptive interaction. As already noted, this abnormal shift toward interoceptive processing may promote increased bodily awareness and subsequent distressful bodily symptoms. At the same time, the decreased exteroceptive processing may be accompanied by reduced awareness of and concern with environmental changes, especially positive events that could beneficially impact depression. This means that, phenomenally, one may want to speak not only of an increased self-focus but also of an increased bodily focus and a decreased environmental focus (Northoff et al., 2011).

Why, though, are rest–extero interaction and external awareness reduced when compared to rest–intero interaction and internal (i.e., bodily and self-) awareness? Recall that I assumed that the increased self-focus and increased self-specificity during stimulus-induced activity could be traced back to the increased resting-state activity in the anterior regions of the inner ring, the midline network. At the same time, however, the resting-state data also showed decreased resting-state activity in the lateral regions of the outer ring. The question is how such decreased resting-state activity in the outer ring is manifest in stimulus-induced activity.

We already know that in MDD, stimulus-induced activity is reduced during exteroceptive stimuli. This may go along with decreased external awareness, which phenomenally can be described as decreased environmental focus (which corresponds more or less to decreased environmental awareness). The question now arises how such decreased stimulus-induced activity in lateral regions and the decreased environmental focus are related to the abnormally low resting-state activity in the very same regions?

The preintentional organization of the resting state may be associated with the neural balance between midline and lateral networks. If this neural balance is shifted toward the midline regions, as seems to be the case in depression, the associated balance between self- and nonself-specific processing will also shift. More specifically, the resting state's self-nonself balance will shift toward self-specific processing (and the own or internal self) and away from nonself-specific processing of external environmental stimuli. Any subsequent phenomenal consciousness would then be predisposed or biased toward increased self-specificity, along with the decreased external directedness of intentionality.

This is exactly what one observes in depression: The resting state's abnormally strong self-specific organization is manifested in increased self-specificity and increased directedness toward internal contents at the expense of external contents.

The Neural Basis of Self-Experience in Schizophrenia

Recent studies have investigated the DMN in schizophrenia (Kuhn & Gallinat, 2013). Imaging studies have found abnormal resting-state activity and functional connectivity in the anterior cortical midline structures (aCMS). One study demonstrated that the aCMS (and posterior CMS, like the PCC/precuneus) show decreased task-induced deactivation (TID) during a working memory task, indicative of decreased task-related suppression and possibly increased resting-state activity (Whitfield-Gabrieli et al., 2009). This was observed in both patients with schizophrenia and their relatives, when compared to healthy subjects, suggesting that it may reflect a vulnerability or risk factor.

Furthermore, the same patients with schizophrenia also showed increased functional connectivity of the aCMS with other posterior regions of the CMS, such as the PCC. Functional hyperconnectivity and TID were negatively correlated with each other: the less task-related suppression, the greater the degree of functional connectivity. In short, external tasks can induce less change in the brain because of the brain's increased functional connectivity. Finally, both decreased TID and increased functional connectivity in aCMS correlated with psychopathology, that is, the predominantly positive symptoms.

Decreased TID in aCMS was also observed in an earlier study that investigated working memory (Pomarol-Clotet et al., 2008). Similar to the study described earlier, patients with schizophrenia who performed a working memory task showed decreased TID in aCMS when compared to healthy subjects. Abnormal task-related activation in the right dorsolateral prefrontal cortex was also observed in patients with schizophrenia. Another study reported abnormal TID in aCMS, as well as abnormal functional connectivity from aCMS and posterior CMS to the insula in schizophrenic patients (Mannell et al., 2010; see also Calhoun, Maciejewski, Pearlson, & Kiehl, 2008; Jafri, Pearlson, Stevens, & Calhoun, 2008; Park, 2009; Williamson, 2007). In addition to TID and functional connectivity, another measure of abnormal resting-state activity involves its temporal features, more specifically fluctuations or oscillations in certain temporal frequencies. For instance, Hoptman and colleagues (2010) found that low-frequency fluctuations in the resting state were increased in the aCMS (and the parahippocampal gyrus) in patients with schizophrenia, while they were decreased in other regions like the insula. Abnormally increased low-frequency oscillations (<0.06 Hz) in the aCMS (as well as posterior CMS regions and the auditory network) and their correlation with positive symptom severity were also observed in another study on schizophrenic patients (Rotarska-Jagiela et al., 2010). This means that abnormal low-frequency fluctuations in the CMS are directly related to the abnormal phenomenal features, as they are most apparent in positive symptoms like auditory hallucinations and delusions. In both cases (auditory hallucinations and delusions), either internal (hallucination) or external (delusions) contents are processed in an abnormal way in that they are associated with phenomenal features.

Let us sketch the case of auditory hallucinations. Internal contents that are usually not associated with phenomenal features – and thus are not experienced as such as contents of consciousness – become linked to phenomenal features and are experienced as voices, resulting in what we call auditory hallucinations. A similar process may occur in the case of delusions. Here, external contents from the environment are abnormally linked with each other, and phenomenal features then surface as abnormal contents in consciousness. Since both auditory hallucinations and delusions are typical positive symptoms of schizophrenia, their correlation with low-frequency fluctuations in CMS support its role in linking neural and phenomenal features with respect to internal (hallucination) and external (delusions) mental contents.

Self-Specificity in Schizophrenia

In addition to alterations in the resting-state activity, there are changes in stimulus-induced activity in patients with schizophrenia that may be related to self-experience. A recent imaging study by Holt and colleagues (2011) found that abnormal anterior-to-posterior midline connectivity is related to self-specificity. They investigated patients with schizophrenia performing a word task in which subjects had to judge trait adjectives according to their degree of self-specificity (and also two other tasks: other-reflection, i.e., relation of that adjective to another person; and perception-reflection, i.e., whether the word is printed in uppercase or lowercase letters). Patients with schizophrenia showed significantly elevated activity in posterior midline regions like the mid- and posterior cingulate cortex during self-reflection, whereas signal changes in the anterior midline regions like the medial prefrontal cortex were significantly reduced when compared to healthy subjects. Finally, functional connectivity was abnormally elevated from the posterior to the anterior midline regions. Analogous results of altered midline activity with a dysbalance between anterior and posterior midline regions are also observed in other studies on self-specificity in schizophrenia (Taylor, Welsh, Chen, Velander, & Liberzon, 2007). Taken together, these results demonstrate abnormal resting-state activity in especially the anterior and posterior midline network in schizophrenia (for a recent meta-analysis, see Kuhn & Gallinat, 2013). The same network also shows alterations in the balance between anterior and posterior midline regions when probing for self-specific stimuli.

Studies that test linkage between resting-state abnormalities and self-specific stimuli are needed to support the argument for the resting state's self-specific organization influence on subsequent stimulus-induced activity and the associated phenomenal state of consciousness. Although we currently do not have such neuronal evidence, there is plenty of phenomenal evidence of patients with schizophrenia suffering from an abnormality in self-specificity. This makes it likely that abnormal self-specific organization in the resting state may be transferred onto the subsequent stimulus-induced activity and its associated phenomenal states.

Basic Disturbance of the Self in Schizophrenia

How do these findings relate to the psychopathological and phenomeno-logical descriptions of patients with schizophrenia? What the early psychiatrists described as "the peculiar destruction of the inner coherence of the personality" or "basic alteration of self-consciousness" may correspond to changes in the resting state's self-specific organization.

Following the early descriptions, the basic disturbance in the self in schizophrenia is assumed to impact on all subsequent functions and domains of the personality. Analogously, the resting state's self-specific organization may also affect any subsequent stimulus-induced activity and associated functions, including sensory, motor, affective, and cognitive processes. In the same way that the basic disturbance of the self is present everywhere, the resting state, metaphorically speaking, "has its hands" in all kinds of neural processing. The resting state's abnormal self-specific organization would therefore be carried over or transferred to subsequent stimulus-induced activity and all of its associated functions (see Figure 4.4).

The resting state's abnormal self-specific organization ultimately may be traced back to an abnormal encoding of environmental stimuli's statistical frequency distribution by the resting state's neural activity (Northoff 2014a). This, in turn, leads to an abnormal "environment brain unity," which in turn affects the resting state's self-specific organization. The resting state's abnormal self-specific organization then would to lead to abnormal experiences on the phenomenal level of consciousness.

Therefore, the phenomenal descriptions of abnormal self-experience in schizophrenia may reflect an abnormal self-specific organization in the

NEURONAL

| Stimulus-Rest Interaction: Disruption in the **encoding** of the stimulus's **natural statistics** | Rest-Rest Interaction: Abnormal **functional connectivity** and low **frequency fluctuations** | Rest-Stimulus Interaction: Abnormal **recruitment** of functional connectivity and low frequency fluctuations |

BODY

ENVIRONMENT

Altered resting state activity → Abnormal self-specific organization → Altered sense of self

PRE-PHENOMENAL

| Disruption in and **Environment-Brain Unity** | Abnormal **pre-phenomenal structures** in the resting state | **Carry-over and transfer** of abnormal pre-phenomenal structures into phenomenal states |

PSYCHOPATHOLOGICAL

| **Neurodevelopmental** abnormalities | **Basic** Disturbance of the **Self** | Ego-disturbances as **blurry distinction** of the self from body and environment |

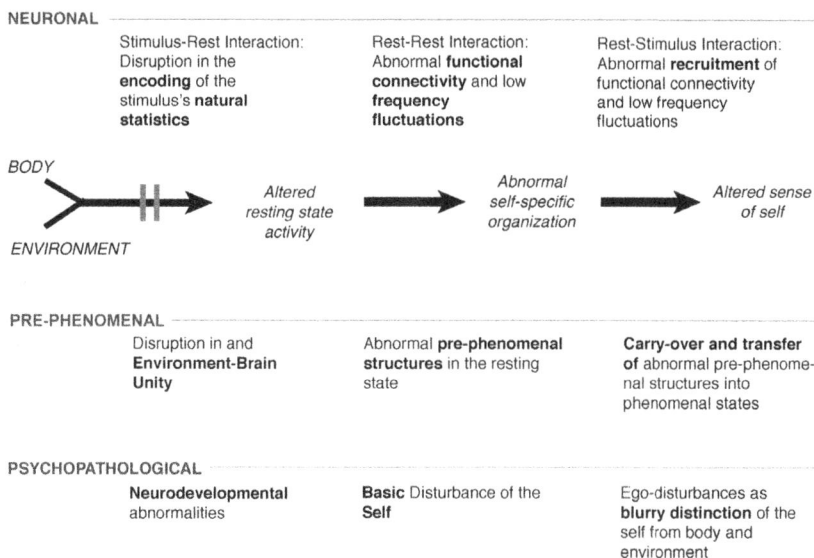

Figure 4.4. Basic disturbance of self in schizophrenia. The figure shows different stages in the constitution of an altered sense of self in schizophrenia. I assume the encoding of stimuli and their natural statistics to be abnormal in schizophrenia during stimulus-rest interaction. That leads to abnormal resting state activity with abnormal prephenomenal structures. The abnormal resting state will then affect subsequent rest-rest interaction which leads to abnormal self-specific organisation in the resting state. Any encounter with stimuli during rest-stimulus interaction will be affected by that which results in the consecutive experience of an abnormal sense of self. I indicated three levels, neuronal (upper), phenomenal (middle low), and psychopathological (lower). I assume that the neuronal mechanisms described earlier correspond to the respective phenomenal and psychopathological features. From *Unlocking the Brain: Volume II – Consciousness* (p. 396), by G. Northoff, 2014, New York, NY: Oxford University Press. By permission from Oxford University Press, USA.

resting state that it is carried over and transferred to subsequent stimulus-induced activity. Due to the resting-state abnormalities, the stimulus cannot be properly integrated into the resting state's prephenomenal self-specific organization. The lack of the stimulus's integration into the resting state's self-specific organization then leads to a lack of self-specificity of the stimulus itself during stimulus-induced activity. This decreased or lack of assignment of self-specificity to the stimulus is then phenomenally manifest in what is described as decreases in both self-affection and sense of mineness and belongingness. This corresponds to the way Parnas and others characterize experience in schizophrenia.

Conclusion

In this chapter, I have suggested the value of a neurophenomenal approach to self-disturbances in psychiatric disorders like schizophrenia and depression. Methodologically, the neurophenomenal approach aims to directly link neural and phenomenal features, rather than viewing them as mediated by contents, as is usually the case in neurocognitive theories. Empirically, I have focused on the abnormalities of brain resting-state activity across different regions in MDD and schizophrenia. The recent findings of resting-state hyper- and hypoactivity can be viewed in a wider neuroanatomical context, which suggests that there are multiple radial-concentric and vertical integrations between subcortical and cortical regions. In MDD, the inner-middle ring of subcortical core-paracore and cortical paralimbic-midline regions shows abnormal resting-state hyperactivity, while the outer ring of the lateral subcortical and lateral cortical region is relatively hypoactive. Because the different subcortical-cortical systems include different functional systems (e.g., systems for affect, bodily perception, reward, cognition), abnormal resting-state activity leads to abnormal rest-stimulus interaction and consequently to the different kinds of symptoms seen in MDD. Schizophrenia is also associated with abnormal neural activity in anterior and posterior cortical midline structures, as well as in the resting state, which seem to be related to the characteristic abnormal experiences of the self.

Neurophenomenal studies of both disorders point to the central role of the resting state in abnormalities of self-experience. However, the exact neural mechanisms underlying the self in general and its abnormal changes in psychiatric disorders remain unclear. Future investigations will reveal the neural mechanisms underlying psychopathological experience and may then yield diagnostic and therapeutic markers that allow for new modes of diagnostic assessment and intervention.

Some doubts may be raised, however, concerning the validity of the neurophenomenal approach and its clinical utility. The main challenge to validity rests on the question of correlation versus causality. To provide a valid explanation of psychiatric symptoms and experience, the neurophenomenal approach would need to establish causal, rather than merely correlational, linkages between neuronal and phenomenal features. More specifically, it would need to show how the resting-state neuronal features directly predispose phenomenal features such that the latter can be predicted from the former. I believe that this is indeed possible, and that causally relevant (rather than merely correlational) neurophenomenal hypotheses can be developed. Many such hypotheses are presented in Northoff (2014b), which require extensive future experimental study.

The current chapter provides some indirect evidence for causal linkages between neuronal and phenomenal features by showing how certain neural abnormalities in the resting state could account for specific features of self-experience in MDD and schizophrenia. Psychiatric disorders may be regarded as paradigmatic cases for identifying causal links between the brain's intrinsic activity and phenomenal features of consciousness. The neurophenomenal approach thus can contribute to our search for the mechanisms and basis of consciousness.

For clinicians, the neurophenomenal approach will make possible the detection of direct causal linkages between neuronal and phenomenal features of psychiatric symptoms. If proven valid, this approach may ultimately yield specific diagnostic markers for the different symptoms and clarify the co-occurrence of core sets of symptoms in psychiatric disorders. Ultimately, this may lead not only to more refined diagnostic methods, but also to the development of novel forms of therapeutic interventions that target the modulation of the as yet unknown spatial and temporal features of the brain's resting-state activity in psychopathology.

Acknowledgments

The work was supported by grants to the author from the Hope for Depression Research Foundation (HDRF/ISAN), and G.N. from the German Research Foundation DFG/SFB 776 A6, the EJLB Michael Smith Foundation, and CRC Canada Research Chair. I also thank Constance Cummings and Laurence Kirmayer for some excellent suggestions on a prior draft of this chapter.

REFERENCES

Alcaro, A., Panksepp, J., Witczak, J., Hayes, D. J., & Northoff, G. (2010). Is subcortical-cortical midline activity in depression mediated by glutamate and GABA? A cross-species translational approach. *Neuroscience & Biobehavioral Reviews, 34*(4), 592–605. http://dx.doi.org/10.1016/j.neubiorev.2009.11.023

Bleuler, E. (2010). [Dementia praecox or the group of schizophrenias]. *Vertex, 21*(93), 394–400. (Original work published 1911)

Boker, H., Budischewski, K., Eppel, A., Hartling, F., Rinnert, J., von Schmeling, C., ... Schoeneich, F. (2000). [Self concept and object relations of patients with affective disorders: Individual-centered diagnosis with the repertory-grid technique]. *Psychotherapie, Psychosomatik, Medizinische Psychologie, 50*(8), 328–34. http://dx.doi.org/10.1055/s-2000-9094

Buckner, R. L., Andrews-Hanna, J. R., & Schacter, D. L. (2008). The brain's default network: anatomy, function, and relevance to disease. *Annals of the New York Academy of Sciences, 1124*, 1–38. http://dx.doi.org/10.1196/annals.1440.011

Calhoun, V. D., Maciejewski, P. K., Pearlson, G. D., & Kiehl, K. A. (2008). Temporal lobe and "default" hemodynamic brain modes discriminate between schizophrenia and bipolar disorder. *Human Brain Mapping, 29*(11), 1265–75. http://dx.doi.org/10.1002/hbm.20463

Christoff, K., Cosmelli, D., Legrand, D., & Thompson, E. (2011). Specifying the self for cognitive neuroscience. *Trends in Cognitive Sciences, 15*(3), 104–12. http://dx.doi.org/10.1016/j.tics.2011.01.001

D'Argembeau, A., Collette, F., Van der, L. M., Laureys, S., Del Fiore, G., Degueldre, C., ... Salmon, E. (2005). Self-referential reflective activity and its relationship with rest: a PET study. *Neuroimage, 25*(2), 616–24. http://dx.doi.org/10.1016/j.neuroimage.2004.11.048

de Greck, M., Enzi, B., Prosch, U., Gantman, A., Tempelmann, C., & Northoff, G. (2010). Decreased neuronal activity in reward circuitry of pathological gamblers during processing of personal relevant stimuli. *Human Brain Mapping, 31*(11), 1802–12. http://dx.doi.org/10.1002/hbm.20981

de Greck, M., Supady, A., Thiemann, R., Tempelmann, C., Bogerts, B., Forschner, L., ... Northoff, G. (2009). Decreased neural activity in reward circuitry during personal reference in abstinent alcoholics: A fMRI study. *Human Brain Mapping, 30*(5), 1691–1704. http://dx.doi.org/10.1002/hbm.20634

Doering, S., Burgmer, M., Heuft, G., Menke, D., Baumer, B., Lubking, M., ... Schneider, G. (2013). Assessment of personality functioning: Validity of the operationalized psychodynamic diagnosis Axis IV (Structure). *Psychopathology, 47*, 185–93. http://dx.doi.org/10.1159/000355062

Feinberg, T. E. (2009). *From axons to identity: Neurological explorations of the nature of the self.* Norton Series on Interpersonal Neurobiology. New York, NY: W. W. Norton.

Feinberg, T. E. (2011). Neuropathologies of the self: Clinical and anatomical features. *Consciousiousness and Cognition, 20*(1), 75–81. http://dx.doi.org/10.1016/j.concog.2010.09.017

Feinberg, T. E., Venneri, A., Simone, A. M., Fan, Y., & Northoff, G. (2010). The neuroanatomy of asomatognosia and somatoparaphrenia. *Journal of Neurology, Neurosurgery, & Psychiatry, 81*(3), 276–81. http://dx.doi.org/10.1136/jnnp.2009.188946

Fitzgerald, P. B., Oxley, T. J., Laird, A. R., Kulkarni, J., Egan, G. F., & Daskalakis, Z. J. (2006). An analysis of functional neuroimaging studies of dorsolateral prefrontal cortical activity in depression. *Psychiatry Research, 148*(1), 33–45. http://dx.doi.org/10.1016/j.pscychresns.2006.04.006

Gillihan, S. J., & Farah, M. J. (2005). Is self special? A critical review of
    evidence from experimental psychology and cognitive neuroscience.
    Psychological Bulletin, 131(1), 76–97. http://dx.doi.org/10.1037/0033-
    2909.131.1.76
Grimm, S., Ernst, J., Boesiger, P., Schuepbach, D., Boeker, H., & Northoff, G.
    (2011). Reduced negative BOLD responses in the default-mode network
    and increased self-focus in depression. *World Journal of Biological Psychiatry,
    12*(8), 627–37. http://dx.doi.org/10.3109/15622975.2010.545145
Grimm, S., Ernst, J., Boesiger, P., Schuepbach, D., Hell, D., Boeker, H., &
    Northoff, G. (2009). Increased self-focus in major depressive disorder is
    related to neural abnormalities in subcortical-cortical midline structures.
    Human Brain Mapping, 30(8), 2617–27. http://dx.doi.org/10.1002/
    hbm.20693
Grunebaum, M. F., Keilp, J., Li, S., Ellis, S. P., Burke, A. K., Oquendo, M. A., &
    Mann, J. J. (2005). Symptom components of standard depression scales and
    past suicidal behavior. *Journal of Affective Disorders, 87*(1), 73–82. http://dx.
    doi.org/10.1016/j.jad.2005.03.002
Hasler, G., & Northoff, G. (2011). Discovering imaging endophenotypes for
    major depression. *Molecular Psychiatry, 16*(6), 604–19. http://dx.doi.org/
    10.1038/mp.2011.23
Holt, D. J., Cassidy, B. S., Andrews-Hanna, J. R., Lee, S. M., Coombs, G.,
    Goff, D. C., . . . Moran, J. M. (2011). An anterior-to-posterior shift in
    midline cortical activity in schizophrenia during self-reflection. *Biological
    Psychiatry, 69*(5), 415–423. http://dx.doi.org/10.1016/j.
    biopsych.2010.10.003
Hoptman, M. J., Zuo, X. N., Butler, P. D., Javitt, D. C., D'Angelo, D.,
    Mauro, C. J., & Milham, M. P. (2010). Amplitude of low-frequency
    oscillations in schizophrenia: A resting state fMRI study. *Schizophrenia
    Research, 117*(1), 13–20. http://dx.doi.org/10.1016/j.schres.2009.09.030
Huang, Z., Dai, R., Wu, X., Yang, Z., Liu, D., Hu, J., . . . Northoff, G. (2013).
    The self and its resting state in consciousness: An investigation of the
    vegetative state. *Human Brain Mapping, 35*(5), 1997–2008. http://dx.doi.org/
    10.1002/hbm.22308
Ingram, R. E. (1990). Self-focused attention in clinical disorders: Review and a
    conceptual model. *Psychological Bulletin, 107*(2), 156–76. http://dx.doi.org/
    10.1037/0033-2909.107.2.156
Jafri, M. J., Pearlson, G. D., Stevens, M., & Calhoun, V. D. (2008). A method
    for functional network connectivity among spatially independent resting-
    state components in schizophrenia. *Neuroimage, 39*(4), 1666–81.
    http://dx.doi.org/10.1016/j.neuroimage.2007.11.001
Jaspers, K. (1964). *General psychopathology.* Chicago, IL: University of Chicago
    Press.
Kraeplin, E. (1913). *Ein Lehrbuch für Studierende und Ärzte.* Leipzig, Germany:
    Barth.
Kuhn, S., & Gallinat, J. (2013). Resting-state brain activity in schizophrenia
    and major depression: A quantitative meta-analysis. *Schizophrenia Bulletin,
    39*(2), 358–65. http://dx.doi.org/10.1093/schbul/sbr151

Ladouceur, C. D., Versace, A., & Phillips, M. L. (2015). Understanding the neural circuitry of emotion regulation: White matter tract abnormalities and psychiatric disorder. In L. J. Kirmayer, R. Lemelson, & C. A. Cummings (Eds.), *Re-visioning psychiatry: Cultural phenomenology, critical neuroscience, and global mental health* (pp. 236–72). New York, NY: Cambridge University Press.

Legrand, D., & Ruby, P. (2009). What is self-specific? Theoretical investigation and critical review of neuroimaging results. *Psychological Review, 116*(1), 252–82. http://dx.doi.org/10.1037/a0014172

Lemogne, C., Bergouignan, L., Piolino, P., Jouvent, R., Allilaire, J. F., & Fossati, P. (2009). Cognitive avoidance of intrusive memories and autobiographical memory: Specificity, autonoetic consciousness, and self-perspective. *Memory, 17*(1), 1–7. http://dx.doi.org/10.1080/09658210802438466

Lemogne, C., Delaveau, P., Freton, M., Guionnet, S., & Fossati, P. (2012). Medial prefrontal cortex and the self in major depression. *Journal of Affective Disorders, 136*(1–2), e1–e11. http://dx.doi.org/10.1016/j.jad.2010.11.034

Lemogne, C., le Bastard, G., Mayberg, H., Volle, E., Bergouignan, L., Lehericy, S., . . . Fossati, P. (2009). In search of the depressive self: Extended medial prefrontal network during self-referential processing in major depression. *Social Cognitive & Affective Neuroscience, 4*(3), 305–12. http://dx.doi.org/10.1093/scan/nsp008

Lemogne, C., Mayberg, H., Bergouignan, L., Volle, E., Delaveau, P., Lehericy, S., . . . Fossati, P. (2010). Self-referential processing and the prefrontal cortex over the course of depression: A pilot study. *Journal of Affective Disorders, 124*(1–2), 196–201. http://dx.doi.org/10.1016/j.jad.2009.11.003

Lou, H. C., Gross, J., Biermann-Ruben, K., Kjaer, T. W., & Schnitzler, A. (2010). Coherence in consciousness: Paralimbic gamma synchrony of self-reference links conscious experiences. *Human Brain Mapping, 31*(2), 185–92. http://dx.doi.org/ 10.1002/hbm.20855

Lou, H. C., Joensson, M., Biermann-Ruben, K., Schnitzler, A., Ostergaard, L., Kjaer, T. W., & Gross, J. (2011). Recurrent activity in higher order, modality non-specific brain regions: A Granger causality analysis of autobiographic memory retrieval. *PLOS One, 6*(7), e22286. http://dx.doi.org/10.1371/journal.pone.0022286

Lou, H. C., Kjaer, T. W., Friberg, L., Wildschiodtz, G., Holm, S., & Nowak, M. (1999). A 15O-H2O PET study of meditation and the resting state of normal consciousness. *Human Brain Mapping, 7*(2), 98–105.

Lou, H. C., Luber, B., Crupain, M., Keenan, J. P., Nowak, M., Kjaer, T. W., . . . Lisanby, S. H. (2004). Parietal cortex and representation of the mental Self. *Proceedings of the National Academy of Sciences of the United States of America, 101*(17), 6827–32. http://dx.doi.org/10.1073/pnas.0400049101

Lou, H. C., Luber, B., Stanford, A., & Lisanby, S. H. (2010). Self-specific processing in the default network: a single-pulse TMS study. *Experimental Brain Research, 207*(1–2), 27–38. http://dx.doi.org/10.1007/s00221-010-2425-x

Lou, H. C., Nowak, M., & Kjaer, T. W. (2005). The mental self. *Progress in Brain Research, 150*, 197–204. http://dx.doi.org/10.1016/S0079-6123(05)50014-1

Lutz, A., & Thompson, E. (2003). Neurophenomenology integrating subjective experience and brain dynamics in the neuroscience of consciousness. *Journal of Consciousness Studies, 10*(9–10), 31–52.

Mannell, M. V., Franco, A. R., Calhoun, V. D., Canive, J. M., Thoma, R. J., &
    Mayer, A. R. (2010). Resting state and task-induced deactivation:
    A methodological comparison in patients with schizophrenia and healthy
    controls. *Human Brain Mapping, 31*(3), 424–37. http://dx.doi.org/10.1002/
    hbm.20876
Mayberg, H. S. (2002). Depression, II: Localization of pathophysiology.
    American Journal of Psychiatry, 159(12), 1979. http://dx.doi.org/10.1176/
    appi.ajp.159.12.1979
Mayberg, H. S. (2003). Modulating dysfunctional limbic-cortical circuits in
    depression: Towards development of brain-based algorithms for diagnosis
    and optimised treatment. *British Medical Bulletin, 65*, 193–207. http://dx.doi.
    org/10.1093/bmb/65.1.193
Mayberg, H. S. (2009). Targeted electrode-based modulation of neural circuits
    for depression. *Journal of Clinical Investigation, 119*(4), 717–725. http://dx.
    doi.org/10.1172/JCI38454
Metzinger, T. (2003). *Being no one: The self-model theory of subjectivity.*
    Cambridge, MA: MIT Press.
Nelson, B., Whitford, T. J., Lavoie, S., & Sass, L. A. (2014a). What are the
    neurocognitive correlates of basic self-disturbance in schizophrenia?
    Integrating phenomenology and neurocognition. Part 1 (Source monitoring
    deficits). *Schizophrenia Research, 152*(1), 12–19. http://dx.doi.org/10.1016/j.
    schres.2013.06.022
Nelson, B., Whitford, T. J., Lavoie, S., & Sass, L. A. (2014b). What are the
    neurocognitive correlates of basic self-disturbance in schizophrenia?
    Integrating phenomenology and neurocognition. Part 2 (Aberrant salience).
    Schizophrenia Research, 152(1), 20–7. http://dx.doi.org/10.1016/j.
    schres.2013.06.033
Northoff, G. (2004). *Philosophy of the brain: The brain problem.* Amsterdam,
    The Netherlands: John Benjamins.
Northoff, G. (2007). Psychopathology and pathophysiology of the self in
    depression: Neuropsychiatric hypothesis. *Journal of Affective Disorders,
    104*(1–3), 1–14. http://dx.doi.org/10.1016/j.jad.2007.02.012
Northoff, G. (2011). Self and brain: What is self-related processing? *Trends in
    Cognitive Sciences, 15*(5), 186–7. http://dx.doi.org/10.1016/j.
    tics.2011.03.001
Northoff, G. (2013a). What the brain's intrinsic activity can tell us about
    consciousness? A tri dimensional view. *Neuroscience and Biobehavioral
    Reviews, 37*(4), 726–38. http://dx.doi.org/10.1016/j.neubiorev.2012.12.004
Northoff, G. (2013b). Gene, brains, and environment-genetic neuroimaging of
    depression. *Current Opinion in Neurobiology, 23*(1), 133–42. http://dx.doi.
    org/10.1016/j.conb.2012.08.004
Northoff, G. (2014a). *Unlocking the brain: Volume 1 – Coding.* New York, NY:
    Oxford University Press.
Northoff, G. (2014b). *Unlocking the brain: Volume 2 – Consciousness.* New York,
    NY: Oxford University Press.
Northoff, G., Heinzel, A., de Greck, M., Bermpohl, F., Dobrowolny, H., &
    Panksepp, J. (2006). Self-referential processing in our brain: A meta-analysis
    of imaging studies on the self. *Neuroimage, 31*(1), 440–57. http://dx.doi.org/
    10.1016/j.neuroimage.2005.12.002

Northoff, G., & Panksepp, J. (2008). The trans-species concept of self and the subcortical-cortical midline system. *Trends in Cognitive Sciences, 12*(7), 259–64. http://dx.doi.org/10.1016/j.tics.2008.04.007

Northoff, G., Qin, P., & Nakao, T. (2010). Rest-stimulus interaction in the brain: A review. *Trends in Neurosciences, 33*(6), 277–84. http://dx.doi.org/10.1016/j.tins.2010.02.006

Northoff, G., Schneider, F., Rotte, M., Matthiae, C., Tempelmann, C., Wiebking, C., . . . Panksepp, J. (2009). Differential parametric modulation of self-relatedness and emotions in different brain regions. *Human Brain Mapping, 30*(2), 369–82. http://dx.doi.org/10.1002/hbm.20510

Northoff, G., Wiebking, C., Feinberg, T., & Panksepp, J. (2011). The "resting-state hypothesis" of major depressive disorder: A translational subcortical-cortical framework for a system disorder. *Neuroscience & Biobehavioral Reviews, 35*(9), 1929–45. http://dx.doi.org/10.1016/j.neubiorev.2010.12.007

Panksepp, J. (1998). *Affective neuroscience: The foundations of human and animal emotions*. New York, NY: Oxford University Press.

Panksepp, J., & Northoff, G. (2009). The trans-species core SELF: The emergence of active cultural and neuro-ecological agents through self-related processing within subcortical-cortical midline networks. *Consciousness and Cognition, 18*(1), 193–215. http://dx.doi.org/10.1016/j.concog.2008.03.002

Park, I. G., Kim, J. J., Chun, J., Jung, Y. C., Seok, J. H., Park, H. J., & Lee, J. D. (2009). Medial prefrontal default-mode hypoactivity affecting trait physical anhedonia in schizophrenia. *Psychiatric Research, 171*(3),155–65. http://dx.doi.org/10.1016/j.pscychresns

Parnas, J. (2003). Self and schizophrenia: A phenomenological perspective. In T. Kircher & A. David (Eds.), *The self in neuroscience and psychiatry* (pp. 217–41). Cambridge, England: Cambridge University Press. http://dx.doi.org/10.1017/CBO9780511543708.012

Parnas, J., Vianin, P., Saebye, D., Jansson, L., Volmer-Larsen, A., & Bovet, P. (2001). Visual binding abilities in the initial and advanced stages of schizophrenia. *Acta Psychiatrica Scandinavica, 103*(3), 171–80. http://dx.doi.org/10.1034/j.1600-0447.2001.00160.x

Phillips, M. L. (2003). Understanding the neurobiology of emotion perception: implications for psychiatry. *British Journal of Psychiatry, 182*, 190–2. http://dx.doi.org/10.1192/bjp.182.3.190

Phillips, M. L., Drevets, W. C., Rauch, S. L., & Lane, R. (2003). Neurobiology of emotion perception II: Implications for major psychiatric disorders. *Biological Psychiatry, 54*(5), 515–28. http://dx.doi.org/10.1016/S0006-3223(03)00171-9

Pomarol-Clotet, E., Salvador, R., Sarro, S., Gomar, J., Vila, F., Martinez, A., . . . McKenna, P. J. (2008). Failure to deactivate in the prefrontal cortex in schizophrenia: dysfunction of the default mode network? *Psychological Medicine, 38*(8), 1185–93. http://dx.doi.org/10.1017/S0033291708003565

Price, J. L., & Drevets, W. C. (2010). Neurocircuitry of mood disorders. *Neuropsychopharmacology, 35*(1), 192–216. http://dx.doi.org/10.1038/npp.2009.104

Qin, P., Di, H., Liu, Y., Yu, S., Gong, Q., Duncan, N., ... Northoff, G. (2010). Anterior cingulate activity and the self in disorders of consciousness. *Human Brain Mapping, 31*(12), 1993–2002. http://dx.doi.org/10.1002/hbm.20989

Qin, P., & Northoff, G. (2011). How is our self related to midline regions and the default-mode network? *Neuroimage, 57*(3), 1221–33. http://dx.doi.org/10.1016/j.neuroimage.2011.05.028

Raichle, M. E., MacLeod, A. M., Snyder, A. Z., Powers, W. J., Gusnard, D. A., & Shulman, G. L. (2001). A default mode of brain function. *Proceedings of the National Academy of Sciences of the United States of America, 98*(2), 676–82. http://dx.doi.org/10.1073/pnas.98.2.676

Raz, A., & Macdonald, E. (2015). Paying attention to a field in crisis: Psychiatry, neuroscience, and functional systems of the brain. In L. J. Kirmayer, R. Lemelson, & C. A. Cummings (Eds.), *Re-visioning psychiatry: Cultural phenomenology, critical neuroscience, and global mental health* (pp. 273–304). New York, NY: Cambridge University Press.

Rimes, K. A., & Watkins, E. (2005). The effects of self-focused rumination on global negative self-judgements in depression. *Behaviour Research and Therapy, 43*(12), 1673–81. http://dx.doi.org/10.1016/j.brat.2004.12.002

Rotarska-Jagiela, A., van, d. V., V, Oertel-Knochel, V., Uhlhaas, P. J., Vogeley, K., & Linden, D. E. (2010). Resting-state functional network correlates of psychotic symptoms in schizophrenia. *Schizophrenia Research, 117*(1), 21–30. http://dx.doi.org/10.1016/j.schres.2010.01.001

Sass, L. A., & Parnas, J. (2003). Schizophrenia, consciousness, and the self. *Schizophrenia Bulletin, 29*(3), 427–44. http://dx.doi.org/10.1093/oxfordjournals.schbul.a007017

Savitz, J. B., & Drevets, W. C. (2009a). Bipolar and major depressive disorder: Neuroimaging the developmental-degenerative divide. *Neuroscience & Biobehavioral Reviews, 33*(5), 699–771. http://dx.doi.org/10.1016/j.neubiorev.2009.01.004

Savitz, J. B., & Drevets, W. C. (2009b). Imaging phenotypes of major depressive disorder: genetic correlates. *Neuroscience, 164*(1), 300–330. http://dx.doi.org/10.1016/j.neuroscience.2009.03.082

Schneider, F., Bermpohl, F., Heinzel, A., Rotte, M., Walter, M., Tempelmann, C., ... Northoff, G. (2008). The resting brain and our self: Self-relatedness modulates resting state neural activity in cortical midline structures. *Neuroscience, 157*(1), 120–31. http://dx.doi.org/10.1016/j.neuroscience.2008.08.014

Taylor, S. F., Welsh, R. C., Chen, A. C., Velander, A. J., & Liberzon, I. (2007). Medial frontal hyperactivity in reality distortion. *Biological Psychiatry, 61*(10), 1171–8. http://dx.doi.org/10.1016/j.biopsych.2006.11.029

Treynor, W., Gonzalez, R., & Nolen-Hoeksema, S. (2003). Rumination reconsidered: A psychometric analysis. *Cognitive Therapy and Research, 27*(3), 247–59. http://dx.doi.org/10.1023/A:1023910315561

van der Meer, L., Costafreda, S., Aleman, A., & David, A. S. (2010). Self-reflection and the brain: A theoretical review and meta-analysis of neuroimaging studies with implications for schizophrenia. *Neuroscience & Biobehavioral Reviews, 34*(6), 935–46. http://dx.doi.org/10.1016/j.neubiorev.2009.12.004

Whitfield-Gabrieli, S., Thermenos, H. W., Milanovic, S., Tsuang, M. T., Faraone, S. V., McCarley, R. W., . . . Seidman, L. J. (2009). Hyperactivity and hyperconnectivity of the default network in schizophrenia and in first-degree relatives of persons with schizophrenia. *Proceedings of the National Academy of Sciences of the United States of America, 106*(4), 1279–84. http://dx.doi.org/10.1073/pnas.0809141106

Wiebking, C., Bauer, A., de Greck, M., Duncan, N. W., Tempelmann, C., & Northoff, G. (2010). Abnormal body perception and neural activity in the insula in depression: An fMRI study of the depressed "material me." *World Journal of Biological Psychiatry, 11*(3), 538–49. http://dx.doi.org/10.3109/15622970903563794

Williamson, P. (2007). Are anticorrelated networks in the brain relevant to schizophrenia? *Schizophrenia Bulletin, 33*(4), 994–1003. http://dx.doi.org/10.1093/schbul/sbm043

5 Cultural Phenomenology and Psychiatric Illness

Thomas J. Csordas

The title of this chapter evokes the common ground between anthropology and psychiatry, and by extension suggests Edward Sapir's (1932) enduringly astute essay on this topic, written already eighty years ago, as a starting point for defining a cultural phenomenology of psychiatric illness.[1] Sapir was a close collaborator of Harry Stack Sullivan, based in part on the concordance of Sullivan's interpersonal psychiatry and Sapir's anthropological understanding that the locus of culture is in the interaction of specific individuals. Sapir begins by observing that cultural anthropology emphasizes the group and its traditions, and the testimony of discrete individuals is of interest only insofar as they can be assumed typical of their community. Despite the presence in ethnography of "a kaleidoscopic picture of varying degrees of generality" from the broadly shared to the idiosyncratic, the individual note creates "disquieting interruptions to the impersonality of his [the anthropologist's] thinking" (1932, p. 230). Psychiatry's concern for individual pathology tends to be dominated by a need to magnify the biological approach in order to maintain legitimacy in the medical profession, even though "attempts to explain a morbid suspiciousness of one's companions or delusion as to one's status in society by some organically definable weakness of the nervous system or of the functioning of endocrine glands may be no more to the point than to explain the habit of swearing by the absence of a few teeth or by a poorly shaped mouth" (1932, p. 232). Psychiatric morbidity is "not a morbidity of organic segments or even organic functions but of experience itself," and it is unrealistic to "assume that all experience is but the mechanical sum of physiological processes lodged in isolated individuals" (1932, p. 232).

Sapir's argument, perhaps ironically, is that anthropology and psychiatry most fruitfully overlap precisely at their respective blind spots: the individual for anthropology, experience for psychiatry. Culture as

---

[1] See also Sapir's related 1938 article reprinted with commentaries (Sapir, 2001; Kleinman, 2001; Darnell, 2001; Kirmayer, 2001).

"superorganic" or abstracted from individual experience is a deterrent to "the more dynamic study of . . . cultural patterns because these cannot be disconnected from those organizations of ideas and feelings which constitute the individual" (1932, p. 233). The locus of psychiatry cannot be "the human organism at all in any fruitful sense of the word but the more intangible, and yet more intelligible, world of human relationships and ideas that such relationships bring forth" (1932, p. 231). Both critiques are as relevant now as they were eighty years ago, and perhaps more so. The critical point is that culture is neither an abstract system nor located in an abstract entity called society, but that "[t]he true locus of culture is in the interactions of specific individuals and, on the subjective side, in the world of meanings which each one of these individuals may unconsciously abstract for himself from his participation in these interactions" (1932, p. 236). Furthermore, the individual of whom we speak is not simply a biological organism but "that total world of form, meaning, and implication of symbolic behavior which a given individual partly knows and directs, partly intuits and yields to, partly is ignorant of and is swayed by" (1932, p. 238).

In this context, the most valuable contribution of anthropology to the understanding of psychiatric illness is that "it is constantly rediscovering the norm . . . for personalities are not conditioned by a generalized process of adjustment to 'the normal' but by the necessity of adjusting to the greatest variety of idea patterns and action patterns according to the accidents of birth and biography" (1932, p. 235). Here Sapir gives his famous examples of the psychological difference in engaging cultural forms: Of two men registered as members of a municipal ward, one who is in contact with civic officials may hold his identity as a ward member in equal salience to his definition as father of a family, whereas the other may not even be aware that the town is divided into wards and that membership offers potential duties and privileges (1932, pp. 236–7); the movie actress and the physicist may exist in equally intense but mutually marginal worlds of values, while the hard-headed business-man may consider them as "lively" (actress) and "sleepy" (physicist) representatives of a cultural zone defined as "triviality" (1932, p. 239). General culture patterns can have greater or lesser salience and vividness, with distinct and even contradictory meanings, depending on how they are taken up by individuals as idea complexes and integrated with their physical and psychological needs. In this context, "adjustment" is not just to the behavioral requirements of the group but also to the meanings that have developed in the experience of the individual. Pathology can result if these two forces are not balanced, as well as if a cultural pattern once integrated into the personality is relinquished without another to replace its symbolic work.

Recognizing the diversity this entails could allow psychiatrists to be not just good surgeons of the psyche who guide patients back to performance of social rituals, but to be "profoundly sympathetic students of the mind who respect the fundamental intent and direction of every personality organization" (1932, p. 242). Sapir grants credit to the psychoanalysis of his day for advocating the importance of experience in this respect, but he expresses discomfort about how psychoanalysts took up the data of cultural anthropology to support a theory of the racial inheritance of ideas, to assert equivalence between "primitive mentality" and certain forms of psychopathology, and to posit that contemporary nonindustrial peoples exhibit the same psychological processes as archaic humans. Even from a contemporary standpoint, psychoanalysis may not be the most productive bridge between anthropology and psychiatry, both because since Sapir's time it has not managed to hold its own against biological psychiatry and because its trajectory in anthropology has been toward a literary hermeneutic rather than a hermeneutic of psychopathology. It is precisely at this point that phenomenology becomes relevant, not necessarily to displace psychoanalysis, but to be its complement. In particular, phenomenology highlights the elements of the individual and experience so important to Sapir in a manner that elaborates the individual in intersubjective relations and experience in vivid immediacy.

This, then, is the starting point of a cultural phenomenology of psychiatric illness. The critical point in this endeavor is that the "phenomenon" of interest is not a psychiatric disorder, for the nosological denomination is an abstraction from lived experience. Neither is it a symptom, because the phenomenon described as a symptom was likely already present before having been identified as a symptom. What is at issue is the modulation of phenomena that exist for a person, where the description of these phenomena sheds light on the nature of affliction. Here, there is an affinity between phenomenological psychiatry (Binswanger, 1963; Boss, 1963; Fuchs, 2005, 2007; Minkowski, 1970; Ratcliffe, 2008; Stanghellini, 2004) with its commitment to suspend attribution of clinical meaning in a way that requires the methodological *epoché* or bracketing of phenomena, and a cultural phenomenology of psychiatric disorder with its commitment to suspend attribution of cultural meaning to phenomena in a way that demands at least a starting point in cultural relativism. The practice of cultural phenomenology consists on the one hand of using phenomenological methods, phenomenological concepts, and phenomenological sensibility in the interpretation of ethnographic data, and on the other using ethnographic instances as the concrete data for phenomenological reflection (Csordas, 1994, 1999, 2012). Work at this level of analysis emphasizes (1) experiential immediacy, (2) intersubjective specificity, (3) modulations of temporality, and (4) nuances of intentionality. I will briefly suggest how these elements of analysis can be deployed to elaborate a cultural phenomenology of psychiatric disorder, using my own work with adolescent psychiatric inpatients.

Immediacy and Intersubjectivity

By experiential immediacy, I mean direct contact with a phenomenon, that is, with an appearance in reality. For our purposes, immediacy includes both the temporal sense of experience in the moment and the sense in which experience is unmediated by reflection. Intersubjectivity is critical, both in the sense that experience is co-constructed through interpersonal interaction and in the sense that our phenomenological reconstruction of that experience is based on our own research encounter with a patient. An emphasis on immediacy and intersubjectivity does not allow us to answer the question, "What is it like to be someone else?" but instead enables us to ask the question, "What is it like for someone else to be?" (cf. Linger, 2010). The first question implies that what we want to know is what it would be like *for me* to be another person; the second is about what it is like for that person to be him or herself. This understanding has to be an inferential process because it is based on empathy and intuitive listening, rather than our identity with that person; intersubjectivity is not shared subjectivity but, as Merleau-Ponty (1962) observed, the recognition that an interlocutor is "another myself." It is also inferential both because a person is unlikely to be able to respond to a direct question about what it is like to be him or her, and because such an answer in any case would already be in the register of reflexivity and not immediacy.

Given these considerations, and guided by contemporary work in cultural phenomenology and phenomenological anthropology (Csordas, 1990; Desjarlais & Throop, 2011; Jackson, 1996; Katz & Csordas, 2003; Parnas & Gallagher, Chapter 3, *this volume*; Throop & Hollan, 2008; Willen & Seeman, 2012), several elementary methodological rules not unlike what might be applied in therapeutic listening can abet an intuitive listening that allows for the intersubjective inference of experiential immediacy:

1. Observe word choice, which can reveal both contextual features of the social situation and nuances of interpersonal relationships.
2. Anticipate surprises, which can reveal presuppositions and taken-for-granted ideas different from those of the interlocutor/interviewer.

3. Attend to affect, expressed both in narrative and by tone of voice, which informs about intensity of distress and style of engagement.
4. Respect reflexivity, the expression of which indicates complexity of experience and the content of which is a motivationally consequential interpretation.

Several abbreviated examples of how these rules can be applied can be excerpted from material gathered in our research project "Southwest Youth and the Experience of Psychiatric Treatment" (SWYEPT), a study of adolescent psychiatric inpatients and their families in the southwest United States.[2] These fragments of experiential immediacy are drawn from interviews of participants who met diagnostic criteria for major depression or dysthymia (see Csordas, 2013, for a fuller account).

One young person said, "I just get in these moods where I don't want to move. I hate that." Here the reference is not to a capacity but to a mood, not to an inability but to a lack of motivation, and not to accomplishment of any task but to any physical movement at all. The affective tone is unambiguous, and in vivid contrast to what one might conclude is lethargy, "hate" connotes an active and energetic resistance to incapacitation.

Another young person commented that "Eh, the medication controls me (laughs) like depression-wise." What we can infer from the choice to say that "the medication controls me" rather than "it controls my depression," and from the reflexive laughter in response to this phrase, is a self-aware ambivalence about the notion of control. There is an overtone of embarrassment about needing to be controlled, an acknowledgment of the medication's beneficial efficacy, and an element of resignation at having surrendered some autonomy to the medication.

Again, we heard "I felt like I had to be perfect and if I wasn't, I was the devil or something." Here the patient's experience of depression is related to the pressure of behavioral standards imposed by parents, but sufficiently internalized to be experienced as oppressive. It is likely this sense of condemnatory oppressiveness that is indexed by choice of the word "devil," a word with negative implications for self-esteem at the least and literal insinuations of demonic evil at the most.

A statement during a follow-up interview in response to a question about how a young person's situation had changed since our last encounter was that the problem was "[j]ust anger, basically. I'm not depressed

[2] Southwest Youth and the Experience of Psychiatric Treatment was funded by National Institute of Mental Health grant RO1 MH071781, Thomas J. Csordas and Janis H. Jenkins, Co-Principal Investigators.

anymore. I'm pretty happy, actually." Here there is a clear sense expressed that there has been improvement, with depressed or sad feeling having given way to happiness, but with the addition of "actually" suggesting that this might be an awareness occurring as an insight in the moment of the interview itself. At the same time, there is from the observer's standpoint an apparent incongruity in the persistence of anger as an underlying emotional state independent of depression, particularly since in the clinical view anger and depression can be intertwined.

Finally, consider the comment from another participant that "I kinda realized that I don't really have a good distinction between depression and anger." Here is an example of reflexivity in which depression is clearly again understood as an emotion rather than a disorder, and as a distinct emotion in relation to anger. The implication is both that the two are distinct and that they should be distinguished, with a subtext that failure to distinguish them also complicates being able to distinguish between normal occurrences and pathological exaggerations of either.

Temporality and Intentionality

Temporality, the sense of time, is a dimension that is subject to alteration in psychiatric disorder. The experience of duration as the slow or fast passage of time is relevant here, as is what Jenkins (2015) has identified as the rhythm of life. Attention to time frame is implicated as well, with respect to whether the temporal horizon is experientially fixed on the immediate, mediate, or remote future (Minkowski, 1970). Intentionality enters to the extent that the future is conditioned by becoming and even striving, that it can be governed by events or subject to plans, and that it is possible to articulate possibilities and goals. Again we can draw on material from the SWYEPT project to focus on the phenomenology of temporality and intentionality. These very condensed glimpses of temporal orientation are formulated attitudes toward the future, expressed at three interview points during a year-long participation in the project, and as an intersubjective construction of patient and parent viewpoints. Independent of diagnosis, they are intended to outline the range of temporal possibilities among this group of adolescent psychiatric inpatients.

- *Jenny* expressed the desire of becoming a social worker. At the second interview she had expectations of Behavioral Management Services and attending a different school, but felt she might be "on the verge of going back" to Childrens' Psychiatric Hospital. At this time, her goals were either to attend beauty school, become a social worker, or music because "I sing." At final follow-up, she said, "I know I need treatment but don't know if I'm ready for it." She said she has many things to live for but can't handle school, was interested in cosmetology, and would go "wherever life takes me." Her mother initially said that only God can help and high hopes are unrealistic, that Jenny would never get better. At the first follow-up, she was afraid of her daughter's going to jail, and particularly that having her picked up by the police without warning would violate the trust in their relationship. At the final interview, she was oriented toward a residential treatment center for her daughter but didn't want to have to drive far to visit.

- *Ted* had a constrained ability to interact with others, but was sufficiently aware of this as a problem that he articulated increased sociability as an explicit goal. He wanted to earn a General Educational Development (GED) high school equivalency degree, become capable of living independently of his grandmother, and enter the Job Corps. He noted having come to realize that his life was destined for more than the disease with which he was afflicted, a realization that both defined his situation in terms of disease and resisted the implication of disease as a foreclosed horizon for his future trajectory.

- *Susan* in her initial interview acknowledged having wanted to become a veterinarian but, in part because of her own experience of emotional distress, had decided she was now interested in psychology. Her mother expressed confidence that she would completely recover and go to college in psychology. At the first follow-up, Susan and her mother together expressed her immediate desire to transfer back to a regular high school from the "short-cut school" where she was making up missed credits. Her mother expressed the view that psychotherapy is good not only for the psychiatric illness her daughter had experienced, but in general for relaxing, and Susan acknowledged that she had always been encouraged to engage in therapy by her mother. By the time of the final interview, she had identified the local college in which she wanted to enroll to study social developmental or counseling psychology, saying that although she used to worry, there were a lot of ways to go toward the future. Her mother said she thought her daughter would do well, though "probably not as well as I think she can."

Even these radically abbreviated vignettes exhibit a range of phenomenological dimensions of temporality and intentionality. Foremost is the degree to which the temporal horizon appears as foreclosed/constricted or as open to a future of plans and possibilities, whether it is bound to the immediate future prescribed by the illness or whether there exists a mediate future of hope and desire. Critically in the SWYEPT data, and evident in these three vignettes, this dimension of open or closed

temporal horizon is independent of whether the illness is understood
as a permanent condition or as episodic, whether it is something that
must be lived with indefinitely or whether it can be considered an
interruption in developmental and life trajectory. Less evident here, but
equally relevant, are the dimensions defined by *minimal vs. elaborated* and
realistic vs. unrealistic orientations toward the future.

Cross-Cultural Exemplars

This brief exposition points to the possibility of a cultural phenomenology of psychiatric illness based on current work in psychiatric anthropology. In the remainder of this chapter, I take up the question of
extending this approach into distinct cultural settings, and more particularly the question of the extent to which extant literature is addressed
to concerns that can generally be said to fall within the scope of or be
compatible with a cultural phenomenology of psychiatric illness. Given
the lack of space to examine the full range of relevant studies, I will
concentrate on two works that constitute gold standards for anthropological studies of major psychiatric disorders: *Culture and Depression*,
edited by Kleinman and Good (1985), and *Schizophrenia, Culture, and
Subjectivity*, edited by Jenkins and Barrett (2004).

Depression

In their introduction, the editors of *Culture and Depression* move almost
immediately past the problem of defining depression as a universal
disease, a discrete disorder, or a nosological category. The problem of
variation in the experience of depression leads directly to a broadly
phenomenological stance:

So dramatic are the differences in the cultural worlds in which people live that
translation of emotional terms requires much more than finding semantic
equivalents. Describing how it feels to be grieved or melancholy in another
society leads straightway into analysis of different ways of being a person in
radically different worlds. (1985, p. 3)

Such a stance problematizes the validity of depression as a clinical and
ontological entity insofar as such validity is predicated on Western "tacit
cultural knowledge concerning emotion, interior experience, and psychological disorders" (1985, p. 6). This goal represents the classical
anthropological impulse to relativize the universal by foregrounding an
understanding of culture as that which we take for granted about human
experience, and insisting on a reflexive critique of how the taken-for-

granted contributes to the formation of cultural categories including those of psychiatric diagnosis. In situating the volume's intellectual approach, the editors (1) place anthropology in dialogue with psychiatry and psychology "to relate meaning with experience, symbol with soma, culture with nature" (1985, p. 8); (2) place ethnography in relation to the clinical and epidemiological approaches to distinguish between depression as an emotion and as a disorder, as sometimes normal as well as often pathological, and with the recognition that ethnography is characterized by an interpretive methodology that bears a kinship to that used in "psychoanalytic, existential, and phenomenological clinical research" (1985, p. 11); and (3) place social reality and the social sources of depression in relation to the lived experience of individual persons as the critical underpinning for clinical understanding of depression in cross-cultural perspective. Although waiting until the book's epilogue to do so, they also make the critically important distinction between phenomenology as a clinical description of subjective symptoms and an interpretive description of lifeworlds (1985, pp. 496–7).

One contribution that explicitly evokes phenomenology in the latter sense is Shweder's (1985) discussion of depression as an emotion rather than a disorder. The tone is set by the statement that "To speak of the emotional life is to talk about *felt* experiences" (p. 183; emphasis in original). Across cultural settings, this is to be understood in terms of the types of feelings that people experience, the situations that people find most emotion-laden, the implications of feelings for lived experience, how feelings are expressed and communicated, the propriety of feeling or displaying certain emotions, and how people handle emotions even when they are not expressed. Shweder describes the subjective experience of depression in terms of soul loss: "When you feel depressed you feel as though your soul has left your body" (1985, p. 193). Shweder resists treating the notion of soul loss as metaphorical, arguing that there is a way to define the soul and its departure from the body without theological commitment and in recognition that the idea of soul loss is widespread across cultures. In terms of experiential immediacy, Shweder's point is that "When your soul leaves your body you feel empty" (1985, p. 194), and the exposition focuses on identifying linguistic expressions of that emptiness that specify its meaning, such that for him the semantic and phenomenological are synonymous.

Lutz (1985) critiques the contemporary category of depression with wariness of cultural assumptions that emotions are natural and universal, and that the categories of emotion and cognition are dichotomous. Her premise is that depression as either state or syndrome is an emotion, and that an emotion is a culturally constructed judgment that defines events and relationships, and thus people's roles and behaviors within them. Furthermore, in this view "[a]nalytic and phenomenological priority is given ... to the terms in which people themselves construe their experience" (1985, pp. 66–7). Such terms are "fundamental symbolic forms through which people perceive and experience themselves" (pp. 67–8) and constitute a more or less systematic indigenous theory of persons and selves, or ethnopsychology; but most important for a cultural phenomenology is that they may comprise not only explicit belief but tacit, taken-for-granted presuppositions unavailable for explicit articulation or discussion. Different cultures entertain different theories about inner life with respect to what can be known and what should be known, whether the internal is positively or negatively valued, and whether it is relevant or irrelevant to the problem at hand. Lutz takes an analytical giant step back from depression per se to outline the North American ethnopsychology of emotion in which it is embedded, and that characterizes emotion as essentially an unintended and subjective physical event, a precultural energy or natural substrate on which culture has a secondary influence. She contrasts this with the ethnopsychology of the tiny Pacific atoll of Ifaluk (population 430), where the term *nunuwan* designates the integrated thoughts/feelings of psychic and moral life, interpersonal relationships are dense and multilayered, and the notion of privacy is nonexistent. Such differences pose a challenge for the translation of emotional life across cultures, insofar as "[e]motions may be grouped with moral values rather than (or as much as) with internal disruption, they may be linked with logical thoughts as much as or more than internal conflict, and they may be seen as characteristics of situations or relationships rather than as the property of individuals" (1985, p. 91).

It is evident from our review thus far that in these writings, phenomenological description of experience is subordinate to the epistemological status of depression as a disease category, which is in turn subordinate to the manner in which the disease category is understandable in terms of the broader category of emotion/affect, which finally itself is subject to cultural critique insofar as it is based on Western presuppositions and admits of historical and cultural variability at its most fundamental level. This is strongly a function of the move within anthropology in the 1980s to reconceptualize the locus of emotion in systems of cultural knowledge and patterns of social relations. Drawing on Bateson's concept of ethos to describe the emotional milieu of a society, Schieffelin (1985) makes this same move by examining the central dynamic between (1) personal dynamism and assertiveness expressed as anger, and (2) dependency and appeal expressed as grief among the Kaluli people of New Guinea. The structure of affective immediacy in Kaluli society is epitomized by the transformation of grief into anger in situations of loss, compensated for by ceremonial reciprocity. This leads Schieffelin to suggest that if there is in fact a Kaluli form of depression (there is no equivalent term in their language), it would not come as a response to loss or disappointment, since loss is overtly managed, but through "being placed unwillingly into a long-term life situation in which his or her assertive moves were regularly rebuffed or frustrated and in which there were no socially acceptable grounds for expressing anger or feeling owed" (1985, p. 117). Throughout his time spent with the Kaluli, the only instance he observed approximating depression was the unhappily married third wife of an older man. In this society, where happiness is not typically recognized as an emotional goal of marriage, any therapeutic intervention would have to have been an improvised variant of traditional ceremonies, the form of which is compensation for a loss – in this case, the wife's loss of her freedom and youthful "sparkle."

Obeyesekere (1985) takes up the issue of loss in a manner that shows how experiential immediacy is given a meaningful valence by the manner in which affect is anchored to an ideology. Citing the argument by Brown and Harris (1978) that loss can lead to hopelessness, which in turn underlies depression as a disorder, Obeyesekere suggests that in Buddhist and other societies, the sorrow of hopelessness is structured into cosmology, along with the religious means to overcome it, whereas in Western civilization and its psychiatry, such affects are "free-floating" and thus conducive to being labeled as illness. In Sinhalese Buddhist society, hopelessness is generalized into an ontological problem of existence defined as suffering, and tradition provides "special occasions for ontological reflection on despair" (1985, p. 140), not only for monks but for laypeople as well, through practices of *sil* (observance of the ten precepts) and meditation. Meditation to evoke revulsion at the impermanent and feces-filled nature of the body and the universality of sorrow and hopelessness gives a radically different experiential configuration to what is called depression in the West, a configuration that is moreover deeply inculcated in domains of cultural practice, ranging from myth to child-rearing. This has critical pragmatic implications for experience, regardless of whether similar constellations of symptoms can be identified across cultures.

In counterpoint, Keyes (1985) attempts to find common ground for a cross-cultural understanding of depression by elaborating concepts of mood and mind as subject to predispositions inherent in the human condition that are conducive to depression. Like Obeyesekere, he cites Brown and Harris, but focuses on their broader conception of depression's source in the "meaningful relationship between self and the world" and the "loss of important sources of value" (1985, p. 158). With this broader stance, Keyes is comfortably able to apply the term depression to a case he encountered during fieldwork in Thailand. The case involved an instance of bereaved depression following a violent death, which was exacerbated by both the circumstance of the event and the cultural practice of a protracted time period of several years for completing the funeral of those who die violently. In the end, the depressed mood was resolved through the same kind of ritual work of culture that Obeyesekere described by contextualizing the mood within the broader cosmological and existential meaning of human suffering.

Critical to a cultural phenomenology is a stance wherein the task is not simply the interpretation of cultural meanings *associated* with dysphoric affect and depressive illness, but a recognition that dysphoric affect is inherently *shaped* by those cultural meanings. Good, DelVecchio Good, and Moradi (1985) emphasize that this task be carried out within an awareness of the limits both of psychiatry's ability to generalize its diagnostic categories, and of anthropology's questionable assumption that physical diseases are culturally interpreted natural entities, while mental disorders are purely products of cultural production. This meaning-centered approach is conducive to phenomenological understanding insofar as the notion of interpretation encompasses (1) attention to contextualized depressive discourse and its symbolic and rhetorical structure; (2) cultural differences in attention to and perception of personal realities and social conditions; (3) interpretive errors along the lines described by Beck et al. (1979), but reflecting variant cultural patterning of cognition; and (4) comparison of psychiatric and indigenous discourses of depression and their relation to alternative ways of life, rather than attempting to discover one-to-one correspondence in symptoms or direct semantic equivalents of descriptive categories. Good and colleagues demonstrate this approach with respect to the Iranian Shi'ite ethos, in which dysphoric affect is charged with symbolic meaning at both religious and personal levels. The occurrence and experiential contours of depression can be expected to be conditioned by an ethos in which sadness is associated with personal depth and the capacity to experience grief is highly valued. A collectively shared sense of tragedy and despair is evident in religious commemoration of the martyrdom of Hossein and contemporary literary works, but is also elaborated in the experience of patients, especially those displaced in the aftermath of the Iranian revolution. This circumstance does not mute the distinction between acceptable sadness and pathological depression, but endows it with a particular phenomenological form articulated in distinctively Iranian idioms such as distress of the heart or nerves.

In the book's final chapter, Arthur Kleinman and Joan Kleinman (1985) offer a phenomenologically salient account of somatization in Chinese society that, while recognizing depression as a universally identifiable disorder, shows how it is experientially articulated in terms of the "sociosomatic reticulum" or symbolic bridge "that connects individuals to each other and to their life world" (1985, p. 429). They situate their analysis of the relation among depression, neurasthenia, and chronic pain in relation to the dynamic of somatization and psychologization of experience in historical and cross-cultural perspective. Their data show that symptoms classified as different types of neurasthenia in China correspond to those distributed across depression, anxiety, and chronic pain disorders in North America. Here, the emphasis is on cultural variation in the organization of a constellation of psychobiological symptoms into different diagnostic categories – most evidently relevant for how patients are treated, but also, by implication, for how their experience is configured both prior to and as a consequence of treatment. Over the course of three years, Kleinman's study determined that severity of symptoms was ameliorated in accord with the amelioration of social situations, but also that overall there was a shift toward a higher proportion of Chinese patients who regarded their problems as psychological rather than somatic in nature, and that pain itself was endowed with a substantial amount of symbolic social significance in both psychiatric and primary-care settings. Critical to grasping experiential immediacy in this setting are the sociopolitical milieu of post–Cultural Revolution China; cultural norms for dealing with loss; an array of interpretive schemata for expressing distress; and patterned relationships among morality, feeling, self-concept, communication, action, ideology, and power (Kleinman, 1986).

Schizophrenia

Examining the immediacy of experience in schizophrenia is not complicated by the overlap between depression as an emotion ("I feel depressed") and as a disorder ("I have depression"). Although its emotional sequelae are significant and much debated, schizophrenia is more clearly demarcated as a pathological state both clinically and in everyday understanding; and if one says "I feel schizophrenic," it is more likely to be a colloquialized misuse of the term to mean "I am torn in two directions" or "I am of two minds" than "I am delusional" or "I am hallucinating." In their introduction, while recognizing the biological factors involved in schizophrenia and taking contemporary research diagnostic criteria as a touchstone for cross-cultural analysis, the editors

of *Schizophrenia, Culture, and Subjectivity* recognize not only that schizophrenia is cross-culturally variable but also that even in Euro-American
society, it exists as a family of disorders rather than a single disorder,
and they assert the value of taking "the complex phenomenal reality of
subjective experience as a starting point" (Jenkins & Barrett, 2004, p. 2)
for analysis. With this as the leitmotif, they emphasize the understanding
of culture as emergent from human interaction rather than as a quantifiable factor or variable. At the level of experience, culture merges with
intersubjectivity insofar as both are constituted by meaning structures
and interpretive processes for interactive sense-making; hence, "culture
is critical in nearly *every* aspect of schizophrenic illness experience"
(2004, p. 6). A phenomenologically inflected reassertion of the clinical
and ethnographic importance of subjectivity uses this cultural foundation
to emphasize the primacy of lived experience, intersubjectivity, and the
active engagement of subjects in the cultural construction of reality via
agency and intentionality.

In the opening chapter, Jenkins (2004) offers an analytic framework
that simultaneously asserts the centrality of subjective experience for
understanding schizophrenia and the importance of schizophrenia as a
paradigm case for a broader understanding of fundamental and ordinary
human processes. Rather than being so far outside the norm that their
experience is irrelevant or unintelligible, those afflicted with schizophrenia face the same issues as the nonafflicted in terms of culture and
agency, desire and attachment, shared meaning and social communication, but in ways that are fraught and filled with daily struggle rather
than taken for granted, such that in certain ways they are "just like
everyone else, only more so" (2004, p. 30). Invoking Canguilhem's
(1978) notion of a continuum between normal and pathological, Jenkins
argues that with respect to the immediacy of experience in schizophrenia,
strict differentiation between the two states is not possible. She elaborates
this position in relation to processes of everyday life in four domains: self
processes, emotion, social engagement, and cultural orientation. *Self
processes*, which in a "theoretical retreat" were eliminated from the formulation of schizophrenia in the revision that produced *DSM-IV*, must
be reinstated in analysis as capacities of orientation to the world and
others characterized by effort and reflexivity. Here, Jenkins introduces
a phenomenological account of hearing voices as discontinuous from
ordinary experience but not from the self, and in terms of the relationship
among intentionality, agency, and meaning. In the domain of *emotion*,
Jenkins addresses the clinical presumption of either a disorganized
intensification or a flattening and blunting of affect in schizophrenia.
She points out that when one attends to the subjective feel of the illness,

it is observable that linguistic devices and poetic elements of schizophrenic speech are continuous with those of ordinary language and often implicate a highly nuanced emotional sensitivity even in the face of muted expression. In the domains of *social engagement* and *cultural orientation*, Jenkins shows how attunement to intersubjectivity allows understanding of the lifeworld of schizophrenia with respect to expressed emotion in families, patients' conceptualization of their illness, patterns of socioemotional distancing, gender identity and expression, and immediate residential milieu.

The task of elaborating the centrality of subjectivity and intersubjectivity from the standpoint of phenomenological psychiatry faces a challenge when linguistic and cultural differences are so great as to call into question how experience can be described or the identification of symptoms as such. Barrett (2004) takes up this challenge in his approach to the experience of schizophrenia or *sakit gila* (mad sickness) among the Iban people of Sarawak. He begins with translating the Present State Exam, a structured psychiatric assessment, into terms culturally intelligible to the Iban, and using it as data for a comparative cultural phenomenology of Schneider's first-rank symptoms of schizophrenia. Barrett's account of the translation process is itself an exercise in the phenomenology of language, taking into account stylistic and sociolinguistic incommensurabilities between Iban and English, as well as the fact that while the Iban readily recognize the phenomenon of auditory hallucinations, they hardly understand concepts such as thought insertion or broadcasting, constituted as they are on the cultural presupposition of an autonomous mental realm characterized by the presence of silent and uniquely personal thought. The overlap between thought and speech in Iban culture belies the relevance of distinction between internal/external, mind/body, and public/private. A commensurable cultural phenomenology of auditory hallucination was borne out in Barrett's comparisons of Iban and Australian patients' experience. Iban patients were considerably less likely than their Australian counterparts to report experience classifiable as subjective thought disorder, and the three instances of such reports were all women who were deeply influenced by Christianity and its cultural elaboration of internal mental and spiritual life. Although disturbances in speech occur in both groups, the Iban material metaphor of such speech being "off track" and the Australian mental metaphor of it as "nonsense" may be consequential, both experientially and clinically. Barrett's analysis also suggests differentiation among first-rank symptoms along the lines that some symptoms, like auditory hallucinations, may be more cross-culturally robust, whereas others, such as thought disorder, may be intrinsically more variable.

An equally fine-grained analysis of how psychotic experience is expressed and can be understood across significant cultural differences is Wilce's (2004) case study of *pāgalāmi* (madness) in Bangladesh, which approaches experiential immediacy through a focus on language and nonverbal interaction, based on videotaped interviews with patients and their family members. Although Wilce confirmed that the patients with whom he worked also met the psychiatric criteria for schizophrenia, cultural meaning significantly inflects their experience. Thus, *pāgalāmi* has ritual aspects associated with the divine and spirit possession, while the uncontrolled behavior of those afflicted is also analogized to the behavior of goats. This is in the context of a self culturally oriented toward collective values, such that madness is interpreted as a form of self-indulgence and is "constructed largely in terms of morally deviant attention to the self" (2004, p. 201). Moreover, insofar as schizophrenia involves a loss of natural self-evidence, close attention to consequently disrupted communicative interaction "reveals how repeated failure to achieve intersubjectivity can cause suffering, exacerbated when high expectations for this achievement are upheld" (2004, p. 205). Wilce describes a young afflicted woman whose speech reveals a struggle for culturally valued "beauty" in expression, while her utterances focused on word play with Bangladeshi homonyms and verb conjugations instead of conversational engagement.

Casting their approach to experiential immediacy in terms of the phenomenological analysis of the life world (*lebenswelt*), Corin, Thara, and Padmavati (2004) describe research in South India that addresses how culture mediates psychosis, or more precisely how subjective experience is framed and articulated among people with schizophrenia. They argue that experience is a critical concept in understanding cross-cultural variation in the course of schizophrenia, bringing together psychological anthropology, psychoanalysis, and phenomenological psychiatry and applying the method of phenomenological reduction (the *epoché* or bracketing of assumptions in order to grasp the phenomenon's essence) to place affect, cognition, and meaning in the context of broader social and cultural frames. Their focus is neither on symptoms per se nor on specific utterances, but on the sometimes nuanced alteration in the lived worlds of the afflicted at the onset of schizophrenia among patients in their twenties. These alterations include experiences of fear and transparency, confusion and indeterminacy, the loss of mundane behavioral markers, and the presence of disturbing bodily sensations. In the onset of schizophrenia, the attention of family and of the afflicted person is gradually drawn to these changes, and a search ensues for their cause and significance. Religion provides a repertoire of symbolic resources and ritual practices (e.g., healing, pilgrimage, renunciation) that people draw on, sometimes being absorbed into an all-encompassing religious universe and sometimes therapeutically framing the experience. Withdrawal takes the form of solitude or secrecy, and can be positive in allowing a safe space away from the overloaded intersubjectivity of others or the oversignified world of meaning. To their credit, the authors pose the epistemological question of whether inquiry at this level of experiential immediacy can avoid perpetrating interpretive violence or seductively promulgating its fascinating fearfulness, and the ethical question of whether such inquiry risks exacerbating the intensity of suffering for the afflicted.

Although not invoking the classic notion of a culture-bound syndrome, Good and Subandi (2004) offer a cultural phenomenology of a brief, acute psychosis they identified as typical of some patients in the city of Yogyakarta, central Java. They present a case study of an afflicted Muslim woman in her thirties, weaving together descriptions of illness episodes and life history, romantic attachments and religious commitments, psychiatric treatment and ritual healing. Their approach emphasizes self processes insofar as psychosis involves the destruction of self and subjectivity in a specific social setting, the ineffable or extraordinary experiences of psychoses and their interpenetration with the ordinary perceptual world of everyday life, and the experiential milieu of families inhabited by intimates with intertwined life histories, developmental trajectories, and personal relationships. Experiential immediacy resides in a vitalistic lifeworld undergirded by a sense of all-pervasive power present across and undermining any explicit divide between organic and inorganic, sentient corporal or insensible material. The self is cultivated to be reserved and refined in the face of this power, but its behavioral environment is defined in part by a culturally elaborated experience of magic and spirits, such that there is "less of a disjuncture between the everyday world and the lifeworlds of those who are psychotic than in some societies" (2004, p. 186). Here the experiential specificity of the patient's affliction becomes intelligible with respect to psychocultural themes of corporal defilement thematized in terms of an Islamic notion of purity, healing enacted in terms of Islamic prayer practices, and an experiential rhythm of withdrawal/solitude and wandering/flight in the context of a conflicted relationship with her mother, loss of her father, and a history of romantic disappointment. The authors rightly suggest that this level of analysis contributes to comparative understanding of types of psychosis, as well as to the understanding of the relationship of broad sociocultural processes to experientially specific self processes.

Lucas (2004) carries the claim of culture further by showing how ethnography can enrich the understanding of the ways that a diagnosis of schizophrenia affects peoples' daily lives, working with Australian patients through ethnographic interviews and following them through everyday activities like riding a bus, shopping, or sitting in a waiting room. He observes that the ineffable strangeness and atmospheric otherness of schizophrenia, combined with unaccountable bodily sensations in the face of an obscure physical locus of the illness, contribute to its placement virtually outside or beyond culture. This is evident in images of schizophrenia as the persistence or resurfacing of the primitive state of human mental evolution, and as an alienation that at the same time is produced by and constitutes a critique of contemporary society, or as an experiential domain analogous to art where the emphasis is on creativity and genius within madness. However, on the level of immediate experience, these images themselves are part of the cultural milieu of modernity that patients engage in a process of finding a multiplicity of touchstones or points of reference for their experience. Thus, people grappling with psychotic experience may use the Bible as an "operator's manual for hearing voices" (2004, p. 157), reinvent images found in works of modernist literature without necessarily being familiar with such works themselves, and mobilize the symbolic resources of popular culture through music and movies.

The theme of modernity appears again in Sass's (2004) phenomenological account of schizophrenia's negative symptoms. He suggests that these are not essentially a kind of neurological shutting down: following Minkowski (1970), they are better described as disengagement from vital contact with reality, such that it becomes difficult to grant priority to and achieve orientation among the multiplicity of features in the world; following Blankenburg (1971), the fundamental alteration of the lived world in schizophrenia is better described as a loss of natural self-evidence, such that what is taken for granted becomes fundamentally problematic. In this circumstance, one becomes hyperreflexive and immediately conscious of both alterations of perception and interaction with the surrounding world, and develops a somatic mode of attention highly attuned to cenesthetic bodily experiences. The coherence of the cultural milieu that guarantees what normally remains tacit and what becomes explicit, what is presupposed and what must be articulated, is challenged; however, withdrawal and alienation from the consequent overstimulation does not place the afflicted person outside culture, but in a vexed relation to it. Taking the case of the artist Antonin Artaud as emblematic, Sass suggests that the intensity of this experience is amplified by a synergy between schizoid tendencies and schizotypal disturbance, on the one hand, and the tendency of modernity to thematize introspection, doubt, self-detachment, meta-awareness, and relativism, on the other.

The problem of modernity appears again in Sadowsky's (2004) contribution, which analyzes the self-reported experience of two Yorùbá asylum inmates in southwest Nigeria during the late colonial period and transition to independence. He endorses Jenkins's assertion of continuity between "insane" and "normal" in treating the content of psychotic raving as a valid object of social analysis, especially salient at the blurry boundary between persecutory delusion and anticolonial sentiment in patients' writing. In contrast, Estroff (2004) examines published contemporary first-person accounts and poetry by people who self-categorize as "consumer/survivor/ex-patients (c/s/x)" (2004:283) of schizophrenia. Experience is here both politicized and narrativized, as writings by c/s/x authors challenge professional and clinical understandings and recategorize experience by giving equal weight to symptoms of illness and symptoms of treatment, rejecting the legitimacy of "side effects" as a category.

Finally, although patients with schizophrenia have often been characterized as exhibiting "flat affect," two contributions in contrasting ways highlight the place of emotion in the experience of schizophrenia. McGruder (2004) reports on three former inpatients treated for schizophrenia in a mental hospital in Zanzibar, a predominantly Muslim society with Swahili culture, in which madness is widely held to be caused by spirits. Taking into account an indigenous conception of self as composed of body, vitality, heart, soul, and reason, and a conception of emotion that values self-control and reserve, her case studies suggest the applicability in Zanzibar of the Expressed Emotion paradigm, which identifies the effect of hostility, criticism, and emotional overinvolvement on the course of schizophrenia. Kring and Germans (2004) draw on studies using standardized instruments to discuss how intra- and interpersonal processes are undermined by disturbances in the way expressive, experiential, and physiological components of emotion are coordinated. In particular, they review research that distinguishes the apparent "flat affect" in the expressive dimension from the actual intensity of emotion experientially, sort out elements of anhedonia such as the difference between being able to experience pleasure and the actual engagement in pleasurable activity, and raise the question of emotional response by the afflicted to the very situation of having the illness.[3]

Conclusion

In this chapter I have emphasized the importance of the alliance between psychiatry and anthropology, taking Sapir's classic article both as a foundation text and the jumping-off point for a cultural phenomenology of psychiatric illness. I proposed that such an approach would include specific attention to the modulation of experience with respect to immediacy, intersubjectivity, temporality, and intentionality. Drawing on data from the SWYEPT project, I presented a brief example of such an analysis focused on adolescent patients' experience of depression and their orientation toward the future. From the standpoint of psychiatry, I suggest that this approach is relevant to the clinical encounter insofar as it is conducive to a more thorough understanding of patient experience and sensitive to cultural variation in that experience. From the standpoint of anthropology, it is relevant insofar as it leads to a more thorough understanding of the cultural patterning of experience beyond the elaboration of indigenous cultural categories of affliction.

I have also reconsidered two books that stand as pillars of the study of major mental disorder in psychiatric anthropology. Both include contributions that explicitly elaborate the cultural phenomenology of psychiatric illness, others that approach experiential specificity and immediacy from different directions, and still others that are a step removed from immediate experience. If there is a difference in their overall approaches, it is less attributable to the empirical difference between depression and schizophrenia than to developments in the field during the nearly twenty years that separate their publication, across the divide created by the challenge of biological psychiatry throughout the 1990s. *Culture and*

---

[3] Several other chapters treat elements of experiential immediacy relevant to our concerns without employing explicitly phenomenological approaches. Hopper (2004) focuses on the role of culture in WHO studies of the course of schizophrenia settings in various parts of the globe, with a critique that points to how experiential specificity could be introduced, particularly with respect to the prospects for and ameliorating effects of marriage for the afflicted. Diaz, Fergusson, and Strauss (2004) discuss a therapeutic community for the homeless mentally ill in Bogota, Colombia, that targets "developmental arrest" along with issues of personal independence and autonomy among the mentally ill. They describe the experience of six patients in response to the stability of urban and rural living and work environments provided by the clinic. Important in this respect are gendered cultural meanings of assertiveness and submissiveness, street survival skills, and the acquisition of work-related skills, religious frameworks of understanding, and changes in patients' explanations for illness that made it possible for them to accept treatment.

Depression was a product of the "new cross-cultural psychiatry" that resulted from a creative synthesis of interpretive anthropology and psychiatry. It was part critique and part reinvigoration of a way of thinking about the meaning of experience and the significance of cultural diversity in the study of psychiatric disorder, the golden era of which was the period characterized by Sapir. This movement was placed on the defensive during the 1990's "Decade of the Brain," which heralded the consolidation of the dominance of biological psychiatry in the national mental health research agenda, the orientation of academic departments of psychiatry, and clinical practice defined as medication management.

The publication of *Schizophrenia, Culture, and Subjectivity* in 2004 marked the resurgence of an emphasis on experience with an explicit theorization of and empirical emphasis on subjectivity. The collective voice of its contributors constitutes an overt assertion and elaboration of the methodological relevance of phenomenological analysis, sometimes drawing explicitly on the tradition of phenomenological psychiatry and steadfastly introducing ethnographic and ethnological sensibility to forge a mature cultural phenomenology. Taken together, these two volumes can serve as touchstones for researchers and clinicians concerned with the cultural phenomenology of psychiatric disorder that places experiential specificity and immediacy at the center of analysis. We can justly follow their lead toward determining clinically and intellectually consequential relations between emotion and mental illness, among fundamental human processes linking pathological and nonpathological experience, and between anthropology and psychiatry as sister disciplines.

REFERENCES

Barrett, R. J. (2004). Kurt Schneider in Borneo: Do first rank symptoms apply to the Iban? In J. H. Jenkins & R. L. Barrett (Eds.), *Schizophrenia, culture, and subjectivity: The edge of experience* (pp. 87–109). Cambridge, England: Cambridge University Press.

Beck, A. T., Rush, A. J., Shaw, B. F., & Emery, G. (1979). *Cognitive Therapy of Depression.* New York, NY: Guilford Press.

Binswanger, L. (1963). *Being-in-the-world: Selected papers of Ludwig Binswanger (J. Needleman, Trans. and Introduction).* New York, NY: Basic Books.

Blankenburg, W. (1971). *Der Verlust der Naturlichen Selnstverstandlichkeit: Ein Beitrag zur Psychopathologie Symptomarmer Schizophrenien.* Stuttgart, Germany: Ferdinand Enke Verlag.

Boss, M. (1963). *Psychoanalysis and daseinanalysis.* New York, NY: Basic Books.

Brown, G., & Harris, T. (1978). *Social origins of depression: A study of psychiatric disorder in women.* London, England: Tavistock.

Canguilhem, G. (1978). *On the normal and the pathological.* Dordrecht, Germany: D. Reidel. http://dx.doi.org/10.1007/978-94-009-9853-7

Corin, E., Thara, R., & Padmavati, R. (2004). Living through a staggering world: The play of signifiers in early psychosis in South India. In J. H. Jenkins & R. L. Barrett (Eds.), *Schizophrenia, culture, and subjectivity: The edge of experience* (pp.110–45). Cambridge, England: Cambridge University Press.

Csordas, T. J. (1990). Embodiment as a paradigm for anthropology. 1988 Stirling Award Essay, *Ethos, 18*, 5–47. http://dx.doi.org/10.1525/eth.1990.18.1.02a00010

Csordas, T. J. (1994). *The sacred self: A cultural phenomenology of charismatic healing.* Berkeley: University of California Press.

Csordas, T. J. (1999). Embodiment and cultural phenomenology. In G. Weiss & H. Haber (Eds.), *Perspectives on embodiment* (pp. 143–62). New York, NY: Routledge.

Csordas, T. J. (2012). Psychoanalysis and phenomenology. In S. Willen & D. Seeman (Eds.), Horizons of experience: Reinvigorating dialogue between phenomenological and psychoanalytic anthropologies [Special issue]. *Ethos, 40(1)*, 54–74.

Csordas, T. J. (2013). Inferring immediacy in adolescent accounts of depression. In M. Ratcliffe & A. Stephan (Eds.), Emotional experience in depression [Special issue]. *Journal of Consciousness, 20(7–8)*, 239–53.

Desjarlais, R., & Throop, C. J. (2011). Phenomenological approaches in anthropology. *Annual Review of Anthropology, 40*, 87–102. http://dx.doi.org/10.1146/annurev-anthro-092010-153345

Diaz, E., Fergusson, A., & Strauss, J. S. (2004). Innovative care for the homeless mentally ill in Bogota, Colombia. In J. H. Jenkins & R. L. Barrett (Eds.), *Schizophrenia, culture, and subjectivity: The edge of experience* (pp. 219–37). Cambridge, England: Cambridge University Press.

Estroff, S. (2004). Subject/subjectivities in dispute: The poetics, politics, and performance of first-person narratives of people with schizophrenia. In J. H. Jenkins & R. L. Barrett (Eds.), *Schizophrenia, culture, and subjectivity: The edge of experience* (pp. 282–302). Cambridge, England: Cambridge University Press.

Fuchs, T. (2005). Corporealized and disembodied minds. A phenomenological view of the body in melancholia and schizophrenia. *Philosophy, Psychiatry & Psychology, 12*, 95–107.

Fuchs, T. (2007). Psychotherapy of the lived space: A phenomenological and ecological concept. *American Journal of Psychotherapy, 61*, 432–9.

Good, B. J., DelVechio Good, M.-J., & Moradi, R. (1985). The interpretation of Iranian depressive illness and dysphoric affect. In A. Kleinman & B. Good (Eds.), *Culture and depression: Studies in the anthropology and cross-cultural psychiatry of affect and disorder* (pp. 369–428). Berkeley: University of California Press.

Good, B. J., & Subandi, M. A. (2004). Experiences of psychosis in Javanese culture: Reflections on a case of acute, recurrent psychosis in contemporary Yogyakarta, Indonesia. In J. H. Jenkins & R. L. Barrett (Eds.), *Schizophrenia, culture, and subjectivity: The edge of experience* (pp. 167–95). Cambridge, England: Cambridge University Press.

Hopper, K. (2004). Interrogating the meaning of "culture" in the WHO international studies of Schizophrenia. In J. H. Jenkins & R. L. Barrett (Eds.), *Schizophrenia, culture, and subjectivity: The edge of experience* (pp. 62–86). Cambridge, England: Cambridge University Press.

Jackson, Michael, (Ed.). (1996). *Things as they are: New directions in phenomenological anthropology*. Bloomington: Indiana University Press.

Jenkins, J. H. (2004). Schizophrenia as a paradigm case for understanding fundamental human processes. In J. H. Jenkins & R. J. Barrett (Eds.), *Schizophrenia, culture, and subjectivity: The edge of experience* (pp. 29–61). Cambridge, England: Cambridge University Press.

Jenkins, J. H. (2015). *Extraordinary conditions: Culture and experience in mental illness*. Berkeley: University of California Press.

Jenkins, J. H., & Barrett, R. J. (Eds.). (2004). *Schizophrenia, culture, and subjectivity: The edge of experience*. Cambridge, England: Cambridge University Press.

Katz, J., & Csordas, T. (Eds.). (2003). Phenomenology and ethnography [Theme issue]. *Ethnography 4*(3). http://dx.doi.org/10.1177/146613810343001

Keyes, C. (1985). The interpretive basis of depression. In A. Kleinman & B. Good (Eds.), *Culture and depression: Studies in the anthropology and cross-cultural psychiatry of affect and disorder* (pp. 153–74). Berkeley: University of California Press.

Kirmayer, L. J. (2001). Sapir's vision of culture and personality. *Psychiatry, 64*(1), 23–30.

Kleinman, A. (1986). *Social origins of distress and disease: depression, neurasthenia, and pain in modern China*. New Haven, CT: Yale University Press.

Kleinman, A., & Good, B. (Eds.). (1985). *Culture and depression: Studies in the anthropology and cross-cultural psychiatry of affect and disorder*. Berkeley: University of California Press.

Kleinman, A., & Kleinman, J. (1985). Somatization: The interconnections in Chinese society among culture, depressive experiences, and the meanings of pain. In A. Kleinman & B. Good (Eds.), *Culture and depression: Studies in the anthropology and cross-cultural psychiatry of affect and disorder* (pp. 429–90). Berkeley: University of California Press.

Kring, A., & Germans, M. K. (2004). Subjective experience of emotion in schizophrenia. In J. H. Jenkins & R. L. Barrett (Eds.), *Schizophrenia, culture, and subjectivity: The edge of experience* (pp. 329–48). Cambridge, England: Cambridge University Press.

Linger, D. (2010). What is it like to be someone else? *Ethos, 38*(2), 205–29. http://dx.doi.org/10.1111/j.1548-1352.2010.01136.x

Lucas, R. (2004). In and out of culture: Ethnographic means to interpreting schizophrenia. In J. H. Jenkins & R. L. Barrett (Eds.), *Schizophrenia, culture, and subjectivity: The edge of experience* (pp. 146–65). Cambridge, England: Cambridge University Press.

Lutz, C. (1985). Depression and the translation of emotional worlds. In A. Kleinman & B. Good (Eds.), *Culture and depression: Studies in the anthropology and cross-cultural psychiatry of affect and disorder* (pp. 63–100). Berkeley: University of California Press.

McGruder, J. H. (2004). Madness in Zanzibar: An exploration of lived experience. In J. H. Jenkins & R. L. Barrett (Eds.), *Schizophrenia, culture, and subjectivity: The edge of experience* (pp. 255–81). Cambridge, England: Cambridge University Press.

Merleau-Ponty, M. (1962). *Phenomenology of perception* (C. Smith, Trans.). London, England: Routledge and Kegan Paul.

140   *Thomas J. Csordas*

Minkowski, E. (1970). *Lived time: Phenomenological and psychopathological studies* (N. Metzel, Trans.). Evanston, IL: Northwestern University Press.

Obeyesekere, G. (1984). Depression and the work of culture in Sri Lanka. In A. Kleinman & B. Good (Eds.), *Culture and depression: Studies in the anthropology and cross-cultural psychiatry of affect and disorder* (pp. 134–52). Berkeley: University of California Press.

Parnas, J., & Gallagher, S. (2015). Phenomenology and the interpretation of psychopathological experience. In L. J. Kirmayer, R. Lemelson, & C. A. Cummings (Eds.), *Re-visioning psychiatry: Cultural phenomenology, critical neuroscience, and global mental health* (pp. 65–80). New York, NY: Cambridge University Press.

Ratcliffe, M. (2008). *Feelings of being: Phenomenology, psychiatry and the sense of reality.* New York, NY: Oxford University Press. http://dx.doi.org/10.1093/med/9780199206469.001.0001

Sadowsky, J. (2004). Symptoms of colonialism: Content and context of delusion in Southwest Nigeria, 1945–60. In J. H. Jenkins & R. L. Barrett (Eds.), *Schizophrenia, culture, and subjectivity: The edge of experience* (pp. 238–53). Cambridge, England: Cambridge University Press.

Sapir, E. (1932). Cultural anthropology and psychiatry. *The Journal of Abnormal and Social Psychology, 27*(3), 229–42. http://dx.doi.org/10.1037/h0076025

Sapir, E. (1938/2001). Why cultural anthropology needs the psychiatrist. *Psychiatry, 64*(1), 2–10. Reprinted from 1938 with new commentaries by Stephen Anderson, Arthur Kleinman, Regna Darnell, and Laurence Kirmayer.

Sass, L. A. (2004). "Negative symptoms," commonsense, and cultural disembedding in the modern age. In J. H. Jenkins & R. L. Barrett (Eds.), *Schizophrenia, culture, and subjectivity: The edge of experience* (pp. 303–28). Cambridge, England: Cambridge University Press.

Schieffelin, E. (1985). The cultural analysis of depressive affect: An example from New Guinea. In A. Kleinman & B. Good (Eds.), *Culture and depression: Studies in the anthropology and cross-cultural psychiatry of affect and disorder* (pp. 101–33). Berkeley: University of California Press.

Shweder, R. (1985). Menstrual pollution, soul loss, and the comparative study of emotions. In A. Kleinman & B. Good (Eds.), *Culture and depression: Studies in the anthropology and cross-cultural psychiatry of affect and disorder* (pp. 182–215). Berkeley: University of California Press.

Stanghellini, G. (2004). *Disembodied spirits and deanimated bodies: The psychopathology of common sense.* New York, NY: Oxford University Press. http://dx.doi.org/10.1093/med/9780198520894.001.0001

Throop, C. J., & Hollan, D. (Eds.). (2008). Whatever happened to empathy? [Theme issue]. *Ethos, 36*(4). http://dx.doi.org/10.1111/j.1548-1352.2008.00023.x

Wilce, J. M. (2004). To "speak beautifully" in Bangladesh: Subjectivity as *pāgalāmi.* In J. H. Jenkins & R. L. Barrett (Eds.), *Schizophrenia, culture, and subjectivity: The edge of experience* (pp. 196–218). Cambridge, England: Cambridge University Press.

Willen, S. S., & Seeman, D. (Eds.). (2012). Horizons of experience: Reinvigorating dialogue between phenomenological and psychoanalytic anthropologies [Theme issue]. *Ethos, 40*(1), 1–23. http://dx.doi.org/10.1111/j.1548-1352.2011.01228.x

6   Empathy and Alterity in Psychiatry

Laurence J. Kirmayer

Introduction

At the center of psychiatry as a clinical discipline is the human encounter between patient and clinician. Although we can imagine forms of psychiatry in the future that might eliminate this relationship in favor of self-management or interactions with artificial intelligence, there are arguments for insisting that the interaction of two human beings allows unique forms of communication, understanding, and intervention. What is distinctive about this embodied encounter are the dynamics of interpersonal interaction, which include processes of empathy, identification, and emotional connection based on similarity, but also the recognition of difference, otherness, or alterity. In some ways, the construct of empathy stands in for larger questions about the nature of the relationship between patient and clinician. Of course, this relationship involves much more than empathy, but thinking about empathy provides a way to begin to explore the phenomenology and dynamics of the clinical encounter.

Contemporary mental health practitioners rely on empathy to understand patients' experiences and to maintain the interpersonal relatedness that facilitates helping and healing. Various forms of psychopathology, unusual or extreme experiences, and differences in cultural background or social position all present challenges to clinicians' ability to empathize. Failures of empathy may undermine the working alliance, but they may also convey diagnostic information about psychopathological processes or the status of the clinician–patient relationship. When empathy reaches its limits, the other may be experienced as alien, uncanny, and unknown. Theories of psychopathology, which may include structural models and causal mechanisms, offer alternative ways to explain alien or inaccessible experience (Glover, 2014). Clinicians learn to use these models to guide their response to patients, and, in some circumstances, such technical models or explanations may enhance or restore empathy. But cultural difference also demands that we learn to use our imagination in disciplined ways to build bridges between different worlds of experience and to respect the limits of our understanding of the other.

Forms of Knowledge in the Clinical Encounter

Clinical understanding demands attention to multiple sources of knowledge, each with its own epistemology and methods of inquiry (McHugh & Slavney, 1998). Recognizing the kinds of knowledge needed for clinical work has implications for psychiatric theory, research, and practice. Figure 6.1 depicts three basic ways of knowing that are employed in current psychiatric practice and their counterparts in the phenomenological and social science literature.

The central line involves empathy (*Einfühlung*), that is, knowledge of the other based on emotional feeling, in which both verbal and nonverbal communication – including facial expression, bodily stance, gesture,

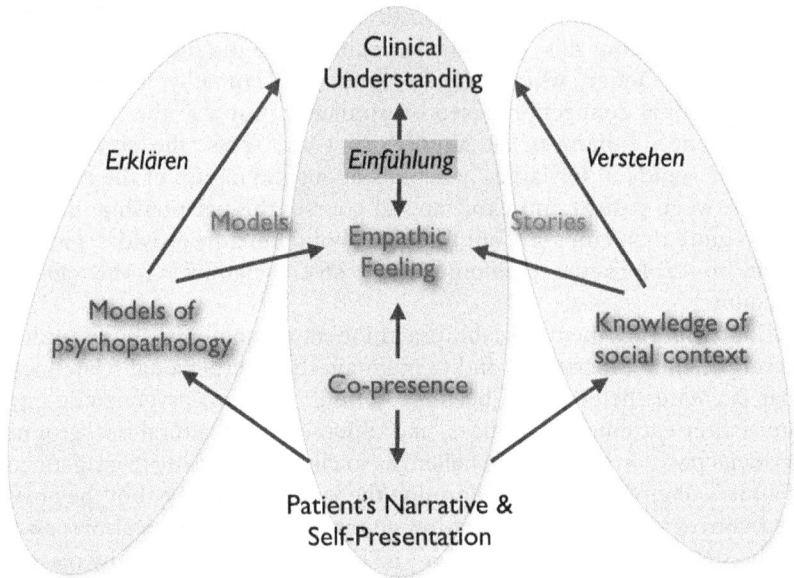

Figure 6.1. Forms of knowledge in the clinical encounter. The clinical encounter makes use of multiple forms of knowledge, including empathy (*Einfühlung*) through interaction and emotional resonance; explanations (*Erklären*) through models and mechanism of psychopathology; and understanding (*Verstehen*) through constructing narratives that situate the patients experience in a lifeworld. Each way of knowing has its own epistemology, modes of inquiry, and limits.

tone of voice or prosody, and other sensory modalities, such as olfaction (Semin & Groot, 2013) – serve to convey particular feelings and call forth an answering response. When clinicians monitor their own response to the patient as a way of gaining diagnostic information and tracking the process of clinical interaction and treatment, this way of knowing has been called " autognosis" (Lazare, Putnam, & Lipkin, 1995). Empathy involves feedback loops between the participants that are influenced by their immediate goals and intentions, as well as the demands of the clinical context. This interactive process can be thought of as a kind of *co-presence* in which being together gives rise to intersubjective experience (Zahavi, 2001). Rudimentary empathic attunement can occur without verbal communication, but more complex understanding depends on reconstructing the perspective of the other, which requires knowing about the person's lifeworld, either through narrative accounts or observation.

The right side of the figure represents what the sociologist Max Weber called *Verstehen*, that is, understanding human action by taking the other's perspective through vicarious experiencing or imaginative recon-struction (Abel, 1957). Learning about patients' lifeworlds, motivations, and predicaments provides knowledge of their experience and intentions in relation to the social contexts that give actions and emotions particular meaning. Appreciating these meanings depends on having sufficient background knowledge of the patient's history and social world to make sense of the narrative. In this way, information about context not only contributes directly to clinical knowledge, but also deepens empathic understanding by allowing the clinician to construct a narrative, story or scenario that situates the patient as an actor in a meaningful social world (Gallagher, 2012). Imagining oneself in the same scenario may evoke thoughts and feelings that are analogous to those felt by the patient.

Of course, not all of the causes of individuals' behavior and experience are included in their self-understanding and narrative accounts. Weber contrasted *Verstehen* with *Erklären*, or causal explanations of behavior in terms of underlying mechanisms (represented on the left side of Figure 6.1). Many causal factors may be outside of patients' awareness, either because they involve subpersonal physiological or cognitive processes or because they result from social structural determinants that may be distant or difficult to discern because they are tacit and taken-for-granted, or even actively hidden and denied by others. These physiological, psychological, and social determinants of behavior and experience can be used to construct causal models or mechanistic explanations. Clinicians use causal models to explain symptoms and behaviors in ways that may diverge from the patient's self-understanding. In many instances, these models are presented to patients to foster greater self-understanding, better adaptation, or provide a rationale for particular kinds of treatment. The explanatory models of biological psychiatry, psychoanalysis, and cognitive-behavioral therapy can all be considered from this point of view. Each provides a conceptual framework that allows clinician and patient to make sense of suffering and points toward potential solutions. The clinician's aim, though, is not just to convey knowledge but to emotionally engage, support, motivate, change, and empower the patient. The success of this process of interpersonal influence may depend crucially on mutual understanding, empathic connection, and rapport between clinician and patient.

From Aesthetic Resonance to Empathic Concern

To empathize is to understand another's experience through feeling or thinking something similar oneself. Although it commonly occurs without any deliberate plan or intention, empathy is facilitated by the willingness to meet, engage, and be moved by the other.

The concept of empathy has its roots in the experience of "feeling-into," which can refer to aesthetic appreciation, as when one is drawn into and moved by a work of art, as well as interpersonal communication. Indeed, there are important historical and conceptual links between empathy as aesthetic engagement and as the ground of emotional attunement and concern for the other (Jahoda, 2005). Perhaps, aesthetic experience provides an instructive instance of empathy because its obvious artifice encourages us to become aware of our own imaginative capacity to inhabit a fictional place and feel the feelings of others (or of ourselves, as though we were living in another place and time). In fact, there is evidence that reading fiction can improve empathic capacity (Oatley, 2011). However, there are important differences between empathy as an aesthetic response to an object and interpersonal empathy, where the temporal dynamics, power, and politics of relatedness are central to the experience.

The term *empathy* was derived from the notion of sympathy, which took on something like its current emotional meaning in the seventeenth century, but prior to that denoted an affinity, not only between people but also in relation to things, especially in medical contexts (Jahoda, 2005). In Renaissance medicine, the concept of sympathy served as a metaphor for the physical phenomenon of resonance (e.g., sympathetic vibrations), implying that there was a coupling or cooperative effect between medicine and illness, as in the homeopathic doctrine of "like curing." The psychological meaning of sharing the feelings of another person or being affected by their suffering existed in parallel with this physical meaning. "Empathy" entered the English language psychology literature in 1909 as a translation for German psychologist Theodor Lipps's notion of *Einfühlung* (lit., "feeling-into"). British psychologist Edward Titchener coined the term expressly to set *empathy* apart from *sympathy* (Jahoda 2005). For Lipps, however:

the concept of Einfühlung took on a quite general significance as the avenue of human understanding of nature. He considered empathy the primitive connection to the world that admitted of no further explanation; all other modes of knowledge and interaction were parasitic on it. . . . It also accounts for relations among human beings . . . Lipps differed with his main explanatory rival on this issue, Benno Erdmann, in rejecting an *analogical* approach, which understood the recognition of others' existence and behaviors as dependent on a mental parallelism with one's own. (Moyn, 2005, p. 59)

Although this parallelism of experience recalls the earlier notion of "resonance," it points to the modern conception of empathy as based on analogical reasoning or imagination. But empathy is not simply conceptual analogy; it can involve bodily feelings or "resonance" with another at several levels: adopting similar bodily stances, postures, or gestures; experiencing similar emotions; and imagining oneself in similar situations through images, stories, or scenarios.

In Karl Jaspers's early text on psychopathology, he recognized empathy as a privileged way of understanding the psychological dynamics of another person by entering that person's psychology. By this, Jaspers meant the affective and meaning-saturated structures of experience, which, he argued, differed from the logical structures of rational argument or association:

Rational understanding always leads to a statement that the psychic content was simply a rational connection, understandable without the help of any psychology. Empathic understanding, on the other hand, always leads directly into the psychic connection itself. Rational understanding is merely an aid to psychology, empathic understanding brings us to psychology itself. (Jaspers, 1913/1997, p. 304)

The notion that empathy allows access to what is specifically "psycho"-logical recognizes the central role of emotion in shaping psychic life. From the 1950s onward, empathy became a keyword in the professional worlds of psychiatry and clinical psychology, spurred on by the recognition that the effort to listen closely and track another's experience was a key element in successful psychotherapy (Rogers, 1957). This positive effect may be due to the knowledge of the other's experience empathy affords, but also might occur because empathic tracking or attunement can convey a sense of presence, warmth, closeness, solidarity, and concern.

Components of Empathy

Empathy can be decomposed into several distinct but interacting processes: sensorimotor synchrony (mirroring facial expressions, breathing or moving in synchrony with another person); vicarious emotion (or emotional contagion – feeling the same kind of emotion as another person); perspective taking (seeing or understanding things as if from the other's point of view); and imaginative elaboration (constructing scenarios to situate others' actions and experiences in their life context). Some of these effects may occur through relatively simple mechanisms of perception-action coupling but others require more complex cognitive functions and enactments that depend, to varying degrees, on previous experience or detailed knowledge of particular social worlds.

For example, a built-in link between action and perception leads people to automatically mimic the postures, mannerisms, facial expressions, and behaviors of others (Chartrand & Bargh, 1999). This "chameleon effect" is unintentional and usually not conscious (although we may notice it after the fact or have it brought to our attention by others). The effect is stronger when paying close attention to the other (Chartrand & Laskin, 2013). Even when subtle and unnoticed, mimicry and synchronous behavior may convey important information about the other. Imitating another's facial expression, for example, may lead us to experience some of the same sensations or emotions. We may not be aware of the source of our feeling, but find ourselves anxious, sad, or uncomfortable in response to another's facial expression of fear, grief, or pain. More complex forms of "inner imitation" may subserve empathic understanding of others' thoughts and feelings. Mimicry is associated with feelings of being like another person and a tendency toward helpful or compassionate action on the other's behalf (Valdesolo & DeSteno, 2011).

Theories of empathy reflect concepts of emotion. If emotions are universal bodily experiences, then we can empathize simply by having much the same feeling. In response to someone who is pacing anxiously and hyperventilating, we find ourselves feeling restless, anxious, and breathing rapidly. We can read off knowledge of the other by recognizing our own emotional state – although to avoid confusing our own feelings with those of the other we need some additional recognition that our feeling originated in the other.

This theory of empathy is sometimes used to explain the contagious spread of basic emotions from one person to another. If empathic mirroring evokes multiple elements in the right proportion, we can extend this notion to emotions that involve more complex blends of feelings. To the extent that more complex emotions involve sequences or configurations of feelings related to specific contexts or responses from others, empathy requires matching the same temporal trajectory or spatial deployment across a social landscape. Finally, for the most complex (and culture-specific) emotions, which involve narrative constructions that are anchored in personal history and social contexts, empathy requires understanding particular scenarios, which, in turn, depends on a shared fund of cultural knowledge and experience.

Cognitive theories of emotion emphasize that complex sentiments involve not simply bodily dispositions to respond in particular ways but appraisals of the personal and social meaning of situations (Oatley, 1992). Some of these meanings are encoded in representations of past events, some are enacted in one's stance or disposition to respond, still others present as possible courses of actions with their anticipated consequences and response from others. In this way, an emotion is embedded in a web of meaning that links past, present, and future, through multiple processes, including: embodied learning (habits, conditioned responses); cognitive representational structures (memories, images and schemas); and a social context that exerts ongoing influence on experience. Thus, emotions involve bodily, cognitive, and socially situated enactments.

To achieve accurate empathy, these basic bodily and cognitive-emotional actions must be sustained over time to yield the layering, sequence, and texture of complex emotions. However, from the moment one has an emotional response to another (empathic or otherwise) it is caught up in one's own inner dynamics of identity and emotion, eliciting countervailing feelings and reactions that may intensify, change, or displace the original empathic response. In fact, it is easy to mistake a reactive emotion for an understanding of the other. For example, a paranoid patient might evoke fear in a clinician when the patient is mainly experiencing anger. Fear and anger are reciprocally related responses to threat (Cannon's [1929/1963] "fight or flight"), and the balance between the two is modulated by perceptions of relative power, safety, and position that have an internal economy as well as interpersonal dynamics. In a sense, fear and anger form a larger affective system that involves both participants. The recognition of danger might be shared, but the causes and responses may be quite divergent, leading the clinician to fail to understand the patient's predicament.

In the encounter with another, then, we may feel a complementary or reactive feeling that actually makes it harder to track their experience. This is especially challenging with strong feelings, both negative and positive. Vicarious emotion can lead to distancing from feelings that are too intense, or else to obscuring the experience of the other with one's own thoughts and feelings. Thus, empathy requires modulating one's own emotional reactions to the other in order to remain open and track the other's feelings.

Clinically, empathy is expected to motivate compassionate concern. However, this is not an automatic outcome of empathy. Empathic concern requires an optimal level of empathy, coupled with socially scripted ways to communicate, acknowledge, and respond to the distress of the other. Empathy combined with knowledge of the causes of suffering leads to compassion. Empathy allows us to feel something like what the other is feeling, but because this feeling occurs in the midst of our own struggles, striving, and commitments, it immediately acquires new meaning and consequence. The initial moment of empathic attunement is not sufficient to stay on track with another – we must have conceptual models of their predicament and an equally acute awareness of difference. Nor does a moment of feeling the other's feeling guarantee our kindness and concern: Empathy can serve sadism as well as compassion (Decety, 2014; Decety & Ickes, 2011). To lead to compassionate action, empathy must be coupled with moral commitments and translated into action, guided by detailed knowledge of specific pragmatic social and cultural contexts.

Empathy can go well beyond engaging with others' emotions to include other dimensions of subjectivity. Understanding the nature of subjectivity, therefore, is crucial for understanding the dynamics, prospects, and limits of empathy. For example, how we frame empathy depends on whether we view child development as starting from an autonomous self, which only gradually over time comes to know of the existence of others, or we give primacy to a relational self that can only be formed in the presence and through the actions of others. Most current outlines of the developmental history of the self hold that interaction between the nascent self and the other allows the construction of progressively more complex representations, accompanied by self-reflexive awareness. In this view, empathy is a consequence of the social origins and embedding of the self.

Empathy may also require a social response from the other. Accurate or sustained empathy depends on a process of error correction, in which failures to track the other's feelings are recognized, and one's attention, stance, or interpretive frame is shifted and realigned in response to feedback. Empathy as a communicative process is dialogical: both participants must work to achieve some shared understanding and experience (Vreeke & van der Mark, 2003). In this process, the clinician's ongoing commitment to understanding the other, including how they handle moments of failure, may be as important for empathic rapport as the initial experience of affective attunement.

The Biology of Empathy

As a psychological construct, empathy covers a range of capacities and behaviors, with possible evolutionary roots in several distinct, adaptive functions: the ability to imitate, learn from, and understand the perspectives of others; the rapid communication of emotional states and expectations; and the motivating effect of experiencing another's predicament as one's own (Preston & de Waal, 2002). Recent research has identified several brain regions and mechanisms that may contribute to the process of empathizing with another, including systems at the levels of the brainstem, the autonomic nervous system (ANS), the hypothalamic-pituitary-adrenal axis (HPA), and endocrine systems, which are involved in attachment and social affiliation, emotion regulation, and reactivity (Decety, 2011; Bernhardt & Singer, 2012; Decety & Fotopoulu, 2015). Although capacities for empathic concern may have evolved originally as a way to ensure parental care and attachments with family or members of a social group (Decety, 2014; Decety & Ickes, 2011), empathy functions more broadly to allow understanding, trust, and social cooperation with people from different backgrounds.

Research on social cognition has approached empathy as a process that involves either the simulation of others' experiences through vicarious activation of networks involved in emotion and action imitation, or the construction of a theory of the other's experience by building a cognitive model or representation (Goldman, 2011). Models of empathy based purely on a cognitive theory of the other ignore the obvious role that bodily feeling plays in everyday experiences of empathy. Moreover, affective and cognitive-social processes mediated by bodily enactments may also contribute directly to sensitivity to interpersonal communication, empathic accuracy, and empathic concern (Decety & Fotopoulu, 2015). However, "simulation" and "theory-based" theories of empathy are not entirely distinct notions. To the extent that building a theory of the other requires knowledge of particular contexts or scenarios, the two approaches to empathy converge on the notion that we may need to use of our own capacities for action, imagination, and emotional response to generate a sense of what others must be feeling given their specific circumstances.

Current social neuroscience perspectives on empathy suggest that we understand others' experience through at least two processes: (1) vicarious activation of the similar neural networks that are part of own action systems, as well as (2) a more cognitive (i.e., top-down or "representational") process involving mentalizing or theory of mind. Of course, even the cognitive approach – in which we create "representations of the others' potential mental state" (Engen & Singer, 2013, p. 276) – will activate action observation networks.

We may understand the quality of others' actions, intentions, and experiences by simulating them at various levels, both bodily or sensorimotor and more conceptual or abstract. Action simulation, for example, gives us access to another's emotional experience and its associational logic through activation of our own emotion-related networks. This model immediately raises questions about the extent to which this emotional logic is hardwired and universal, acquired only through specific developmental experiences, or emergent from ongoing interactions with others in specific social contexts or local worlds.

The observation of "mirror neurons" in macaque monkeys was thought to provide a biological basis for action understanding and imitation learning (Rizzolati & Craighero, 2004). It was suggested that a similar common coding of motor action and perception in humans might subserve understanding of others' actions, and even intentions (Gallese, Keysers, & Rizzolatti, 2004). Several imaging studies have attempted to show that an analogous system underlies empathy, which is based at least in part on shared representations of emotions. Although there is still debate about the significance of these systems, evidence does suggest an overlap in several neural circuits, including those involved in "sensorimotor resonance," that are activated during first-person experience of emotions and observing emotions in others (Bernhardt & Singer, 2012; Decety 2011).

In particular, pain-related circuitry shows similar activation during one's own experience of pain and when observing another person in pain (Jackson, Rainville, & Decety, 2006). As well, the social pain we experience firsthand – the pain of rejection, separation, and loss – activates some of the same neural circuitry as physical pain (Eisenberger, 2012; Eisenberger, Lieberman, & Williams, 2003). This grounding of basic interpersonal events in bodily responses to pain provides anchor points for a shared empathic understanding of suffering. Similarly, the brain regions that activate in response to another's display of emotions, such as fear, anxiety, happiness, or disgust, may overlap with regions that activate when we experience those feelings ourselves. For example, the anterior insula activates both at the sight of a disgusted expression on the face of another and when one personally feels disgust; the amplitude of the activation correlates with the degree of felt disgust (Wicker et al.,

2003). Similarly, happiness and anxiety may evoke parallel patterns of activation in a witness (Fan, Duncan, de Greck, & Northoff, 2011).

Although much was made of the existence of a mirror-neuron system in the decade following its discovery in monkeys, subsequent research has tempered initial claims for its explanatory power (Hickok, 2014). Mirror neuron networks may represent an evolutionary prerequisite for acquiring culture through imitative learning (Arbib, 2011). But the functional systems that contribute to empathy also have a developmental history that occurs within a cultural world. Emotions are not just bodily actions or dispositions but cognitive responses to complex social scenarios. Empathy for complex feelings, therefore, requires the close coordination of action simulation and other processes underlying social cognition, including "theory of mind" that is, "the ability to make attributions about mental states such as intentions, desires or beliefs to others (and oneself) and to understand that others have beliefs, desires and intentions that are different from one's own" (Singer, 2012). Moreover, the simulation of another's experience cannot stop with their inner theater; it must extend outward to include a simulation of the social world that gives meaning and consequence to the other's concepts, values and actions.

The notions of mirror neurons, mimcry, and vicarious emotion take us only a short distance toward explaining empathy for complex feelings and their corresponding social predicaments, which are constituted by whole social worlds. Empathy for another via the route of bodily mirroring or resonance depends in part on a shared developmental history. When that fails we must go the long route – constructing imaginative scenarios or more abstract theories of what might be going on for the other. In effect, the mirror is empty until it is held up to the social world.

Although empathy is a potential bridge to understanding, fellow-feeling, and connection, it also depends on our level of identification with the other. Our empathic response to others is modulated by whether we view them as similar to ourselves or as somehow foreign or alien (Engen & Singer, 2013). Indeed, empathic arousal may be reduced in response to people from a different ethnic group, and this effect likely occurs early in information processing (Decety, 2011). Empathic attunement thus reflects the stance toward the other that we bring to the encounter, making it easier to empathize with those with whom we identify, and difficult to empathize with those we view as strange or disturbing. This poses an important challenge for psychiatry.

Psychopathology and Empathic Understanding

Some forms of psychopathology render people difficult to understand or empathize with. Difficulties of empathy and understanding may be due to their unfamiliar or bizarre experiences, altered logic or thought disorder, or inappropriate or strange emotional responses and behaviors. These differences may impede empathy in several ways: (1) by leading to experiences that are difficult to simulate or imagine because they have no common correlate in everyday life or clear relation to familiar cultural norms and conventions (e.g., bizarre hallucinations or disorganized thinking), (2) by changing the organization of behavior in ways that make it difficult to intuit the person's goals (e.g., pursuing self-destructive behaviors with no apparent motive or rationale), (3) by changes in emotional expression that make it hard to track the person's feeling state (e.g., the blunted or inappropriate affect of schizophrenia), or (4) by presenting situations that are simply too terrible to imagine in any detail (e.g., the suffering of survivors of torture) (Kirmayer, 2001).

Technical models of psychopathology – and of the process of therapeutic communication itself – allow the clinician to move past these difficulties by interpreting the rupture in terms of specific kinds of symptoms (e.g., thought disorder, blunted affect, dissociation). Psychiatric diagnosis maps the suffering of the person onto specific types of "disorder," which allows the clinician to fill in gaps in understanding or rapport with models of psychopathological process. The technical model then serves as a partial substitute for empathic understanding of the patient's experience. The model can be used to make predictions about the patient's experience and behavior and allows the clinician to cordon off areas of incomprehension as "symptoms" in their own right.

The prototype of the strange is psychosis, which is defined in terms of nonconsensual, bizarre, and incoherent experience. As Jaspers put it:

> The affective illnesses appear to us to be open to empathy and natural but the various types of 'madness' do not seem open to empathy and appear unnatural. The theory, which so far seems the aptest, explains the various features of this ununderstandable psychic life in terms of a split in the psychic life. (Jaspers, 1913/ 1997, p. 578)

This hypothetical split, enshrined in Bleuler's (1911/1950) term "schizophrenia," means that there are causal or structuring elements of psychology outside of experience – and hence, beyond the possibility of knowing by empathy. Only explanation can allow us to approximate, by rational reconstruction, the underlying logic of such psychotic experience.

Of course, it might be possible to understand odd experiences like hallucinations or the thought disorder of schizophrenia by altering normal experience to simulate psychosis. For example, one could take a hallucinogenic drug to try to gain some appreciation of what it is like to hallucinate and then call up the memory of this experience when faced with a hallucinating patient (Klüver, 1966). Indeed, in the 1950s and 1960s, psychiatrists Abram Hoffer, Humphrey Osmond, and colleagues followed just this route, taking LSD in an effort to understand the nature of psychotic experience in schizophrenia and to find clues to its underlying mechanism (Dyck, 2006). But if specific attributions or misattributions of cause are part of the psychosis, then it would be crucial to be unaware of having taken the drug in order to experience something akin to the confusion, malaise, anxiety, panic, loss of control, and desperate effort to impute meaning that can occur with acute psychosis.

Similarly, although reading autobiographical accounts of psychotic experience can tutor empathy, such accounts tend to impose coherence through narrative smoothing and secondary emplotment, resulting in a tamed and tidied version of what was originally deeply perplexing, confusing, chaotic and terrifying (Humpston, 2014). Here is where aesthetics can conflict with clinical and ethical demands for accurate representation. Accounts of illness that are closer to lived experience may be difficult to read, though, either because they are disorganized and confusing, or because they are filled with mundane detail, repetitious, and emotionally flat. In some instances, the nonnarrative organization and evocative power of metaphor and imagery in lyric poetry may provide a better vehicle for conveying the texture of illness experience (Kirmayer, 2007).

Efforts in psychiatry to make sense of incomprehensible experiences by explanation have followed several routes. Phenomenological psychology offers a way to characterize the underlying structures of experience (Henriksen, 2013; Parnas & Gallagher, Chapter 3, *this volume*). Thus, the thought disorder and delusions of schizophrenia can be viewed as resulting from a kind of solipsism, in which the patient experiences others as products of his own mind (Sass, 1994). Neurobiology can also provide ways to make sense of anomalous and incomprehensible experience. For example, the delusions of schizophrenia may be explained as a consequence of heightened salience of stimuli (Kapur, 2003). Again, the Capgras delusion of familiar people being replaced by imposters can be explained by a functional disconnection between brain circuits involved in facial recognition and the feeling of emotional familiarity (Ellis & Lewis, 2001). Both phenomenological and neurobiological approaches can be combined, as Northoff (Chapter 4, *this volume*) illustrates in his conjectures about the role of the default mode network in the experience of self in schizophrenia and depression.

By themselves, the explanatory constructs of phenomenology and neurobiology cannot yield the experience of rapport and connection to the other that comes from empathy, but they can be used to supplement empathic experience, allowing the clinician to stay in touch with the perspective and concerns of the patient (Ratcliffe, 2012). In practice, empathy works both ways: maintaining a human connection with the patient, while contributing to clinical understanding.

In the case of mood disorders, there is an affective logic that can be followed by analogy to our own moments of emotional extremity, but the difference between an experience of extreme joy or despair that lasts a moment and one of much longer duration may be crucial to the quality of the experience and, as with the experience of chronic pain, it may be hard to extrapolate from the common acute experience to the unending expanse of feeling characteristic of mania or severe depression (Ratcliffe, 2014). The temporal duration and unrelieved intensity of a manic or depressive episode is crucial to its experience and, once again, may be hard to communicate through narrative or bodily means.

It may be particularly difficult to empathize with the experience of individuals with personality disorders, who exhibit recurrent maladaptive patterns of behavior with little recognition of the ways in which their own actions contribute to their difficulties. The affective instability of borderline personality disorder challenges empathy, not simply because of the intensity or abruptness of changes in affect, but because the emotional shifts may occur in response to idiosyncratic cues and elicit self-destructive behaviors. Further, it may be difficult to empathize with an experience that is centered on an absence, and this may account for our difficulty empathizing with individuals who we believe are exhibiting denial or dissociative symptoms. We must enter into the world of "as if," yet we retain some awareness of the "as if" nature of our experience, which places us in an ironic position that undercuts accurate empathy. Describing denial and dissociation as self-deception may reflect this failure of empathy.

Psychodynamic theories function may contribute to clinical empathy by identifying a developmental history, persistent schema, or recurring scenario in which the patient's emotional experience and behavior make sense. They also introduce models of gradations of awareness and volition that may accord better with patients' experience than folk psychological models that dichotomize all behavior into voluntary or involuntary, intention or accident.

Psychodynamic clinicians have accorded a privileged status to empathy as a way of understanding others, not only through the emotional meaning it conveys but also by characterizing patterns of response to failures of empathy in the clinical alliance (Akhtar, 2007). Patients enact their own emotional and interpersonal conflicts in the microcosm of psychotherapy. Of course, clinicians have their own conflicts, and empathy is vulnerable to distortion by the therapist's personal associations and emotional responses, which may be projected onto the patient or bias interpretation in other ways. Clinicians, therefore, need to become aware of their own personal history as a source of both conscious and unconscious biases, and take these biases explicitly into account. According to psychodynamic theory, removing or accounting for the distortions of such countertransference should allow more accurate access to the experience of the other.

The epistemic problem of distinguishing empathy from projection is complicated by several factors: (1) the intensity and immediacy of one's own feelings places them in the foreground of perception; (2) the tacit, habitual, taken-for-granted, and unquestioned quality of one's own perspective is woven into the background of perception; (3) defensive processes work against uncovering one's own biases and concerns that may be sources of conflict because they are anxiety-laden or they conflict with one's ideals; (4) the mutual influence or looping effect in interpersonal dyads, in which participants work toward a consensual view, so that an empathic response that is initially inaccurate becomes accurate after the fact; and (5), in a wider instance of this same process, the larger social forces that project onto the clinical dyad itself shape and constrain the imagination of both participants. This last process occurs in ways that can create pseudo-mutuality, or pseudo-empathy, as both individuals are drawing from a limited range of options for self-understanding. In this instance, participants do not really tune into each other's initial experience but simply rewrite their joint experience in a way that conforms to a conventional narrative. This dilemma also points to the problem of seeking some notion of personal authenticity through empathy, when collective norms and ways of understanding the self may occlude, suppress, displace, and transform individual experiences. There is a politics of experience that governs what kinds of self-understanding are available in the moment and viable in the social worlds of patients and clinicians.

Empathy in the Intercultural Clinical Encounter

The many forms of odd or unusual experience that impede empathy pose a particular challenge in intercultural clinical work. Patients and clinicians with different cultural backgrounds and social positions must do additional work to build bridges between their experiential worlds in order to reach some mutual understanding and collaboration. Although empathic feeling may give the illusion of occurring in the moment without conscious mediation, it results from the confluence of extended narratives, stories told from different points of view. Understanding these stories depends on a fund of cultural and historical background knowledge and an appreciation of the current contexts or lifeworld of the patient. This is the type of knowledge produced by ethnography, which relies on both participant observation and empathic understanding to gain a picture of others' social worlds.

In the typical ethnographic study, the anthropologist lives in the community and has access to groups of people who are related to one another and who can provide context for one another's actions and experiences. Cultural background knowledge is recounted or displayed in everyday activities and efforts at self-presentation and justification. All of this helps the ethnographer make sense of individuals' experience. In the clinical setting, however, the patient's lifeworld is not present and can only be imagined or investigated through explicit questions.

Experiencing a close approximation to another's feelings requires imaginatively reconstructing and inhabiting some portion of a similar social world, which of necessity means bracketing off or de-centering from our own position. Failures of empathy thus can occur because our emotional experience does not fit the experience of the other or because we lack the social background knowledge and experience to construct the correct model or imagine the right responses in a particular situation. Social and cultural barriers to empathy are evident, for example, in clinical encounters when patient and clinician differ in racialized identity, socio-economic class, or education. Understanding the social world of the other requires that we have the right mental furniture.

Ethnographic reflections on empathy have tended to view it either as a privileged mode of access to others' experience and hence an effective way to gain knowledge of other cultures, or else as a difficult – if not impossible – achievement, the outcome of deep cultural knowledge that is attained rarely and only through prolonged and intensive participation in another's way of life. On the first view, empathy gives us ready access to a universal core of human experience inscribed in our nervous system by evolutionary history or acquired anew in each person's encounter with the existential givens of life; the second view holds that empathy's limits and failures serve to reveal the radical alterity and incommensurability of cultural worlds.

Cultural-interpretive approaches to empathy emphasize the social construction and cultural embedding of all experience, which limits the ability of those who do not share the same history and social position to fully understand and enter into each other's experience (Geertz 1983, 1984; Rosaldo 1980). Only "thick description," building up a densely layered model or scenario replete with cultural associations, can offer a way toward a semblance of the other's experience. An empathic response depends on accessing a system of associations governed by multiple logics: (1) an affective logic of how one emotion is linked to and follows another in a pattern of response that is partly "hard-wired" and partly acquired and (2) a social logic of the meaning of specific situations, predicaments, and scenarios that involve patterns of response acquired through learning the rules, roles, and practices of a social world.

The clinician's ability to elicit and understand social and cultural context is at the core of the notion of "cultural competence" in clinical care (Kleinman & Benson, 2006). Cultural competence begins with the clinician's self-knowledge and an appreciation of how historical circumstances situate the encounter with the patient. The histories of colonialism, slavery, racism, and discrimination that precede the clinical encounter give each word and gesture added meaning. The burden of this history raises particular obstacles to clinical empathy that have to do with the social and cultural embedding of clinician and patient. The effects of this history have been approached through the notions of cultural transference and countertransference (Adams, 1996; Comas-Dias & Jacobsen, 1991). Working through these potential distortions requires knowledge of the larger social contexts of the patient.

Culturally competent clinicians consider the potential impact of these larger social and political contexts on their own feelings and those of their patients and employ a set of strategies for monitoring and managing the subsequent interaction. But the language of competence implies a kind of mastery and control that belies the vulnerability and uncertainty of the clinical encounter in which empathy must sometimes fail.

A social-psychological perspective might argue that, in principle, empathy has no limits because experience itself is fundamentally interpersonal and intersubjective in origin. However, the intersubjective nature of experience does not guarantee the possibility of empathy in every encounter for several reasons: (1) there is plenty of inarticulate experience that precedes, exists to one side, or transcends the limits of language and hence remains compelling yet difficult to communicate explicitly; (2) although social construction may create a shared reality, pockets of idiosyncratic and unique experience always arise in the private theater of the mind, which may be enacted at the margins of culturally prescribed roles, rules, and practices; and (3) most importantly for intercultural settings, people occupy different social and cultural worlds. These three facts ensure that there are substantial practical and epistemic limits to empathy.

Empathy's limits may be particularly severe in intercultural clinical work. First, linguistic differences may make it difficult to communicate, and, even where interpreters are used effectively, cultural differences may challenge the tacit assumption that words mean much the same thing for patient and clinician. Narratives are interpreted against a backdrop of shared meaning, and because of divergent life experiences and cultural frames of reference, an account that seems clear to the clinician may have markedly different meaning for the patient.

There may also be issues of safety that prevent patients from disclosing aspects of their experience due to concern about the trustworthiness of the clinician or the institution (Kirmayer, 2001). Even where patients feel a high degree of trust and confidence in the safety of the clinical setting and relationship, they may still fear exposure to their community with the risk of shame and stigmatization.

An additional source of ambiguity arises from the fact that patients may only have limited awareness of their own social and cultural context, since much of it is so familiar that it is taken for granted and constitutes background knowledge that is not usually talked about or reflected on. Often, it is only with moving across cultures, through migration or interaction with people from very different backgrounds, that one becomes aware of this tacit dimension of experience.

Then too, patients see the world from their own perspectives and may not be able to provide crucial information about interpersonal, family, or community issues that contribute to their problems, constrain their options or, conversely, represent important resources and opportunities for recovery. These larger social contexts may exert influences across great geographic distances, through a broader electronic community, and over long periods of time, through historical memory that is transmitted through collective practices of commemoration, or in the ways that communities view others. Moreover, these social-interactional processes may constitute significant clinical issues in their own right so that adequate clinical assessment requires attention to historical ecological, and political contexts.

These issues have both practical and ethical implications. The practical implications include the need to take time to build a relationship of sufficient trust to elicit relevant information and the need to involve members of patients' families or others in their entourage to understand the context. These pragmatic considerations for the clinician–patient relationship require changes in institutional practices to make the clinical setting safe and familiar in ways that inspire confidence and allow patients and their families to engage in clinical dialogue and collaboration. The ethical dilemmas that remain concern what stance to take when empathy fails or, since – as we have argued – empathy is inherently limited and unreliable, how to address the other at the limits of empathy.

Ethics at the Limits of Empathy

The work of the philosopher Emannuel Levinas represents a concerted effort to found an ethical stance on the very fact of the limits of empathy. Human subjectivity is rooted in alterity; this is not only a developmental fact, but the origin of an ethical imperative. For Levinas, our humanity resides precisely in our actions at the limits of empathy, in the encounter with the other. Many recent authors have recognized the relevance of Levinas's philosophy for thinking through the ethics of the clinical encounter in both psychiatry and psychology (Freeman, 2014; Gantt & Williams, 2002; Orange, 2011), as well as medicine more generally (Tauber, 1999).

Levinas describes the confrontation with the "face" of the other, by which he means not only the literal face, but the reality of the other's human presence, as the root of the emergence of the self as an ethical being (Bergo, 2011). This recognition of the other's presence transcends culture. "The nudity of the face is a stripping with no cultural ornament – an absolution – a detachment of its form in the heart of production of form" (Levinas, 2003, p. 32). Although the face is the medium through which we encounter others' personal identity and emotional state, this expression is always incomplete, so the face is also a constant reminder of otherness. Levinas sees the ultimate unknowability of the other as both the first impetus and an ongoing call to an urgent ethical awareness.

The face of the person before us, in its nakedness, requires that we acknowledge both their difference from us and their human vulnerability. "Levinas takes the key to embodiment to lie in its vulnerability, a vulnerability that opens the human to the suffering of others" (Cohen, 2003, p. xxxiii) – and empathy can be understood as the process of this opening to the other. This vulnerability, in turn, calls our own moral self into being as an agent responsible for the other. Levinas views responsibility for the other as "the essential, primary and fundamental structure of subjectivity" (Levinas, 1985, p. 95). The demand that issues from this presence of others in their separateness is asymmetrical: It asks us to adopt an open stance toward the other regardless of his or her stance toward us, as the basis on which any ethical response begins (Critchley, 2007).

As a philosopher in the phenomenological tradition, Levinas brackets the historical and political realities of the social world, attempting to frame his argument in a general way. What is largely missing from his writing is a developmental psychological account and, along with that, attention to the social and cultural situatedness and historical particularity of the individual who is the other (Gallagher, 2014). Certainly, Levinas recognizes the centrality of culture, along with embodiment, as the medium through which any realization of self and other must occur. However, his discussions of alterity lack consideration of the politics and pragmatics of culture, identity, and ethnicity. For Levinas,

Although in principle the Other is always a singular being – and hence the one to one rather than communal nature of the ethical relation – s/he is devoid of any concrete identity, unmarked by gender, age, religion or ethnicity. The only defining characteristic is vulnerability, the state of being abandoned, persecuted and in need, which take human form in the figures of the widow, stranger and orphan only as kind[s] of archetypes, personifications existing through history and across culture. (Klaushofer, 2000, p. 62)

This lack of attention to the particular is ironic, given Levinas's steadfast concern with the other, but it arises from his philosophical and theological aims (Moyn, 2004). It is crucial for the universality of his argument that it be framed without reference to any specific language, ethnicity or religion. In recognizing the necessity of responsibility for the other, which includes hospitality toward the stranger, Levinas resists any attempt to divide humanity into two classes based on empathy or election. "The ambiguity of Levinas' treatment of the 'absolutely foreign', then is a reflection of an ethics that responds to a difficult reality in which ethnocentrism is always a possibility while retaining its commitment to welcome the stranger" (Klaushofer, 2000, p. 70).

The implication of Levinas's ethics of encounter for clinical work is to always remind us of both our enduring responsibility for the other and their ultimate unknowability. In clinical settings where we value our capacity for empathy and may be quick to assume that we understand patients with very different backgrounds and experiences, we are encouraged to accept those differences and so recognize the other as a person – distinct in face, voice, and agency – who commands our attention, openness, and hospitality.

In reality, of course, empathy is never truly the result of an encounter between two culturally naked human beings, but always a chapter in an ongoing historical confrontation between peoples of different backgrounds, experiences, and identities. Adopting the basic ethical stance at the center of Levinas's work opens the way for clinicians to develop an awareness and analysis of the many specific forms of difference and their practical, psychological, and political consequences in the clinical encounter and the wider social world.

In psychiatry, this was the unfinished project of Frantz Fanon (1982). Colonial psychiatry argued for a fundamental difference between the psyches of Europeans and non-Europeans. This argument not only created a profound divide between patient and clinician, and justified the privilege and domination of the colonizers, it also contributed to the painful self-estrangement that was a primary effect of colonialism. For Fanon, psychiatry was an attempt to relieve (or transcend) this self-estrangement as well as alienation from the other:

Fanon's contribution as a psychiatrist in the colony was to insist on the importance of the cultural context in which symptoms appear, to demonstrate that therapeutic institutions need to maintain a concrete link and a structural similarity to the local culture of the patients. The condition for a successful therapy was that there existed, he said, a common culture, shared by the patient and the practitioner. (Vergès, 1996, p. 85)

The legacy of colonialism persists in the conceptual models and institutional practices of psychiatry (Kirmayer, 2006) and in the continuing struggles of individuals and communities to come to terms with the gross inequities of power and status in our "postcolonial," globalizing world (Gibson, 2011). In the flux of the contemporary world, clinicians often have the added challenge of finding common ground where there is no common culture. Recognizing the violent histories and structural inequalities that frame our practice is an essential preliminary to creating a safe space of the clinical encounter. Within the safety of this space – founded on mutual recognition and respect for difference – we can pursue the work of learning the other's language and working with them to transform suffering.

Conclusion: A Pedagogy of Empathy?

Psychiatric care is rooted in the empathic encounter with suffering others in all their individuality and strangeness. Clinicians' relationship to their own emotional wounds and vulnerability and their knowledge of psychopathology both serve to maintain a stance of openness, respect and concern that sustains the helping relationship (Kirmayer, 2003). Intercultural work in psychiatry makes it clear, however, that empathy depends on detailed knowledge of the other's social world in both its individual and collective dimensions. This requires imaginative engagement with the other's personal history, willingness to experience strong affect, and the self-reflexivity to distinguish one's own emotional reactions from those of the other. Empathy involves an interactional process of emotional attunement that requires a communicative situation in which both parties are free to be open to mutual influence and to tolerate ambiguity and uncertainty. Even when these conditions obtain, however, there are limits to what can be known about another.

The failure, fracture, or even radical impossibility of empathy has crucial things to teach us about the nature of our humanity generally, and about the contours and possibilities of subjectivity and relatedness. It also underscores the importance of phenomenology to map the contours of psychopathological experience, and ethnographic work to explicate the contexts that constitute diverse lifeworlds, which are the only reliable roads to mutual understanding.

What sort of pedagogy can ensure the development and deployment of the clinician's capacity for empathy, particularly when facing others in extremis? Literature, film, the visual and performing arts all provide ways to get a glimpse of others' experience or touch the other in our selves. Recognizing the performative or enacted nature of empathy, some have argued for the value of training in method acting as a way to practice imagining another's world and to better appreciate another's emotional experience and moral predicament (Larson & Yao, 2005; Verducci, 2000). We might also advocate "method listening" – cultivating the ability to tolerate the sometimes dark and tangled emotions evoked by poetic language and imagery (Kirmayer, 2007). The aim is not to aestheticize experience but to become attuned to the resonances of everyday language and "rhetoric without eloquence" (Levinas, 1993, p. 135). This listening depends on a fund of knowledge about the world so that words are anchored in their sensual, social, and political meanings in context. To achieve this, psychiatry must move beyond the consulting room or the clinic to engage with the communities, both local and global, virtual and embodied, that constitute the lifeworlds of patients.

An empathic stance must include some acceptance of the limits, failure, and even the impossibility of empathy. If nothing human is alien to me then nothing alien will be recognized as essentially human. Cultural and psychological (mis)appropriation, narcissism, collusion, and submission to the powerful can create the illusion of empathy when something radically different is at play: the effacement or erasure of the other through the imposition of some generic feeling, cultural emblem, or formulaic account. In psychiatry, diagnostic labels, psychodynamic interpretations, and biological explanations can all serve this function of effacing the other. When the clinician can set aside these technical models and explanations to encounter the suffering person, a new kind of dialogue can be built on the recognition of the co-presence of sameness and difference. Acknowledging the limits of empathy then becomes a path toward mutual recognition, respect, and collaboration.

Acknowledgment

Portions of this chapter are adapted from "Empathy and alterity in cultural psychiatry" by L. J. Kirmayer, 2008, *Ethos, 36*(4). Copyright 2008 by the Society for Psychological Anthropology. Adapted with permission.

REFERENCES

Abel, T. (1957). The operation called *Verstehen*. *American Journal of Sociology, 54*(3), 211–18. http://dx.doi.org/10.1086/220318

Adams, M. V. (1996). *The multicultural imagination: Race, color, and the unconscious*. New York, NY: Routledge.

Akhtar, S. (Ed.) (2007). *Listening to others: Developmental and clinical aspects of empathy and attunement*. Lanham, MD: Jason Aronson.

Arbib, M. A. (2011). From mirror neurons to complex imitation in the evolution of language and tool use. *Annual Review of Anthropology, 40*, 257–73. http://dx.doi.org/10.1146/annurev-anthro-081309-145722

Bergo, B. (2011). The face in Levinas: Toward a phenomenology of substitution. *Angelaki: Journal of the Theoretical Humanities, 16*(1), 17–40. http://dx.doi.org/10.1080/0969725X.2011.564362

Bernhardt, B. C., & Singer, T. (2012). The neural basis of empathy. *Annual Review of Neuroscience, 35*, 1–23. http://dx.doi.org/10.1146/annurev-neuro-062111-150536

Bleuler, E. (1950). *Dementia praecox or the group of schizophrenias* (J. Zenkin, Trans.). New York, NY: International Universities. (Original work published 1911)

Cannon, W. B. (1963). *Bodily changes in pain, hunger, fear and rage*. New York, NY: Harper and Row. (Original work published 1929)

Chartrand, T. L., & Bargh, J. A. (1999). The chameleon effect: The perception–behavior link and social interaction. *Journal of Personality and Social Psychology, 76*(6), 893. http://dx.doi.org/10.1037/0022-3514.76.6.893

Chartrand, T. L., & Lakin, J. L. (2013). The antecedents and consequences of human behavioral mimicry. *Annual Review of Psychology, 64*, 285–308. http://dx.doi.org/10.1146/annurev-psych-113011-143754

Cohen, R. A. (2003). Introduction: Humanism and anti-humanism – Levinas, Cassirer, and Heidegger. In E. Levinas, E., & Poller, N. *Humanism of the other* (N. Poller, Trans.; pp. viii–xliv). Champaign, IL: University of Illinois Press.

Comas-Diaz, L., & Jacobsen, F. M. (1991). Ethnocultural transference and countertransference in the therapeutic dyad. *American Journal of Orthopsychiatry, 61*(3), 392–402. http://dx.doi.org/10.1037/h0079267

Critchley, S. (2007). *Infinitely demanding: Ethics of commitment, politics of resistance*. London, England: Verso.

Decety, J. (2011). Dissecting the neural mechanisms mediating empathy. *Emotion Review, 3*, 92–108. http://dx.doi.org/10.1177/1754073910374662

Decety, J. (2014). The neuroevolution of empathy and caring for others: Why it matters for morality. In J. Decety & Y. Christian (Eds.), *New frontiers in social*

neuroscience (pp. 127–51). New York, NY: Springer. http://dx.doi.org/
10.1007/978-3-319-02904-7_8

Decety, J., & Fotopoulou, A. (2015). Why empathy has a beneficial impact on others in medicine: unifying theories. *Frontiers in Behavioral Neuroscience, 8*, 457. http://dx.doi.org/10.3389/fnbeh.2014.00457

Decety, J., & Ickes, W. (2011). *The social neuroscience of empathy.* Cambridge, MA: MIT Press.

Dyck, E. (2006). Prairie psychedelics: Mental health research in Saskatchewan, 1951–1967. In J. E. Moran & D. Wright (Eds.), *Mental health and Canadian society* (pp. 221–44). Montreal, Canada: McGill–Queen's University Press.

Eisenberger, N. I. (2012). The pain of social disconnection: Examining the shared neural underpinnings of physical and social pain. *Nature Reviews Neuroscience, 13*, 421–34. http://dx.doi.org/10.1038/nrn3231

Eisenberger, N. I., Lieberman, M. D., & Williams, K. D. (2003). Does rejection hurt? An fMRI study of social exclusion. *Science, 302*, 290–2. http://dx.doi.org/10.1126/science.1089134

Ellis, H. D., & Lewis, M. B. (2001). Capgras delusion: A window on face recognition. *Trends in Cognitive Sciences, 5*(4), 149–56. http://dx.doi.org/10.1016/S1364-6613(00)01620-X

Engen, H. G., & Singer, T. (2013). Empathy circuits. *Current Opinion in Neurobiology, 23*(2), 275–82. http://dx.doi.org/10.1016/j.conb.2012.11.003

Fan, Y., Duncan, N. W., de Greck, M., & Northoff, G. (2011). Is there a core neural network in empathy? An fMRI based quantitative meta-analysis. *Neuroscience & Biobehavioral Reviews, 35*(3), 903–11. http://dx.doi.org/10.1016/j.neubiorev.2010.10.009

Fanon, F. (1982). *Black skin, white masks.* New York, NY: Grove Press.

Freeman, M. P. (2014). *The priority of the other: Thinking and living beyond the self.* New York, NY: Oxford University Press.

Gallagher, S. (2012). Empathy, simulation, and narrative. *Science in Context, 25*(3), 355–81. http://dx.doi.org/10.1017/S0269889712000117

Gallagher, S. (2014). In your face: Transcendence in embodied interaction. *Frontiers in Human Neuroscience, 8*(1) 495. http://dx.doi.org/10.3389/fnhum.2014.00495

Gallese, V., Keysers, C., & Rizzolatti, (2004). A unifying view of the basis of social cognition. *Trends in Cognitive Neuroscience, 8*(9), 396–403. http://dx.doi.org/10.1016/j.tics.2004.07.002

Gantt, E. E., & Williams, R. N. (2002). *Psychology for the other: Levinas, ethics and the practice of psychology.* Pittsburgh, PA: Duquesne University Press.

Geertz, C. (1983). *Local knowledge.* New York, NY: Basic Books.

Gibson, N.C. (2011). *Living Fanon: Global perspectives.* New York, NY: Palgrave Macmillan.

Glover, J. (2014). Alien landscapes?: Interpreting disordered minds. Cambridge, MA: Harvard University Press. http://dx.doi.org/10.4159/harvard.9780674735743

Goldman, A. (2011). Two routes to empathy: Insights from cognitive neuroscience. In A. Coplan & P. Goldie, *Empathy: Philosophical and psychological perspectives* (pp. 31–44). New York, NY: Oxford University Press. http://dx.doi.org/10.1093/acprof:oso/9780199539956.003.0004

Henriksen, M. G. (2013). On incomprehensibility in schizophrenia. *Phenomenology and the Cognitive Sciences, 12*(1), 105–29. http://dx.doi.org/10.1007/s11097-010-9194-7

Hickok, G. (2014). *The myth of mirror neurons: The real neuroscience of communication and cognition.* New York, NY: W. W. Norton.

Humpston, C. (2014). Perplexity and meaning: Toward a phenomenological "core" of psychotic experiences. *Schizophrenia Bulletin, 40*(2): 240–3. http://dx.doi.org/10.1093/schbul/sbt074

Jackson, P. L., Rainville, P. & Decety, J. (2006). To what extent do we share the pain of others? Insight from the neural bases of pain empathy. *Pain, 125,* 5–9. http://dx.doi.org/10.1016/j.pain.2006.09.013

Jahoda, G. (2005). Theodor Lipps and the shift from "sympathy" to "empathy." *Journal of the History of the Behavioral Sciences, 41*(2), 151–63. http://dx.doi.org/10.1002/jhbs.20080

Jaspers, K. (1997). *General psychopathology* (J. Hoenig & M. W. Hamilton, Trans.). Baltimore, MD: Johns Hopkins University Press. (Original work published 1913)

Kapur, S. (2003). Psychosis as a state of aberrant salience: A framework linking biology, phenomenology, and pharmacology in schizophrenia. *American Journal of Psychiatry, 160*(1), 13–23. http://dx.doi.org/10.1176/appi.ajp.160.1.13

Kirmayer, L. J. (2001). Failures of imagination: The refugee's narrative in psychiatry. *Anthropology & Medicine, 10*(2), 167–85. http://dx.doi.org/10.1080/1364847032000122843

Kirmayer, L. J. (2003). Asklepian dreams: The ethos of the wounded-healer in the clinical encounter. *Transcultural Psychiatry, 40*(2), 248–77.

Kirmayer, L. J. (2006). Beyond the "new cross-cultural psychiatry": Cultural biology, discursive psychology and the ironies of globalization. *Transcultural Psychiatry, 4*(1), 126–44. http://dx.doi.org/10.1177/1363461506061761

Kirmayer, L. J. (2007). Celan's poetics of alterity: Lyric and the understanding of illness experience in medical ethics. *Monash Bioethics Review, 26*(4), 21–35. http://dx.doi.org/10.1007/BF03351290

Kirmayer, L. J. (2008). Empathy and alterity in cultural psychiatry. *Ethos, 36*(4), 457–74. http://dx.doi.org/10.1111/j.1548-1352.2008.00027.x

Klaushofer, A. (2000). The foreignness of the other: Universalism and cultural identity in Levinas' ethics. *Journal of the British Society for Phenomenology, 31*(1), 55–73. http://dx.doi.org/10.1080/00071773.2000.11007279

Kleinman, A., & Benson, P. (2006). Anthropology in the clinic: The problem of cultural competency and how to fix it. *PLOS Medicine, 3*(10), e294. http://dx.doi.org/10.1371/journal.pmed.0030294

Klüver, H. (1966). *Mescal and mechanisms of hallucinations.* Chicago, IL: University of Chicago Press.

Larson, E. B., & Yao, X. (2005). Clinical empathy as emotional labor in the patient-physician relationship. *Journal of the American Medical Association, 293*(9), 1100–1106. http://dx.doi.org/10.1001/jama.293.9.1100

Lazare, A., Putnam, S. M., & Lipkin, Jr, M. (1995). Three functions of the medical interview. In M. Lipkin, Jr., S. M. Putname, & A. Lazare (Eds.), *The medical interview: Clinical care, education and research* (pp. 3–19). New York, NY: Springer. http://dx.doi.org/10.1007/978-1-4612-2488-4_1

Levinas, E. (1985). *Ethics and infinity: Conversations with Philippe Nemo.* Pittsburgh, PA: Duquesne University Press.

Levinas, E. (1993). *Outside the subject.* Stanford, CA: Stanford University Press.

Levinas, E. (2003). *Humanism of the other* (N. Poller, Trans.). Chicago: University of Illinois Press.

McHugh, P. R., & Slavney, P. R. (1998). *The perspectives of psychiatry* (2nd ed.). Baltimore, MD: Johns Hopkins University Press.

Moyn, S. (2005). *Origins of the other: Emmanuel Levinas between revelation and ethics.* Ithaca, NY: Cornell University Press.

Northoff, G. (2015). How the self is altered in psychiatric disorders: A neurophenomenal approach. In L. J. Kirmayer, R. Lemelson, & C. A. Cummings (Eds.), *Re-visioning psychiatry: Cultural phenomenology, critical neuroscience, and global mental health* (pp. 81–116). New York, NY: Cambridge University Press.

Oatley, K. (1992). *Best laid schemes: The psychology of emotion.* Cambridge, England: Cambridge University Press.

Oatley, K. (2011). *Such stuff as dreams: The psychology of fiction.* Malden, MA: Wiley-Blackwell. http://dx.doi.org/10.1002/9781119970910

Orange, D. M. (2011). *The suffering stranger: Hermeneutics for everyday clinical practice.* New York, NY: Routledge.

Parnas, J., & Gallagher, S. (2015). Phenomenology and the interpretation of psychopathological experience. In L. J. Kirmayer, R. Lemelson, & C. A. Cummings (Eds.), *Re-visioning psychiatry: Cultural phenomenology, critical neuroscience, and global mental health* (pp. 65–80). New York, NY: Cambridge University Press.

Preston, S. D., & de Waal, F. B. (2002). Empathy: Its ultimate and proximate bases. *Behavioral and Brain Sciences, 25*(1), 1–20; Discussion, 20–71.

Ratcliffe M. (2012). Phenomenology as a form of empathy. *Inquiry, 55*(5), 473–95. http://dx.doi.org/10.1080/0020174X.2012.716196

Ratcliffe, M. (2014). The phenomenology of depression and the nature of empathy. *Medicine, Health Care and Philosophy, 17*(2), 269–80. http://dx.doi.org/10.1007/s11019-013-9499-8

Rizzolatti, G., & Craighero, L. (2004). The mirror-neuron system. *Annual Review of Neuroscience, 27,* 169–92. http://dx.doi.org/10.1146/annurev.neuro.27.070203.144230

Rogers, C. R. (1957). The necessary and sufficient conditions of therapeutic personality change. *Journal of Consulting and Clinical Psychology, 21*(6), 95–103. http://dx.doi.org/10.1037/h0045357

Rosaldo, M. Z. (1980). *Knowledge and passion: Ilongot notions of self and social life.* Cambridge, England: Cambridge University Press. http://dx.doi.org/10.1017/CBO9780511621833

Sass, L. A. (1994). *The paradoxes of delusion: Wittgenstein, Schreber, and the schizophrenic mind.* Ithaca, NY: Cornell University Press.

Semin, G. R., & de Groot, J. H. (2013). The chemical bases of human sociality. *Trends in Cognitive Sciences, 17*(9), 427–9. http://dx.doi.org/10.1016/j.tics.2013.05.008

Singer, T. (2012). The past, present and future of social neuroscience: A European perspective. *NeuroImage, 61*(2), 437–49. http://dx.doi.org/10.1016/j.neuroimage.2012.01.109

Singer, T., Seymour, B., O'Doherty, J., Kaube, H., Dolan, R. J., & Frith, C. D. (2004). Empathy for pain involves the affective but not sensory components of pain. *Science, 303*(5661), 1157–62. http://dx.doi.org/10.1126/science. 1093535

Tauber, A. I. (1999). *Confessions of a medicine man: An essay in popular philosophy.* Cambridge, MA: MIT Press.

Titchener, E. B. (1909). *A text-book of psychology.* New York, NY: Macmillan. http://dx.doi.org/10.1037/12224-000

Valdesolo, P., & DeSteno, D. (2011). Synchrony and the social tuning of compassion. *Emotion, 11*(2), 262–6. http://dx.doi.org/10.1037/a0021302

Verducci, S. (2000). A moral method? Thoughts on cultivating empathy through method acting. *Journal of Moral Education, 29*(1), 87–99. http://dx.doi.org/ 10.1080/030572400102952

Vergès, F. (1996). To cure and to free: The Fanonian project of "decolonized psychiatry." In L. R. Gordon, T. D. Sharpley-Whiting, & R. T. White (Eds.), *Fanon: A critical reader* (pp. 85–99). Oxford, England: Blackwell.

Vreeke, G. J., & van der Mark, I. L. (2003). Empathy, an integrative model. *New Ideas in Psychology, 21*(3), 177–207. http://dx.doi.org/10.1016/j. newideapsych.2003.09.003

Wicker, B., Keysers, C., Plailly, J., Royet, J. P., Gallese, V., & Rizzolatti, G. (2003). Both of us disgusted in my insula: The common neural basis of seeing and feeling disgust. *Neuron, 40*(3), 655–64. http://dx.doi.org/10.1016/ S0896-6273(03)00679-2

Zahavi, D. (2001). Beyond empathy. Phenomenological approaches to intersubjectivity. *Journal of Consciousness Studies, 8*(5–7), 151–67.

Zaki, J., & Ochsner, K. N. (2012). The neuroscience of empathy: Progress, pitfalls and promises. *Nature Neuroscience, 15*(5), 675–80. http://dx.doi.org/ 10.1038/nn.3085

Reflections
The Community Life of Objects
Beyond the Academic Clinic

Nev Jones

The four chapters that comprise this section of *Re-Visioning Psychiatry* collectively call for a reconsideration of the methods of psychiatry and allied fields (including neuroscience and psychiatric anthropology). The authors ask that we think more carefully and critically about the ways in which psychiatry produces its objects and structures the relationship between levels of analysis and explanation (including the brain, subject-ive phenomena, the intentional subject, and diverse social and cultural vectors). In this commentary, I want to extend some of this work by reflecting on the complications occasioned by a more radical decentering of psychiatry (as scholarly discipline and locus of clinical practice). Throughout this discussion, I draw on mixed-methods fieldwork in community-based mental health settings across geopolitically diverse regions of the United States.

Decentering Psychiatry

There would be little purpose in denying the power and reach of the psychiatric research establishment, understood to encompass psychotropic drug discovery and testing in pharmaceutical settings; investigations of the epidemiology, genetics, and neurobiology of mental disorders; psychi-atric phenomenology and nosology; and the evaluation of psychological and rehabilitative, as well as physiological, treatments and interventions. Psychiatrists – rather than social workers or counselors – also direct the vast majority of inpatient mental health facilities and university-based psychiatric clinics, at least in the United States. Outside the hospital and laboratory doors, however, there exists an expansive network of community and gov-ernmental institutions and actors in and through which not only patients, but a wide variety of dis-aggregated psychiatric objects and practices (includ-ing diagnosis, symptoms, medications, and disability as a legal category), materialize, settle, and sediment in powerful and often far-reaching ways.

In the United States, patients diagnosed with a "serious mental illness" and accorded governmentally sanctioned disability status, will typically spend the substantive majority of their "clinical" time interacting not with researchers or "highly credentialed" clinicians (i.e., psychiatrists or doctoral-level psychologists) but rather front-line providers and para-professionals (i.e., peer specialists who may or may not have ever attended college, case managers, social workers, and counselors). Frequent entanglements with the criminal justice, physical health-care, and welfare systems are likely to prompt additional interactions with parole officers, representative payees, employment specialists, healthcare coordinators, judges, and public defenders. "Home" might be a shelter, a halfway house, single-room occupancy hotel (SRO), or institute for mental disease (IMD) – a nursing facility providing around-the-clock care to individuals with psychiatric disabilities, regardless of age. In addition to entanglements with professional and/or governmental organizations and agencies, service users may also engage with mental health advocacy organizations and/or other "alternative" support settings.

In these (often complex) assemblages of services, settings, and systems, the status and function of psychiatric objects such as diagnosis, symptoms, metrics (including the semistructured clinical interview), and various pedagogical and epistemological tactics, frequently diverge from those of the university clinic or laboratory. Over the course of multiyear mixed methods fieldwork conducted in Illinois and Oregon, I rarely encountered front-line providers whose clinical training involved more than a single course on more severe psychopathology (particularly psychosis); instead, most reported entering their first clinical place-ments with only a vague understanding of specific diagnostic criteria, and little or no targeted clinical training in more severe mood and thought disorders. Experience administering formal diagnostic inter-views was equally uncommon. Instead, providers reported learning both clinical strategies and (mostly informal) case formulation on the ground: visiting clients in their homes, walking them through a grocery store, or sitting with them in waiting rooms for ancillary health or welfare appointments. Both learning to work with and to conceptualize specific psychiatric experiences were described as inextricably embodied, immanent, intersubjective processes. As one community support team (CST) member put it:

[T]here's no learning experience at all like driving around with somebody in your car during a psychotic episode. There's nothing that prepares you for that. I think that being in the field – and I could sit through so many classes and so many hours of classwork – [but] to actually be with somebody out in the community in their environment . . . going through it all – there's nothing that you'll learn more from than that.

Even when providing more conventional office-based services, such as medication management, clinical informants often described the practice of formal diagnosis as perfunctory, even trivial. One of the psychiatric nurse practitioners I interviewed ("Erika") described the assignment of specific diagnostic codes as "total bullshit," requisite only as a means of fulfilling the billing criteria required by clients' health insurers. She continued:

> In terms of whether or not [a particular disorder] – like, I don't care what we call it, it really doesn't [matter to me], I don't care. It doesn't have to have a name.

Rather than segue into a discussion of the *validity* of diagnostic practices, including any question of how such practices might be improved, Erika oriented to real-world effects: how diagnoses are taken up internally and intersubjectively; what they do. And here there is significant heterogeneity:

> Some people find that diagnosis, having a word for something helps them feel less alone, because it's a common thread of the human experience and they find it helpful. Other people feel like "the experience that I'm having is unique to me. It doesn't have shit to do with anything else and it doesn't need a name" and I can go either way.

The goal of the clinician is not to enforce particular identities but, rather, to respect the different choices patients make, some of which may help fuel – but others defuse – a more academic preoccupation with nosological validity.

Erika's pointed comments mirrored many conversations with service users – some of whom identified strongly with a particular diagnosis or formulation, some of whom did not. The narratives behind particular identifications typically had little to do with ontological veridicality and much more to do with the cultural politics of the community spaces and systems patients traversed. Whereas a diagnosis of "schizophrenia," for example, might be understood as more stigmatized and likely to engender fear and social distancing, it could also endow the bearer with the unspoken gravitas of "severity" and access to a broader array of services. The experience of voices, similarly, might be narrativized as something that has "happened" to the patient, but also as part of an identity that she actively enters into or "becomes," a constructivist "becoming" that extends well beyond any clinical or academic delineation of auditory hallucinations.

As in many other domains and walks of life more generally, some individuals I observed or interacted with "naturally" oriented to the phenomenological nuances of particular symptoms – the interplay of sensation and imagination in the development of unusual beliefs, for example – whereas others gravitated much more strongly toward broader narratives of recovery and resilience or disability (cf. Frank, 2013; Strawson, 2004). Still others instead emphasized linkages between "symptoms" and particular streams of cultural or religious discourse; a voice might be the voice of God, or a sudden diffuse, tangible presence the breath of a demon. In a cosmic battle of good and evil, debates concerning the validity of particular diagnoses or formulations may be irrelevant or be of only minor interest. Similarly, histories of trauma and marginalization might supersede more proximal variables with sexual abuse, structural racism, or parental incarceration crowding out other ways of thinking about identity and "mental illness" (see also Jones, Kelly, & Shattell, in review; Luhrmann, 2012; Woods, 2011).

The import of particular ways of describing experience may also diverge from concerns central to academic psychiatry. The phenomenological nuances of individual agency in the (re)structuring of symptoms, for instance, might matter most not by virtue of its implications vis-à-vis ipseity or a patients' sense of self, but rather in terms of its moral and ethical implications. One young woman, for example, ruminated at length about the extent to which she might have "actively caused" her own psychosis:

> I knew I was very sort of on the line [of becoming psychotic] anyway. I think that I – from the things I was reading – made it a point to develop a relationship with somebody who didn't exist in my head and I also made it a point to think to myself in the third person. . . . I don't know if I wrote this list of things I needed to do [to become psychotic] and then did them. Or if they were starting and then I was trying to make it feel as if I had control over it.

If, on the one hand, she had actively engendered her own symptoms, did she have the "right" to represent herself as having had experiences similar to patients whose psychoses were "forced" on them? If she claimed the identity of a "voice hearer" would she be misrepresenting herself; inappropriately coopting an identity that, while discrediting in many ways, might also prove advantageous in particular contexts?

Implications

How do the community scenes and individual experiences briefly described here relate to the themes of the chapter in Section 1? As is perhaps already implicit in these narratives, attention to the broader lives of psychiatric objects and practices outside disciplinary psychiatry (the clinic and the laboratory), may prompt us to ask different questions and attend to different effects. Some objects and practices may also turn out to matter more, or matter differently, when unburdened of the structures and limits of a particular academic gaze. In the remainder of this commentary, I focus on implications across three general domains: (1) focal objects, (2) authority and expertise, (3) policy. Notably, while there is clear overlap between the ethos of these questions and Berrios and Marková's important critique (here and elsewhere, e.g., Berrios & Marková, 2012; Marková & Berrios, 2012), my concern is less with the history and/or larger body of scholarly discourse and more with the particular (potential) implications of the chapters in this volume.

Focal Objects

The five chapters in this section broadly cluster around the investigation of symptoms, although certainly with not-insignificant variations. For Csordas, for example, at issue more specifically is "the *modulation* of phenomena that exist for a person" (including, but not limited to symptomatology) and for Parnas and Gallagher, "the [disordered] human *as an extended system*." Berrios and Marková, while formally retaining the "symptom" as focal object, nevertheless underscore the degree of oversimplification of such phenomena in the existing academic literature.

In spite of these complications and caveats, however, there are notable absences in the ground these chapters ultimately do and do not cover (and perhaps even more so the discourses within which they are each situated and to which they are responding). These include, for example, the arguably structuring role of psychotropic medications – particularly antipsychotics and mood stabilizers – across the domains of symptomatology, physical health and integrity, social response, and cultural emplotment. If we examine the gray and qualitative literatures on patients' experiences, however, the ostensibly "epiphenomenal" may in fact occupy a (for some *the*) central role: reconfiguring a centrifugal assemblage spanning phenomenal experiences of the body, social discourse and extended biopolitical infrastructures (*Mad in America* [www.madinamerica.com/]; Martin, 2010; Moncrieff, Cohen, & Mason, 2009). Medication effects may also structurally alter both symptomatology and the brain.

Similarly, were we to focus on "indigenous" or emic ways of configuring identity, resisting categorization on the basis of *illness*, we might identify (and ultimately center) critical strands of the "human as extended system" motivated not by symptoms but instead particular assemblages of mental health *service* experiences, including those accrued in the absence of actual symptoms or disorders (as for individuals who were misdiagnosed, or whom have long since recovered from a brief, initial episode) or grounded primarily in experiential intersections with the criminal justice, disability and/or welfare systems. Across these categories, the implications of what objects we do or do not hone are not limited to sociological or epidemiological aspects of psychiatric disorder, but extend to more basic clinical and neurobiological projects. As Berrios and Marková (this volume) underscore, that is, "internal" processes such as identification as well as external influences such as "treatment" continuously influence neurobiological structure and function (as well as particular cultural configurations of illness).

Authority and Expertise

In a Foucauldian vein, another set of fundamental questions concerns the implications of particular objects and foci with respect to the kinds and types of expertise they established (or reinforce). Who, that is, according to a particular body of discourse or research, is or will be accorded the socially-sanctioned right to speak on particular topics (such as diagnosis or phenomenology) with authority, to carry out or supervise specific practices, to make this or that claim in such a way that he or she is publicly "heard'?

Returning to the brief ethnographic vignettes described above, two obvious *potential* "speakers," often excluded from more theoretically driven academic scholarship and clinical research, are patients and the cross-disciplinary array of nondoctoral front-line providers (social workers, case managers, counselors, and para-professionals) who ultimately provide the majority of psychiatric services. My point in invoking these actors is not so much to make a values-based claim regarding inclusion, but rather to press the importance of interrogating any and all psychiatric scholarship with respect to its implications vis-à-vis expertise. As is true of the particular psychiatric objects selected, as well as the ways in which they are defined, these implications are arguably expansive. If we follow Foucault's (1969/ 2012) iteration of similar issues, for instance, specific implications may include tacit "criteria of competence and knowledge" (including legal, political, and pedagogical norms), particular "differentiations" from and with other experts or authorities (between the psychiatrist and the medical anthropologist, for example, or the social worker or judge of a mental health court), and, finally, the broader role and (in some cases) societal expectations of the "expert" in question. These norms, differences and roles are, of course, reciprocal. Thus, discussions of methods or topics such as those included in this volume, irreducibly both reflect and tacitly challenge or reinforce these vectors in some way.

Policy

In the often silo-ed worlds of psychiatric research and training, discussions of – and attempts to intervene directly in – policy are often cursory, with the tacit expectation that the "actual" work of policy change takes place largely outside the purview of clinically-focused academic scholarship. Ultimately, however, whether the immediate focus is neuroimaging or phenomenology, both the constraints and contingencies of existing policy, as well as the implications of particular clinical research trajectories *with respect to policy*, must be considered. Here I define "policy" very broadly as the net of procedures, rules, norms, and decision-making structures that determine, among other things, whether and how public moneys can be used to fund particular interventions, the particular legal and economic role of psychiatric practices such as diagnosis, and the conceptual delimitations between areas of service delivery such as the legal, institutional, and clinical division(s) between behavioral and physical health.

As earlier, my purpose is less to suggest a particular critique, and more to underscore the importance of thinking through both influences (across the domains of objects, experts, and policy) and implications of the academic scholarship in question with respect to these same domains. Another set of questions, more ethical in motivation, might also concern strategies for intervening in more specific ways. For instance, given a concern for particular clinical outcomes or effects, what can or should be done to a/effect such changes in the "real world" of policy-driven community mental health? Ultimately, depending on the aims of a given intervention in the literature (and in practice) there are both performative and normative stakes in particular configurations of objects, actors, and policies; while these are never under anyone's 'control' in a straightforward sense, critical reflexivity nevertheless seems warranted.

In his review of Jenkins and Barrett's *Schizophrenia, Culture and Subjectivity*, Jaime Saris (2004) concludes that although the volume "accomplishes its goal of reinvigorating a century-long conversation between psychiatry and various social sciences ... [i]t remains to be seen whether both sides are talking about the same issues and according to whose agenda the meeting will be run." In these reflections, we have sought to foreground actors and stakeholders beyond academic psychiatrists and social scientists. Saris's concerns regarding the real-world effects of more critical discourse, and the stubborn hierarchies involved, however, hold.

REFERENCES

Berrios, G. E., & Marková, I. S. (2012). The construction of hallucination: History and epistemology. In J. D. Blom & I. E. C. Sommer (Eds.), *Hallucinations: Research and practice* (pp. 55–71). New York, NY: Springer. http://dx.doi.org/10.1007/978-1-4614-0959-5_5

Berrios, G. E., & Marková, I. S. (2015). Toward a new epistemology of psychiatry. In L. J. Kirmayer, R. Lemelson, & C. A. Cummings (Eds.), *Re-visioning psychiatry: Cultural phenomenology, critical neuroscience, and global mental health* (pp. 41–64). New York, NY: Cambridge University Press.
Csordas, T. J. (2015). Cultural phenomenology and psychiatric illness. In L. J. Kirmayer, R. Lemelson, & C. A. Cummings (Eds.), *Re-visioning psychiatry: Cultural phenomenology, critical neuroscience, and global mental health* (pp. 117–40). New York, NY: Cambridge University Press.
Foucault, M. (2012). *The archaeology of knowledge* (R. Swyer, Trans.). New York, NY: Vintage Books. (Original work published 1969)
Frank, A. W. (2013). *The wounded storyteller: Body, illness, and ethics.* Chicago, IL: University of Chicago Press.
Jones, N., Kelly, T., & Shattell, M. (2014). God in the brain: Reimagining psychosis in the postsecular United States. Manuscript submitted for publication.
Luhrmann, T. M. (2012, July). Living with voices. *The American Scholar.* Retrieved from http://theamericanscholar.org/
Marková, I. S., & Berrios, G. E. (2012). Epistemology of psychiatry. *Psychopathology, 45*(4), 220–7. http://dx.doi.org/10.1159/000331599
Martin, E. (2010). Self-making and the brain. *Subjectivity, 3*(4), 366–81. http://dx.doi.org/10.1057/sub.2010.23
Moncrieff, J., Cohen, D., & Mason, J. P. (2009). The subjective experience of taking antipsychotic medication: A content analysis of Internet data. *Acta Psychiatrica Scandinavica, 120*(2), 102–11. http://dx.doi.org/10.1111/j.1600-0447.2009.01356.x
Parnas, J., & Gallagher, S. (2015). Phenomenology and the interpretation of psychopathological experience. In L. J. Kirmayer, R. Lemelson, & C. A. Cummings (Eds.), *Re-visioning psychiatry: Cultural phenomenology, critical neuroscience, and global mental health* (pp. 65–80). New York, NY: Cambridge University Press.
Saris, J. (2004). [Review of the book *Schizophrenia, culture and subjectivity: The edge of experience*, edited by by J. H. Jenkins & R. J. Barrett]. *Culture, Medicine, and Psychiatry, 28*(3), 427–9. http://dx.doi.org/10.1023/B:MEDI.0000046457.83897.1b
Strawson, G. (2004). Against narrativity. *Ratio, 17*(4), 428–52.
Woods, A. (2011). The limits of narrative: Provocations for the medical humanities. *Medical Humanities, 37*, 73–8. http://dx.doi.org/10.1136/medhum-2011-010045

Biosocial Mechanisms in Mental Health and Illness

8 Dimensional and Categorical Approaches to Mental Illness
Let Biology Decide

Robert M. Bilder

There are two kinds of people in the world: those who divide the world into two kinds of people and those who don't.
— Robert Charles Benchley (1889–1945)

Introduction

Psychiatric disorders can be thought of as discrete categories or as reflecting extremes on dimensions of states, traits, or functions. There has long been an inherent conflict between dimensional and categorical models of mental disorders. Psychiatry is hardly unique in this respect and similar controversies are found throughout the long history of disease classification. According to Rounsaville and colleagues, dimensions are theoretically attractive in general, but categorical taxonomies are preferred by practicing clinicians (Rounsaville et al., 2002). Others have pointed out that most sciences start with a categorical classification of their subject matter, but often replace this approach with dimensions as more accurate measurement becomes possible (Hempel, 1961). In this chapter, I consider the history and current state of play of dimensional and categorical views of mental disorders and their implications for the future of psychiatry.

A Brief Historical Overview of Categorical and Dimensional Approaches to Psychiatry

Some of the earliest schemes for describing mental disorders were dimensional. Consider, for example, the ancient theory specifying four humors (blood, yellow bile, black bile, and phlegm) and their associated characteristics (courage/hope, anger, despondency/irritability, and calm/unemotionality, respectively). This theory was popular around the time of Hippocrates (460–370 BCE) and probably had earlier origins in Egypt and/or Mesopotamia; it may also be linked to similar theories from Ayurvedic medicine (c. 1000 BCE; Subbarayappa, 2001). These themes continued well into the Middle Ages, as represented, for example, in Islamic medicine and the Canon of Medicine attributed to Avicenna in 1025 CE (Finger, 2001). The passion for classification also has ancient roots. It has been said that taxonomy is as old as human language; Chinese classification systems are documented as early as 3000 BCE, and Aristotle is credited with classifying all plants and animals in the fourth century BCE (Manktelow, 2010).

The history of taxonomy has been divided, however, into pre-Linnean and post-Linnean eras (Manktelow, 2010), based on the publication of *Species Plantarum* (1753) and the tenth edition of *Systema Naturae* (1758). The eighteenth century also provided a fertile climate for the classification of mental illnesses, an extreme example of which was the treatise *Nosologia Methodica* by François Boissier de Sauvages de Lacroix (1706–1767), which was published posthumously in 1771. This work, reportedly inspired by French alienist Philippe Pinel and reflecting the taxonomic *zeitgeist* in biology (de Sauvage was a botanist as well as a physician), defined 10 "classes," 44 "orders," 315 "genera," and 2400 "species" of diseases (Millon & Simonsen, 2010). Although controversy may be common in all areas of medical taxonomy, psychiatry has witnessed some spectacular swings between dimensional and categorical extremes in its theories of "madness," as noted by Karl Menninger and colleagues (Menninger, Ellenberger, Pruyser, & Mayman, 1959). Thus, paralleling the classificatory systems of Pinel and colleagues was the complementary and alternative view of German alienist Ernst von Zeller, who saw all mental illnesses as reflecting variation on a set of dimensions or *Zustandsbilder* (i.e., "state pictures" = syndromes). These Zustands-bilder included: *Schwermut* = Melancholia; *Tollheit* = Mania; *Verrucktheit* = Paranoia; and *Blödsinn* = Dementia.

Where do we stand today? If we consider the currently used diagnostic definitions and boundaries between schizophrenia and "manic depressive" or bipolar disorders, we find they are generally similar to those identified in 1899 by Kraepelin and his colleagues (Kraepelin, 1896, 1919). These definitions included the division of schizophrenia into paranoid, catatonic, and disorganized (hebephrenic) subtypes, which have proven to have little external validity in terms of biological bases, treatment response, or prognosis, and therefore have been abandoned in *DSM-5* (APA, 2013), with the exception of a "catatonia specifier" that preserves this feature as a characteristic but not a category. In the face of a relatively static view that mental illnesses possessed a categorical structure, a view that has persisted for more than a century, there have also emerged some champions of a dimensional approach to psychopathology. As Menninger and colleagues argued, "names do not create illness forms; they only comfort the doctors and impress the relatives" (Menninger et al., 1959).

Menninger and his Spanish contemporary, Bartolomé Llopis, arrived at similar dimensional formulations following parallel investigations. Each of these investigators examined the psychological consequences of diffuse, systemic illnesses. Menninger studied victims of the influenza epidemic in the United States. Llopis studied victims of pellagra following the black fever epidemic in Spain (Llopis, 1954). Both Menninger and Llopis prepared detailed observations of the mental states experienced by the ill at various stages of disease. Menninger (1959) observed that there was an "empirical series" of compensations, which included the following consecutive stages: nervousness; neurotic phenomena; episodic and explosive discharges; and, finally, persistent and severe disorganization. These characteristics, similarly noted by Llopis, incorporated the classically observed phenomenology of neurosis, depression, mania, positive symptoms, and negative symptoms that parallel the severity spectrum of mental illness spanning virtually all mental disorders. Menninger and Llopis further noted that these signs could all be observed *within the same person*, and as a consequence of *the same diffuse pathological process*. It was further noted that a patient with one of these systemic illnesses who continued to worsen, would further progress from severe disorganization to coma and then death. But if they were fortunate enough to recover, their symptoms would regress (in reverse order) through all these stages again on the path back to well-being. These observations across two continents make it clear that the remarkable heterogeneity of mental disorders does not require the operation of specific neuroanatomically localized or neurochemically distinctive dysfunctions, although this concept has been the holy grail of researchers for most of the last century and persists today as the dogma of discrete psychiatric disease states.

While the categorical view of mental disorders has been the prevailing view in modern psychiatry, there are notable modern exceptions. For example, Cloninger argued that "there is no empirical evidence for natural boundaries between major syndromes" and suggested the categorical approach is "fundamentally flawed" (Cloninger, 1999, pp. 174–5). Other respected scholars in psychiatric research have noted that the "prototypical mental disorders (major depressive disorder, anxiety disorders, schizophrenia, and bipolar disorder) merge imperceptibly both into one another and into normality with no demonstrable natural boundaries or zones of rarity in between" (Kendler & Gardner, 1998). In reviews of genetic and environmental factors underlying these syndromes, risks were noted to be most often nonspecific (Brown, 1996; Kendler, 1996).

But as ardent as some of these comments may be, there have been similarly strong statements opposing any move to dimensional models. For example, Lawrie and colleagues argue that "rejecting time-tested and progressively refined clinical concepts is at best premature and at worst wrong scientifically, and that a continuous approach to psychosis would be time consuming and quite possibly disastrous in clinical practice" (Lawrie, Hall, McIntosh, Owens, & Johnstone, 2010). Interestingly, Lawrie and colleagues start with the assumption that the categorical scheme is appropriate until proven otherwise. In contrast, it is argued here that both science and ultimately practice will be better served by adopting the null hypothesis that diagnostic boundaries do *not* exist, until demonstrated to possess validity of etiology, pathophysiology, treatment specificity, or distinctive prognosis.

The latter position acknowledges that phenomenological differences between individuals are the rule, not the exception, but it actively questions the utility of these distinctions as the basis for diagnostic formulations that are then used to guide research and treatment. If our goal is to promote research on the causes of mental illness or identify optimal treatments, then the latter approach is more direct. The only circumstance in which continued use of these phenomenological distinctions appears warranted is to increase the consistency with which different observers can label individuals who suffer from these problems. This was the advance enabled by development of the *DSM-III* criteria. However, once we have stronger biological hypotheses or evidence of differential treatment efficacy, it will be of value to see if we can develop models that show us how the observed symptoms relate to their biological substrates.

The widespread adoption of the current diagnostic taxonomy can be seen as an active impediment to progress in research on both the causes and treatments of mental disorders. Particularly problematic is the fact that the vast majority of research on psychopathology is conducted using these categories. This prevents determination of the possible relevance of dimensional measures because boundary conditions are frequently excluded so that unnaturally distinctive groups are studied. The natural overlap of dimensions across the syndromal boundaries is artificially constrained by eliminating "comorbid" disorders. The current diagnostic taxonomies solve these problems largely by fiat. For example, *DSM-5* frequently resorts to adding exclusionary criteria – a particular diagnosis is permitted only if the signs and symptoms "are not better explained" by another disorder, thus requiring application of a categorical boundary regardless of the empirically observed symptoms. These categories are required in virtually all research studies. This ends up generating additional evidence that further reifies the distinctions among the categories because overlapping groups are avoided, so the only "positive" evidence is accrued about group differences (Hyman, 2010). This approach increases the likelihood of finding evidence for group differences even if they are not true group differences. The more narrowly the groups are defined, the greater the risk of bias. This is a well-recognized problem with "extreme group designs," which systematically overestimate effect sizes (Preacher, Rucker, MacCallum, & Nicewander, 2005). Thus, the conventional approach is biased to "validate" diagnoses even if groups are truly on a continuum and differ only in severity. New strategies are needed that avoid making prior assumptions about the validity of diagnostic categories and instead document symptoms and functional impairments that define these diagnoses in order to evaluate their validity on a level field with other behavioral dimensions and categories.

Current Status

The third edition of the *DSM* (*DSM-III*; APA, 1980) helped improve agreement among diagnosticians, but was explicitly considered by its authors to be "atheoretical" with respect to etiological or pathophysiological bases. The categorical structure of the *DSM-III* has persisted with mostly cosmetic changes over the last three decades. There was no clear empirical basis for the categories or the criteria used to distinguish them. Instead, the disorders were defined based on prevailing views, sometimes involving the work of committees and largely depending on the insights of Robert Spitzer, "a psychoanalytically trained biometrician" who chaired the *DSM-III* task force (Shorter & Fink, 2010, p. 7; Spiegel, 2005). The first revision (*DSM-III-R*; APA, 1987) incorporated some substantive changes in the definition of personality disorders (Widiger, Frances, Spitzer, & Williams, 1988), but changes to major mental disorder classifications were more modest. The fourth edition and subsequent text revision (*DSM-IV* and *DSM-IV-TR*; APA, 1994, 2000) changed little with respect to the principle categories and criteria, but the criteria for significant distress or impairment were more systematically incorporated into a range of diagnoses.

The planning process for *DSM-5* – now designated with an Arabic numeral in anticipation of more timely updates (e.g., *DSM-5.1*; Kupfer, Kuhl, & Wulsin, 2013) – began in 1999, involving discussions among leaders of the National Institute of Mental Health (NIMH) and the APA; a series of "white papers" that emanated from this work (and were subsequently published in a monograph entitled *A Research Agenda for DSM-V)* considered multiple goals for the fifth edition of the manual (Kupfer, First, & Regier, 2002). In their introduction, the monograph's editors suggested that "research exclusively focused on refining the *DSM*-defined syndromes may never be successful in uncovering their underlying etiologies. For that to happen, an as yet unknown paradigm shift may need to occur" (2002, p. xix). A major topic for consideration was a more dimensional approach to psychopathology.

While the *DSM-5* was under development, a separate work group was convened to study dimensional approaches (Helzer et al., 2008), but these ideas were not actually incorporated into the final product. Despite extensive discussion of how dimensional strategies might replace or supplement the existing categorical structure, most of the primary diagnostic categories in *DSM-5* remain essentially similar to the *DSM-IV-TR*, and only some supplemental dimensional scales are recommended for optional use (see Section III: Emerging Measures and Models). It remains to be seen how widely used and valuable these assessments will be. The entire process of revision for *DSM-5* has been criticized on multiple grounds, including unsatisfactory reliability of its field trials, lack of transparency, and efforts to burnish the image of the product via public relations rather than through applying customary scientific criteria (Frances, 2012).

The International Statistical Classification of Diseases and Related Health Problems (ICD-10; http://www.who.int/classifications/icd/en/) is currently in its tenth edition and work groups are actively pursuing the eleventh edition, scheduled for release in 2015. Comparisons of the *ICD-10* and *DSM-IV* suggest that the differences in categories and criteria are relatively subtle, reflecting some of the differences between views in the United States and Europe (especially the United Kingdom; Andrews, Slade, & Peters, 1999). Harsher critics such as Allen Frances, chair of the *DSM-IV* task force, contend that the differences are "trivial and arbitrary" and urge that the systems be fully reconciled to avoid meaningless disagreements (Frances, 2012). Because the two systems reflect very similar taxonomic structures, we will refer to these systems throughout the rest of this chapter as "*DSM/ICD.*"

Psychometric Evidence for Categories and Dimensions

Psychometric research has challenged the categorical models. Psychometric evidence can inform us about the degree to which the symptoms used to make diagnoses actually support the existence of discrete classes or may better be explained as dimensions. The most straightforward example of this approach is to examine a distribution of trait scores from some symptom and determine if the distribution shows clear evidence of bimodality, with an obvious clustering of some scores at high extreme levels and the rest of the distribution lower, and a clear zone of rarity between the two. This is an intuitively appealing approach, but it is overly stringent and unreliable (Meehl, 1999). True group differences may easily be missed by this approach, given that measurements seldom provide a complete representation of group characteristics (Haslam, 2003; Murphy, 1964).

A somewhat more sophisticated approach uses *cluster analytic procedures*. These methods are designed to identify clusters using statistical criteria, but will do so even if clusters do not truly exist. They also have a relatively poor track record in simulation studies (Grove, 1991; Haslam, 2003). Paul Meehl developed a set of methods known as *taxometrics*, which has a better track record and is more intuitively appealing; but it assumes independent indicators, and only works if there are no more than two classes (Beauchaine, 2003, 2007; Cole, 2004; Meehl, 1995, 2004; Waller, 2006). *Finite mixture modeling* is capable of identifying more groups of cases if these exist, but it demands large samples and assumptions about underlying distributions that are generally unknown. More modern methods are derived from *latent class analysis* (Lazarsfeld & Henry, 1968), which is designed to find subtypes from multivariate categorical data. This method may be considered a parallel of *latent variable modeling*, which has become popular, for example, in *structural equation modeling* (An & Bentler, 2011; Bentler & Bonnett, 1980; Jöreskog & Sörbom, 1985; Yuan & Bentler, 2010). Recent developments have brought together the methods for modeling with latent variables and latent classes simultaneously; one example of this approach is *factor mixture modeling* (Muthen, Asparouhov, & Rebollo, 2006). This approach requires large samples, and is variably effective depending on multiple factors including the size of subgroups, and their separation.

Haslam (2003) reviewed taxometric studies of mental disorder categories and found little support for categorical structure; only a modest number of true "groups" appeared to exist, while almost all other psychopathological traits appeared to be better represented by dimensions. In brief, he found evidence that "melancholia" may be a discrete category but other forms of depression appeared better represented by a continuum. Some evidence existed in support of social phobia and inhibited temperament in childhood as discrete categories, but all other kinds of anxiety appeared to be on a continuum. There was also some evidence that bulimia nervosa (BN) and anorexia nervosa (AN) may be categories. (*DSM-IV* criteria inappropriately identified binge-eating/purging as a subtype of AN, but a binge-eating disorder is now recognized as an entirely separate category in *DSM-5*). Further support was found for the categorical structure of dissociative identity disorder (with a narrow definition), and a subgroup of individuals who show high hypnotic susceptibility. Evidence for categorical structure was also found for schizotypal personality disorder, albeit the *DSM* category represents only the most severe subset of this taxon. A systematic review and supplementary analyses support the identification of a latent class of individuals with - vulnerability to schizophrenia but this latent class includes about 11 percent of the entire population and this is more than ten times greater than the number of people who ever receive the diagnosis in their lifetimes (Linscott & van Os, 2010). Finally, there is evidence that antisocial personality disorder may be a discrete class (Harris, Rice, & Quinsey, 1994; Skilling, Harris, Rice, & Quinsey, 2001; Skilling, Quinsey, & Craig, 2001).

By contrast, virtually every other category within the *DSM* is better understood as reflecting dimensional traits. A cardinal example is depression, for which all kinds and putative subtypes other than melancholia are best represented as dimensional. Similarly posttraumatic stress disorder, generalized anxiety, avoidant attachment style, anxiety sensitivity, and panic disorders all are better understood as continuous quantitative traits without categorical substructure. Haslam, Holland, and Kuppens (2012) revisited the taxonic findings for mental illness, and found that more recently accumulated data, with better experimental designs, decreased the likelihood of taxonic findings, and concluded that true categories are relatively rare in psychopathology.

Similarly, the personality disorders are almost all better described dimensionally, so that all interpersonal and affective components of psychopathy are dimensional, as is borderline personality disorder. Beyond the *DSM* descriptions of disorders, there are the well-known results of other personality assessments, which have yielded consistent findings of dimensionality (for example, the Five Factor Model that specifies dimension of openness, conscientiousness, extraversion, agreeableness, and neuroticism or negative affectivity), and the addition of categorical structure adds no additional robust information to the dimensional characterization (Costa Jr. & McCrae, 2008; Eaton, Krueger, South, Simms, & Clark, 2010). Lacking a sharp line to distinguish pathology from healthy variation on the trait dimensions, the diagnoses of personality disorders are made by clinicians who associate significant social-vocational dysfunction with identified personality characteristics.

Recent applications of factor mixture modeling (FMM) are beginning to shed more light on how combinations of dimensional and categorical structures will ultimately be important to understand psychopathology. For example, FMM was used to examine the primary symptoms of attention deficit hyperactivity disorder (ADHD) from the SWAN rating scale (Lubke et al., 2007). The authors reported "the best fitting models support two continuous factors representing severity of inattentiveness and hyperactivity with considerable variability on both dimensions" (p. 1591). Furthermore, they found that the two dimensions of "inattentiveness and hyperactivity are positively correlated" (p. 1591) and concluded, "We see no support of qualitatively distinct ADHD subtypes in these analyses" (p. 1588). Recent results further suggest that cannabis use disorder is best represented by a single latent factor, without any latent categories (Gillespie, Neale, Legrand, Iacono, & McGue, 2012). Application of FMM to borderline personality disorder traits found that the *DSM* criteria were best fit by a single dimension and only two latent classes of affected and unaffected individuals; but among affected individuals, evidence of four subgroups was also found, suggesting that both latent dimensions and categories may be important in some domains (Hallquist & Pilkonis, 2012). It is important to recognize, however, that categorical structure may be found even though categories may differ primarily in severity of symptoms. For example, an FMM study of autism spectrum disorders revealed two latent dimensions reflecting social communication deficits and fixated interests and repetitive behaviors, and then identified three latent classes that differed primarily in severity of these dimensions (Georgiades et al., 2012).

It is also critical to recognize that most studies conducted so far have focused on selected symptom scales, which in turn are generally derived from prior conventional wisdom about the syndromes, so there is an inherent bias in the psychometric approaches to recover the same structure that was originally used to inform scale construction. Thus, for example, it may be considered unsurprising that an FMM study of ADHD symptoms recovered evidence supporting the existence of "impulsivity" and "inattentiveness" latent variables, given that these constructs were used to select items for the scale in the first place. Future research will need to avoid the circularity of these approaches. One way to do so is to sample more broadly across phenotypic traits (i.e., what would be found in ADHD if we asked questions more broadly). In genetics research, a more agnostic approach has been used to examine the entire "genome" and determine associations empirically. Can the "-omics" approach be applied to studying symptoms? Could we define a universe of symptoms as the "symptome"? There are relatively broad symptom surveys (for example, the old Present State Examination), but do even these capture all relevant symptoms? How do we know when behaviors are important and relevant, even if they are not "unusual" or "atypical"? If we could define such a universe of symptoms or behaviors, would it be practical to assess these? Another way to escape circularity is to examine more external variables, and preferably those that may link the high-level symptoms and syndromes to deeper biological roots. This is essentially the "phenomics" approach, which aims to characterize behavior along with other putative relevant neural system, cellular, and molecular processes simultaneously, with the goal of assembling mechanistic models of neuropsychiatric syndromes (Bilder, Howe, & Sabb, 2013; Bilder et al., 2009).

Neuropsychology

Neuropsychological assessment has long been widely used for the assessment of brain dysfunction, and informative early work focused on the degree to which these test scores might enable us to distinguish "organic" from "functional" psychiatric syndromes. In a landmark review of the literature, Heaton and colleagues summarized findings about the ability of neuropsychological batteries to succeed in making this distinction (Heaton, Baade, & Johnson, 1978). Interestingly, they found that some groups (people with "neurotic" disorders) could easily be distinguished from the "organics," but as the severity of psychiatric disturbance increased – and included more individuals with affective disorders and more people with psychotic disorders – the "hit rate" decreased (see Table 8.1). In the most severely affected groups of psychiatric patients – people classified as having chronic or process schizophrenia – the hit rate was near 50 percent; in other words, the tests could not distinguish these patients from other patients with known brain damage. They concluded that these patients may "look organic" because a "significant proportion of such patients are organic" (Heaton, Baade, & Johnson, 1978, p. 141). This conclusion hardly seems surprising today, now that we have ample evidence of structural and other functional abnormalities of the brain well documented in these groups. But at the time it was news and was part of the breaking wave of discovery that patients with severe psychopathology had clearcut evidence of neuropathology. What is even more striking in retrospect, and in the current context, is that the severity of neuropsychological impairment clearly follows the overall severity spectrum identified by Menninger and Llopis that led to their unitary dimensional models of psychopathology.

In addition to these findings suggesting that the ranking of effect sizes for generalized deficit follow the overall severity continuum that has

Table 8.1 *"Hit Rate" for Successful Classification of Different Psychiatric Groups from Patients with Known Brain Damage*

Group	Classification Rate (%)
Nonpsychotic psychiatric disorders	82
Mixed psychiatric disorders	77
Mixed affective disorders	77
Mixed psychotic disorders	70
Acute or reactive schizophrenia	77
Mixed schizophrenic disorders	69
Chronic or process schizophrenia	54

Note. Adapted from Heaton, Baade, and Johnson (1978). The classification rates are the percent of patients correctly assigned to the psychiatric group based on neuropsychological test results.

been observed along the spectrum of major psychiatric syndromes, there is a striking lack of functional specificity in the neuropsychological findings across these syndromes. Despite considerable effort focused on identifying more specific patterns of neuropsychological deficit that might distinguish different psychiatric syndromes, most research has found relatively consistent impairment of the same "fluid" cognitive abilities (including learning and memory functions, "executive" or "cognitive control" functions, attentional functions, and speed of processing) across the syndromes, with the greatest differences between diagnostic groups being differences of severity rather than pattern of deficit (Bora, Yücel, & Pantelis, 2010; Daban et al., 2006; Hill et al., 2009; Krabbendam, Arts, van Os, & Aleman, 2005).

This does not appear to be a limitation of tests to detect more specific pathology. The tests that best distinguish syndromes from healthy groups and from other syndromes tend to be more general and to include more complex "polyfactorial" coverage of cognitive domains than the more functionally specific tests, which tap more pure "domain-specific" processes and tend to be less discriminating (Dickinson, Goldberg, Gold, Elvevag, & Weinberger, 2011; Hill et al., 2009). Although it remains possible that some syndrome-specific dysfunctions will one day be discovered, the lack of positive findings to date is telling, given that virtually all research on the topic has been seeking to identify "signature" patterns of deficit based on the best prevailing theory of dysfunction within each syndrome. At this point, it seems likely that there are major overlapping causes of brain dysfunction that yield vulnerability to neuropsychiatric syndromes, and that, from a neurocognitive perspective, severity of generalized deficit explains more about psychopathology than does the specific pattern of cognitive dysfunction.

Neuroimaging

When CT-scans first revealed diffuse neuropathology in schizophrenia, there was excitement that we at last had found the "smoking gun" for this syndrome, and that this finding would lead to identifying a biological basis for the Kraepelinian distinction between schizophrenia and bipolar disorder (Johnstone, Crow, Frith, Husband, & Kreel, 1976; Johnstone et al., 1978). Research rapidly accumulated showing that the pathology was "graded" in schizophrenia, and while we could observe correlations among indications of neuropathology and symptoms (particularly "negative" and "disorganization" symptoms), this appeared to reflect discrete processes but not discrete "subtypes" (Crow, 1980, 1982, 1985). A large literature based on MRI, now including multiple reviews and meta-analyses, reveals ventricular enlargement and widespread gray- and white-matter deficits cortically, subcortically, and in limbic structures in schizophrenia and bipolar disorder, with schizophrenia being distinguished primarily by severity of deficits (Arnone et al., 2009; McDonald et al., 2005; McIntosh et al., 2008; Rimol et al., 2010). Some studies suggest specificity of deficits to schizophrenia relative to bipolar disorder (McDonald et al., 2005), but this appears primarily due to the perception that deficits in bipolar disorder are more subtle. A more persuasive argument would be based on the identification of a regional deficit in bipolar disorder relative to schizophrenia that would not be predicted on simple severity. This was suggested, for example, to be true of gray-matter deficits in the anterior cingulate gyrus, and contrasted to all other anomalies of brain structure that were interpreted as nonspecific (Ellison-Wright & Bullmore, 2010). One recent study attempted to tease apart structural anomalies that are shared and that distinguish schizophrenia from bipolar disorders, and to determine the degree to which these anomalies are due to shared genetic or environmental influences, using a family design (Pol et al., 2012). This study identified shared genetic influences underlying common deficits in cortical gray matter and white matter; a generally larger intracranial volume distinguished bipolar disorder, while a thicker parietal cortex distinguished schizophrenia. It will be interesting to see if these findings can be replicated in other samples and using other research designs.

Although most comparative studies have focused on schizophrenia and bipolar disorder, some sparse information also enables comparison of brain abnormalities across other groups of mental disorders. Unipolar depression is associated with similar widespread deficits if the syndrome is sufficiently severe (for example, in major depression with psychotic features), but in general, there are no structural anomalies with sufficient sensitivity and specificity to be useful in distinguishing unipolar from bipolar mood disorders (Drevets, Price, & Furey, 2008). Drevets and colleagues (2008) suggest that the failure of research so far to reveal syndrome-specific abnormalities is due to heterogeneity of the syndromes, and that if more specific "subtypes" are found, these may be associated with more specific structural anomalies. Again, however, it remains unclear to what extent behavioral observations alone will fruitfully distinguish unique forms of neuropathological compromise.

There are suggestions that molecular imaging may yield greater specificity and inform us about the structure of true "endophenotypes" – phenotypes that are more closely related to the genetic vulnerability of the disease, even if these are not perfectly correlated with disease phenotypes (Gottesman & Gould, 2003). For example, there are claims that magnetic resonance spectroscopy (MRS) can be used to obtain measures of gamma amino butyric acid (GABA), and that decreases in GABA concentration may be typical of depression (and possibly also panic disorder and alcohol dependence), but not schizophrenia or bipolar disorder (Hasler & Northoff, 2011). MRS signals for glutamate and glutamine (Glx) may also distinguish unipolar from bipolar depression (Hasler & Northoff, 2011). These studies so far have not been widely replicated, however, leaving it unclear to what extent these are robust findings from which further phenomenological characterization might proceed.

It is clearly an important target for future research to determine what specific abnormalities of brain structure or function diverge based on unique genetic or experiential factors, and how these may combine to yield syndromal diversity at the cognitive and symptom level. So far, however, there are few compelling examples of unique features of brain structure that follow the current diagnostic taxonomy. Instead, there is abundant evidence that the degree of structural abnormality in the brain follows the same severity gradient of major psychopathology that was identified by Menninger and Llopis as the basis for their unitary dimensional views.

Genetics

The revolution in genetics accompanying the completion of the human genome project and the advent of genome-wide association studies (GWAS) has led to remarkable progress in certain areas of biomedicine. For example, by studying a large number of genetic markers across the entire genome, it has been possible to identify loci reflecting genetic risk for Crohn's disease, Type 1 and Type 2 diabetes, and other common diseases (Wellcome Trust Case Control Consortium, 2007). In contrast, psychiatric genetics has been relatively disappointing, with increasing evidence converging to suggest that most psychiatric syndromes are associated with a large number (from hundreds to thousands) of very small effects from common genetic variants, along with possibly some larger effects from rare genetic variants. It is particularly striking to observe the degree to which genetic risks appear to be shared across many brain diseases, including schizophrenia, bipolar disorder, autism spectrum disorders, and intellectual disability (Cross-Disorder Group of the Psychiatric Genomics Consortium, 2013; Fanous et al., 2012; Owen, 2012; Owen, Craddock, & Jablensky, 2007; Purcell et al., 2009). The familial risk for psychiatric disorders is shared with familial risk for dementia, suggesting that the genetic factors may underlie a broad set of generalized vulnerabilities for brain dysfunction (Narayanaswamy et al., 2011). There is evidence, however, that despite some shared genetic risk for both unipolar and bipolar mood disorders (i.e., 25 percent of liability for bipolar disorder may be explained by shared genetic risks for depression), the risk for bipolar disorder should *not* be seen as simply a more severe form of unipolar depression on the same continuum (McGuffin et al., 2003).

A study from the International Schizophrenia Consortium is particularly interesting in that it estimated the combined risk of many common genetic variants that would not be detected by standard GWAS methods (Purcell et al., 2009). They estimated that at least one third of the total variation in schizophrenia risk is accounted for by a large number (thousands) of common genetic variants, each with very small contributions to risk (genetic risk ratios < 1.05); and that this risk is substantially shared with bipolar disorder. Moreover, they found that these risks were not shared with several nonpsychiatric diseases (coronary artery disease, Crohn's disease, hypertension, rheumatoid arthritis, type I diabetes, type II diabetes).

Although much work using GWAS has failed to reveal many validated candidate common genetic variants for distinctive psychopathological syndromes, several studies already have identified increased numbers of rare variants (copy number variations or *de novo* mutations) in samples of patients with schizophrenia or autism relative to controls (Ingason et al., 2011; Sebat et al., 2007; Stefansson et al., 2008; Tam et al., 2010). One study of ADHD did not find any increase in specific rare variants, but did find that candidates associated with *other* neuropsychiatric illnesses (including autism, schizophrenia, and Tourette's syndrome), appeared to be enriched in the ADHD sample, thus implying some common final neurodevelopmental pathways (Elia et al., 2009).

So far, there have been fewer studies of rare variants in bipolar disorder, and one study found no increase in rare variants, and indeed significantly *fewer* rare variants in bipolar than have been found in schizophrenia samples (Grozeva et al., 2010). The authors suggest the possibility that in the face of shared genetic risk from common variants, individuals who also possess rare variants may be at increased risk for schizophrenia, while those who do not have additional mutations end up with bipolar disorder presentations.

Finally, several other recent studies suggest that genetic bases of mental disorders may be more compatible with several major dimensions rather than with the multiplicity of categories in *DSM* and *ICD* taxonomies. Kendler and colleagues reported that the common mental disorders are modeled best as reflecting four correlated genetic factors: two fundamental dimensions (internalizing disorders and externalizing disorders) and Axis I and Axis II (Kendler et al., 2011). A similar result was obtained in a child and adolescent sample, where the best-fitting model involved three higher-order genetic factors: one "general" factor associated with increased risk for *all* syndromes and two other factors, one representing internalizing and the other representing externalizing syndromes (Lahey, Van Hulle, Singh, Waldman, & Rathouz, 2011).

Overall, the emerging genetic data are highlighting the role of common and rare genetic variations in risk for psychopathology. Current evidence suggests that large numbers of common genetic variants, each with very small effect, contribute to risk for psychopathology in relatively general ways via their effects on diverse neurodevelopmental processes and signaling pathways. Rare variants also play an important role, and sometimes have larger effects, in contributing to overall risk for mental disorders. This evidence is most consistent with a taxonomy of psychopathological syndromes that would ultimately include both categorical and dimensional approaches. To the extent that discrete groups have been identified on genetic grounds, these do not follow traditional *DSM* or *ICD* boundaries.

Informatics

We are at a critical juncture in the development of major health information resources, as the Affordable Care Act is leading most large medical centers across the United States to implement electronic medical record systems. The centralization of these records will ultimately enable large-scale data mining of information about symptoms, diagnostic test results, clinical care, and treatments received. It is likely that at some point, whole genome-sequencing data will also be part of comprehensive, life-long medical records. Although the potential of this informatics revolution is vast, there already are some examples of the utility of these records, including their relevance to psychiatric syndromes. For example, 161 illnesses described in 1.5 million patient records were analyzed using a statistical model to estimate genetic overlap; results suggested significant overlap among autism, bipolar disorder, and schizophrenia (Rzhetsky, Wajngurt, Park, & Zheng, 2007). The authors were further able to estimate the degree of overlap and suggested: "20–60% of autism-predisposing variations also predispose the bearer to bipolar disorder, and 20–75% of autism-predisposing variations also predispose the bearer to schizophrenia" (p. 11698). In addition to highlighting these specific correlations across traditional diagnostic boundaries, they highlighted a number of other associations spanning a broad range of neurodevelopmental and neurological syndromes. As these informatics strategies are expanded from studies of 1.5 million records to hundreds of millions of records, and the longitudinal patterns of these findings are interrogated, it seems likely that many additional insights and novel patterns of association will be found. So far, there is little evidence that these findings are likely to validate the current diagnostic taxonomy as described in the *DSM* and *ICD* models.

Trends and Future Directions

There is now strong interest in dimensional models in psychopathology to complement the categorical models adopted in the *DSM* and *ICD*. The NIMH has incorporated into its strategic plan a "circuit-neuroscience"-based classification framework with a major emphasis on dimensional approaches within five major domains (positive and negative valence systems, cognitive systems, systems for social processes, and arousal and regulatory systems); this approach is known as the Research Domain Criterion (RDoC) project (Insel & Cuthbert, 2009; Insel et al., 2010; Sanislow et al., 2010). The RDoC initiative (www.nimh.nih.gov/research-priorities/rdoc/) explicitly aims to foster research in psychopathology according to "dimensions of functioning (such as fear circuitry or working memory)" based on evidence spanning "multiple units of analysis" or biological scales, including genes, molecules, cells, circuits, physiology, behavior, and self-reports; and the development of "novel, circuit-based interventions" (Morris, Rumsey, & Cuthbert, 2013; see Table 8.2).

Table 8.2 *NIMH Research Domain Criteria (RDoC)*

Functional Domains (Constructs)				
Negative Valence Systems (e.g., acute threat ["fear"], potential threat ["anxiety"], loss)	Positive Valence Systems (e.g., approach motivation ["reward"], reward learning, habit)	Cognitive Systems (e.g., attention, perception, declarative memory, language, cognitive control)	Systems for Social Processes (e.g., affiliation and attachment, social communication, perception and understanding of self/others)	Arousal and Regulatory Systems (e.g., arousal, circadian rhythms, sleep-wakefulness)

Units of Analysis
Genes   Molecules   Cells   Circuits   Physiology   Behavior   Self-Reports   Paradigms

Source. Adapted with permission from "Rethinking Psychiatric Diagnosis on the Eve of *DSM-5*: A New Paradigm for NIMH" by T. Doug, May 7, 2013. Retrieved from http://www.behavioral.net/blogs/tom-doub/rethinking-psychiatric-diagnosis-eve-dsm-5-new-paradigm-nimh

In the Consortium for Neuropsychiatric Phenomics at UCLA (http://www.phenomics.ucla.edu/), we have articulated a similar seven-level hierarchy including: genome, proteome, cellular systems/ signaling pathways, neural systems, cognitive phenotypes, symptoms, and syndromes (Bilder, Howe, & Sabb, 2013; Bilder, Parker, & Sabb, 2010; Bilder, Howe, Novak, Sabb, & Parker, 2011; Bilder et al., 2009; see Table 8.3). The challenge faced by these initiatives is profound, however, insofar as the conduct of research spanning all of these biological scales calls for transdisciplinary work that is likely well beyond the scope of what is currently feasible within the budgetary limits of most research projects. There is hope, however, that the shift in strategic emphasis will: (a) induce investigators to develop innovative research designs that actively challenge existing taxonomic conventions, (b) develop new evidence that will test the validity of new dimensions and categories with respect to strong biological roots, and (c) promote the deposition of research data into repositories that will facilitate the pooling of results and investigation of hypotheses with adequate sample sizes.

Table 8.3 *Levels of Analysis for Investigation of Mechanistic Links from Neuropsychiatric Syndrome to Genome*

Level of Analysis	Description
Syndrome	Clusters of symptoms that tend to co-occur within individuals (usually diagnosed by clinician)
Symptom	Patients' self-reports and/or clinicians' judgments of behavioral problems or idiosyncrasies (usually determined by a clinician based on interview)
Cognitive-Behavioral	Measurable aspects of behavior, perception, cognition, affect, or emotion (usually assessed with rating scales or psychometric tests)
Neural System	Activity of cell populations, from small circuits to large-scale networks (usually assessed with electrophysiological or other neuroimaging methods)
Cellular Systems & Signaling Pathways (Metabolome)	Intracellular activities including metabolic processes, signaling pathways; and extracellular modulating effects (usually assessed with in vitro neurophysiology or other neurobiological procedures)
Proteome	Proteins (~500K–2M; usually assessed by chromatography, crystallography or biochemical methods)
Genome	Genes (three billion base pairs in human genome, associated with ~20K "genes," i.e., segments of DNA that code for proteins)

   In addition, some developments in healthcare reform may promote the development of more accurate taxonomies of mental illness. For example, many patients with mental illness have their first encounter with the health system in primary care settings, where the complex algorithms used to diagnose mental disorders following *DSM* or *ICD* models are too cumbersome and require too much additional training. *The International Classification of Primary Care (ICPC)* was first published in 1987 and primary care versions of *DSM* and *ICD* systems were promulgated in 1995 (Gask, Klinkman, Fortes, & Dowrick, 2008). These systems reduce the complexity of the *DSM/ICD* systems to eleven "clusters," which include "internalizing" and "externalizing" disorders, along with "psychosis," "neurocognitive," "developmental," and "bodily function" syndromes. The primary care system also embraces the use of dimensional ratings to complement any of its categorical assignments. By "simplifying" the frameworks developed for *DSM/ICD*, it may be that these systems will provide methods better suited to determine the natural boundaries of mental disorders on an empirical basis.

Ultimately, these strategies will need to work in concert to revolutionize the diagnostic taxonomy of neuropsychiatric disorders and promote better understanding of the causes of these syndromes, which could lead to the development of novel and more effective treatments. NIMH director Thomas Insel once remarked that completion of the human genome project gave us the "edge pieces" of the jigsaw puzzle representing all of human biology. The more we learn, however, the more likely it seems that these are the "center pieces" of a puzzle that is built from the inside out, and we do not yet know exactly how big it is. In the face of this complexity, we will need to amass large quantities of data – on lots of people, across diverse levels of analysis, and across time – in order to detect subtle patterns of association that can help us assemble mechanistic links from one level to the next. This would seem impossible if it were not for the dramatic acceleration of information sciences, including capacities to store and manipulate data and discern patterns in data that far exceed the capacity of individual humans. We are now beginning to aggregate data – through health records; massive warehouses of genomic data; and personal records of our travels, keystrokes, search topics, and social networks being accumulated by providers of web and social media services. Major efforts already are underway, aiming to effectively "harvest" information from these Big Data repositories. We must hope and strive to maximize the use of these data for the advancement of the common good and alleviation of suffering.

Acknowledgments

This work was supported by the Consortium for Neuropsychiatric Phenomics (NIH Roadmap for Medical Research grants UL1-DE019580 and PL1MH083271) and the Michael E. Tennenbaum Family Center for the Biology of Creativity.

REFERENCES

American Psychiatric Association. (1980). *Diagnostic and statistical manual of mental disorders* (3rd ed.). Washington, DC: Author.

American Psychiatric Association. (1987). *Diagnosis and statistical manual of mental disorders* (3rd ed., revised). Washington, DC: Author.

American Psychiatric Association. (1994). *Diagnostic and statistical manual of mental disorders* (4th ed.). Washington, DC: Author.

American Psychiatric Association. (2000). *Diagnostic and statistical manual of mental disorders* (4th ed., text rev.). Washington, DC: Author.

198   *Robert M. Bilder*

American Psychiatric Association. (2013). *Diagnostic and statistical manual of mental disorders* (5th ed.). Washington, DC: Author.

An, X., & Bentler, P. M. (2011). Extended mixture factor analysis model with covariates for mixed binary and continuous responses. *Statistics in Medicine, 30*(21), 2634–47. http://dx.doi.org/10.1002/sim.4310

Andrews, G., Slade, T., & Peters, L. (1999). Classification in psychiatry: *ICD-10* versus *DSM-IV*. *British Journal of Psychiatry, 174*, 3–5. http://dx.doi.org/10.1192%2Fbjp.174.1.3

Arnone, D., Cavanagh, J., Gerber, D., Lawrie, S., Ebmeier, K., & McIntosh, A. (2009). Magnetic resonance imaging studies in bipolar disorder and schizophrenia: Meta-analysis. *British Journal of Psychiatry, 195*(3), 194–201. http://dx.doi.org/10.1192%2Fbjp.bp.108.059717

Beauchaine, T. P. (2003). Taxometrics and developmental psychopathology. *Developmental Psychopathology, 15*(3), 501–27. http://dx.doi.org/10.1017%2FS0954579403000270

Beauchaine, T. P. (2007). A brief taxometrics primer. *Journal of Clinical Child & Adolescent Psychology, 36*(4), 654–76. http://dx.doi.org/10.1080/15374410701662840

Bentler, P. M., & Bonnett, D. G. (1980). Significance tests and goodness-of-fit in the analysis of covariance structures. *Psychological Bulletin, 88*, 588–606. http://dx.doi.org/10.1037%2F%2F0033-2909.88.3.588

Bilder, R. M., Howe, A., Novak, N., Sabb, F. W., & Parker, D. S. (2011). The genetics of cognitive impairment in schizophrenia: A phenomic perspective. *Trends in Cognitive Sciences, 15*(9), 428–35. http://dx.doi.org/10.1016/j.tics.2011.07.002

Bilder, R. M., Howe, A. S., & Sabb, F. W. (2013). Multilevel models from biology to psychology: Mission impossible? *Journal of Abnormal Psychology, 122*(3), 917–27. http://dx.doi.org/10.1037/a0032263

Bilder, R. M., Parker, D. S., & Sabb, F. W. (2010). Modeling cognitive Phenotypes from circuit to syndrome. *Biological Psychiatry, 67*(9), 254.

Bilder, R. M., Poldrack, R., Parker, D. S., Reise, S. P., Jentsch, J. D., Cannon, T., ... Freimer, N. (2009). Cognitive phenomics. In S. Wood, N. Allen, & C. Pantelis (Eds.), *Handbook of neuropsychology of mental disorders* (pp. 271–82). Cambridge, England: Cambridge University Press.

Bilder, R. M., Sabb, F. W., Cannon, T. D., London, E. D., Jentsch, J. D., Parker, D. S., ... Freimer, N. B. (2009). Phenomics: The systematic study of phenotypes on a genome-wide scale. *Neuroscience, 164*(1), 30–42. http://dx.doi.org/10.1016/j.neuroscience.2009.01.027

Bora, E., Yücel, M., & Pantelis, C. (2010). Cognitive impairment in schizophrenia and affective psychoses: implications for *DSM-V* criteria and beyond. *Schizophrenia Bulletin, 36*(1), 36–42. http://dx.doi.org/10.1093%2Fschbul%2Fsbp094

Brown, G. W. (1996). Genetics of depression: A social science perspective. *International Review of Psychiatry, 8*(4), 387–401. http://dx.doi.org/10.3109%2F09540269609051554

Cloninger, C. R. (1999). A new conceptual paradigm from genetics and psychobiology for the science of mental health. *Australian and New Zealand Journal of Psychiatry, 33*(2), 174–86. http://dx.doi.org/10.1046%2Fj.1440-1614.1999.00533.x

Cole, D. A. (2004). Taxometrics in psychopathology research: an introduction to some of the procedures and related methodological issues. *Journal of Abnormal Psychology, 113*(1), 3–9. http://dx.doi.org/10.1037/0021-843X.113.1.3

Costa Jr., P. T., & McCrae, R. R. (2008). The revised NEO Personality Inventory (NEO-PI-R). *The SAGE handbook of personality theory and assessment, 2,* 179–98.

Cross-Disorder Group of the Psychiatric Genomics Consortium. (2013). Identification of risk loci with shared effects on five major psychiatric disorders: A genome-wide analysis. *Lancet, 381*(9875), 1371–9. http://dx.doi.org/10.1016/S0140-6736(12)62129-1

Crow, T. J. (1980, January 12). Molecular pathology of schizophrenia: more than one disease process? *British Medical Journal,* 66–8. http://dx.doi.org/10.1136%2Fbmj.280.6207.66

Crow, T. J. (1982). Two syndromes in schizophrenia? *Trends in Neuroscience,* 351–4. http://dx.doi.org/10.1016%2F0166-2236%2882%2990202-8

Crow, T. J. (1985). The two-syndrome concept: Origins and current status. *Schizophrenia Bulletin, 11*(3), 471–86. http://dx.doi.org/10.1093%2Fschbul%2F11.3.471

Daban, C., Martinez-Aran, A., Torrent, C., Tabarés-Seisdedos, R., Balanzá-Martínez, V., Salazar-Fraile, J., ... Vieta, E. (2006). Specificity of cognitive deficits in bipolar disorder versus schizophrenia. *Psychotherapy and Psychosomatics, 75*(2), 72–84. http://dx.doi.org/10.1159/000090891

Dickinson, D., Goldberg, T. E., Gold, J. M., Elvevag, B., & Weinberger, D. R. (2011). Cognitive factor structure and invariance in people with schizophrenia, their unaffected siblings, and controls. *Schizophrenia Bulletin, 37*(6), 1157–67. http://dx.doi.org/10.1093/schbul/sbq018

Drevets, W. C., Price, J. L., & Furey, M. L. (2008). Brain structural and functional abnormalities in mood disorders: Implications for neurocircuitry models of depression. *Brain Structure and Function, 213*(1), 93–118. http://dx.doi.org/10.1007%2Fs00429-008-0189-x

Eaton, N. R., Krueger, R. F., South, S. C., Simms, L. J., & Clark, L. A. (2010). Contrasting prototypes and dimensions in the classification of personality pathology: Evidence that dimensions, but not prototypes, are robust. *Psychological Medicine, 41*(6), 1151–63. http://dx.doi.org/10.1017/S0033291710001650

Elia, J., Gai, X., Xie, H., Perin, J., Geiger, E., Glessner, J., & D'arcy, M. (2009). Rare structural variants found in attention-deficit hyperactivity disorder are preferentially associated with neurodevelopmental genes. *Molecular Psychiatry, 15*(6), 637–46. http://dx.doi.org/10.1038%2Fmp.2009.57

Ellison-Wright, I., & Bullmore, E. (2010). Anatomy of bipolar disorder and schizophrenia: A meta-analysis. *Schizophrenia Research, 117*(1), 1–12. http://dx.doi.org/10.1016%2Fj.schres.2009.12.022

Fanous, A. H., Middleton, F. A., Gentile, K., Amdur, R. L., Maher, B. S., Zhao, Z., . . . Ferreira, S. R. (2012). Genetic overlap of schizophrenia and bipolar disorder in a high-density linkage survey in the Portuguese Island population. *American Journal of Medical Genetics Part B: Neuropsychiatric Genetics.* http://dx.doi.org/10.1002%2Fajmg.b.32041

Finger, S. (2001). *Origins of neuroscience: A history of explorations into brain function.* New York, NY: Oxford University Press.

Frances, A. (2012). *DSM-5* in distress [Blog post]. Retrieved from www.psychologytoday.com/blog/dsm5-in-distress

Gask, L., Klinkman, M., Fortes, S., & Dowrick, C. (2008). Capturing complexity: The case for a new classification system for mental disorders in primary care. *European Psychiatry, 23*(7), 469–76. http://dx.doi.org/10.1016%2Fj.eurpsy.2008.06.006

Georgiades, S., Szatmari, P., Boyle, M., Hanna, S., Duku, E., Zwaigenbaum, L., . . . Thompson, A. (2012). Investigating phenotypic heterogeneity in children with autism spectrum disorder: A factor mixture modeling approach. *J Child Psychol Psychiatry.* http://dx.doi.org/10.1111/j.1469-7610.2012.02588.x

Gillespie, N. A., Neale, M. C., Legrand, L. N., Iacono, W. G., & McGue, M. (2012). Are the symptoms of cannabis use disorder best accounted for by dimensional, categorical, or factor mixture models? A comparison of male and female young adults. *Psychol Addict Behav, 26*(1), 68–77. http://dx.doi.org/10.1037/a0026230

Gottesman, I. I., & Gould, T. D. (2003). The endophenotype concept in psychiatry: etymology and strategic intentions. *American Journal of Psychiatry, 160*(4), 636–45. http://dx.doi.org/10.1176%2Fappi.ajp.160.4.636

Grove, W. M. (1991). Validity of taxometric inferences based on cluster analysis stopping rules. *Thinking Clearly About Psychology, 2*, 313–29.

Grozeva, D., Kirov, G., Ivanov, D., Jones, I. R., Jones, L., Green, E. K., . . . Farmer, A. E. (2010). Rare copy number variants: a point of rarity in genetic risk for bipolar disorder and schizophrenia. *Archives of General Psychiatry, 67*(4), 318–27. http://dx.doi.org/10.1001%2Farchgenpsychiatry.2010.25

Hallquist, M. N., & Pilkonis, P. A. (2012). Refining the phenotype of borderline personality disorder: Diagnostic criteria and beyond. *Personal Disord, 3*(3), 228–46. http://dx.doi.org/10.1037/a0027953

Harris, G. T., Rice, M. E., & Quinsey, V. L. (1994). Psychopathy as a taxon: Evidence that psychopaths are a discrete class. *Journal of Consulting and Clinical Psychology, 62*, 387–97. http://dx.doi.org/10.1037%2F%2F0022-006X.62.2.387

Haslam, N. (2003). Categorical versus dimensional models of mental disorder: The taxometric evidence. *Australian and New Zealand Journal of Psychiatry, 37*(6), 696–704. http://dx.doi.org/10.1111%2Fj.1440-1614.2003.01258.x

Haslam, N., Holland, E., & Kuppens, P. (2012). Categories versus dimensions in personality and psychopathology: A quantitative review of taxometric research.

Psychological Medicine, 42(05), 903–20. http://dx.doi.org/10.1017/S0033291711001966

Hasler, G., & Northoff, G. (2011). Discovering imaging endophenotypes for major depression. *Molecular Psychiatry, 16*(6), 604–19. http://dx.doi.org/10.1038%2Fmp.2011.23

Heaton, R. K., Baade, L. E., & Johnson, K. L. (1978). Neuropsychological test results associated with psychiatric disorders in adults. *Psychological Bulletin, 85*, 141–62. http://dx.doi.org/10.1037%2F%2F0033-2909.85.1.141

Helzer, J. E., Kraemer, H. C., Krueger, R. F., Wittchen, H.-U., Sirovatka, P. J., & Regier, D. A. (Eds.). (2008). *Dimensional approaches in diagnostic classification: Refining the research agenda for "DSM-V."* Arlington, VA: American Psychiatric Association.

Hempel, C. G. (1961). Introduction to problems of taxonomy. *Field Studies in the Mental Disorders, 5*, 3–22.

Hill, S. K., Reilly, J. L., Harris, M. S. H., Rosen, C., Marvin, R. W., DeLeon, O., & Sweeney, J. A. (2009). A comparison of neuropsychological dysfunction in first-episode psychosis patients with unipolar depression, bipolar disorder, and schizophrenia. *Schizophrenia Research, 113*(2–3), 167–75. http://dx.doi.org/10.1016%2Fj.schres.2009.04.020

Hyman, S. E. (2010). The diagnosis of mental disorders: the problem of reification. *Annu Rev Clin Psychol, 6*, 155–79. http://10.1146/annurev.clinpsy.3.022806.091532

Ingason, A., Rujescu, D., Cichon, S., Sigurdsson, E., Sigmundsson, T., Pietilainen, O. P., . . . St Clair, D. M. (2011). Copy number variations of chromosome 16p13.1 region associated with schizophrenia. *Molecular Psychiatry, 16*(1), 17–25. http://dx.doi.org/10.1038/mp.2009.101

Insel, T. R., & Cuthbert, B. N. (2009). Endophenotypes: Bridging genomic complexity and disorder heterogeneity. *Biological Psychiatry, 66*(11), 988–9. http://dx.doi.org/10.1016/j.biopsych.2009.10.008

Insel, T., Cuthbert, B., Garvey, M., Heinssen, R., Pine, D. S., Quinn, K., . . . Wang, P. (2010). Research domain criteria (RDoC): Toward a new classification framework for research on mental disorders. *American Journal of Psychiatry, 167*(7), 748–51. http://dx.doi.org/10.1176/appi.ajp.2010.09091379

Johnstone, E. C., Crow, T. J., Frith, C. D., Husband, J., & Kreel, L. (1976). Cerebral ventricular size and cognitive impairment in chronic schizophrenia. *Lancet*, 924–6. http://dx.doi.org/10.1016%2FS0140-6736%2876%2990890-4

Johnstone, E. C., Crow, T. J., Frith, C. D., Stevens, M., Kreel, L., & Husband, J. (1978). The dementia of dementia praecox. *Acta Psychiatrica Scandinavica, 57*, 305–24. http://dx.doi.org/10.1111%2Fj.1600-0447.1978.tb06899.x

Jöreskog, K. G., & Sörbom, D. (1985). *LISREL VI. Analysis of linear structural relationships by maximum likelihood, instrumental variables, and least squares methods.* Unpublished manuscript. University of Uppsala, Sweden.

Kendler, K. S. (1996). Major depression and generalised anxiety disorder: Same genes, (partly) different environments – revisited. *British Journal of Psychiatry, 168*(Suppl. 30), 68–75.

Kendler, K. S., Aggen, S. H., Knudsen, G. P., Røysamb, E., Neale, M. C., & Reichborn-Kjennerud, T. (2011). The structure of genetic and environmental risk factors for syndromal and subsyndromal common *DSM-IV* Axis I and all Axis II disorders. *American Journal of Psychiatry, 168*(1), 29–39. http://dx.doi.org/10.1176%2Fappi.ajp.2010.10030340

Kendler, K. S., & Gardner, C. O., Jr. (1998). Boundaries of major depression: an evaluation of *DSM-IV* criteria. *American Journal of Psychiatry, 155*(2), 172–7.

Krabbendam, L., Arts, B., van Os, J., & Aleman, A. (2005). Cognitive functioning in patients with schizophrenia and bipolar disorder: a quantitative review. *Schizophrenia Research, 80*(2), 137–49. http://dx.doi.org/10.1016%2Fj.schres.2005.08.004

Kraepelin, E. (1896). *Psychiatrie: Ein Lehrbuch fur Studirende und Aerzte. Funfte, vollstandig umgearbeitete Auflage*. Leipzig, Germany: Barth.

Kraepelin, E. (1919). *Dementia praecox and paraphrenia*. Edinburgh, Scotland: E and S Livingstone.

Kupfer, D. J., First, M. B., & Regier, D. A. (2002). Introduction. In D. J. Kupfer, M. B. First, & D. A. Regier (Eds.), *A research agenda for "DSM-V."* Washington, DC: American Psychiatric Association.

Kupfer, D. J., Kuhl, E. A., & Wulsin, L. (2013). Psychiatry's integration with medicine: The role of *DSM-5. Annual Review of Medicine, 64*, 385–92. http://dx.doi.org/10.1146/annurev-med-050911-161945

Lahey, B. B., Van Hulle, C. A., Singh, A. L., Waldman, I. D., & Rathouz, P. J. (2011). Higher-order genetic and environmental structure of prevalent forms of child and adolescent psychopathology. *Archives of General Psychiatry, 68*(2), 181–9. http://dx.doi.org/10.1001/archgenpsychiatry.2010.192

Lawrie, S. M., Hall, J., McIntosh, A. M., Owens, D. G., & Johnstone, E. C. (2010). The "continuum of psychosis": Scientifically unproven and clinically impractical. *British Journal of Psychiatry, 197*(6), 423–5. http://dx.doi.org/10.1192/bjp.bp.109.072827

Lazarsfeld, P. F., & Henry, N. W. (1968). *Latent structure analysis*. Boston, MA: Houghton Mifflin.

Linscott, R. J., & van Os, J. (2010). Systematic reviews of categorical versus continuum models in psychosis: Evidence for discontinuous subpopulations underlying a psychometric continuum. Implications for *DSM-V, DSM-VI,* and *DSM-VII. Annual Review of Clinical Psychology, 6*, 391–419. http://dx.doi.org/10.1146%2Fannurev.clinpsy.032408.153506

Llopis, B. (1954). La psicosis única. *Archivos de Neurobiología, 17*, 1–34.

Lubke, G. H., Muthen, B., Moilanen, I. K., McGough, J. J., Loo, S. K., Swanson, J. M., ... Smalley, S. L. (2007). Subtypes versus severity differences in attention-deficit/hyperactivity disorder in the Northern Finnish Birth Cohort. *Journal of the American Academy of Child and Adolescent*

Psychiatry, 46(12), 1584–93. http://dx.doi.org/10.1097/
chi.0b013e31815750dd

Manktelow, M. (2010). *History of taxonomy.* [Lecture.] Department of
Systematic Biology, Uppsala University, Uppsala, Sweden.

McDonald, C., Bullmore, E., Sham, P., Chitnis, X., Suckling, J.,
MacCabe, J., ... Murray, R. M. (2005). Regional volume deviations of
brain structure in schizophrenia and psychotic bipolar disorder. *British
Journal of Psychiatry, 186*(5), 369–77. http://dx.doi.org/10.1192%
2Fbjp.186.5.369

McGuffin, P., Rijsdijk, F., Andrew, M., Sham, P., Katz, R., & Cardno, A.
(2003). The heritability of bipolar affective disorder and the genetic
relationship to unipolar depression. *Archives of General Psychiatry, 60*(5),
497–502. http://dx.doi.org/10.1001%2Farchpsyc.60.5.497

McIntosh, A. M., Maniega, S. M., Lymer, G. K. S., McKirdy, J., Hall, J.,
Sussmann, J. E. D., ... Lawrie, S. M. (2008). White matter tractography
in bipolar disorder and schizophrenia. *Biological Psychiatry, 64*(12),
1088–92. http://dx.doi.org/10.1016%2Fj.biopsych.2008.07.026

Meehl, P. E. (1995). Bootstraps taxometrics. Solving the classification problem
in psychopathology. *American Psychologist, 50*(4), 266–75. http://dx.doi.org/
10.1037%2F%2F0003-066X.50.4.266

Meehl, P. E. (1999). Clarifications about taxometric method. *Applied and
Preventive Psychology, 8*(3), 165–74. http://dx.doi.org/10.1016%2FS0962-
1849%2805%2980075-7

Meehl, P. E. (2004). What's in a taxon? *Journal of Abnormal Psychology, 113*(1),
39–43. http://dx.doi.org/10.1037/0021-843X.113.1.39

Menninger, K. (1959). Toward a unitary concept of mental illness. In B. H. Hall
(Ed.), *A psychiatrist's world* (pp. 516–28). New York, NY: Viking.

Menninger, K., Ellenberger, H., Pruyser, P., & Mayman, M. (1959). The unitary
concept of mental illness. *Pastoral Psychology, 10*(4), 13–19. http://dx.doi.
org/10.1007%2FBF01741038

Millon, T., & Simonsen, E. (2010). A précis of psychopathological history. In
T. Millon, R. F. Krueger, & E. Simonsen (Eds.), *Contemporary directions in
psychopathology: Scientific foundations of the "DSM-V" and "ICD-11"* (pp. 3–52).
New York, NY: Guilford Press.

Morris, S. E., Ramsey, J. M., & Cuthbert, B. N. (2013). Rethinking mental
disorders: The role of learning and brain plasticity. *Restorative Neurology
and Neurosciences, 32*(1), 5–23. http://dx.doi.org/10.3233/RNN-139015

Murphy, E. A. (1964). One cause? Many causes? The argument from the
bimodal distribution. *Journal of Chronic Disease, 17*, 301–24. http://dx.doi.
org/10.1016%2F0021-9681%2864%2990117-1

Muthen, B., Asparouhov, T., & Rebollo, I. (2006). Advances in behavioral
genetics modeling using Mplus: Applications of factor mixture modeling to
twin data. *Twin Research and Human Genetics, 9*(3), 313–24. http://dx.doi.
org/10.1375/183242706777591317

Narayanaswamy, J. C., Varghese, M., Jain, S., Sivakumar, P. T., Prakash, O.,
Bharath, S., & Kandavel, T. (2011). Is there a familial overlap between

dementia and other psychiatric disorders? *International Psychogeriatrics,*
23(5), 749–55. http://dx.doi.org/10.1017/S1041610210001572

Owen, M. J. (2012). Intellectual disability and major psychiatric disorders:
A continuum of neurodevelopmental causality. *British Journal of Psychiatry,*
200(4), 268–9. http://dx.doi.org/10.1192%2Fbjp.bp.111.105551

Owen, M. J., Craddock, N., & Jablensky, A. (2007). The genetic deconstruction
of psychosis. *Schizophrenia Bulletin, 33*(4), 905–11. http://dx.doi.org/
10.1093%2Fschbul%2Fsbm053

Pol, H. E. H., van Baal, G. C. M., Schnack, H. G., Brans, R. G. H., van der
Schot, A. C., Brouwer, R. M., . . . Evans, A. C. (2012). Overlapping and
segregating structural brain abnormalities in twins with schizophrenia or
bipolar disorder. *Archives of General Psychiatry, 69*(4), 349–59. http://dx.doi.
org/10.1001/archgenpsychiatry.2011.1615

Preacher, K. J., Rucker, D. D., MacCallum, R. C., & Nicewander, W. A. (2005).
Use of the extreme groups approach: A critical reexamination and new
recommendations. *Psychological Methods, 10*(2), 178–92. http://dx.doi.org/
10.1037%2F1082-989X.10.2.178

Purcell, S. M., Wray, N. R., Stone, J. L., Visscher, P. M., O'Donovan, M. C.,
Sullivan, P. F., . . . Morris, D. W. (2009). Common polygenic variation
contributes to risk of schizophrenia and bipolar disorder. *Nature, 460*(7256),
748–52. http://dx.doi.org/10.1038%2Fnature08185

Rimol, L. M., Hartberg, C. B., Nesvåg, R., Fennema-Notestine, C., Hagler,
D. J., Pung, C. J., . . . Nakstad, P. H. (2010). Cortical thickness and
subcortical volumes in schizophrenia and bipolar disorder. *Biological
Psychiatry, 68*(1), 41–50. http://dx.doi.org/10.1016%2Fj.
biopsych.2010.03.036

Rounsaville, B. J., Alarcón, R. D., Andrews, G., Jackson, J. S., Kendell, R. E., &
Kendler, K. (2002). Basic nomenclature issues for *DSM-V.* In D. J.
Kupfer, M. B. First, & D. A. Regier (Eds.), *A research agenda for "DSM-V."*
(pp. 1–29). Washington, DC: American Psychiatric Association.

Rzhetsky, A., Wajngurt, D., Park, N., & Zheng, T. (2007). Probing genetic
overlap among complex human phenotypes. *Proceedings of the National
Academy of Sciences of the United States of America, 104*(28), 11694–9. http://
dx.doi.org/10.1073/pnas.0704820104

Sanislow, C. A., Pine, D. S., Quinn, K. J., Kozak, M. J., Garvey, M. A.,
Heinssen, R. K., . . . Cuthbert, B. N. (2010). Developing constructs for
psychopathology research: Research domain criteria. *Journal of Abnormal
Psychology, 119*(4), 631–9. http://dx.doi.org/10.1037%2Fa0020909

Sebat, J., Lakshmi, B., Malhotra, D., Troge, J., Lese-Martin, C., Walsh, T., . . .
Wigler, M. (2007). Strong association of de novo copy number mutations
with autism. *Science, 316*(5823), 445–9. http://dx.doi.org/10.1126/
science.1138659

Shorter, E., & Fink, M. (2010). *Endocrine psychiatry: Solving the riddle of
melancholia.* New York, NY: Oxford University Press.

Skilling, T. A., Harris, G. T., Rice, M. T., & Quinsey, V. L. (2001). Identifying
persistently antisocial offenders using the Hare Psychopathy Checklist and

DSM antisocial personality disorder criteria. *Psychological Assessment, 14*(1), 27–38. http://dx.doi.org/10.1037/1040-3590.14.1.27

Skilling, T. A., Quinsey, V. L., & Craig, W. M. (2001). Evidence of a taxon underlying serious antisocial behavior in boys. *Criminal Justice and Behavior, 28*, 450–70. http://dx.doi.org/10.1177%2F009385480102800404

Spiegel, A. (2005). The dictionary of disorder. *New Yorker, 80*(41), 56–63.

Stefansson, H., Rujescu, D., Cichon, S., Pietilainen, O. P., Ingason, A., Steinberg, S., ... Stefansson, K. (2008). Large recurrent microdeletions associated with schizophrenia. *Nature, 455*(7210), 232–6. http://dx.doi.org/10.1038/nature07229

Subbarayappa, B. (2001). The roots of ancient medicine: An historical outline. *Journal of Biosciences-Bangalore, 26*(2), 135–43. http://dx.doi.org/10.1007%2FBF02703637

Tam, G. W., van de Lagemaat, L. N., Redon, R., Strathdee, K. E., Croning, M. D., Malloy, M. P., ... Grant, S. G. (2010). Confirmed rare copy number variants implicate novel genes in schizophrenia. *Biochemical Society Transactions, 38*(2), 445–51. http://dx.doi.org/10.1042/BST0380445

Waller, N. G. (2006). Carving nature at its joints: Paul Meehl's development of taxometrics. *Journal of Abnormal Psychology, 115*(2), 210–15. http://dx.doi.org/10.1037/0021-843X.115.2.210

Widiger, T. A., Frances, A., Spitzer, R. L., & Williams, J. B. (1988). The *DSM-III-R* personality disorders: An overview. *American Journal of Psychiatry, 145*(7), 786–95.

Wellcome Trust Case Control Consortium. (2007). Genome-wide association study of 14,000 cases of seven common diseases and 3,000 shared controls. *Nature, 447*(7145), 661–78. http://dx.doi.org/10.1038/nature05911

Yuan, K. H., & Bentler, P. M. (2010). Finite Normal Mixture SEM Analysis by Fitting Multiple Conventional SEM Models. *Sociological Methodology, 40*(1), 191–245. http://dx.doi.org/10.1111/j.1467-9531.2010.01224.x

9   Early-Life Adversity and Epigenetic Changes
      Implications for Understanding Suicide

Benoit Labonté, Adel Farah, and Gustavo Turecki

Introduction

Every year more than eight hundred thousand people die by suicide, and more than twenty times that number attempt suicide (World Health Organization [WHO], 2014). In addition to the confusion and pain generated by the loss of a beloved family member or friend, suicide has major consequences for society. The WHO estimates the actual burden of suicide to be twenty million life-years and predicts that, by 2020, suicide could be responsible for 2.4 percent of the total burden of disease (WHO, 2006). These statistics not only clearly show the importance suicide has on society but also highlight our inability to properly implement prevention strategies.

Suicide represents the extreme of a behavioral continuum comprising different forms and severities of self-injurious behaviors (van Heeringen, 2001). It is generally assumed that suicide is a complex behavior resulting from the interaction of different distal and proximal risk factors. Distal risk factors such as familial history of suicide, genetic and epigenetic factors, early life adversity, and personality traits confer vulnerability to suicide, while proximal risk factors like psychopathology, recent life events, hopelessness, and acute substance intoxication are better understood as precipitants of the suicidal crisis. The presence of comorbid major depressive disorder (MDD) and substance abuse are among the strongest proximal risk factors. Indeed, studies suggest that 50 to 70 percent of suicide completers die during an episode of MDD (Arsenault-Lapierre, Kim, & Turecki, 2004; Cavanagh, Carson, Sharpe, & Lawrie, 2003), although most individuals who are affected by MDD and other mood disorders will not die by suicide (F. Angst, Stassen, Clayton, & Angst, 2002; J. Angst, Angst, & Stassen, 1999; J. Angst, Degonda, & Ernst, 1992; Blair-West, Cantor, Mellsop, & Eyeson-Annan, 1999). Age and other sociodemographic factors such as educational level, employment, and income moderate the impact of proximal factors on suicide risk (Brezo, Paris,

Tremblay, et al., 2007; Brezo, Paris, & Turecki, 2006; van den Bos, Harteveld, & Stoop, 2009).

Among risk factors influencing suicide more distally are personality traits and familial history of suicidal behavior, both considered strong predictors of suicide (Hawton & van Heeringen, 2009; Suominen et al., 2004). Genetic variation, which consistently has been identified in genetic-epidemiological studies as an important contributor to suicide risk (Ernst, Mechawar, & Turecki, 2009), accounts in part for the familial aggregation of suicide. This appears to be partly independent of the familial transmission of underlying Axis-I disorders (McGirr et al., 2009); rather, it seems to be explained by the familial transmission of personality traits, particularly those characterized by emotional and behavioral dysregulation (Brezo et al., 2006; Jollant, Lawrence, Olie, Guillaume, & Courtet, 2011).

Among the strongest distal predictors of suicide risk is early-life adversity (ELA), such as child abuse (sexual and physical) and parental neglect (Brezo, Paris, Vitaro, et al., 2008; Fergusson, Horwood, & Lynskey, 1996). Between 10 and 40 percent of individuals displaying suicidal behaviors experienced abuse during childhood (Brezo, Klempan, & Turecki, 2008; Fergusson, Boden, & Horwood, 2008), and a positive history of ELA is associated with higher odds of self-harm (Akyuz, Sar, Kugu, & Dogan, 2005; Fliege, Lee, Grimm, & Klapp, 2009; Gladstone et al., 2004; Hawton, Rodham, Evans, & Weatherall, 2002; Spinhoven, Slee, Garnefski, & Arensman, 2009); suicidal ideation (Brezo, Paris, Vitaro, et al., 2008; Fergusson et al., 2008); and suicide attempts (Andover, Zlotnick, & Miller, 2007; Brezo, Paris, Vitaro, et al., 2008; Fergusson et al., 2008; Joiner et al., 2007; McHolm, MacMillan, & Jamieson, 2003; Molnar, Berkman, & Buka, 2001), with an estimated twelvefold overall increase in risk (Bensley, Van Eenwyk, Spieker, & Schoder, 1999; Molnar et al., 2001). Moreover, the prevalence of suicidal ideation and suicide attempts increases with the severity and intensity of the abuse (Brezo, Paris, Vitaro, et al., 2008; Fergusson et al., 2008; Joiner et al., 2007), and ELA strongly associates with negative predictors of several proximal risk factors for suicide, including increased psychiatric comorbidity, earlier age of onset of depression, chronic course, and more severe depressive outcome (Dinwiddie et al., 2000; Evans, Hawton, & Rodham, 2005; Gladstone et al., 2004; Jaffee et al., 2002; Widom, DuMont, & Czaja, 2007; Ystgaard, Hestetun, Loeb, & Mehlum, 2004). The impact of ELA on suicide risk depends on the frequency of the abuse and the identity of the abuser, both important moderators of the relationship between ELA and suicide risk. Abuse perpetrated by a close family member and taking place more often is a stronger predictor of suicidal behavior (Brezo, Paris, Vitaro, et al., 2008). Close family members such as parents are essential for establishing appropriate emotional and behavioral patterns (Cole, Michel, & Teti, 1994), and repeated acts of abuse by parental figures or other close family members may signal an adverse environment to which an individual may respond by adapting key processes involved in emotional regulation and stress reactivity. These processes may be adaptive in hostile environments, but, as we will discuss in this chapter, they may also increase susceptibility for suicidal behaviors when facing stressful events.

How does an individual respond to ELA, what molecular processes take place, and how stable are these changes are fascinating questions that we are only now starting to understand. Growing evidence suggests that epigenetic mechanisms may mediate the effects of stress on behavior. In this chapter, we present and discuss recent findings showing that the behavioral consequences of ELA and stress are, at least in part, mediated via epigenetic mechanisms. With this in mind, we propose a model in which the neurobiological consequences of ELA build into long-lasting and stable behavioral patterns characterized by certain personality traits, which in turn may increase suicide risk.

Defining Epigenetics

Epigenetics refers to the study of the epigenome, a term used to describe the complete set of chemical and physical properties associated with DNA. As such, epigenetic regulation involves changes in the activity of a gene caused by mechanisms independent of modifications to the DNA sequence, but that generally lead to tissue-specific changes in gene expression. These chemical and physical modifications, which are highly responsive to changes in the organism's environment via chemical activation of cell-signaling pathways, dynamically control the access of a cell's transcriptional machinery to regulatory sequences, and consequently the level of gene expression. Epigenetic mechanisms comprise primarily histone modifications and DNA methylation (Klose & Bird, 2006; Kouzarides, 2007).[1]

In order to fit inside the cell nucleus, DNA is packaged into chromatin, which is composed of smaller units called nucleosomes. Each nucleosome consists of DNA wrapped around a core unit made up of eight histone proteins (two copies each of H2A, H2B, H3, and H4). Each

---

[1] Recently, noncoding RNA, such as microRNA, and hydroxymethylation have also been categorized as epigenetic mechanisms (Kriaucionis & Heintz, 2009; Schratt, 2009). However, the latter mechanisms will not be discussed in the present chapter.

of the core histones is characterized by a unique "tail" of amino acids. Histone tails are susceptible to modifications via enzymes that add or remove amino acid residues, which can in turn modify the structure of chromatin (Kouzarides, 2007). These modifications are induced by proteins that recognize specific residues on the histone tails and carry further enzymatic activity. In terms of structure, chromatin primarily adopts one of two configurations: heterochromatin, the compacted form of chromatin associated with repression of gene expression, and euchromatin, the open form of chromatin associated with gene expression. Changing the structure of the chromatin allows various DNA-based tasks (DNA replication, repair, and gene expression) to be executed.

Although more than eight chromatin modifications have been characterized, most of the attention has focused on methylation and acetylation processes (Kouzarides, 2007). Although histone acetylation has been almost exclusively associated with activation of gene expression by making DNA "accessible" for transcription, some histone methylation effects are associated with gene activation and others with gene silencing, depending on their location on the histone tail (Kouzarides, 2007; Szyf, McGowan, Turecki, & Meaney, 2010). Indeed, histone modifications are organized into a codelike fashion allowing DNA-based tasks to be accomplished depending on cellular context. This code is still far from being decoded, but recent evidence suggests that the combination of various histone modifications following a sequence-dependent context organizes the structure of the chromatin and exerts a control over gene expression (J. Ernst et al., 2011).

DNA methylation – the chemical addition of a methyl group (CH_3) – is mainly found on the cytosine ring of a CpG dinucleotide.[2] In somatic cells, 80 percent of the genome is methylated (Tucker, 2001). This holds true for regions between genes (intergenic regions) and within the gene itself. Gene promoters, noncoding sequences of DNA that initiate gene transcription, are an exception, as only 5 to 10 percent of promoters are methylated. As such, DNA methylation in gene promoters has a major role in regulating gene expression. Classically, DNA methylation in gene promoters has been associated with transcriptional repression, although some studies have shown opposite effects (Klose & Bird, 2006; Meaney & Ferguson-Smith, 2010). DNA methylation in gene promoters is expected to repress gene expression by interfering with the binding of transcription factors and transcriptional

---

[2] Recent studies suggest that DNA methylation may also be found on other nucleotides, however, although this may be particularly prevalent in stem cells and progenitors and less in somatic cells (Lister et al., 2009; Meissner et al., 2008; Xie et al., 2012; Ziller et al., 2011).

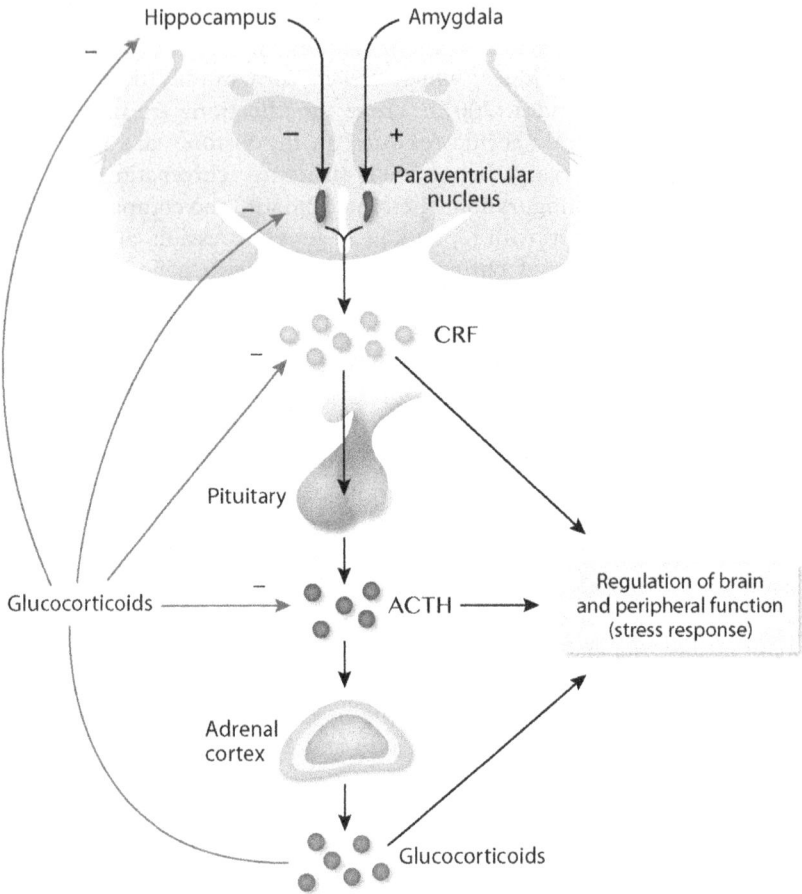

Figure 9.1. The hypothalamic-pituitary-adrenal (HPA) axis. In the
hypothalamus, the paraventricular nucleus releases CRF, which is
transported to the anterior pituitary, where it causes the release of
ACTH into the blood stream. ACTH stimulates the adrenal cortex to
synthesize and release the glucocorticoids cortisol (humans) or
corticosterone (rodents). Glucocorticoids feed back at the level of the
hippocampus, hypothalamus, and pituitary to dampen excess
activation of the HPA axis. Reprinted by permission from
Macmillan Publishers Ltd: *Nature Neuroscience* ("How Adversity Gets
Under the Skin") by Steven E. Hyman, 2009, *12*(3), p. 242,
Copyright (2009).

machinery to the regulatory sequences of DNA. The situation is the opposite in gene bodies, as exemplified, for instance, in studies of the X chromosome (Hellman & Chess, 2007). Accordingly, DNA methylation in gene bodies is associated with active transcription and alternative transcript expression (Aran, Toperoff, Rosenberg, & Hellman, 2011; Maunakea et al., 2010; Rauch, Wu, Zhong, Riggs, & Pfeifer, 2009).

Epigenetic processes are complex and not yet fully understood, and while DNA methylation and histone modifications have been described separately, it is unlikely that they act in an independent fashion. Changes in levels of methylation may modify the binding of DNA methyl-binding proteins, which, on their own, possess histone-modifying properties and are also known to recruit histone-modifying enzymes to the DNA (Deplus et al., 2002; Fuks, Burgers, Brehm, Hughes-Davies, & Kouzarides, 2000; Fuks, Burgers, Godin, Kasai, & Kouzarides, 2001; Geiman, Sankpal, Robertson, Zhao, & Robertson, 2004). Gene expression is thus likely to be regulated by a complex epigenetic interplay between DNA methylation and chromatin modifications that impact each other.

Molecular Consequences of Early-Life Adversity: Transcriptional Regulation by Epigenetic Mechanisms

As discussed earlier, epigenetic mechanisms play a major role in the regulation of gene expression and, by extension, may have an important regulatory impact on behavior. Changes in epigenetic marks occur in response to a number of environmental events, including the social environment. Epigenetic mechanisms are best understood as plastic changes that take place in the genome to better help an organism adapt to the particular environment in which it lives. Although this idea is appealing and is gaining growing support from empirical data, the precise molecular mechanisms mediating these epigenetic changes in response to environmental/social events remain largely unknown. Nevertheless, some important insights into this critical issue have been made through animal studies, and more recently, in humans. The following sections will describe these findings and integrate them into a comprehensive model that aims to understand how the environment impacts behavioral development and mental health by altering epigenetic mechanisms.

The Impact of Early-Life Adversity on the Hypothalamic-Pituitary Adrenal Axis

The hypothalamic-pituitary adrenal (HPA) axis is the main stress regulatory system in mammals, and its dysfunction has long been associated with psychopathology characterized primarily by mood and anxiety symptoms (Heim, Newport, Mletzko, Miller, & Nemeroff, 2008; Heim, Shugart, Craighead, & Nemeroff, 2010). Under normal conditions, stress induces the synthesis and release of corticotropin releasing hormone (CRH) and arginine vasopressin (AVP) in the paraventricular nucleus (PVN) of the hypothalamus, both of which activate the release of adrenocorticotropic hormone (ACTH) from the anterior pituitary into the blood stream. ACTH migrates through the blood to the adrenal cortex, where it triggers the synthesis and the release of stress hormones (glucocorticoids; GCs) into the blood – corticosterone in rats and cortisol in humans. GCs migrate to the hippocampus (HPC), where they bind to glucocorticoid receptors (GR). The activation of GR in the HPC exerts an inhibitory feedback on the activity of the HPA axis and brings it back to baseline levels.

Regulation of the HPA axis baseline activity seems to take place early in development. For instance, prolonged stressors occurring early in life are associated with extensive and seemingly stable abnormal activation of the HPA axis. Importantly, these effects have been reported both in animals and humans. For instance, variation in maternal care in rats, measured by frequency of licking and grooming (LG), has been associated with variation in levels of GR in the HPC (Francis, Diorio, Liu, & Meaney, 1999; Liu et al., 1997), as well as different corticosterone and ACTH plasma levels (Francis et al., 1999) in offspring. More specifically, low LG mothers have offspring with lower HPC GR levels and higher cortisol and ACTH plasma levels when compared to offspring of high LG mothers. These molecular alterations were associated with depressive-like behaviors when offspring become adults (Caldji et al., 1998; Francis et al., 1999). Similarly, early-life maternal separation in mice was associated with stress-coping alterations in pups and a long-lasting increase in corticosterone secretion with higher AVP and proopiomelanocortin (POMC) expression in the PVN of the hypothalamus (Murgatroyd et al., 2009). Furthermore, higher CRH expression in the PVN of chronically stressed mice and in low LG offspring has been associated with multiple behavioral alterations (Elliott, Ezra-Nevo, Regev, Neufeld-Cohen, & Chen, 2010; Liu et al., 1997).

These findings in animals have correlates in humans. Individuals who were victims of child abuse have higher plasmatic ACTH and cortisol levels (Heim et al., 2000) following stressful conditions and lower cerebrospinal fluid (CSF) oxytocin levels (Heim et al., 2009), compared to nonabused controls. Individuals who died by suicide and had histories of childhood abuse have lower GR expression levels in the HPC, compared to suicides with no history of childhood abuse and to healthy controls

(Labonte, Yerko, et al., 2012; McGowan et al., 2009). Higher POMC pituitary mRNA levels (J. F. Lopez et al., 1992) and elevated CSF CRH levels (Nemeroff et al., 1984) are also common features in suicide. Indeed, suicide completers exhibit hyperactivation of CRH neurons in the PVN, as suggested by increased CRH mRNA levels and increased numbers of CRH-positive neurons (Raadsheer, Hoogendijk, Stam, Tilders, & Swaab, 1994; Raadsheer et al., 1995; Wang, Kamphuis, Huitinga, Zhou, & Swaab, 2008). Moreover, several brain regions in suicide completers have been found to have decreased CRH binding sites (Nemeroff, Owens, Bissette, Andorn, & Stanley, 1988), altered CRH receptor type ratios (Hiroi et al., 2001), and elevated CRH immunoreactivity and mRNA levels (Austin, Janosky, & Murphy, 2003; Merali et al., 2006), although some evidence has suggested that alcohol-use disorders, which are frequently observed among individuals who died by suicide, could dysregulate these ratios as well, regardless of history of childhood abuse (Richardson, Lee, O'Dell, Koob, & Rivier, 2008). Furthermore, people who die by suicide have increased adrenal gland weight, which seems to be accounted for by cortical hypertrophy (Dumser, Barocka, & Schubert, 1998; Szigethy, Conwell, Forbes, Cox, & Caine, 1994), also suggesting chronic HPA axis hyperactivity (Nemeroff & Vale, 2005; Pfennig et al., 2005). Thus, variation in the early environment changes the expression of genes involved in the function of the HPA axis in both animals and humans. This variability is associated with functional alterations of the HPA axis and with the development of behaviors in animals that parallel aspects of human mood-related psychopathology.

Molecular Impact of Early-Life Environment
and Early-Life Adversity

From a molecular point of view, it has been challenging to conceptualize how events occurring early in life can lead to persistent changes in behavior. A series of elegant groundbreaking studies in rodents provided major insight into the molecular mechanisms by which early-life stress can induce long-lasting behavioral alterations.

One of the first studies addressing this important question focused on the transcriptional regulation of GR in the brain of offspring from low LG mothers. This work showed that pups raised by low LG mothers, when compared to those raised by high LG mothers, exhibit lower hippocampal expression of an untranslated exon 1 variant of the GR gene – the exon 1_7 variant – which is important in the regulation of GR expression in the hippocampus (Weaver et al., 2004). This was associated with significantly higher DNA methylation levels in the GR 1_7 promoter. Importantly, this region of hypermethylation was found to overlap a binding site for a nerve growth transcription factor (NGF1-A), which is important in the regulation of GR expression. (Briefly, the level of LG affects the level of serotonin turnover and the expression of NGF1-A in the HPC – the lower the LG, the lower the level of serotonin receptor binding in the HPC, which can inhibit NGF1-A binding and activation of the GR gene [Nr3c1] and, consequently, lower GR expression.) Lower expression of other GR variants (GR1_5, 1_6, 1_8, 1_9, 1_{10}, and 1_{11}) associated with alterations in DNA methylation patterns has also been recently reported in the HPC of offspring of low versus high LG mothers (McGowan et al., 2011).

Interesting molecular parallels can be traced between rodents and human in the regulation of the HPC GR activity by methylation. Indeed, studies investigating ELA in the human brain found lower levels of both GR_{total} and $GR1_F$ (the human homologue of GR1_7 in rats) expression in the HPC of individuals who died by suicide and had a history of ELA compared to individuals with no history of ELA who died by suicide and controls (McGowan et al., 2009). As in the rodent model, these gene expression differences were associated with sites of hypermethylation in the promoter region of $GR1_F$, precisely within an NGFI-A binding site. Functional experiments showed that methylation at this precise site represses the binding of NGFI-A to DNA and decreases the transcriptional activity of the promoter, providing a potential explanation for the lower expression of GR found in the brain of abused suicide completers. Follow-up work showed that other GR variants (GR1_B, 1_C and 1_H) are also downregulated in the HPC of abused suicide completers, and this was associated with several sites of differential methylation in respective promoters (Labonte, Yerko, et al., 2012).

More recently, these findings were supported by a series of studies investigating both clinical and community samples with histories of ELA. For instance, the infants of mothers reporting intimate partner violence during their pregnancy showed higher levels of methylation in the promoter of $GR1_F$ compared to infants of mothers not exposed to this kind of violence (Radtke et al., 2011). Another study reported correlation between $GR1_F$ promoter methylation levels in leukocytes from healthy adults and history of parental loss, child maltreatment, and parental care (Tyrka, Price, Marsit, Walters, & Carpenter, 2012). Furthermore, DNA methylation levels in $GR1_F$ promoter were shown to be positively correlated with childhood sexual abuse, its severity, and the number of maltreatment types in individuals with MDD, and with repetition of severe types of abuse in patients with bipolar disorders (Perroud et al., 2011). These interesting findings suggest that the GR gene region, in both animals and humans, may be poised for epigenetic regulation by ELA, which increases the odds of exhibiting mood disorders and suicide later in life.

As mentioned previously, early-life stress has been shown to alter other constituents of the HPA axis activity such as CRH, oxytocin, POMC, and AVP. Although no study in humans has yet assessed the molecular effects of early-life stress on the epigenetic regulation of related genes, two recent studies in mice revealed complex epigenetic alterations in the regulation of CRH (Elliott et al., 2010) and AVP (Murgatroyd et al., 2009) in animals that faced ELA. In one of these studies, which focused on the relationship between chronic social stress and social avoidance, the higher CRH expression found in the PVN of chronically stressed mice was associated with a significant site-specific hypomethylation in the CRH gene promoter (Elliott et al., 2010). Specifically, hypomethylation was found within a cyclic adenosine monophosphate (cAMP) response element (CRE) binding site, the importance of which was further confirmed by *in vitro* functional studies using luciferase. These assays showed that mutating a single base in the CRE binding site substantially reduced cAMP-induced CRH promoter activity in chronically stressed mice that displayed social avoidance (Elliott et al., 2010). These alterations were also accompanied by modifications in the levels of enzymes responsible for adding (DNMT3b) and removing (Gadd45b) DNA methylation on the DNA. Interestingly, chronic treatment with the tricyclic imipramine attenuated the behavioral, transcriptional, and epigenetic changes induced by social stress (Elliott et al., 2010).

The other recent study investigated perinatal maternal deprivation in rats and its effects on CRH promoter methylation patterns and subsequent CRH expression in response to stress in adulthood. Eight weeks after maternal deprivation (MD), these rats expressed higher levels of corticosterone and CRH than did rats not so deprived. The investigators found a decrease in the methylation of the CRE region of the promoter of CRH in the MD rats. This study shows how stable methylation effects are. Their impacts on gene expression and behavior can be observed in adulthood after adversity was experienced early in life (J. Chen et al., 2012).

In sum, these studies clearly suggest that the early environment plays a key role in regulation of the HPA axis activity through epigenetic mechanisms, and particularly by DNA methylation. Although most of the work to date has focused on the regulation of GR, there is also evidence that other important components of the HPA axis are similarly regulated by the early environment through epigenetic mechanisms.

Neurotrophic Factors

Brain derived neurotrophic factor (BDNF), a growth factor associated with brain development and plasticity, has been extensively investigated in psychiatric disorders, particularly as a potential mediator of the interaction between stress and physiological and structural changes (Hashimoto, 2010). Low serum and brain BDNF expression has been reported in patients with major depression (Brunoni, Lopes, & Fregni, 2008; Dwivedi et al., 2003; Pandey et al., 2008), and these alterations were reversed by antidepressant treatment (B. Chen, Dowlatshahi, MacQueen, Wang, & Young, 2001; Matrisciano et al., 2009; Sen, Duman, & Sanacora, 2008). In addition, BDNF depletion in mice induces depression-like behaviors (Chan, Unger, Byrnes, & Rios, 2006), while in rats chronic stress reduces BDNF expression in the hippocampus (Duric & McCarson, 2005; Gronli et al., 2006), effects that are counteracted by antidepressant treatment (Duric & McCarson, 2006; Rogoz, Skuza, & Legutko, 2005; Xu et al., 2006). Thus, it seems clear that BDNF has a role in mediating stress responses in the brain. However, this effect is probably dynamic, complex, and nonlinear.

Recently, interest in BDNF has been directed to the relationship between BDNF expression levels, epigenetic regulation, and response to stress in rodents. Chronic social stress in mice, as well as maternal maltreatment and traumatic stress in rats, were shown to decrease the expression of BDNF transcripts III and IV in the HPC (Roth, Zoladz, Sweatt, & Diamond, 2011; Tsankova et al., 2006) and the prefrontal cortex (PFC) (Roth, Lubin, Funk, & Sweatt, 2009; Roth et al., 2011), respectively. Although similar, these transcriptional alterations are induced by different epigenetic mechanisms. Whereas chronic stress in mice increases histone H3K27 dimethylation levels at the BDNF promoter in the HPC, resulting in a more compacted, and thus less active chromatin (Tsankova et al., 2006), traumatic stress in rats was shown to alter DNA methylation patterns. Hypermethylation has been reported in the promoter of BDNF transcript IV both in the dorsal dentate gyrus and CA3 regions of the HPC, but the same promoter region was hypomethylated in the ventral CA1 region (Roth et al., 2011). Similarly, maternal maltreatment in rats was associated with site-specific hypermethylation in the promoters of transcripts IV and IX in the PFC (Roth et al., 2009).

Similar alterations have been associated with suicide completion and depression in humans. For instance, hypermethylation at four sites within the promoter of BDNF IV was reported in the Wernicke area of the cortex of people who died by suicide (Keller et al., 2010). Interestingly, the authors reported an inverse correlation between BDNF expression and promoter methylation, supporting the repressive effects of methylation on transcription. Based on previous evidence in mice (Tsankova et al., 2006), our group provided evidence suggesting that antidepressants promote open chromatin structure (i.e., lower H3K27me3 level) in the promoter of BDNF in the PFC (E. S. Chen, Ernst, & Turecki, 2011). Follow-up studies in depressed patients revealed higher BDNF expression in the blood of citalopram treatment responders compared to nonresponders (J. P. Lopez et al., 2013) Interestingly, H3K27me3 levels were inversely correlated with both BDNF IV expression levels and with the severity of symptoms.

Tyrosine receptor kinase B (TrkB), the receptor for BDNF, has also been strongly associated with mood disorders. For instance, lower TrkB expression has been reported in the PFC of depressed subjects (Aston, Jiang, & Sokolov, 2005; Nakatani et al., 2006), and antidepressant treatment has been shown to increase its expression in cultured astrocytes (Mercier et al., 2004). The astrocytic variant of TrkB, TrkB.-T1, was also shown to be downregulated in the PFC of a subset of suicide completers. Interestingly, an inverse correlation was found between TrkB.T1 expression and TrkB promoter methylation, particularly with two CpG sites that were hypermethylated in suicide completers (Ernst, Deleva, et al., 2009). In addition, suicides with low TrkB.T1 expression showed enrichment of H3K27 methylation in the TrkB promoter (Ernst, Chen, & Turecki, 2009), suggesting the presence of a dual epigenetic control over the expression of the astrocytic variant of TrkB. Interestingly, recent data showed that mice overexpressing the TrkB.T1 variant are more vulnerable to manifest avoidance behaviors when exposed to chronic social stress than wildtype mice (Razzoli et al., 2011). This is consistent with studies in humans indicating that a functional 11 base pair deletion of the TrkB gene that leads to decreased activity of the gene is associated with the development of anxiety traits (C. Ernst et al., 2011).

More recent data suggest that the epigenetic regulation of the glial cell-derived neurotrophic factor (GDNF), as well as genetic background and environmental factors, may contribute to the behavioral responses to stress in different strains of mice (Uchida et al., 2011). Indeed, low GDNF levels, as well as a closed chromatin conformation in the GDNF promoter (i.e., less histone acetylation and methylation), have been associated with a depression-like phenotype in a stress-susceptible mouse strain (BALB) and a stress-resilient one (B6) that faced chronic stress. This lower level of GDNF following chronic stress was correlated with higher levels of methylation in GDNF promoter that enhanced the binding of the transcriptional repressor meCP2. Although there were similarities in the findings between the two mouse strains, GDNF methylation and expression was more consistent in the stress-susceptible strain (Uchida et al., 2011). This suggests that the behavioral effects of chronic stress arise from epigenetic modifications.

Together, these data suggest that epigenetic changes in genes coding for different components of the neurotrophic system, and primarily in BDNF/TrkB, may be regulated by the early environment and lead to stable changes in gene expression associated with behavioral phenotypes.

Investigating Genome-Wide DNA Methylation Patterns

Overall, environmental factors seem to target the epigenetic regulation of genes involved in key regulatory processes such as the HPA axis and neurotrophic factors. This is also supported by numerous other studies looking at genes involved in neurotransmission (Abdolmaleky et al., 2006; Abdolmaleky, Smith, Zhou, & Thiagalingam, 2008; Abdolmaleky et al., 2011; Dammann et al., 2011; De Luca, Likhodi, Kennedy, & Wong, 2007; De Luca, Viggiano, Dhoot, Kennedy, & Wong, 2009; Poulter et al., 2008); polyamines (Fiori, Gross, & Turecki, 2012; Fiori & Turecki, 2010); and protein synthesis (McGowan et al., 2008). However, although a growing body of evidence supports the contribution of epigenetic factors translating the effects of ELA on the human genome, there is a real need for large-scale comprehensive studies assessing genome-wide epigenetic patterns in the context of different environmental factors. A few of these studies recently reported interesting findings, suggesting that environmental factors, while targeting critical genes, may also induce genome-wide reprogramming of epigenetic patterns.

Our group recently assessed the impact of child abuse on genome-wide DNA methylation signature in gene promoters (Labonte, Suderman, Maussion, Navaro, et al., 2013). In this study, we compared hippocampal DNA methylation patterns between suicide completers with a severe history of child abuse (sexual and/or physical) and healthy controls. We identified hundreds of sites that were differentially methylated, both hyper- and hypomethylated, in the HPC of severely abused suicide completers. Interestingly, DNA methylation levels in gene promoters were inversely correlated with gene expression at the genome-wide level, and differential methylation in abused suicide completers was enriched in genes involved in neuroplasticity, a finding consistent with the notion that abuse experienced during childhood can lead to plastic changes in the brain as a response to these negative environmental stimuli. Similar observations have been made in suicide completers (Labonte, Suderman, Maussion, Lopez, et al., 2012), who present methylation enriched in genes related to learning and memory, and in PTSD patients (Uddin et al., 2010). However, in the study of PTSD patients, the analysis of DNA methylation levels was not restricted to promoters but, rather, to fourteen thousand CpGs across the genome. The analysis revealed an overrepresentation of differentially methylated CpGs in genes related to immune function. This may be translated into the development of different psychopathological processes. Furthermore, a previous study comparing the PFC of psychotic and bipolar patients reported differential methylation in numerous sites that were involved in glutamatergic and GABAergic neurotransmission, brain development, and response to stress (Mill et al., 2008). It is important to note that these studies were conducted in different tissues (blood versus brain) and different brain regions (HPC versus PFC), which may account for the discrepancies between studies, as different tissues (Ladd-Acosta et al., 2007) and cell types (Deaton et al., 2011; Iwamoto et al., 2011) have been shown to exhibit specific DNA methylation signatures.

Toward an Integrative Model of Stress-Induced Psychopathology

As discussed earlier, the early-life environment plays an important role regulating critical brain and behavioral functions, including mechanisms of stress response. Experiences of ELA lead to hyperactivity of such systems, which behaviorally correlate with states of hypervigilance. One may speculate that the organism is trying to adapt to a hostile environment in which increased attention and readiness to react may be key for appropriate adaptation. These early-life experiences induce long-lasting molecular changes in the brain by altering the epigenetic regulation of genes. These changes have been shown to affect particular functions such as the HPA axis (Labonte, Yerko, et al., 2012; McGowan et al., 2009; McGowan et al., 2011; Perroud et al., 2011; Radtke et al., 2011; Tyrka et al., 2012; Weaver et al., 2004) and neurotrophins (Ernst, Chen, et al., 2009; Ernst, Deleva, et al., 2009; Keller et al., 2010; Roth et al., 2009; Roth et al., 2011), as well as genes involved in cellular plasticity (Champagne et al., 2008; Labonte, Yerko, et al., 2012); learning and memory (Day & Sweatt, 2010, 2011); and the immune system (Uddin et al., 2010). However, it remains to be better understood how these molecular effects impact behavioral development and increase the risk for suicide.

In addition to the molecular alterations described earlier, ELA also induces brain structural changes that may be associated with sustained neurobiological alterations. Indeed, ELA has been associated with significant changes in gray-matter volume in various brain regions, including the anterior cingulate gyrus, dorsolateral, and medial PFC (Kitayama, Quinn, & Bremner, 2006; Tomoda et al., 2009); superior temporal gyrus (Tomoda et al., 2011); amygdala (Weniger, Lange, Sachsse, & Irle, 2008); hippocampus (Vythilingam et al., 2002; Weniger et al., 2008); and corpus callosum (Vythilingam et al., 2002). Functionally, these structural changes would be expected to have a significant impact on the development of personality traits, leading to emotional and behavioral dysregulation and cognitive impairments, which have been associated with increased risk for suicidal behaviors (Brezo et al., 2006). Of particular interest are results from longitudinal studies suggesting that developmental trajectories of anxiousness or disruptiveness (impulsivity and aggression) mediate the relationship between histories of child abuse and suicidal behaviors in adulthood (Boden, Fergusson, & Horwood, 2007; Brezo, Barker, et al., 2008; Brezo, Paris, Barker, et al., 2007; Brezo, Paris, Hebert, et al., 2008; Yen et al., 2009). Furthermore, ELA has been associated with cognitive impairments such as decision-making and problem-solving deficits (Bremner, Vermetten, Afzal, & Vythilingam, 2004; Navalta, Polcari, Webster, Boghossian, & Teicher, 2006; Perez & Widom, 1994; Yen et al., 2009), which are expected to increase the vulnerability toward suicidal behaviors (Cha, Najmi, Park, Finn, & Nock, 2010; Jollant et al., 2005; Jollant et al., 2008; Keilp et al., 2001; Speckens & Hawton, 2005). For instance, exposure to stressful situations has been shown to impact decision-making and problem-solving skills in individuals with suicidal behaviors displaying dysfunctional responses to stress (Grover et al., 2009; Sinclair, Crane, Hawton, & Williams, 2007; van den Bos et al., 2009; Williams, Barnhofer, Crane, & Beck, 2005; Yang & Clum, 2000).

With this in mind, one may hypothesize that ELA may increase risk of suicidal behaviors by epigenetically regulating certain genes, such as those coding for components of the HPA axis and neurotrophic factors, among others, which in turn would lead to the development of behavioral traits characterized by high levels of anxiousness and impulsivity. Such traits are well-known vulnerabilities for suicidal behavior, acting as distal risk factors and increasing suicide risk when combined with precipitants such as depressive psychopathology and substance use disorders (see Figure 9.2).

It is tempting to speculate on the clinical implications of these findings. The characterization of these epigenetic changes could eventually lead to the development of tools for identifying individuals at risk, but most importantly, to the development of preventive interventions. However, current knowledge is significantly limited, and there are major challenges in the potential implementation of tools for specific modification of epigenetic marks at a given histological and genetic locus level. An

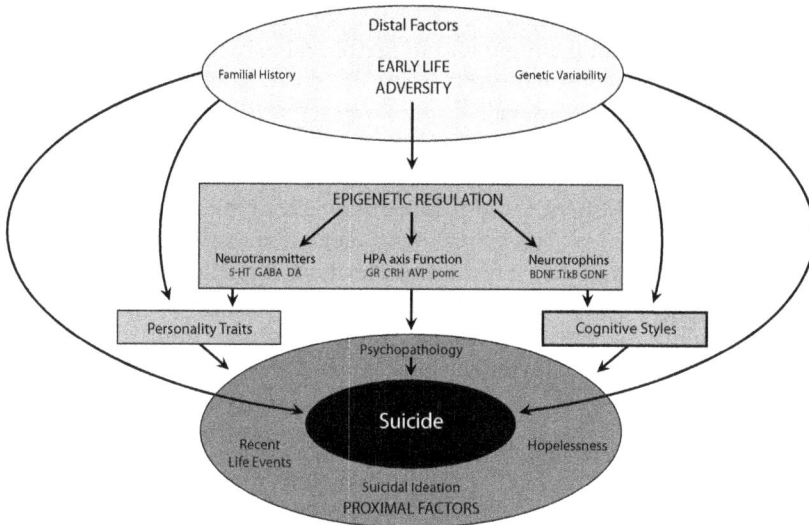

Figure 9.2. Proximal and distal factors: Early life adversity and suicide. Schematic model of the mechanisms by which early-life adversity is thought to increase risk of psychopathology and suicide. Early-life adversity probably interferes with the epigenetic control of genes coding for components of the HPA axis and neurotrophic factors. This, in turn, may lead to the development of high levels of anxiousness and impulsivity. These behavioral traits enhance vulnerability to suicidal behavior by acting as distal risk factors, which increase suicide risk when combined with precipitants such as depressive psychopathology and substance disorders. 5-HT: Serotonin, GABA: Gamma-Aminobutryic acid; DA: Dopamine, GR: Glucocorticoid receptor, CRH: Corticotropin-releasing hormone, AVP: Arginine-vasopressin, pomc: Pro-opiomelanocortin, BDNF: Brain-derived neurotropic factor, TrkB: Tyrosine receptor kinase B, GDNF: Glial-derived neurotrophic factor.

important methodological question concerns the extent to which epigenetic changes observed in brain tissue are reflected in peripheral tissue. Research would be greatly facilitated if alterations in more accessible tissue, such as blood or saliva, paralleled changes in brain tissue. DNA methylation patterns are tissue-specific, and what is found in the brain may not necessarily be the same in other tissues. However, there is evidence suggesting that there is some level of correlation between epigenetic marks associated with psychiatric phenotypes in peripheral and brain tissues. For instance, there are important parallels in GR locus DNA methylation patterns observed in the HPC and peripheral samples (Perroud et al., 2011; Radtke et al., 2011; Tyrka et al., 2012). It remains to be shown whether, in general, there is a correlation between epigenetic changes observed in the brain and in peripheral tissues for the same loci, and therefore, whether peripheral samples can reliably be used as proxy markers of mental disorders.

Given the novelty of this research in psychiatry, additional studies are required to better address this and other important questions. Such approaches should benefit from integrating DNA methylation, histone modifications, genetic variations, and gene expression to provide a more comprehensive view on the complexity of the relationship between ELA and psychopathology. As the science evolves, we will gain a better understanding of the mechanisms through which the environment impacts on the development of psychopathology.

Acknowledgement

Originally submitted October 9, 2012. For more recent work on epigenetics by Turecki and colleagues, see http://www.mgss.ca.

REFERENCES

Abdolmaleky, H. M., Cheng, K. H., Faraone, S. V., Wilcox, M., Glatt, S. J., Gao, F., ... Thiagalingam, S. (2006). Hypomethylation of MB-COMT promoter is a major risk factor for schizophrenia and bipolar disorder. *Human Molecular Genetics, 15*(21), 3132–45. http://dx.doi.org/10.1093/hmg/ddl253

Abdolmaleky, H. M., Smith, C. L., Zhou, J. R., & Thiagalingam, S. (2008). Epigenetic alterations of the dopaminergic system in major psychiatric disorders. *Methods in Molecular Biology, 448*, 187–212. http://dx.doi.org/10.1007/978-1-59745-205-2_9

Abdolmaleky, H. M., Yaqubi, S., Papageorgis, P., Lambert, A. W., Ozturk, S., Sivaraman, V., & Thiagalingam, S. (2011). Epigenetic dysregulation of HTR2A in the brain of patients with schizophrenia and bipolar disorder. *Schizophrenia Research, 129*(2–3), 183–90. http://dx.doi.org/10.1016/j.schres.2011.04.007

Akyuz, G., Sar, V., Kugu, N., & Dogan, O. (2005). Reported childhood trauma, attempted suicide and self-mutilative behavior among women in the general population. *European Psychiatry, 20*(3), 268–73. http://dx.doi.org/10.1016/j.eurpsy.2005.01.002

Andover, M. S., Zlotnick, C., & Miller, I. W. (2007). Childhood physical and sexual abuse in depressed patients with single and multiple suicide attempts. *Suicide and Life-Threatening Behavior, 37*(4), 467–74. http://dx.doi.org/10.1521/suli.2007.37.4.467

Angst, F., Stassen, H. H., Clayton, P. J., & Angst, J. (2002). Mortality of patients with mood disorders: Follow-up over 34–38 years. *Journal of Affective Disorders, 68*(2–3), 167–81. http://dx.doi.org/10.1016/S0165-0327(01)00377-9

Angst, J., Angst, F., & Stassen, H. H. (1999). Suicide risk in patients with major depressive disorder. *Journal of Clinical Psychiatry*, *60*(Suppl. 2), 57–62; Consensus discussion, 113–16.

Angst, J., Degonda, M., & Ernst, C. (1992). The Zurich Study: XV. Suicide attempts in a cohort from age 20 to 30. *European Archives of Psychiatry and Clinical Neuroscience*, *242*(2–3), 135–41. http://dx.doi.org/10.1007/BF02191561

Aran, D., Toperoff, G., Rosenberg, M., & Hellman, A. (2011). Replication timing-related and gene body-specific methylation of active human genes. *Human Molecular Genetics*, *20*(4), 670–80. http://dx.doi.org/10.1093/hmg/ddq513

Arsenault-Lapierre, G., Kim, C., & Turecki, G. (2004). Psychiatric diagnoses in 3275 suicides: A meta-analysis. *BMC Psychiatry*, *4*, 37. http://dx.doi.org/10.1186/1471-244X-4-37

Aston, C., Jiang, L., & Sokolov, B. P. (2005). Transcriptional profiling reveals evidence for signaling and oligodendroglial abnormalities in the temporal cortex from patients with major depressive disorder. *Molecular Psychiatry*, *10*(3), 309–22. http://dx.doi.org/10.1038/sj.mp.4001565

Austin, M. C., Janosky, J. E., & Murphy, H. A. (2003). Increased corticotropin-releasing hormone immunoreactivity in monoamine-containing pontine nuclei of depressed suicide men. *Molecular Psychiatry*, *8*(3), 324–32. http://dx.doi.org/10.1038/sj.mp.4001250

Bensley, L. S., Van Eenwyk, J., Spieker, S. J., & Schoder, J. (1999). Self-reported abuse history and adolescent problem behaviors. I. Antisocial and suicidal behaviors. *Journal of Adolescent Health*, *24*(3), 163–72. http://dx.doi.org/10.1016/S1054-139X(98)00111-6

Blair-West, G. W., Cantor, C. H., Mellsop, G. W., & Eyeson-Annan, M. L. (1999). Lifetime suicide risk in major depression: Sex and age determinants. *Journal of Affective Disorders*, *55*(2–3), 171–8. http://dx.doi.org/10.1016/S0165-0327(99)00004-X

Boden, J. M., Fergusson, D. M., & Horwood, L. J. (2007). Anxiety disorders and suicidal behaviors in adolescence and young adulthood: Findings from a longitudinal study. *Psychological Medicine*, *37*(3), 431–40. http://dx.doi.org/10.1017/S0033291706009147

Bremner, J. D., Vermetten, E., Afzal, N., & Vythilingam, M. (2004). Deficits in verbal declarative memory function in women with childhood sexual abuse-related posttraumatic stress disorder. *Journal of Nervous and Mental Disease*, *192*(10), 643–9. http://dx.doi.org/10.1097/01.nmd.0000142027.52893.c8

Brezo, J., Barker, E. D., Paris, J., Hebert, M., Vitaro, F., Tremblay, R. E., & Turecki, G. (2008). Childhood trajectories of anxiousness and disruptiveness as predictors of suicide attempts. *Archives of Pediatrics & Adolescent Medicine*, *162*(11), 1015–21. http://dx.doi.org/10.1001/archpedi.162.11.1015

Brezo, J., Klempan, T., & Turecki, G. (2008). The genetics of suicide: A critical review of molecular studies. *Psychiatric Clinics of North America*, *31*(2), 179–203. http://dx.doi.org/10.1016/j.psc.2008.01.008

Brezo, J., Paris, J., Barker, E. D., Tremblay, R., Vitaro, F., Zoccolillo, M., ... Turecki, G. (2007). Natural history of suicidal behaviors in a population-based sample of young adults. *Psychological Medicine*, *37*(11), 1563–74. http://dx.doi.org/10.1017/S003329170700058X

Brezo, J., Paris, J., Hebert, M., Vitaro, F., Tremblay, R., & Turecki, G. (2008). Broad and narrow personality traits as markers of one-time and repeated suicide attempts: A population-based study. *BMC Psychiatry, 8*, 15.

Brezo, J., Paris, J., Tremblay, R., Vitaro, F., Hebert, M., & Turecki, G. (2007). Identifying correlates of suicide attempts in suicidal ideators: A population-based study. *Psychological Medicine, 37*(11), 1551–62. http://dx.doi.org/10.1017/S0033291707000803

Brezo, J., Paris, J., & Turecki, G. (2006). Personality traits as correlates of suicidal ideation, suicide attempts, and suicide completions: A systematic review. *Acta Psychiatrica Scandinavica, 113*(3), 180–206. http://dx.doi.org/10.1111/j.1600-0447.2005.00702.x

Brezo, J., Paris, J., Vitaro, F., Hebert, M., Tremblay, R. E., & Turecki, G. (2008). Predicting suicide attempts in young adults with histories of childhood abuse. *British Journal of Psychiatry, 193*(2), 134–9. http://dx.doi.org/10.1192/bjp.bp.107.037994

Brunoni, A. R., Lopes, M., & Fregni, F. (2008). A systematic review and meta-analysis of clinical studies on major depression and BDNF levels: Implications for the role of neuroplasticity in depression. *International Journal of Neuropsychopharmacology, 11*(8), 1169–80. http://dx.doi.org/10.1017/S1461145708009309

Caldji, C., Tannenbaum, B., Sharma, S., Francis, D., Plotsky, P. M., & Meaney, M. J. (1998). Maternal care during infancy regulates the development of neural systems mediating the expression of fearfulness in the rat. *Proceedings of the National Academy of Sciences of the United States of America, 95*(9), 5335–40. http://dx.doi.org/10.1073/pnas.95.9.5335

Cavanagh, J. T., Carson, A. J., Sharpe, M., & Lawrie, S. M. (2003). Psychological autopsy studies of suicide: A systematic review. *Psychological Medicine, 33*(3), 395–405. http://dx.doi.org/10.1017/S0033291702006943

Cha, C. B., Najmi, S., Park, J. M., Finn, C. T., & Nock, M. K. (2010). Attentional bias toward suicide-related stimuli predicts suicidal behavior. *Journal of Abnormal Psychology, 119*(3), 616–22. http://dx.doi.org/10.1037/a0019710

Champagne, D. L., Bagot, R. C., van Hasselt, F., Ramakers, G., Meaney, M. J., de Kloet, E. R., Krugers, H. (2008). Maternal care and hippocampal plasticity: Evidence for experience-dependent structural plasticity, altered synaptic functioning, and differential responsiveness to glucocorticoids and stress. *Journal of Neuroscience, 28*(23), 6037–45. http://dx.doi.org/10.1523/JNEUROSCI.0526-08.2008

Chan, J. P., Unger, T. J., Byrnes, J., & Rios, M. (2006). Examination of behavioral deficits triggered by targeting Bdnf in fetal or postnatal brains of mice. *Neuroscience, 142*(1), 49–58. http://dx.doi.org/10.1016/j.neuroscience.2006.06.002

Chen, B., Dowlatshahi, D., MacQueen, G. M., Wang, J. F., & Young, L. T. (2001). Increased hippocampal BDNF immunoreactivity in subjects treated with antidepressant medication. *Biological Psychiatry, 50*(4), 260–5. http://dx.doi.org/10.1016/S0006-3223(01)01083-6

Chen, E. S., Ernst, C., & Turecki, G. (2011). The epigenetic effects of antidepressant treatment on human prefrontal cortex BDNF expression.

International Journal of Neuropsychopharmacology, 14(3), 427–9. http://dx.doi.org/10.1017/S1461145710001422

Chen, J., Evans, A. N., Liu, Y., Honda, M., Saavedra, J. M., & Aguilera, G. (2012). Maternal deprivation in rats is associated with corticotrophin-releasing hormone (CRH) promoter hypomethylation and enhances CRH transcriptional responses to stress in adulthood. *Journal of Neuroendocrinology, 24*(7), 1055–64. http://dx.doi.org/10.1111/j.1365-2826.2012.02306.x

Cole, P. M., Michel, M. K., & Teti, L. O. (1994). The development of emotion regulation and dysregulation: A clinical perspective. *Monographs of the Society for Research in Child Development, 59*(2–3), 73–100. http://dx.doi.org/10.2307/1166139

Dammann, G., Teschler, S., Haag, T., Altmuller, F., Tuczek, F., & Dammann, R. H. (2011). Increased DNA methylation of neuropsychiatric genes occurs in borderline personality disorder. *Epigenetics, 6*(12), 1454–62. http://dx.doi.org/10.4161/epi.6.12.18363

Day, J. J., & Sweatt, J. D. (2010). DNA methylation and memory formation. *Nature Neuroscience, 13*(11), 1319–23. http://dx.doi.org/10.1038/nn.2666

Day, J. J., & Sweatt, J. D. (2011). Epigenetic mechanisms in cognition. *Neuron, 70*(5), 813–29. http://dx.doi.org/10.1016/j.neuron.2011.05.019

De Luca, V., Likhodi, O., Kennedy, J. L., & Wong, A. H. (2007). Differential expression and parent-of-origin effect of the 5-HT2A receptor gene C102T polymorphism: Analysis of suicidality in schizophrenia and bipolar disorder. *American Journal of Medical Genetics Part B: Neuropsychiatric Genetics, 144B*(3), 370–4. http://dx.doi.org/10.1016/j.jpsychires.2008.07.007

De Luca, V., Viggiano, E., Dhoot, R., Kennedy, J. L., & Wong, A. H. (2009). Methylation and QTDT analysis of the 5-HT2A receptor 102C allele: Analysis of suicidality in major psychosis. *Journal of Psychiatric Research, 43*(5), 532–7. http://dx.doi.org/10.1016/j.jpsychires.2008.07.007

Deaton, A. M., Webb, S., Kerr, A. R., Illingworth, R. S., Guy, J., Andrews, R., & Bird, A. (2011). Cell type-specific DNA methylation at intragenic CpG islands in the immune system. *Genome Research, 21*(7), 1074–86. http://dx.doi.org/10.1101/gr.118703.110

Deplus, R., Brenner, C., Burgers, W. A., Putmans, P., Kouzarides, T., de Launoit, Y., & Fuks, F. (2002). Dnmt3L is a transcriptional repressor that recruits histone deacetylase. *Nucleic Acids Research, 30*(17), 3831–8. http://dx.doi.org/10.1093/nar/gkf509

Dinwiddie, S., Heath, A. C., Dunne, M. P., Bucholz, K. K., Madden, P. A., Slutske, W. S., ... Martin, N. G. (2000). Early sexual abuse and lifetime psychopathology: A co-twin-control study. *Psychological Medicine, 30*(1), 41–52. http://dx.doi.org/10.1017/S0033291799001373

Dumser, T., Barocka, A., & Schubert, E. (1998). Weight of adrenal glands may be increased in persons who commit suicide. *American Journal of Forensic Medicine and Pathololology, 19*(1), 72–6. http://dx.doi.org/10.1097/00000433-199803000-00014

Duric, V., & McCarson, K. E. (2005). Hippocampal neurokinin-1 receptor and brain-derived neurotrophic factor gene expression is decreased in rat

models of pain and stress. *Neuroscience, 133*(4), 999–1006. http://dx.doi.org/
10.1016/j.neuroscience.2005.04.002

Duric, V., & McCarson, K. E. (2006). Effects of analgesic or antidepressant
drugs on pain- or stress-evoked hippocampal and spinal neurokinin-1
receptor and brain-derived neurotrophic factor gene expression in the rat.
Journal of Pharmacology and Experimental Therapeutics, 319(3), 1235–43.
http://dx.doi.org/10.1124/jpet.106.109470

Dwivedi, Y., Rizavi, H. S., Conley, R. R., Roberts, R. C., Tamminga, C. A., &
Pandey, G. N. (2003). Altered gene expression of brain-derived
neurotrophic factor and receptor tyrosine kinase B in postmortem brain of
suicide subjects. *Archives of General Psychiatry, 60*(8), 804–15. http://dx.doi.
org/10.1001/archpsyc.60.8.804

Elliott, E., Ezra-Nevo, G., Regev, L., Neufeld-Cohen, A., & Chen, A. (2010).
Resilience to social stress coincides with functional DNA methylation of the
Crf gene in adult mice. *Nature Neuroscience, 13*(11), 1351–3. http://dx.doi.
org/10.1038/nn.2642

Ernst, C., Chen, E. S., & Turecki, G. (2009). Histone methylation and decreased
expression of TrkB.T1 in orbital frontal cortex of suicide completers.
Molecular Psychiatry, 14(9), 830–2. http://dx.doi.org/10.1038/mp.2009.35

Ernst, C., Deleva, V., Deng, X., Sequeira, A., Pomarenski, A., Klempan, T., ...
Turecki, G. (2009). Alternative splicing, methylation state, and expression
profile of tropomyosin-related kinase B in the frontal cortex of suicide
completers. *Archives of General Psychiatry, 66*(1), 22–32. http://dx.doi.org/
10.1001/archpsyc.66.1.22

Ernst, C., Mechawar, N., & Turecki, G. (2009). Suicide neurobiology. *Progress in
Neurobiology, 89*(4), 315–33. http://dx.doi.org/10.1016/j.
pneurobio.2009.09.001

Ernst, C., Wanner, B., Brezo, J., Vitaro, F., Tremblay, R., & Turecki, G. (2011).
A deletion in tropomyosin-related kinase B and the development of human
anxiety. *Biological Psychiatry, 69*(6), 604–7. http://dx.doi.org/10.1016/j.
biopsych.2010.10.008

Ernst, J., Kheradpour, P., Mikkelsen, T. S., Shoresh, N., Ward, L. D., Epstein,
C. B., ... Bernstein, B. E. (2011). Mapping and analysis of chromatin state
dynamics in nine human cell types. *Nature, 473*(7345), 43–9. http://dx.doi.
org/10.1038/nature09906

Evans, E., Hawton, K., & Rodham, K. (2005). Suicidal phenomena and abuse
in adolescents: a review of epidemiological studies. *Child Abuse & Neglect,
29*(1), 45–58. http://dx.doi.org/10.1016/j.chiabu.2004.06.014

Fergusson, D. M., Boden, J. M., & Horwood, L. J. (2008). Exposure to
childhood sexual and physical abuse and adjustment in early adulthood.
Child Abuse & Neglect, 32(6), 607–19. http://dx.doi.org/10.1016/j.
chiabu.2006.12.018

Fergusson, D. M., Horwood, L. J., & Lynskey, M. T. (1996). Childhood
sexual abuse and psychiatric disorder in young adulthood: II. Psychiatric
outcomes of childhood sexual abuse. *Journal of the American Academy of
Child and Adolescent Psychiatry, 35*(10), 1365–74. http://dx.doi.org/10.1097/
00004583-199610000-00024

Fiori, L. M., Gross, J. A., & Turecki, G. (2012). Effects of histone modifications
on increased expression of polyamine biosynthetic genes in suicide.

International Journal of Neuropsychopharmacology, 15(8), 1161–6. http://dx. doi.org/10.1017/S1461145711001520

Fiori, L. M., & Turecki, G. (2010). Genetic and epigenetic influences on expression of spermine synthase and spermine oxidase in suicide completers. *International Journal of Neuropsychopharmacology, 13*, 725–36. http://dx.doi.org/10.1017/S1461145709991167

Fliege, H., Lee, J. R., Grimm, A., & Klapp, B. F. (2009). Risk factors and correlates of deliberate self-harm behavior: A systematic review. *Journal of Psychosomatic Research, 66*(6), 477–93. http://dx.doi.org/10.1016/j. jpsychores.2008.10.013

Francis, D., Diorio, J., Liu, D., & Meaney, M. J. (1999). Nongenomic transmission across generations of maternal behavior and stress responses in the rat. *Science, 286*(5442), 1155–8. http://dx.doi.org/10.1126/ science.286.5442.1155

Fuks, F., Burgers, W. A., Brehm, A., Hughes-Davies, L., & Kouzarides, T. (2000). DNA methyltransferase Dnmt1 associates with histone deacetylase activity. *Nature Genetics, 24*(1), 88–91. http://dx.doi.org/10.1038/71750

Fuks, F., Burgers, W. A., Godin, N., Kasai, M., & Kouzarides, T. (2001). Dnmt3a binds deacetylases and is recruited by a sequence-specific repressor to silence transcription. *EMBO Journal, 20*(10), 2536–44. http://dx.doi.org/10.1093/emboj/20.10.2536

Geiman, T. M., Sankpal, U. T., Robertson, A. K., Zhao, Y., & Robertson, K. D. (2004). DNMT3B interacts with hSNF2H chromatin remodeling enzyme, HDACs 1 and 2, and components of the histone methylation system. *Biochemical and Biophysical Research Communications, 318*(2), 544–55. http://dx.doi.org/10.1016/j.bbrc.2004.04.058

Gladstone, G. L., Parker, G. B., Mitchell, P. B., Malhi, G. S., Wilhelm, K., & Austin, M. P. (2004). Implications of childhood trauma for depressed women: An analysis of pathways from childhood sexual abuse to deliberate self-harm and revictimization. *American Journal of Psychiatry, 161*(8), 1417–25. http://dx.doi.org/10.1176/appi.ajp.161.8.1417

Gronli, J., Bramham, C., Murison, R., Kanhema, T., Fiske, E., Bjorvatn, B., ... Portas, C. M. (2006). Chronic mild stress inhibits BDNF protein expression and CREB activation in the dentate gyrus but not in the hippocampus proper. *Pharmacology Biochemistry and Behavior, 85*(4), 842–9. http://dx.doi.org/10.1016/j.pbb.2006.11.021

Grover, K. E., Green, K. L., Pettit, J. W., Monteith, L. L., Garza, M. J., & Venta, A. (2009). Problem solving moderates the effects of life event stress and chronic stress on suicidal behaviors in adolescence. *Journal of Clinical Psychology, 65*(12), 1281–90. http://dx.doi.org/10.1002/jclp.20632

Hashimoto, K. (2010). Brain-derived neurotrophic factor as a biomarker for mood disorders: An historical overview and future directions. *Psychiatry and Clinical Neurosciences, 64*(4), 341–57. http://dx.doi.org/10.1111/ j.1440-1819.2010.02113.x

Hawton, K., Rodham, K., Evans, E., & Weatherall, R. (2002). Deliberate self harm in adolescents: Self report survey in schools in England. *BMJ, 325*(7374), 1207–11. http://dx.doi.org/10.1136/bmj.325.7374.1207

Hawton, K., & van Heeringen, K. (2009). Suicide. *Lancet, 373*(9672), 1372–81. http://dx.doi.org/10.1016/S0140-6736(09)60372-X

Heim, C., Newport, D. J., Heit, S., Graham, Y. P., Wilcox, M., Bonsall, R., ...
Nemeroff, C. B. (2000). Pituitary-adrenal and autonomic responses to stress
in women after sexual and physical abuse in childhood. *JAMA, 284*(5),
592–7. http://dx.doi.org/10.1001/jama.284.5.592

Heim, C., Newport, D. J., Mletzko, T., Miller, A. H., & Nemeroff, C. B. (2008).
The link between childhood trauma and depression: Insights from HPA axis
studies in humans. *Psychoneuroendocrinology, 33*(6), 693–710. http://dx.doi.
org/10.1016/j.psyneuen.2008.03.008

Heim, C., Shugart, M., Craighead, W. E., & Nemeroff, C. B. (2010).
Neurobiological and psychiatric consequences of child abuse and neglect.
Developmental Psychobiology, 52(7), 671–90. http://dx.doi.org/10.1002/
dev.20494

Heim, C., Young, L. J., Newport, D. J., Mletzko, T., Miller, A. H., &
Nemeroff, C. B. (2009). Lower CSF oxytocin concentrations in women with
a history of childhood abuse. *Molecular Psychiatry, 14*(10), 954–8. http://dx.
doi.org/10.1038/mp.2008.112

Hellman, A., & Chess, A. (2007). Gene body-specific methylation on the active
X chromosome. *Science, 315*(5815), 1141–3. http://dx.doi.org/10.1126/
science.1136352

Hiroi, N., Wong, M. L., Licinio, J., Park, C., Young, M., Gold, P. W., ...
Bornstein, S. R. (2001). Expression of corticotropin releasing hormone
receptors type I and type II mRNA in suicide victims and controls.
Molecular Psychiatry, 6(5), 540–6. http://dx.doi.org/10.1038/sj.mp.4000908

Hyman, S. E. (2009). How adversity gets under the skin. *Nature Neuroscience,
12*(3), 241–3.

Iwamoto, K., Bundo, M., Ueda, J., Oldham, M. C., Ukai, W., Hashimoto, E., ...
Kato, T. (2011). Neurons show distinctive DNA methylation profile
and higher interindividual variations compared with non-neurons.
Genome Research, 21(5), 688–96. http://dx.doi.org/10.1101/
gr.112755.110

Jaffee, S. R., Moffitt, T. E., Caspi, A., Fombonne, E., Poulton, R., & Martin, J.
(2002). Differences in early childhood risk factors for juvenile-onset and
adult-onset depression. *Archives of General Psychiatry, 59*(3), 215–22.
http://dx.doi.org/10.1001/archpsyc.59.3.215

Joiner, T. E., Jr., Sachs-Ericsson, N. J., Wingate, L. R., Brown, J. S., Anestis,
M. D., & Selby, E. A. (2007). Childhood physical and sexual abuse and
lifetime number of suicide attempts: A persistent and theoretically important
relationship. *Behaviour Research and Therapy, 45*(3), 539–47. http://dx.doi.
org/10.1016/j.brat.2006.04.007

Jollant, F., Bellivier, F., Leboyer, M., Astruc, B., Torres, S., Verdier, R., ...
Courtet, P. (2005). Impaired decision making in suicide attempters.
American Journal of Psychiatry, 162(2), 304–10. http://dx.doi.org/10.1176/
appi.ajp.162.2.304

Jollant, F., Lawrence, N. L., Olie, E., Guillaume, S., & Courtet, P. (2011).
The suicidal mind and brain: A review of neuropsychological and
neuroimaging studies. *World Journal of Biological Psychiatry, 12*(5), 319–39.
http://dx.doi.org/10.3109/15622975.2011.556200

Jollant, F., Lawrence, N. S., Giampietro, V., Brammer, M. J., Fullana, M. A., Drapier, D., ... Phillips, M. L. (2008). Orbitofrontal cortex response to angry faces in men with histories of suicide attempts. *American Journal of Psychiatry, 165*(6), 740–8. http://dx.doi.org/10.1176/appi.ajp.2008.07081239

Keilp, J. G., Sackeim, H. A., Brodsky, B. S., Oquendo, M. A., Malone, K. M., & Mann, J. J. (2001). Neuropsychological dysfunction in depressed suicide attempters. *American Journal of Psychiatry, 158*(5), 735–41. http://dx.doi.org/10.1176/appi.ajp.158.5.735

Keller, S., Sarchiapone, M., Zarrilli, F., Videtic, A., Ferraro, A., Carli, V., ... Chiariotti, L. (2010). Increased BDNF promoter methylation in the Wernicke area of suicide subjects. *Archives of General Psychiatry, 67*(3), 258–67. http://dx.doi.org/10.1001/archgenpsychiatry.2010.9

Kitayama, N., Quinn, S., & Bremner, J. D. (2006). Smaller volume of anterior cingulate cortex in abuse-related posttraumatic stress disorder. *Journal of Affective Disorders, 90*(2–3), 171–4. http://dx.doi.org/10.1016/j.jad.2005.11.006

Klose, R. J., & Bird, A. P. (2006). Genomic DNA methylation: The mark and its mediators. *Trends in Biochemical Sciences, 31*(2), 89–97. http://dx.doi.org/10.1016/j.tibs.2005.12.008

Kouzarides, T. (2007). Chromatin modifications and their function. *Cell, 128*(4), 693–705. http://dx.doi.org/10.1016/j.cell.2007.02.005

Kriaucionis, S., & Heintz, N. (2009). The nuclear DNA base 5-hydroxymethylcytosine is present in Purkinje neurons and the brain. *Science, 324*(5929), 929–30. http://dx.doi.org/10.1126/science.1169786

Labonté, B., Suderman, M., Maussion, G., Lopez, J. P., Navarro-Sánchez, L., Yerko, V., ... Turecki, G. (2013). Genome-wide methylation changes in the suicide brain. *American Journal of Psychiatry, 170*(5), 511–20. http://dx.doi.org/10.1176/appi.ajp.2012.12050627

Labonté, B., Suderman, M., Maussion, G., Navaro, L., Yerko, V., Mahar, I., ... Turecki, G. (2012). Genome-wide epigenetic regulation by early-life trauma. *Archives of General Psychiatry, 69*(7), 722–31. http://dx.doi.org/10.1001/archgenpsychiatry.2011.2287

Labonté, B., Yerko, V., Gross, J., Mechawar, N., Meaney, M. J., Szyf, M., & Turecki, G. (2012). Differential glucocorticoid receptor exon 1(B), 1(C), and 1(H) expression and methylation in suicide completers with a history of childhood abuse. *Biological Psychiatry, 72*(1), 41–8. http://dx.doi.org/10.1016/j.biopsych.2012.01.034

Ladd-Acosta, C., Pevsner, J., Sabunciyan, S., Yolken, R. H., Webster, M. J., Dinkins, T., ... Feinberg, A. P. (2007). DNA methylation signatures within the human brain. *American Journal of Human Genetics, 81*(6), 1304–15. http://dx.doi.org/10.1086/524110

Lister, R., Pelizzola, M., Dowen, R. H., Hawkins, R. D., Hon, G., Tonti-Filippini, J., ... Ecker, J. R. (2009). Human DNA methylomes at base resolution show widespread epigenomic differences. *Nature, 462*(7271), 315–22. http://dx.doi.org/10.1038/nature08514

Liu, D., Diorio, J., Tannenbaum, B., Caldji, C., Francis, D., Freedman, A., ... Meaney, M. J. (1997). Maternal care, hippocampal glucocorticoid receptors, and hypothalamic-pituitary-adrenal responses to stress. *Science, 277*(5332), 1659–62. http://dx.doi.org/10.1126/science.277.5332.1659

Lopez, J. F., Palkovits, M., Arato, M., Mansour, A., Akil, H., & Watson, S. J. (1992). Localization and quantification of pro-opiomelanocortin mRNA and glucocorticoid receptor mRNA in pituitaries of suicide victims. *Neuroendocrinology, 56*(4), 491–501. http://dx.doi.org/10.1159/000126266

Lopez, J. P., Mamdani, F., Labonte, B., Beaulieu, M. M., Yang, J. P., Berlim, M. T., . . . Turecki, G. (2013). Epigenetic regulation of BDNF expression according to antidepressant response. *Molecular Psychiatry, 18*, 398–9. http://dx.doi.org/10.1038/mp.2012.38

Matrisciano, F., Bonaccorso, S., Ricciardi, A., Scaccianoce, S., Panaccione, I., Wang, L., . . . Shelton, R. C. (2009). Changes in BDNF serum levels in patients with major depression disorder (MDD) after 6 months treatment with sertraline, escitalopram, or venlafaxine. *Journal of Psychiatric Research, 43*(3), 247–54. http://dx.doi.org/10.1016/j.jpsychires.2008.03.014

Maunakea, A. K., Nagarajan, R. P., Bilenky, M., Ballinger, T. J., D'Souza, C., Fouse, S. D., . . . Costello, J. F. (2010). Conserved role of intragenic DNA methylation in regulating alternative promoters. *Nature, 466*(7303), 253–7. http://dx.doi.org/10.1038/nature09165.

McGirr, A., Alda, M., Seguin, M., Cabot, S., Lesage, A., & Turecki, G. (2009). Familial aggregation of suicide explained by cluster B traits: A three-group family study of suicide controlling for major depressive disorder. *American Journal of Psychiatry, 166*(10), 1124–34. http://dx.doi.org/10.1176/appi.ajp.2009.08111744

McGowan, P. O., Sasaki, A., D'Alessio, A. C., Dymov, S., Labonte, B., Szyf, M., . . . Meaney, M. J. (2009). Epigenetic regulation of the glucocorticoid receptor in human brain associates with childhood abuse. *Nature Neuroscience, 12*(3), 342–8. http://dx.doi.org/10.1038/nn.2270

McGowan, P. O., Sasaki, A., Huang, T. C., Unterberger, A., Suderman, M., Ernst, C., . . . Szyf, M. (2008). Promoter-wide hypermethylation of the ribosomal RNA gene promoter in the suicide brain. *PLOS One, 3*(5), e2085. http://dx.doi.org/10.1371/journal.pone.0002085

McGowan, P. O., Suderman, M., Sasaki, A., Huang, T. C., Hallett, M., Meaney, M. J., & Szyf, M. (2011). Broad epigenetic signature of maternal care in the brain of adult rats. *PLOS One, 6*(2), e14739. http://dx.doi.org/10.1371/journal.pone.0014739

McHolm, A. E., MacMillan, H. L., & Jamieson, E. (2003). The relationship between childhood physical abuse and suicidality among depressed women: results from a community sample. *American Journal of Psychiatry, 160*(5), 933–8. http://dx.doi.org/10.1176/appi.ajp.160.5.933

Meaney, M. J., & Ferguson-Smith, A. C. (2010). Epigenetic regulation of the neural transcriptome: The meaning of the marks. *Nature Neuroscience, 13*(11), 1313–18. http://dx.doi.org/10.1038/nn1110-1313

Meissner, A., Mikkelsen, T. S., Gu, H., Wernig, M., Hanna, J., Sivachenko, A., . . . Lander, E. S. (2008). Genome-scale DNA methylation maps of pluripotent and differentiated cells. *Nature, 454*(7205), 766–70.

Merali, Z., Kent, P., Du, L., Hrdina, P., Palkovits, M., Faludi, G., . . . Anisman, H. (2006). Corticotropin-releasing hormone, arginine vasopressin, gastrin-releasing peptide, and neuromedin B alterations in stress-relevant brain regions of suicides and control subjects. *Biological Psychiatry, 59*(7), 594–602. http://dx.doi.org/10.1016/j.biopsych.2005.08.008

Mercier, G., Lennon, A. M., Renouf, B., Dessouroux, A., Ramauge, M., Courtin, F., & Pierre, M. (2004). MAP kinase activation by fluoxetine and its relation to gene expression in cultured rat astrocytes. *Journal of Molecular Neuroscience, 24*(2), 207–16. http://dx.doi.org/10.1385/JMN:24:2:207

Mill, J., Tang, T., Kaminsky, Z., Khare, T., Yazdanpanah, S., Bouchard, L., ... Petronis, A. (2008). Epigenomic profiling reveals DNA-methylation changes associated with major psychosis. *American Journal of Human Genetics, 82*(3), 696–711. http://dx.doi.org/10.1016/j.ajhg.2008.01.008

Molnar, B. E., Berkman, L. F., & Buka, S. L. (2001). Psychopathology, childhood sexual abuse and other childhood adversities: relative links to subsequent suicidal behavior in the US. *Psychological Medicine, 31*(6), 965–77. http://dx.doi.org/10.1017/S0033291701004329

Murgatroyd, C., Patchev, A. V., Wu, Y., Micale, V., Bockmuhl, Y., Fischer, D., ... Spengler, D. (2009). Dynamic DNA methylation programs persistent adverse effects of early-life stress. *Nature Neuroscience, 12*, 1559–66. http://dx.doi.org/10.1038/nn.2436

Nakatani, N., Hattori, E., Ohnishi, T., Dean, B., Iwayama, Y., Matsumoto, I., ... Yoshikawa, T. (2006). Genome-wide expression analysis detects eight genes with robust alterations specific to bipolar I disorder: Relevance to neuronal network perturbation. *Human Molecular Genetics, 15*(12), 1949–62. http://dx.doi.org/10.1093/hmg/ddl118

Navalta, C. P., Polcari, A., Webster, D. M., Boghossian, A., & Teicher, M. H. (2006). Effects of childhood sexual abuse on neuropsychological and cognitive function in college women. *Journal of Neuropsychiatry & Clinical Neurosciences, 18*(1), 45–53. http://dx.doi.org/10.1176/appi.neuropsych.18.1.45

Nemeroff, C. B., Owens, M. J., Bissette, G., Andorn, A. C., & Stanley, M. (1988). Reduced corticotropin releasing factor binding sites in the frontal cortex of suicide victims. *Archives of General Psychiatry, 45*(6), 577–9. http://dx.doi.org/10.1001/archpsyc.1988.01800300075009

Nemeroff, C. B., & Vale, W. W. (2005). The neurobiology of depression: Inroads to treatment and new drug discovery. *Journal of Clinical Psychiatry, 66* *(Suppl. 7)*, 5–13.

Nemeroff, C. B., Widerlov, E., Bissette, G., Walleus, H., Karlsson, I., Eklund, K., ... Vale, W. (1984). Elevated concentrations of CSF corticotropin-releasing factor-like immunoreactivity in depressed patients. *Science, 226* (4680), 1342–4. http://dx.doi.org/10.1126/science.6334362

Pandey, G. N., Ren, X., Rizavi, H. S., Conley, R. R., Roberts, R. C., & Dwivedi, Y. (2008). Brain-derived neurotrophic factor and tyrosine kinase B receptor signalling in post-mortem brain of teenage suicide victims. *International Journal of Neuropsychopharmacology, 11*(8), 1047–61. http://dx.doi.org/10.1017/S1461145708009000

Perez, C. M., & Widom, C. S. (1994). Childhood victimization and long-term intellectual and academic outcomes. *Child Abuse & Neglect, 18*(8), 617–33. http://dx.doi.org/10.1016/0145-2134(94)90012-4

Perroud, N., Paoloni-Giacobino, A., Prada, P., Olie´, E., Salzmann, A., Nicastro, R., ... Malafosse, A. (2011). Increased methylation of glucocorticoid receptor gen (NR3C1) in adults with a history of childhood maltreatment: A link with the severity and type of trauma. *Translational Psychiatry, 1*(e59). http://dx.doi.org/10.1038/tp.2011.60

Pfennig, A., Kunzel, H. E., Kern, N., Ising, M., Majer, M., Fuchs, B., ... Binder, E. B. (2005). Hypothalamus-pituitary-adrenal system regulation and suicidal behavior in depression. *Biological Psychiatry, 57*(4), 336–42. http://dx.doi.org/10.1016/j.biopsych.2004.11.017

Poulter, M. O., Du, L., Weaver, I. C., Palkovits, M., Faludi, G., Merali, Z., ... Anisman, H. (2008). GABAA receptor promoter hypermethylation in suicide brain: Implications for the involvement of epigenetic processes. *Biological Psychiatry, 64*(8), 645–52. http://dx.doi.org/10.1016/j. biopsych.2008.05.028

Raadsheer, F. C., Hoogendijk, W. J., Stam, F. C., Tilders, F. J., & Swaab, D. F. (1994). Increased numbers of corticotropin-releasing hormone expressing neurons in the hypothalamic paraventricular nucleus of depressed patients. *Neuroendocrinology, 60*(4), 436–44. http://dx.doi.org/10.1159/000126778

Raadsheer, F. C., van Heerikhuize, J. J., Lucassen, P. J., Hoogendijk, W. J., Tilders, F. J., & Swaab, D. F. (1995). Corticotropin-releasing hormone mRNA levels in the paraventricular nucleus of patients with Alzheimer's disease and depression. *American Journal of Psychiatry, 152*(9), 1372–6.

Radtke, K. M., Ruf, M., Gunter, H. M., Dohrmann, K., Schauer, M., Meyer, A., & Elbert, T. (2011). Transgenerational impact of intimate partner violence on methylation in the promoter of the glucocorticoid receptor. *Translational Psychiatry, 1*(e21), 1–6.

Rauch, T. A., Wu, X., Zhong, X., Riggs, A. D., & Pfeifer, G. P. (2009). A human B cell methylome at 100-base pair resolution. *Proceedings of the National Academy of Sciences of the United States of America, 106*(3), 671–8. http://dx. doi.org/10.1073/pnas.0812399106

Razzoli, M., Domenici, E., Carboni, L., Rantamaki, T., Lindholm, J., Castren, E., & Arban, R. (2011). A role for BDNF/TrkB signaling in behavioral and physiological consequences of social defeat stress. *Genes, Brain and Behavior, 10*(4), 424–33. http://dx.doi.org/10.1111/j.1601-183X.2011.00681.x

Richardson, H. N., Lee, S. Y., O'Dell, L. E., Koob, G. F., & Rivier, C. L. (2008). Alcohol self-administration acutely stimulates the hypothalamic-pituitary-adrenal axis, but alcohol dependence leads to a dampened neuroendocrine state. *European Journal of Neuroscience, 28*(8), 1641–53. http://dx.doi.org/10.1111/j.1460-9568.2008.06455.x

Rogoz, Z., Skuza, G., & Legutko, B. (2005). Repeated treatment with mirtazepine induces brain-derived neurotrophic factor gene expression in rats. *Journal of Physiology and Pharmacology, 56*(4), 661–71.

Roth, T. L., Lubin, F. D., Funk, A. J., & Sweatt, J. D. (2009). Lasting epigenetic influence of early-life adversity on the BDNF gene. *Biological Psychiatry, 65*(9), 760–9. http://dx.doi.org/10.1016/j.biopsych.2008.11.028

Roth, T. L., Zoladz, P. R., Sweatt, J. D., & Diamond, D. M. (2011). Epigenetic modification of hippocampal Bdnf DNA in adult rats in an animal model of post-traumatic stress disorder. *Journal of Psychiatric Research, 45*(7), 919–26. http://dx.doi.org/10.1016/j.jpsychires.2011.01.013

Schratt, G. (2009). Fine-tuning neural gene expression with microRNAs. *Current Opinion in Neurobiology, 19*(2), 213–19. http://dx.doi.org/10.1016/j. conb.2009.05.015

Sen, S., Duman, R., & Sanacora, G. (2008). Serum brain-derived neurotrophic factor, depression, and antidepressant medications: Meta-analyses and implications. *Biological Psychiatry, 64*(6), 527–32. http://dx.doi.org/10.1016/ j.biopsych.2008.05.005

Sinclair, J. M., Crane, C., Hawton, K., & Williams, J. M. (2007). The role of autobiographical memory specificity in deliberate self-harm: Correlates and consequences. *Journal of Affective Disorders, 102*(1–3), 11–18. http://dx.doi. org/10.1016/j.jad.2006.12.006

Speckens, A. E., & Hawton, K. (2005). Social problem solving in adolescents with suicidal behavior: A systematic review. *Suicide and Life-Threatening Behavior, 35*(4), 365–87. http://dx.doi.org/10.1521/suli.2005.35.4.365

Spinhoven, P., Slee, N., Garnefski, N., & Arensman, E. (2009). Childhood sexual abuse differentially predicts outcome of cognitive-behavioral therapy for deliberate self-harm. *Journal of Nervous and Mental Disease, 197*(6), 455–7. http://dx.doi.org/10.1097/NMD.0b013e3181a620c8

Suominen, K., Isometsa, E., Suokas, J., Haukka, J., Achte, K., & Lonnqvist, J. (2004). Completed suicide after a suicide attempt: A 37-year follow-up study. *American Journal of Psychiatry, 161*(3), 562–3. http://dx.doi.org/ 10.1176/appi.ajp.161.3.562

Szigethy, E., Conwell, Y., Forbes, N. T., Cox, C., & Caine, E. D. (1994). Adrenal weight and morphology in victims of completed suicide. *Biological Psychiatry, 36*(6), 374–80. http://dx.doi.org/10.1016/0006-3223 (94)91212-2

Szyf, M., McGowan, P. O., Turecki, G., & Meaney, M. J. (2010). The social environment and the epigenome. In C. M. Worthman, P. M. Plotsky, D. S. Schechter, & C. A. Cummings (Eds.), *Formative experiences: The interaction of caregiving, culture, and developmental psychobiology* (pp. 53–81). New York, NY: Cambridge University Press.

Tomoda, A., Sheu, Y. S., Rabi, K., Suzuki, H., Navalta, C. P., Polcari, A., & Teicher, M. H. (2011). Exposure to parental verbal abuse is associated with increased gray matter volume in superior temporal gyrus. *Neuroimage, 54*(Suppl. 1), S280–6. http://dx.doi.org/10.1016/j.neuroimage.2010.05.027

Tomoda, A., Suzuki, H., Rabi, K., Sheu, Y. S., Polcari, A., & Teicher, M. H. (2009). Reduced prefrontal cortical gray matter volume in young adults exposed to harsh corporal punishment. *Neuroimage, 47*(Suppl. 2), T66–71. http://dx.doi.org/10.1016/j.neuroimage.2009.03.005

Tsankova, N. M., Berton, O., Renthal, W., Kumar, A., Neve, R. L., & Nestler, E. J. (2006). Sustained hippocampal chromatin regulation in a mouse model of depression and antidepressant action. *Nature Neuroscience, 9*(4), 519–25. http://dx.doi.org/10.1038/nn1659

Tucker, K. L. (2001). Methylated cytosine and the brain: A new base for neuroscience. *Neuron, 30*(3), 649–52. http://dx.doi.org/10.1016/S0896-6273(01)00325-7

Tyrka, A. R., Price, L. H., Marsit, C., Walters, O. C., & Carpenter, L. L. (2012). Childhood adversity and epigenetic modulation of the leukocyte glucocorticoid receptor: Preliminary findings in healthy adults. *PLOS One, 7*(1), e30148. http://dx.doi.org/10.1371/journal.pone.0030148

Uchida, S., Hara, K., Kobayashi, A., Otsuki, K., Yamagata, H., Hobara, T., ... Watanabe, Y. (2011). Epigenetic status of Gdnf in the ventral striatum determines susceptibility and adaptation to daily stressful events. *Neuron, 69*(2), 359–72. http://dx.doi.org/10.1016/j.neuron.2010.12.023

Uddin, M., Aiello, A. E., Wildman, D. E., Koenen, K. C., Pawelec, G., de Los Santos, R., ... Galea, S. (2010). Epigenetic and immune function profiles associated with posttraumatic stress disorder. *Proceedings of the National Academy of Sciences of the United States of America, 107*(20), 9470–5. http://dx.doi.org/10.1073/pnas.0910794107

van den Bos, R., Harteveld, M., & Stoop, H. (2009). Stress and decision-making in humans: Performance is related to cortisol reactivity, albeit differently in men and women. *Psychoneuroendocrinology, 34*(10), 1449–58. http://dx.doi.org/10.1016/j.psyneuen.2009.04.016

van Heeringen, C. (Ed.). (2001). *Understanding suicidal behavior: The suicidal process approach to research, treatment and prevention*. Chichester, England: Wiley.

Vythilingam, M., Heim, C., Newport, J., Miller, A. H., Anderson, E., Bronen, R., ... Bremner, J. D. (2002). Childhood trauma associated with smaller hippocampal volume in women with major depression. *American Journal of Psychiatry, 159*(12), 2072–80. http://dx.doi.org/10.1176/appi.ajp.159.12.2072

Wang, S. S., Kamphuis, W., Huitinga, I., Zhou, J. N., & Swaab, D. F. (2008). Gene expression analysis in the human hypothalamus in depression by laser microdissection and real-time PCR: The presence of multiple receptor imbalances. *Molecular Psychiatry, 13*(8), 786–99, 741. http://dx.doi.org/10.1038/mp.2008.38

Weaver, I. C., Cervoni, N., Champagne, F. A., D'Alessio, A. C., Sharma, S., Seckl, J. R., ... Meaney, M. J. (2004). Epigenetic programming by maternal behavior. *Nature Neuroscience, 7*(8), 847–54. http://dx.doi.org/10.1038/nn1276

Weniger, G., Lange, C., Sachsse, U., & Irle, E. (2008). Amygdala and hippocampal volumes and cognition in adult survivors of childhood abuse with dissociative disorders. *Acta Psychiatrica Scandinavica, 118*(4), 281–90. http://dx.doi.org/10.1111/j.1600-0447.2008.01246.x

Widom, C. S., DuMont, K., & Czaja, S. J. (2007). A prospective investigation of major depressive disorder and comorbidity in abused and neglected children grown up. *Archives of General Psychiatry, 64*(1), 49–56. http://dx.doi.org/10.1001/archpsyc.64.1.49

Williams, J. M., Barnhofer, T., Crane, C., & Beck, A. T. (2005). Problem solving deteriorates following mood challenge in formerly depressed patients with a history of suicidal ideation. *Journal of Abnormal Psychology, 114*(3), 421–31. http://dx.doi.org/10.1037/0021-843X.114.3.421

World Health Organization. (2006). *Suicide prevention*. Retrieved from www.who.int/mental_health/prevention/suicide/suicideprevent/en/

World Health Organization. (2014). *Preventing suicide: A global imperative.* Retrieved from www.who.int/mental_health/suicide-prevention/world_report_2014/en/

Xie, W., Barr, C. L., Kim, A., Yue, F., Lee, A. Y., Eubanks, J., … Ren, B. (2012). Base-resolution analyses of sequence and parent-of-origin dependent DNA methylation in the mouse genome. *Cell, 148*(4), 816–31. http://dx.doi.org/10.1016/j.cell.2011.12.035

Xu, H., Chen, Z., He, J., Haimanot, S., Li, X., Dyck, L., & Li, X. M. (2006). Synergetic effects of quetiapine and venlafaxine in preventing the chronic restraint stress-induced decrease in cell proliferation and BDNF expression in rat hippocampus. *Hippocampus, 16*(6), 551–9. http://dx.doi.org/10.1002/hipo.20184

Yang, B., & Clum, G. A. (2000). Childhood stress leads to later suicidality via its effect on cognitive functioning. *Suicide and Life-Threatening Behavior, 30*(3), 183–98.

Yen, S., Shea, M. T., Sanislow, C. A., Skodol, A. E., Grilo, C. M., Edelen, M. O., … Gunderson, J. G. (2009). Personality traits as prospective predictors of suicide attempts. *Acta Psychiatrica Scandinavica, 120*(3), 222–9. http://dx.doi.org/10.1111/j.1600-0447.2009.01366.x

Ystgaard, M., Hestetun, I., Loeb, M., & Mehlum, L. (2004). Is there a specific relationship between childhood sexual and physical abuse and repeated suicidal behavior? *Child Abuse & Neglect, 28*(8), 863–75. http://dx.doi.org/10.1016/j.chiabu.2004.01.009

Ziller, M. J., Muller, F., Liao, J., Zhang, Y., Gu, H., Bock, C., … Meissner, A. (2011). Genomic distribution and inter-sample variation of non-CpG methylation across human cell types. *PLOS Genetics, 7*(12), e1002389. http://dx.doi.org/10.1371/journal.pgen.1002389

10 Understanding the Neural Circuitry of Emotion Regulation

White Matter Tract Abnormalities and Psychiatric Disorders

Cecile D. Ladouceur, Amelia Versace, and Mary L. Phillips

Introduction

The ability to effectively process and regulate emotional information is a crucial social skill that undergoes important developmental changes from childhood through adolescence and adulthood. Clinical studies indicate that individuals diagnosed with psychiatric disorders, in particular anxiety and mood disorders, exhibit abnormalities in emotion processing and regulation (Phillips, Ladouceur, & Drevets, 2008). Evidence from epidemiological, genetic, and neuroimaging studies suggests that abnormalities in neural connectivity within and between regions of the brain implicated in emotion processing and regulation may play an important role in the neuropathophysiology of these disorders (Almeida & Phillips, 2012; Hajek, Carrey, & Alda, 2005; Leibenluft, Charney, & Pine, 2003; Merikangas et al., 2011; Phillips et al., 2008; Versace et al., 2015).

Collectively, these neural connections, or networks, constitute the brain's "connectome" (Hagmann, 2005; Sporns, Tononi, & Kötter, 2005). It is possible that altered development of these neural networks might contribute to the developmental trajectories of these disorders in vulnerable youth or youth at familial risk for these disorders.

In this chapter, we will focus particularly on bipolar disorder (BD), a serious and recurrent neuropsychiatric illness that affects 2–5 percent of the population (Merikangas et al., 2007) and ranks as one of the top ten leading causes of disability in the world (WHO, 2001). One of the chief clinical features of BD is the difficulty in regulating a range of emotions. In particular, BD is characterized by a pervasive mood disturbance that involves rapid fluctuations and changes in the valence and intensity of emotional states ranging from episodes of sadness, irritability, and anger to episodes of extreme happiness, elation, increased activity, and risky behavior.

236

The emergence of BD in children and adolescents is of particular concern because early onset of BD has been associated with severe presentation and course, including high rates of hospitalization, psychosis, suicidal behavior, substance abuse, and other psychosocial problems (Birmaher et al., 2006; Geller et al., 2002; Perlis et al., 2004). Moreover, evidence from adoption, twin, high-risk, and family studies indicate that BD is highly heritable (Birmaher et al., 2009; DelBello & Geller, 2001; Goodwin & Jamison, 2007; Tsai, Lee, & CC, 1999; Tsuang & Faraone, 1990). Yet, to date, the single strongest most predictive factor for risk of developing BD is high-family loading for the disorder. Given the impact of BD on the development of children and adolescents and the serious negative consequences on functioning into adulthood, it is crucial that we develop new strategies to detect early signs of the illness – ideally before cognitive, emotional, or behavioral manifestations of BD emerge and contribute to poor functioning. Although there have been some advances in identifying early signs of BD, developmental differences in the presentation of the disorder in youth (e.g., symptoms of inattention, irritability, impulsivity, etc.) can often be misinterpreted for the onset of other forms of psychopathology (e.g., attention deficit disorder, oppositional defiant disorder) and lead to inappropriate or less efficient treatment. Conversely, the developmental stage may affect symptom expression and, as a result, there has been a growing controversy regarding the over-diagnosis and treatment of BD (Biederman et al., 2003; Dickstein & Leibenluft, 2012; Post et al., 2008). One potential explanation for this phenomenon is that diagnostic criteria for mood disorders, including depression and BD, in children and adolescents are essentially the same as those for adults, and categorical classifications are very limited in informing different etiologies account- ing for the different courses and responses to treatment (Aggen, Neale, & Kendler, 2005; APA, 2000; Thapar, Collishaw, Pine, & Thapar, 2012). Thus, it has been suggested to study BD as a spectrum disorder with measurable dimensions (e.g., emotion regulation) that in turn can help identify etiologically based homogenous subgroups (Aggen et al., 2005; Frank, Nimgaonkar, Phillips, & Kupfer, 2015; Seemuller et al., 2010). Indeed, this is one of the approaches that have guided revisions of *DSM-5* (APA, 2013; for more information, see www.dsm5.org, and Kupfer & Regier, 2011; Phillips & Vieta, 2007; Regier, Narrow, Kuhl, & Kupfer, 2009). Such an approach could contribute to the identification of early neural markers of emotional dysregulation in at-risk youth through the use of neuroimaging techniques, including functional neuroimaging paradigms that assess emotion processing and regulation subprocesses, and could lead to earlier identification of young people who are likely to develop the disorder and inform early preventive strategies. More importantly, grounding such research studies within a developmental cognitive and affective neuroscience framework is crucial in order to enhance our ability to identify those neuroanatomical networks that constitute, in each person, the brain's connectome and help us further understand the impact of genes and individual experiences in determining those plastic changes that may contribute to the developmental trajectories toward psychiatric disorders, including BD and other affective disorders, such as anxiety and depression.

Our current work focusing on the identification of neural markers of risk for mood disorders such as BD has been guided by a model that incorporates multiple factors (see Figure 10.1).

In essence, we propose that several factors influence individual developmental trajectories toward mood disorders such as BD and that many of these factors mutually influence each other. Certainly the nature of such mutual influences during development is complex and remains to be determined at various levels (i.e., at the microscale level of neurons and synapses and at the macroscale level of fibers connecting different brain regions). Nevertheless, we propose that several of these

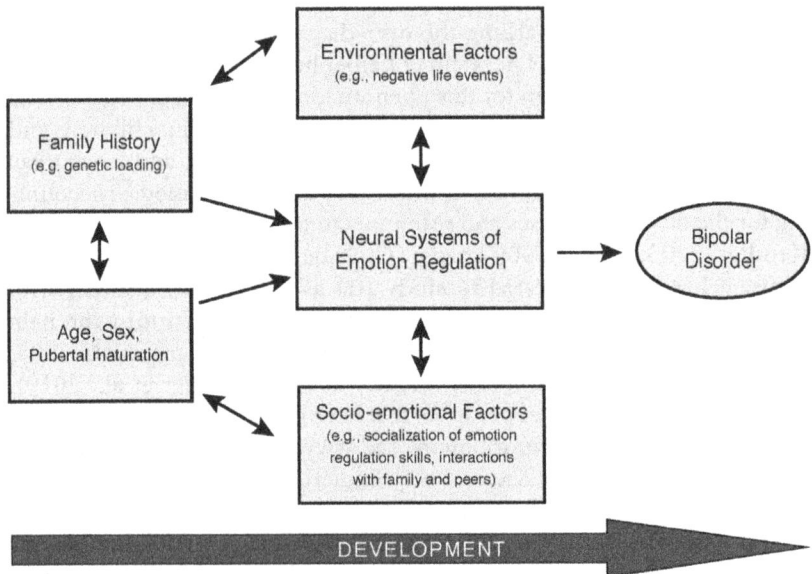

Figure 10.1. Heuristic model of the development of bipolar disorder.

factors – including family history, age, sex, pubertal maturation, and environmental factors, as well as socioemotional factors – influence either directly or indirectly the structural organization and functioning of the brain's "connectome" related to emotion (network of neural regions implicated in emotion processing and regulation). We also propose that the extent of such influences changes across development, thereby creating particular windows of vulnerability and increased risk for the onset of the disorder, but also windows of opportunity for early clinical interventions that could influence the "functional dynamics" (i.e., neural activity) over time. Integrating the study of individual brain plasticity and neurodevelopment is absolutely crucial to defining the structural connectome and its functional dynamics and to foster an individualized approach to the treatment of mental illness.

In this chapter, we will provide a brief overview of our neural model of emotion regulation and describe evidence suggesting that the neural regions implicated in emotion regulation undergo important maturational changes, especially during adolescence. In particular, we will focus on white matter development and describe how deficits in specific white matter regions may represent a pathophysiological marker of BD and a potential vulnerability marker for BD in offspring at familial risk for BD. We will summarize recent neuroimaging data examining white matter structure in clinical samples, including a study that we conducted examining white matter structure in healthy youth at familial risk for BD. "White matter" refers to myelinated and nonmyelinated axons that are bundled into tracts connecting different brain regions. We focus on white matter because of its role in providing the structural architecture of the brain and as the structural network of complex functional neural systems, such as those implicated in supporting emotion regulation. We focus on adolescence because it represents the period with the greatest increase in risk for the development of affective disorders (Angold, Costello, Erkanli, & Worthman, 1995; Angold, Costello, & Worthman, 1998; Angold & Worthman, 1993). It also represents a sensitive period for the development of neural systems supporting emotion regulation, thereby creating a window of vulnerability for the onset of mood disorders in at-risk youth. As a sensitive period for the development of these neural systems, it also represents a period of heightened neuroplasticity, thus offering a window of opportunity for early intervention. We will conclude this chapter by discussing the value of certain methodologies for investigating the neurodevelopment of white matter connectivity in adults and youth and provide recommendations for future research endeavors to advance this area.

Neural Systems Underlying Emotion Regulation

Emotion regulation refers to extrinsic and intrinsic processes involved in the monitoring, evaluation, and modification of an emotional response in order to achieve one's goals (Thompson, 1994). These processes may be "automatic or controlled, conscious or unconscious, and may have their effects at one or more points in the emotion generative process" (Gross & Thompson, 2007, p. 8). Although other definitions of emotion regulation have been proposed, we believe that this definition reflects the complex nature of emotion regulation, including the notion that emotion regulation involves subprocesses that may be either voluntary or automatic.

An increasingly large number of functional neuroimaging studies implicate a network of frontolimbic systems that support processes implicated in the processing and regulation of emotionally salient information. These studies suggest that processing emotionally salient information involves a network of predominantly subcortical, anterior limbic regions, including dorsal and ventral striatal regions, amygdala, hippocampus, and anterior insula (Hariri, Mattay, Tessitore, Fera, & Weinberger, 2003; Morris et al., 1998; Phillips, 2003; Phillips et al., 1997; Surguladze et al., 2003). In order to better understand the nature of neural systems implicated in emotion regulation, we developed a neural model of emotion regulation based on a critical review of the neuroimaging literature and have used this model to guide our studies of individuals diagnosed with or at risk for mood disorders such as BD. Our model emphasizes the roles of two major neural systems in different *voluntary* and *automatic* emotion regulatory subprocesses, described in terms of *behavioral control, attentional control,* and *cognitive change* subprocesses (Phillips et al., 2008; see Table 10.1).

Briefly, *voluntary* emotion regulation subprocesses refer to conscious regulatory processes that serve to modulate an emotional reaction, such as the inhibition of ongoing emotion-expressive behavior (i.e., suppression); alter the emotional meaning of an emotional stimulus (i.e., reappraisal); or modulate attention toward or away an emotional stimulus (i.e., attentional control). Voluntary subprocesses are supported by a lateral prefrontal cortical system that is neocortical in origin and thought to operate by a feedback mechanism[1] (see Figure 10.2). Findings from human neuroimaging studies suggest that voluntary emotion regulation subprocesses are supported by a network of dorsal

---

[1] Process whereby the return of all or part of the output of a neural system is used as input so as to exert some control in the process.

Table 10.1 *Emotion Regulation Subprocesses and Underlying Neural Regions.*

Subprocesses	Neural Regions
Voluntary	
Voluntary Behavioral Control	
Suppression of emotion expression	
	Lateral/Dorsal PFC
Voluntary Attentional Control	bilateral DLPFC (VLPFC)
Avoidance of emotionally salient	bilateral MdPFC
material	bilateral dorsal ACG
Selective attention	(mediated by bilateral OFC)
Inhibition of emotional motor	
responses	
Voluntary Cognitive Change Processes	
Reappraisal	
Automatic	
Automatic Behavioral Control	
Extinction	**Ventral/Medial PFC**
Behavioral regulation	bilateral subgenual ACG
	bilateral OFC
Automatic Attentional Control	left rostral ACG
Cognitive disengagement	bilateral MdPFC
Repressive and avoidant personality	midline dorsal ACG
styles	hippocampus/
	parahippocampus
Automatic Cognitive Change Processes	
Covert appraisal and reappraisal	
Covert response (e.g., error	
monitoring)	
Covert learning that serves to	
automatically adjust behavior	

prefrontal cortical regions, including bilateral dorsolateral prefrontal cortex (DLPFC), bilateral dorsomedial prefrontal cortex (MdPFC), and bilateral dorsal anterior cingulate gyrus (ACG). Activity in these regions may be mediated by bilateral ventromedial prefrontal cortical regions, such as the orbitofrontal cortex (OFC), which have direct connections with subcortical neural regions underlying the identification and initial processing of emotional material.

In parallel, there are *automatic* emotion regulation subprocesses that are involved in the regulation of emotional reactions and behavior. Briefly, *automatic* emotion regulation sub-processes refer to regulatory

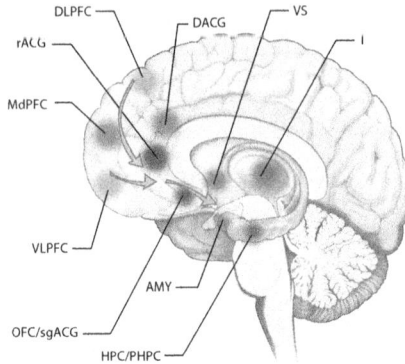

Figure 10.2. Neural model of emotion regulation illustrating neural systems implicated in voluntary subprocesses of emotion regulation. Feedback pathway: lateral prefrontal cortical system, including DLPFC and VLPFC. DLPFC: dorsolateral prefrontal cortex; MdPFC: dorsomedial prefrontal cortex; ACG: anterior cingulate gyrus; VLPFC: ventrolateral prefrontal cortex; OFC: orbital frontal cortex; HPC/PHPC: hippocampus-parahippocampus region; AMY: amygdala; T: thalamus; VS: ventral striatum. Orienting/emotion identification (orange); automatic emotion regulation (green); voluntary emotion regulation (purple); regions implicated in both automatic and voluntary emotion regulation (blue). Adapted from "Neural Systems Underlying Voluntary and Automatic Emotion Regulation" by M. L. Phillips, C. K. Ladouceur, and W. C. Drevets, *Molecular Psychiatry, 13*(9), p. 829, by permission from Macmillan Publishers Ltd., Copyright (2008); and "I Fear for You: A Role for Serotonin in Moral Behavior" by H. Tost and A. Meyer-Lindenberg, *PNAS, 107*(40), p. 17071. (See Color Plate.)

processes that are outside the realm of awareness, such as the extinction of previously acquired behavior, inhibition of the stress response, implicit modulation of attention toward or away emotional material, or implicit appraisal of context or monitoring of behavior. Based on findings from animal as well as human lesion and neuroimaging studies, automatic emotion regulation subprocesses implicate a network of ventromedial neural regions such as bilateral subgenual ACG, bilateral OFC, left rostral ACG and bilateral MdPFC, midline dorsal ACG, as well as hippocampus and parahippocampus (see Figure 10.3). In order to understand how alterations in the functioning of these neural systems may contribute to developmental trajectories of psychiatric disorders such as BD, it is important to briefly consider the normal

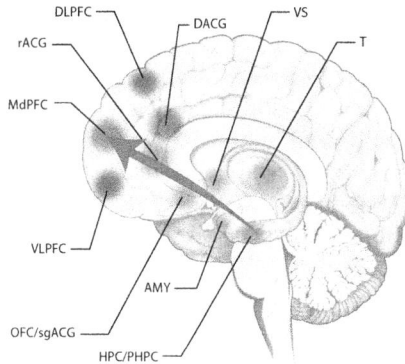

Figure 10.3. Neural model of emotion regulation illustrating neural systems implicated in voluntary subprocesses of emotion regulation. Feedforward pathway: medial prefrontal cortical system, including the OFC, subgenual ACG, rostral ACG, hippocampus and parahippocampus, and MdPFC. DLPFC: dorsolateral prefrontal cortex; MdPFC: dorsomedial prefrontal cortex; ACG: anterior cingulate gyrus; VLPFC: ventrolateral prefrontal cortex; OFC: orbital frontal cortex; HPC/PHPC: hippocampus-parahippocampus region; AMY: amygdala; T: thalamus; VS: ventral striatum. Orienting/emotion identification (orange); automatic emotion regulation (green); voluntary emotion regulation (purple); regions implicated in both automatic and voluntary emotion regulation (blue). Adapted from "Neural Systems Underlying Voluntary and Automatic Emotion Regulation" by M. L. Phillips, C. K. Ladouceur, and W. C. Drevets, *Molecular Psychiatry, 13*(9), p. 829, by permission from Macmillan Publishers Ltd., Copyright (2008); and "I Fear for You: A Role for Serotonin in Moral Behavior" by H. Tost and A. Meyer-Lindenberg, *PNAS, 107*(40), p. 17071. (See Color Plate.)

development of these systems during adolescence – a developmental period during which the occurrence of mood disorders increases dramatically.

Development of Neural Systems Underlying Emotion Regulation

Emotion regulation subprocesses undergo important developmental changes starting in infancy and continuing through childhood and adolescence and into adulthood (Cole, Michel, & O'Donnell Teti, 1994). Although there are important changes in emotion regulation that occur during each of these developmental periods, those that take place during adolescence are particularly relevant (Casey, Jones, & Somerville, 2011; Dahl, 2001; Dahl & Spear, 2004; Ernst, Pine, & Hardin, 2006; Ladouceur, 2012; Steinberg, 2005). Adolescence is a transitional period between childhood and adulthood that encompasses changes in reproductive hormones, physical growth, and socioaffective functioning (Dahl, 2004; Dorn, Dahl, Woodward, & Biro, 2006). Adolescence is one of the healthiest periods of the lifespan with respect to physical health, yet paradoxically, overall morbidity and mortality rates increase by 200–300 percent (Ozer, Macdonald, & Irwin, 2002). For instance, the rate of accidents, suicide, depression, anxiety, and alcohol and substance use all increase drastically during this developmental period (Force, 1996; Ozer et al., 2002). Moreover, several of the most costly, chronic and impairing disorders of adulthood, including mood disorders, typically have their onset during adolescence (Costello et al., 1996; Pine, Cohen, Gurley, Brook, & Ma, 1998). For instance, according to the National Comorbidity Survey – Adolescent Supplement (NCS-A), about 11 percent of adolescents will have a depressive disorder by age eighteen (Kessler, 2011). This increase in mental and behavioral health problems in adolescence is largely associated with difficulties in emotion regulation processes, which undergo important maturational changes during this time. Indeed, during adolescence there are important age-related changes that occur in brain structure relevant to emotion regulation. For instance, a growing number of cross-sectional and longitudinal studies have shown increases in white matter and decreases in grey matter density in the frontal and parietal cortical regions (Barnea-Goraly et al., 2005; Giedd et al., 1999b; Pfefferbaum et al., 1994; Sowell et al., 2003). Recent studies have also documented maturational changes in the structure of particular white matter tracts implicated in emotion regulation (Giedd et al., 1999a; Lebel, Walker, Leemans, Phillips, & Beaulieu, 2008; Schmithorst & Yuan, 2010). For instance, some studies have shown significant age-related changes in the structure of regions such as the uncinate fasciculus, a major tract connecting anterior temporal cortex (including the amygdala) with OFC (Lebel et al., 2008).

With regard to brain function, a large body of work has documented the protracted development in adolescence of prefrontal cortical regions supporting cognitive control processes such as attentional control, response inhibition, and working memory (e.g., Bunge, Dudukovic, Thomason, Vaidya, & Gabrieli, 2002; Luna, Garver, Urban, Lazar, & Sweeney, 2004; Luna, Padmanabhan, & O'Hearn, 2011). Fewer neuroimaging studies, however, have documented adolescent development of neural regions supporting emotion processing and regulation. The majority of these studies have examined age-related changes in emotional face processing. For instance, some have demonstrated greater amygdalar activation to fearful faces in adolescents relative to adults (Guyer et al., 2008; Killgore, Oki, & Yurgelun-Todd, 2001; Monk et al., 2003) and also to both children and adults (Hare et al., 2008). Elevated amygdalar response to emotional stimuli during a response inhibition task has been shown to be negatively correlated with response times to these stimuli, with adolescents overall responding more slowly than adults (Hare et al., 2008). Such findings suggest that adolescents may be more easily distracted by emotionally salient information such as fearful faces, which are known to activate the amygdala (Breiter et al., 1996; Hariri et al., 2003; Hariri, Tessitore, Mattay, Fera, & Weinberger, 2002). They also suggest that such emotional reactivity may influence the regulatory control of behavioral responses, such as response inhibition (Hare et al., 2008). Furthermore, mounting evidence suggests that adolescents tend to be more sensitive to the rewarding properties of stimuli, and this sensitivity is thought to contribute to increased difficulty in regulating approach-related behaviors that contribute to increases in impulsivity and risk-taking in adolescence (Casey, Duhoux, & Cohen, 2010; Ernst et al., 2006; Spear, 2011; Steinberg, 2007; Wahlstrom, White, & Luciana, 2010).

Measures of Developmental Changes in White Matter Integrity

One strategy to begin elucidating alterations in the neurodevelopment of neural systems implicated in emotion processing and regulation is to examine developmental changes in the integrity of white matter tracts. These tracts serve to facilitate communication between neural regions creating neural networks (Paus, 2010). Some of these neural networks implicate cortico-cortical, as well as cortico-subcortical, connections that subserve cognitive and affective functions.

Diffusion tensor imaging (DTI) technique can provide specific information about the integrity of white matter tracts, as it yields information regarding the structural components of white matter, including myelination and axonal organization. DTI provides quantitative information that complements existing findings from volumetric magnetic resonance imaging (MRI) studies by using information about the diffusion of water, which tends to travel more rapidly along highly packed axons (i.e., coherence; Basser & Jones, 2002). Fractional anisotropy (FA) represents the ratio of water diffusion in longitudinally aligned versus transverse directions of white matter tracts. That is, voxels[2] containing water moving predominantly along the principal diffusion direction – rather than across – highly packed axons, have higher FA. FA is sensitive to a number of neurobiological characteristics of white matter such as axonal size, density, and organization, as well as the degree of myelination (Paus, 2005, 2010). Thus, greater FA could reflect greater myelination/diameter of white matter fibers, fiber density, or fiber coherence (ratio of highly packed fibers versus crossing fibers). Other common measures include radial diffusivity (RD) (Hasan, 2006), which is a more specific indirect index of coherence/myelination of the fibers (i.e., greater RD could reflect a context of crossing fibers or de/dysmyelination), than mean diffusivity (MD), which indexes mean overall diffusion.

White Matter Connectivity Studies in Individuals Diagnosed with Bipolar Disorder

Neuropathological studies found cytoarchitectural and neurochemical abnormalities of neuronal and glial cells in adults with BD (for a review, see Harrison, 2002; Rajkowska, 2002). To date, structural white matter abnormalities have been consistently reported in vivo by neuroimaging studies in youth and adults with BD, using DTI. Abnormalities in the corpus callosum and in the white matter of frontal and (anterior) cingulate cortices have also been reported in adults with BD in *region-of-interest (ROI) based analyses* (Adler et al., 2006; Beyer et al., 2005; Haznedar et al., 2005; Macritchie et al., 2010; Wang et al., 2009; Yurgelun-Todd, Silveri, Gruber, Rohan, & Pimentel, 2007); *voxel-based analyses* (Bruno, Cercignani, & Ron, 2008; Chaddock et al., 2009; Mahon et al., 2009; Sussmann et al., 2009; Wessa et al., 2009; Zanetti et al., 2009); *tract-based spatial statistics analyses* (Versace et al., 2008; Wessa et al., 2009); and *tractography-based analyses* (Houenou et al., 2007; Mahon et al., 2009; Matthews & MacLeod, 2002; McIntosh et al., 2008). Taken together, these findings suggest that abnormal white matter integrity may play an important role in the pathophysiology of BD (for reviews, see Heng, Song, & Sim, 2010; Mahon, Burdick, & Szeszko, 2010), and further support the idea that

---

[2] Voxel refers to volumetric pixel or volumetric picture element; it is a volume element, representing a value on a regular grid in three-dimensional space. Voxels are often used to visualize or analyze brain imaging data and as such, the value of a voxel may represent various properties of the imaging data (e.g., intensity in structural MRI, blood oxygenation/deoxygenation in functional MRI, water motility in diffusion MRI).

deficient frontal modulation of subcortical and limbic structures may underlie mood dysregulation in BD (Phillips et al., 2008). Interestingly, a recent meta-analysis of ten selected whole-brain (*voxel-based* or *tract-based spatial statistics analyses*) DTI studies of BD identified one cluster of reduced FA in the right hemisphere, located in the right white matter, close to the parahippocampal gyrus. The most likely pathways crossing this cluster could be identified as the arcuate fasciculus (AF), considered to be part of the superior longitudinal fasciculus (SLF) (Makris et al., 2005); the inferior fronto-occipital fasciculus; the inferior longitudinal fasciculus (ILF); or the posterior thalamic radiations (Vederine, Wessa, Leboyer, & Houenou, 2011).

White Matter Connectivity and Risk for Bipolar Disorder

Fewer studies of white matter integrity have been conducted in pediatric BD and in youth at familial risk for BD. Nevertheless, findings suggest that, similar to adult BD, pediatric BD also implicates white matter abnormalities in temporal (Kafantaris et al., 2009) and occipital (Barnea-Goraly, Chang, Karchemskiy, Howe, & Reiss, 2009; Kafantaris et al., 2009) cortices, as well as in the corpus callosum (Barnea-Goraly et al., 2009; Frazier et al., 2007). More recently, we and others have documented white matter abnormalities in youth at familial risk for BD. These abnormalities were reported in the right ILF (Versace, Ladouceur, et al., 2010) and in the left SLF (Chaddock et al., 2009; Versace, Ladouceur, et al., 2010), as well as in the corpus callosum of healthy relatives of adults with BD. These findings suggest that white matter abnormalities may underlie potential vulnerability for future psychiatric disorders in healthy relatives of adults with BD. We next present data from a DTI study in healthy offspring at familial risk for BD as an example of a research study that is part of a research program dedicated to the investigation of the development of neural networks supporting emotion regulation as a potential path toward the identification of neural markers of risk for BD.

In a more recent diffusion imaging study of 120 youth with behavioral and emotional dysregulation, youth with emotional dysregulation disorders (including youth with bipolar spectrum disorders, depressive disorders, and anxiety disorders) showed lower FA and lower L1 in fibers involved in emotional processing and regulation (i.e., the uncinate fasciculus and the forceps minor), compared to youth with behavioral dysregulation disorders and typically developing age- and gender-matched typically developing youth (Versace et al., 2015). Such a reduction in the number of axons (and/or smaller axonal diameter) in key tracts supporting emotion processing and regulation could represent a potential neural mechanism underlying cross-diagnostic emotional dysregulation in youth. These findings suggest that future longitudinal studies employing a developmental and systems neuroscience approach are needed in order to better understand how altered development of emotion regulation neural circuitry could elucidate potential neural mechanisms underlying symptoms of emotional dysregulation in BD and other affective disorders.

Altered Development of White Matter Connectivity: A Potential Vulnerability Marker for Bipolar Disorder?

In light of evidence that abnormalities in white matter integrity might represent a neuropathophysiological marker of BD, it is possible that such abnormalities might be present before the onset of any symptoms in youth at familial risk for the disorder. Studies in animals (Song et al., 2002) and humans (Giorgio et al., 2007) indicate that age-related increases in FA, with decreases in RD, are considered to reflect developmental changes associated with myelination. As such, identifying alterations in white matter structure in unaffected relatives of individuals with BD could represent a potential vulnerability marker, particularly in younger people before they have reached the typical age of onset.

In this particular study, we compared twenty healthy offspring at high familial risk for BD by virtue of having at least one biological parent diagnosed with BD type I or II, and twenty-five age-matched offspring of healthy parents (for further details about this study, see Versace, Ladouceur, et al., 2010). All participants were between eight and seventeen years old and did not endorse any current *DSM-IV* (APA, 1994, 2000) Axis I diagnosis or history of depression or BD on the K-SADS-PL (Kaufman et al., 1997), a semistructured interview used to assess psychiatric diagnoses in children and adolescents. Exclusion criteria included: IQ < 70, history of head trauma, neurological disorder, or unstable medical illness. Participants and their parents completed a series of questionnaires on the day of the neuroimaging scan to ensure that all participants were free of any current *DSM-IV* Axis I psychiatric diagnoses immediately before the neuroimaging evaluation and to assess the presence of any symptoms of anxiety, depression, or mania.

Diffusion-weighted images were acquired and analyzed using the Functional Magnetic Resonance Imaging of the Brain Software Library (FSL; v.4.1). The primary aim of the study was to examine age-related changes in FA across the two groups. To complement these FA measures, we also explored age-related changes in radial and longitudinal diffusivity and examined main effects of group. Therefore, the preprocessed data were entered into a whole brain, tract-based spatial statistics analysis (TBSS) of FA. Design and inference were based on a general linear model with age as a covariate, and non-parametric independent t-tests.

Briefly, in the healthy comparison group, our results showed increases in FA as a function of increasing age in the left corpus callosum and the right ILF, supporting previously documented age-related changes in FA in normative samples (Figure 10.4).

In offspring at familial risk for BD, however, we observed decreases in FA with age in the left corpus callosum, and no relationship between FA and age in the right ILF. Specifically, we found opposite patterns of age-related changes in the left corpus callosum between the healthy comparison group and the at-risk youth (see Figure 10.5).

Our findings suggest that the unaffected offspring at familial risk for BD did not exhibit the normative changes in structure indices as a function of age in two regions: the corpus callosum and the ILF. The corpus callosum is a major midline white matter tract that is involved in integrating, between hemispheres, sensory-motor functions, attention, language, memory, and emotional states (Gazzaniga, 2000). Developmental studies indicate that the corpus callosum matures through adolescence into adulthood with a posterior-anterior axonal maturation most likely due to increased myelination (Lebel et al., 2008). Our findings of normative increases with age in FA in the corpus callosum in the healthy comparison group are consistent with findings from larger cross-sectional studies indicating normative increases in FA (and decrease in radial diffusivity) with age in adolescence (Lebel et al., 2008). Thus, our findings of decreases in FA (and increase in radial diffusivity) with age in the corpus callosum suggest possible alterations in the white matter development of the corpus callosum in at-risk youth. Our findings also indicate group differences in the pattern of age-related changes in the right ILF. The ILF is a major white matter associative tract connecting occipital and temporal cortices that runs laterally and inferiorly to the lateral wall of the temporal horn. This region is considered part of a "ventral semantic network" with an important role in the visual processing of emotionally salient information, as ILF projections feed information regarding the emotional valence of visual stimuli back to early visual processing cortical regions, thereby enhancing the visual processing of emotionally salient stimuli (Catani, Jones, Donato, & Ffytche, 2003). Our findings of normative increases with age in FA in right ILF in the healthy comparison group are consistent with findings from cross-sectional studies (Lebel et al., 2008). The absence of such age-related changes in FA (and RD) in right ILF in the at-risk group suggests that altered white matter

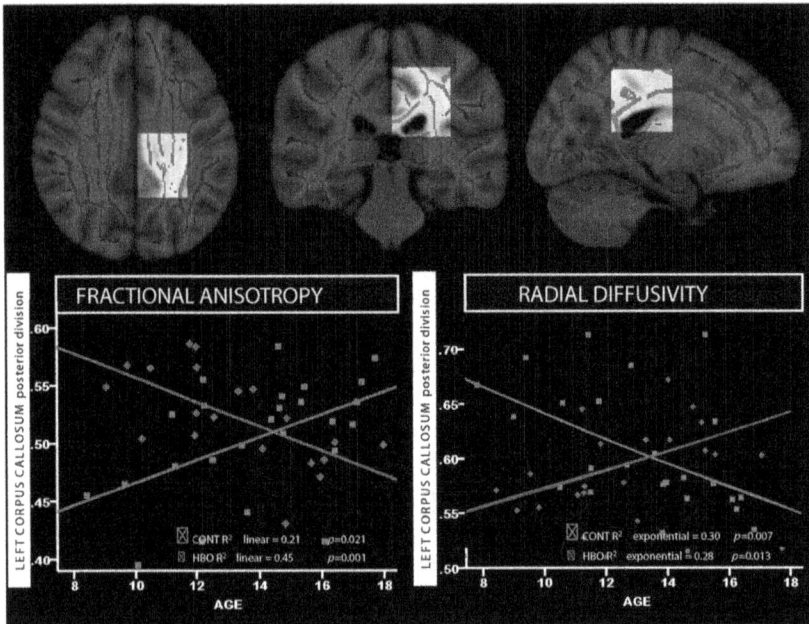

Figure 10.4. Panel A. Fractional Anisotropy (FA) maps depicting (from left to right) coronal, axial, and sagittal views (above) of the left corpus callosum, body division [MNI x, y, z: -18, -30, 34]. Panel B. Radial Diffusivity (RD) maps depicting (from left to right) coronal, axial, and sagittal views (above) of the left corpus callosum, body division [MNI x, y, z: -18, 9, 36]. RD values are reported on the Y axis with a scaling factor of 1000.

The template is the standard MNI-152 1 mm brain template. Colored voxels in red-yellow represent findings significantly different between healthy offspring having a parent with bipolar disorder (HBO) and age-matched control offspring of healthy parents (CONT). Red-yellow indicates higher FA and decreased RD in HBO than CONT ($t > 3$; $p \geq 0.05$, corrected: scale ranging from red to yellow). We determined the most probable anatomical localization of each cluster with the FSL atlas tool, using all anatomical templates. Reprinted from *Journal of the American Academy of Child and Adolescent Psychiatry, 49*, Versace, A., Ladouceur, C. D., Romero, S., Birmaher, B., Axelson, D. A., Kupfer, D. J., Phillips, M.L., "Altered Development of White Matter in Youth at High Familial Risk for Bipolar Disorder: A Diffusion Tensor Imaging Study," p. 1254, Copyright (2010), with permission from Elsevier. (See Color Plate.)

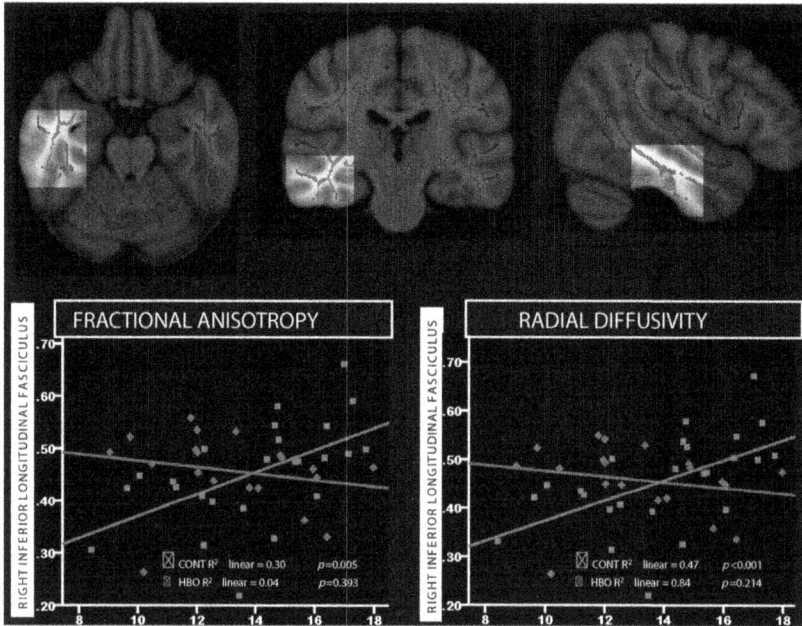

Figure 10.5. Panel A. Fractional Anisotropy (FA) maps depicting (from left to right) coronal, axial, and sagittal views (above) of the right inferior longitudinal fasciculus in the temporal cortex [MNI x, y, z: 49, -23, -22]. Panel B. Radial Diffusivity (RD) maps depicting (from left to right) coronal, axial, and sagittal views (above) of the right inferior longitudinal fasciculus in the temporal cortex [MNI x, y, z: 49, -20, -22]. RD values are reported on the Y axis with a scaling factor of 1000. Panel C. Longitudinal Diffusivity (L1) maps depicting (from left to right) coronal, axial, and sagittal views (above) of the right inferior longitudinal fasciculus in the visual cortex [MNI x, y, z: 24, -59, -1]. L1 values are reported on the Y axis with a scaling factor of 1000.

The template is the standard MNI-152 1 mm brain template. Colored voxels in red-yellow represent findings significantly different between healthy offspring having a parent with bipolar disorder (HBO) and age-matched control offspring of healthy parents (CONT). Red-yellow indicates higher FA, L1 and decreased RD in HBO than CONT ($t > 3$; $p \geq 0.05$, corrected: scale ranging from red to yellow). We determined the most probable anatomical localization of each cluster with the FSL atlas tool, using all anatomical templates. Reprinted from *Journal of the American Academy of Child and Adolescent Psychiatry, 49,* Versace, A., Ladouceur, C. D., Romero, S., Birmaher, B., Axelson, D. A., Kupfer, D. J., Phillips, M.L., "Altered Development of White Matter in Youth at High Familial Risk for Bipolar Disorder: A Diffusion Tensor Imaging Study," p. 1255, Copyright (2010), with permission from Elsevier. (See Color Plate.)

development of this region may represent a vulnerability marker for BD, which would be consistent with findings from a recent meta-analysis in adults with BD (Vederine et al., 2011).

Although these findings may prove interesting, the fact remains that the associations with age were determined using a cross-sectional design. Furthermore, offspring having a parent with BD are at risk not only for BD, but also for other psychiatric disorders such as disruptive disorders, anxiety, and mood spectrum disorders (Birmaher et al., 2009). Our findings therefore also suggest that altered development of these particular white matter tracts may confer, or be associated with, increased vulnerability for subsequent development of BD as well as other psychiatric disorders observed in offspring having a parent with BD. Longitudinal follow-up studies are needed to determine whether such alterations in the development of white matter connectivity represent vulnerability or actual risk markers for BD.

Functional Connectivity and Risk for Bipolar Disorder and Other Affective Disorders

Employing a combination of various neuroimaging techniques (i.e., a multimodal neuroimaging approach) is highly recommended in order to achieve a more comprehensive understanding of the human connectome and its functional dynamics in affective disorders and risk for affective disorders such as BD. For instance, our own findings in adults with BD of abnormal FA in fibers connecting the middle temporal lobe, including the amygdala, with the orbitofrontal cortex (Versace et al., 2008), indicated that those affected individuals, compared to those who were unaffected, showed significantly greater functional connectivity[3] between amygdala and orbitofrontal cortex ($p < .001$) when presented with faces expressing from-neutral-to-intense sad emotions (Versace, Almeida, et al., 2010). We interpreted these findings as indicating that individuals with BD may be "over-appraising" facial expressions depicting sad emotions, and that this could reflect a predisposition

---

[3] Functional connectivity is a type of neuroimaging analysis used to statistically determine the interrelationships of signal changes in distal brain regions. "Functional connectivity" per se refers to statistical associations between remote neurophysiological events. "Effective connectivity" can be considered as a special case of functional connectivity and refers to a statistical analytical approach used to determine the causal associations between distinct neurophysiological events (Friston, 2002). Functional connectivity analysis is conducted with fMRI data collected while the subject is either performing a task or at rest (resting state). As such, these forms of analyses may help elucidate how neural networks process information.

to negative rumination in BD (Van der Gucht, Morriss, Lancaster, Kinderman, & Bentall, 2009). We also found significantly reduced functional connectivity in those individuals with BD, compared to unaffected individuals, between amygdala and orbitofrontal cortex (p = .007) when presented with facial expressions depicting intense happy emotions (Versace, Almeida, et al., 2010). Interestingly, there was a trend effect whereby individuals with BD tended to mislabel "intense" happy facial expressions as neutral.

To date, there have been very few functional connectivity studies in youth at familial risk for BD. Recent work by our group has begun to document differences in patterns of functional connectivity associated with processing and regulation of emotion in youth diagnosed with and at familial risk for BD (Ladouceur et al., 2013; Ladouceur et al., 2011). For instance, eighteen youth diagnosed with BD type I (BD-I); sixteen youth diagnosed with BD Not Otherwise Specified (BD-NOS) (i.e., did not meet full diagnostic criteria, but presented some symptoms of depression and mania); and eighteen healthy control (HC) participants, all between eight and seventeen years old, underwent functional MRI while performing two emotional-face gender labeling tasks (Ladouceur et al., 2011). These tasks involved asking participants to identify the gender of actors depicting happy versus neutral faces and fearful versus neutral faces, respectively. Because of the important role of the ventromedial prefrontal cortex (VMPFC) in implicit emotion regulation and evidence of altered functioning of VMPFC in pediatric BD (Phillips et al., 2008), we focused our analyses on VMPFC connectivity, while processing emotional and neutral faces, and hypothesized reduced VMPFC-amygdala connectivity to emotional faces in both BD-I and BD-NOS youth (vs. HC). Results indicated that youth with BD-I exhibited reduced VMPFC-amygdala functional connectivity to fearful faces, relative to HC and BD-NOS youth. Furthermore, BD-NOS youth showed greater functional connectivity between VMPFC and the dorsal region of the prefrontal cortex (DLPFC) to happy faces, relative to HC and BP-I youth. Given evidence that the DLPFC plays an indirect role in modulating the amygdala through connections via the VMPFC (Phillips et al., 2008; Price, Carmichael, & Drevets, 1996), these patterns of functional connectivity were interpreted as reflecting that BD-NOS may represent an "intermediate" state between being healthy and having BD-I.

In another study, we examined functional connectivity between key neural regions implicated in voluntary attentional control processes in the context of emotional information in fifteen healthy bipolar offspring (eight to seventeen years old) who had at least one parent diagnosed with BD (HBO), and sixteen age-matched HC participants (Ladouceur et al., 2013). Participants performed an emotional working memory task (the Emotional Face N-back task, EFNBACK), which involved performing a visual n-back task[4] while resisting interference from emotionally salient distracters (i.e., fearful, happy, and neutral facial expressions). That is, participants were asked to perform the visual n-back task while ignoring the emotional facial expressions that were presented simultaneously on each side of the letter stimuli. The EFNBACK task was designed to measure functioning of neural systems implicated in voluntary attention control sub-processes (Phillips et al., 2008). Given the role of the ventrolateral prefrontal cortex (VLPFC) in modulating attention in the context of emotional distracters, we focused our analyses on VLPFC connectivity. Results did not yield any significant group differences in behavioral performance (e.g., accuracy rates or reaction times). However, findings suggest that relative to HC, HBO exhibited reduced functional connectivity between the VLPFC and the amygdala while performing the high attentional demand condition of the EFNBACK task in the context of fearful and happy face distracters (vs. no distracters; Figure 10.6 depicts findings with fearful face distracters). There were no group differences in connectivity for the neutral distracters (vs. no distracters). We interpreted these findings as suggesting that alterations in the functioning of frontolimbic systems implicated in voluntary emotion regulation may be present in unaffected offspring with at least one parent diagnosed with BD. Such alterations could be associated with increased risk for future onset of BD or other affective disorders, which are highly prevalent in offspring of parents with BD. However, it will only be possible to address such important developmental questions through the use of follow-up longitudinal studies, which are currently underway. Future studies employing a multimodal neuroimaging approach are needed in order to elucidate how differences in structural and/or functional connectivity contribute to the developmental trajectory of affective disorders such as BD.

---

[4] The n-back task is a continuous performance task that is used to measure an aspect of working memory. The task is often used in neuropsychological and cognitive neuroscience assessments. It consists of visually presenting a pseudorandom sequence of letters and asking participants to respond to a prespecified letter appearing on the computer screen. The "n" represents the number of positions back in the sequence that the target letter appeared. For instance, in a "2-back" condition, participants would press the button to the letter "L" in the sequence L–X–L because "L" appeared two trials back.

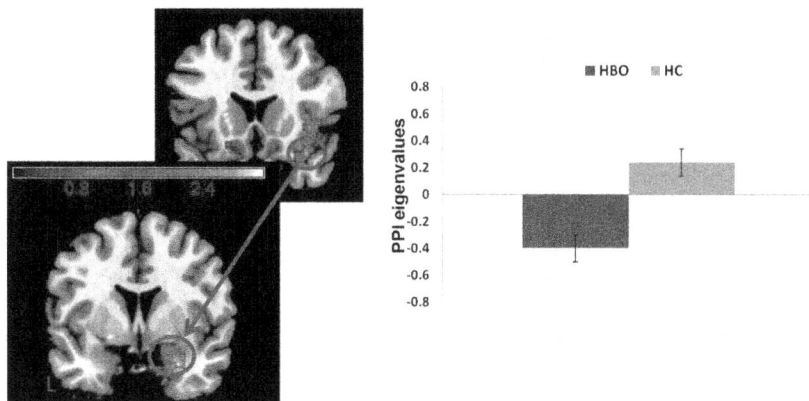

Figure 10.6. PPI results depicting neural connectivity between bilateral ventrolateral prefrontal cortex (VLPFC) and amygdala to fearful face distracters in the 2-back memory condition of the Emotional Face N-back task. Statistical parametric map (SPM-T) displaying a significant between-group contrast. Relative to HC, HBO exhibited significantly reduced positive functional connectivity between right VLPFC seed and right amygdala (MNI x, y, z: 27, 3, -27), T_{29} = 3.19, $p_{corrected}$ < .05, k_E = 46. Histogram on the right displays mean eigenvalues extracted from the peak voxel of the cluster that reached statistical threshold. Color bars ranging from dark blue to yellow represent T statistics. L, left; HBO, Healthy offspring having a parent diagnosed with bipolar disorder (*n* = 16); HC, Healthy control offspring of healthy parents (*n* = 15). Reprinted from *Developmental Cognitive Neuroscience*, 5, Ladouceur, C. D., Diwadkar, V. D., White, R., Bass, J., Birmaher, B., Axelson, D. A., & Phillips, M.L., "Fronto-limbic Function in Unaffected Offspring at Familial Risk for Bipolar Disorder During an Emotional Working Memory Paradigm," p. 191, Copyright (2013), with permission from Elsevier. (See Color Plate.)

Investigation of Structural and Functional Connectivity and Risk for Bipolar Disorder: Important Factors to Consider

Methodological Factors in Developmental Neuroscience

One important challenge to investigating neural markers of risk for BD through the use of neuroimaging methods is the ability to interpret, in a meaningful way, alterations in brain development. For example, changes in white matter FA are thought to reflect changes in anatomical connectivity in particular regions. However, the interpretation of biological mechanisms underlying changes in FA can be challenging. In fact these changes could be explained by a number of factors such as (a) alterations in longitudinally/obliquely-oriented fiber ratios, (b) changes in axonal integrity, (c) changes in tightness of axonal packing, (d) alterations in permeability of myelin sheaths, or (e) abnormalities of one set of fibers in a large group of intersecting fiber pathways (Paus, 2010). Including complementary measures such as radial or longitudinal diffusivity is therefore recommended. Radial diffusivity, for instance, is thought to reflect changes in myelin in white matter, whereas longitudinal diffusivity has been shown to be more sensitive to axonal degeneration (Alexander, Lee, Lazar, & Field, 2007; Hasan & Narayana, 2006; Song et al., 2002). Sophisticated methods of *in vivo* reconstruction of white matter fibers offer an efficient approach to drawing conclusions about structural connectivity in humans (Conturo et al., 1999; Fillard et al., 2011; Mori & Barker, 1999; Mori, Crain, Chacko, & van Zijl, 1999) (for a detailed review on further methodological considerations on DTI, see Fillard et al., 2011; Jones & Cercignani, 2010).

However, several analytical advances are currently under development in the field of MRI. The research field is now shifting from conventional analyses of structural volumes and neural activities to more advanced analyses based on structural-functional integration within specific neural circuitries (Almeida & Phillips, 2012). The combination of different modalities (i.e., structural connectivity, effective connectivity, and resting state connectivity) is now recommended and offers a promising strategy to define the structural connectome and the functional dynamics of healthy human brains, but also those underlying the pathophysiology of major psychiatric disorders, including anxiety and mood disorders.

Issues Associated with the Recruitment of Participants with Psychiatric Disorders

Studies that include patient populations such as adults or youth diagnosed with BD or youth at risk for BD, but exhibiting symptoms of BD or other Axis I disorders are often limited by their sample size. In order to have enough power to detect abnormalities in FA, for instance, studies require sample sizes of at least thirty participants (Wakana et al., 2007). It is therefore difficult to estimate at the neural level the effects of the *heterogeneity of the clinical samples* associated with a primary diagnosis such as BD (e.g., BD type I vs. BD type II, euthymic, depressed, or manic state), or conditions that frequently co-occur with the primary diagnosis (e.g., substance-abuse history, presence of psychosis). Findings from secondary – mainly exploratory – analyses from multiple studies suggest that that these factors may have profound effects on white matter. However, taking a dimensional approach to neuroimaging data analyses and including participants who exhibit mood-related problems could be a way forward in more efficiently elucidating the pathophysiology of mood-related disorders (Frank et al., 2015).

Another important factor to consider when conducting research with clinical samples has to do with effects associated with *medication*. A number of studies have reported data demonstrating the normalizing, rather than confounding, effects of psychotropic medication upon neuroimaging findings in individuals with mood disorders such as BD (Blackhart, Minnix, & Kline, 2006; Haznedar et al., 2005; Henriques & Davidson, 1990; Versace et al., 2008). Therefore, one cannot assume that medication necessarily biases findings in favor of finding group differences. Nevertheless, given the heterogeneity of the various kinds of psychotropic medications used to treat mood disorders and the lack of knowledge regarding their effects on neurodevelopment, one must acknowledge the level of complexity that medications bring to research studies with clinical samples. One avenue that researchers have adopted to avoid these limitations is to focus research studies on healthy youth at familial risk because this kind of sample offers the possibly of identifying potential neurodevelopmental vulnerability markers of the disorder, while eliminating the possible confounding effects on neuroimaging measures of psychopathology and/or psychotropic medication.

Importance of Methodological Designs to Examine Changes in Brain Development

Most research studies aimed at examining brain development and risk for psychiatric disorders have focused on maturational changes associated with age. However, evidence from epidemiological studies of depression suggests that pubertal maturation plays an important role in the development of mood disorders (Angold et al., 1995; Angold et al., 1998). Recently, a number of research studies have documented specific influences of pubertal maturation on the development of white matter (Ladouceur, Peper, & Dahl, 2012; Peper, Pol, Crone, & Van Honk, 2011). For instance, Perrin and colleagues examined the influence of pubertal maturation on white matter volume and magnetization transfer ratio (MTR), which provides information regarding white matter integrity at the macromolecular level and is thought to serve as an indirect proxy of myelination (Perrin et al., 2009). The study involved examining the effects of age, sex, and pubertal maturation and their interaction on measures of white matter density and MTR using a whole-brain approach in a large sample of normally developing adolescents between mid- to late-puberty (n = 408, 204 males, twelve to eighteen years old) (Perrin et al., 2009). Findings indicated that white matter density in frontal, parietal, and temporal lobes increased with pubertal maturation in boys only. MTR, however, was negatively linked to pubertal maturation in parietal and occipital lobes in boys. Also, white-matter density decreased as a function of pubertal maturation in boys in the region of the corticospinal tract. In another study including the same sample of adolescents, Perrin et al. (2008) examined the relationship between white matter density, MTR, and pubertal maturation (Perrin et al., 2008). They also examined the relationship between blood levels of testosterone and white matter volume, and genotyped their participants for a functional polymorphism in the androgen receptor (AR) gene in order to examine the role of the AR in moderating the relationship between testosterone and white matter. Findings from this study revealed a relationship between individual differences in the levels of testosterone and white matter growth in males, but not in females. Furthermore, such a relationship in males appeared to be moderated by the presence of androgen receptors, as this increase in white matter volume in males was greater in those with the shorter versions of the AR gene (i.e., fewer number of CAG-repeats in this gene). Findings from these studies, and others (see Ladouceur et al., 2012, and Peper et al., 2011, for a review), demonstrate associations between hormonal changes with puberty and white matter volume. They also indicate that such associations may be moderated by genetic predispositions.

Because age and puberty are highly correlated in samples of males and females with wide age ranges (e.g., eight to eighteen years of age), it is impossible to determine the specific influence of pubertal maturation without the use of methodological designs aimed at disentangling effects of age versus puberty. One approach is to restrict recruitment to more narrow age ranges (e.g., ten to fourteen years). In addition, it is important to consider the timing of pubertal maturation. Based on epidemiological data on U.S. samples, for instance, adolescent girls reach mid-/late puberty approximately one year earlier than boys (i.e., thirteen to fifteen years old vs. fourteen to sixteen years old for boys) (Karpati, 2002; Wu, Mendola, & Buck, 2002). Thus, it is important that research studies aimed at examining puberty-specific influences on white matter development, for example, recruit samples of males and females within the sex-appropriate age range. The use of such methodological approaches in normative samples of adolescents, as well as those at risk for mood disorders, for instance, will allow researchers to better understand specific contributing factors to alterations in neurodevelopment.

The Richness and Complexities of Models that Incorporate the Influence of Multiple Developmental Factors

Although interpreting data from neuroimaging findings in individuals with psychiatric disorders, at-risk for psychiatric disorders, or those entering sensitive periods of brain development offers a certain level of complexity, it is crucial that the field continues to advance in incorporating factors that may help better predict onset or course of psychiatric illness. Certainly, this area of research will require interdisciplinary work in order to formulate synergistic models able of capturing complex interactions between developmental, environmental, and genetic factors.

A recent study by Whittle et al. (2011) exemplifies nicely the importance of incorporating multiple factors and their interactions in a model of risk for depression. They examined whether individual differences in hippocampal volume (a brain structure implicated in automatic emotion regulation and pathophysiology of depression) might determine sensitivity to environmental context, with respect to vulnerability to the emergence of depressive symptoms during early to mid-adolescence (Whittle et al., 2011). More specifically, they examined the predictive effect of hippocampal volume in adolescents on depressive symptoms as a function of the level of maternal aggressive behavior to which they were exposed. Results from this study showed that girls, not boys, who had larger hippocampal volume were more sensitive to maternal aggressive behavior as it pertains to the future onset of depressive symptoms. Only in these girls did high levels of maternal aggressive behavior appear to increase the risk of depressive symptoms over time, illustrating the complex relationships between brain structure, environmental factors (e.g., parenting style), and sensitivity to (i.e., risk for, and protection from) the emergence of psychiatric disorders such as depression. Although measures of pubertal maturation were not included in this study, the sex differences suggest that changes in sex hormones may be implicated. Such studies can also identify potential windows of opportunity for early intervention by targeting parenting styles for these "vulnerable" girls – who tend to be "more sensitive" to the influence of negative environmental factors. Furthermore, complementary intervention strategies aimed at promoting emotion-regulation skills in these girls could also be particularly beneficial during this developmental period, as these neural structures are undergoing dramatic remodeling and therefore may be more plastic and modifiable by environmental contingencies (Andersen & Teicher, 2008).

Future Directions

There are several ways in which the field of psychiatry can advance with regard to the identification of biomarkers of psychiatric illness such as mood disorders and early markers of risk for these disorders. First, there is a need for research studies to be framed within cognitive and/or affective neuroscience frameworks in order to better delineate specific processes and underlying brain structure and function that may contribute to the neuropathophysiology of the particular disorder. With regard to mood disorders, a growing number of neuroimaging studies have used emotional faces or emotional pictures to investigate neural systems of emotion processing and regulation. Future research is needed to develop more sophisticated methods that would enable researchers to evoke, in a neuroimaging environment, various components of the emotional response, such as action tendencies (e.g., approach, avoidance), physiological correlates, subjective feelings or experiences, and thoughts that accompany feeling (e.g., Immordino-Yang & Singh, 2013; Peake, Dishion, Stormshak, Moore, & Pfeifer, 2013; Saxbe, Yang, Borofsky, & Immordino-Yang, 2012; Silk et al., 2012). The use of such methods would help advance our understanding about the nature of the abnormalities in emotion processing and regulation and underlying neural systems. Furthermore, in order to understand the developmental trajectories toward particular psychiatric disorders such as mood disorders, it will be important to formulate research questions using a developmental framework and to take into account normative neurodevelopmental changes and how such changes may create particular windows of vulnerability (e.g., age versus puberty-specific changes in brain structure and function). Incorporating other relevant factors, such as family and peer interactions, adverse events, and genetics within the realm of longitudinal follow-up studies, will generate more sophisticated predictor models of risk. Such research studies, however, require the collaboration of interdisciplinary research teams and access to large databases.

Moreover, in order to successfully capture alterations in the development of neural systems that support emotion regulation, there is a need to employ multimodal imaging techniques. For instance, by incorporating data from structural, as well as functional, neuroimaging techniques, it would be possible to delineate specific changes in both brain structure (e.g., white matter tracts) and function (e.g., functional connectivity). One promising approach is the use of *tractography-based* studies in youth at high familiar risk for psychiatric disorders. Methodological advances in MRI, including higher-strength magnetic fields, tissue segmentation techniques, and the use of sophisticated algorithms for surface and fiber reconstruction will promote better understanding of white matter (together with gray matter) neurodevelopment and thus allow for a better assessment of alterations in the development of brain circuits underpinning onset and course of mood and other psychiatric disorders and potentially identify biological targets for early interventions.

Conclusion

Our aim in this chapter was to highlight the importance of considering multiple factors when formulating models of the neuropathophysiology of psychiatric disorders such as BD. With regard to understanding the developmental trajectories of BD, framing research questions within developmental cognitive and/or affective neuroscience frameworks will enhance our ability to identify neural markers of risk, as well as potential windows of opportunity for early intervention. This ability will be enhanced further if we build models that incorporate interactions between developmental, social, environmental, and genetic factors. With advances in neuroimaging techniques, it will be possible to test more specific hypotheses about the nature of these interactions, as well as to document with greater specificity the timing of these changes in ways that can inform models of vulnerability and risk for the onset of psychiatric disorders such as BD, as well as models of resilience in the face of adversity. Such endeavors can be achieved only with the collaboration of interdisciplinary research groups dedicated to the study of developmental trajectories of "individual connectomes" and future risk of psychiatric illness.

REFERENCES

Adler, C. M., Adams, J., DelBello, M. P., Holland, S. K., Schmithorst, V., Levine, A., . . . Strakowski, S. M. (2006). Evidence of white matter pathology in bipolar disorder adolescents experiencing their first episode of mania: A diffusion tensor imaging study. *American Journal of Psychiatry, 163*(2), 322–4. http://dx.doi.org/10.1176/appi.ajp.163.2.322

Aggen, S. H., Neale, M. C., & Kendler, K. S. (2005). *DSM* criteria for major depression: Evaluating symptom patterns using latent-trait item response models. *Psychological Medicine, 35*(4), 475–87. http://dx.doi.org/10.1017/S0033291704003563

Alexander, A. L., Lee, J. E., Lazar, M., & Field, A. S. (2007). Diffusion tensor imaging of the brain. *Neurotherapeutics, 4*(3), 316–29. http://dx.doi.org/10.1016/j.nurt.2007.05.011

Almeida, J. R., & Phillips, M. L. (2012). Distinguishing between unipolar depression and bipolar depression: Current and future clinical and neuroimaging perspectives. *Biological Psychiatry, 73*, 111–18. http://dx.doi.org/10.1016/j.biopsych.2012.06.010

American Psychiatric Association. (1994). *Diagnostic and statistical manual of mental disorders* (4th ed.). Washington, DC: Author.

American Psychiatric Association. (2000). *Diagnostic and statistical manual of mental disorders* (4th ed., text rev.). Washington, DC: Author.

American Psychiatric Association. (2013). *Diagnostic and statistical manual of mental disorders* (5th ed.). Washington, DC: Author.

Andersen, S. L., & Teicher, M. H. (2008). Stress, sensitive periods and maturational events in adolescent depression. *Trends in Neurosciences, 31*, 183–91. http://dx.doi.org/10.1016/j.tins.2008.01.004

Angold, A., Costello, E. J., Erkanli, A., & Worthman, C. M. (1995). Pubertal changes in hormone levels and depression in girls. *Psychological Medicine, 29*, 1043–53. http://dx.doi.org/10.1017/S0033291799008946

Angold, A., Costello, E. J., & Worthman, C. M. (1998). Puberty and depression: The roles of age, pubertal status and pubertal timing. *Psychological Medicine, 28*, 51–61. http://dx.doi.org/10.1017/S003329179700593X

Angold, A., & Worthman, C. M. (1993). Puberty onset of gender differences in rates of depression: A developmental, epidemiologic and neuroendocrine perspective. *Journal of Affective Disorders, 29*, 145–58. http://dx.doi.org/10.1016/0165-0327(93)90029-J

Barnea-Goraly, N., Chang, K. D., Karchemskiy, A., Howe, M. E., & Reiss, A. L. (2009). Limbic and corpus callosum aberrations in adolescents with bipolar disorder: A tract-based spatial statistics analysis. *Biological Psychiatry, 66*(3), 238–44. http://dx.doi.org/10.1016/j.biopsych.2009.02.025

Barnea-Goraly, N., Menon, V., Eckert, M., Tamm, L., Bammer, R., Karchemskiy, A., ... Reiss, A. L. (2005). White matter development during childhood and adolescence: A cross-sectional diffusion tensor imaging study. *Cerebral Cortex, 15*, 1848–54. http://dx.doi.org/10.1093/cercor/bhi062

Basser, P. J., & Jones, D. K. (2002). Diffusion-tensor MRI: Theory, experimental design and data analysis: A technical review. *NMR in Biomedicine, 15*, 456–67. http://dx.doi.org/10.1002/nbm.783

Beyer, J. L., Taylor, W. D., MacFall, J. R., Kuchibhatla, M., Payne, M. E., Provenzale, J. M., ... Krishnan, K. R. R. (2005). Cortical white matter microstructural abnormalities in bipolar disorder. *Neuropsychopharmacology, 30*(12), 2225–9. http://dx.doi.org/10.1038/sj.npp.1300802

Biederman, J., Mick, E., Faraone, S. V., Spencer, T., Wilens, T. E., & Wozniak, J. (2003). Current concepts in the validity, diagnosis and treatment of paediatric bipolar disorder. *The International Journal of Neuropsychopharmacology, 6*(3), 293–300. http://dx.doi.org/10.1017/S1461145703003547

Birmaher, B., Axelson, D., Monk, K., Kalas, C., Goldstein, B., Hickey, M. B., ... Brent, D. (2009). Lifetime psychiatric disorders in school-aged offspring of parents with bipolar disorder: The Pittsburgh Bipolar Offspring

study. *Archives of General Psychiatry, 66*(3), 287–96. http://dx.doi.org/
10.1001/archgenpsychiatry.2008.546

Birmaher, B., Axelson, D. A., Strober, M., Gill, M. K., Valeri, S., Chiapetta, L., ... Keller, M.(2006). Clinical course of children and adolescents with bipolar spectrum disorders. *Archives of General Psychiatry, 63*, 175–83. http://dx.doi.org/10.1001/archpsyc.63.2.175

Blackhart, G. C., Minnix, J. A., & Kline, J. P. (2006). Can EEG asymmetry patterns predict future development of anxiety and depression? A preliminary study. *Biological Psychology, 72*(1), 46–50. http://dx.doi.org/
10.1016/j.biopsycho.2005.06.010

Breiter, H. C., Etcoff, N. L., Whalen, P. J., Kennedy, W. A., Rauch, S. L., Buckner, R. L., ... Rosen, B. R. (1996). Response and habituation of the human amygdala during visual processing of facial expression. *Neuron, 17*, 875–87. http://dx.doi.org/10.1016/S0896-6273(00)80219-6

Bruno, S., Cercignani, M., & Ron, M. A. (2008). White matter abnormalities in bipolar disorder: A voxel-based diffusion tensor imaging study. *Bipolar Disorders, 10*(4), 460–8. http://dx.doi.org/10.1111/j.1399-
5618.2007.00552.x

Bunge, S. A., Dudukovic, N. M., Thomason, M. E., Vaidya, C. J., & Gabrieli, J. D. E. (2002). Immature frontal lobe contributions to cognitive control in children: Evidence from fMRI. *Neuron, 33*, 301–11. http://dx.doi.org/
10.1016/S0896-6273(01)00583-9

Casey, B. J., Duhoux, S., & Cohen, M. M. (2010). Adolescence: What do transmission, transition, and translation have to do with it? *Neuron, 67*, 749–60. http://dx.doi.org/10.1016/j.neuron.2010.08.033

Casey, B. J., Jones, R. M., & Somerville, L. H. (2011). Braking and accelerating of the adolescent brain. *Journal of Research on Adolescence, 21*, 21–33. http://dx.doi.org/10.1111/j.1532-7795.2010.00712.x

Catani, M., Jones, D. K., Donato, R., & Ffytche, D. H. (2003). Occipito-temporal connections in the human brain. *Brain, 126*(Pt. 9), 2093–2107. http://dx.doi.org/10.1093/brain/awg203

Chaddock, C. A., Barker, G. J., Marshall, N., Schulze, K., Hall, M. H., Fern, A., ... McDonald, C. (2009). White matter microstructural impairments and genetic liability to familial bipolar I disorder. *British Journal of Psychiatry, 194*, 527–34. http://dx.doi.org/10.1192/bjp.
bp.107.047498

Cole, P. M., Michel, M. K., & O'Donnell Teti, L. (1994). The development of emotion regulation and dysregulation: A clinical perspective. In *Monographs of the Society for Research in Child Development 59* (pp. 73–102). http://dx.doi.
org/10.2307/1166139

Conturo, T. E., Lori, N. F., Cull, T. S., Akbudak, E., Snyder, A. Z., Shimony, J. S., ... Raichle, M. E. (1999). Tracking neuronal fiber pathways in the living human brain. *Proceedings of the National Academy of Sciences of the United States of America, 96*(18), 10422–7. http://dx.doi.org/10.1073/
pnas.96.18.10422

Costello, E., Angold, A., Burns, B., Erkanli, A., Stangl, D., & Tweed, D. (1996). The Great Smoky Mountains Study of Youth: Functional impairment and serious emotional disturbance. *Archives of General*

Psychiatry, 53, 1137–43. http://dx.doi.org/10.1001/
archpsyc.1996.01830120077013

Dahl, R. E. (2001). Affect regulation, brain development, and behavioral/
emotional health in adolescence. *CNS Spectrums, 6*(1), 60–72.

Dahl, R. E., & Spear, L. (2004). Adolescent brain development: A period of
vulnerabilities and opportunities. *Annals of the New York Academy of Sciences,
1021,* 1–22. http://dx.doi.org/10.1196/annals.1308.001

DelBello, M. P., & Geller, B. (2001). Review of studies of child and adolescent
offspring of bipolar parents. *Bipolar Disorders, 3*(6), 325–34. http://dx.doi.
org/10.1034/j.1399-5618.2001.30607.x

Dickstein, D. P., & Leibenluft, E. (2012). Beyond dogma: From diagnostic
controversies to data about pediatric bipolar disorder and children with
chronic irritability and mood dysregulation. *Israel Journal of Psychiatry and
Related Sciences, 49,* 52–61.

Dorn, L. D., Dahl, R. E., Woodward, H. R., & Biro, F. (2006). Defining
boundaries of early adolescence: A user's guide to assessing pubertal status
and pubertal timing in research with adolescents. *Applied Developmental
Science, 10,* 30–56. http://dx.doi.org/10.1207/s1532480xads1001_3

Ernst, M., Pine, D. S., & Hardin, M. (2006). Triadic model of the neurobiology
of motivated behavior in adolescence. *Psychological Medicine, 36,* 299–312.
http://dx.doi.org/10.1017/S0033291705005891

Fillard, P., Descoteaux, M., Goh, A., Gouttard, S., Jeurissen, B., Malcolm, J., . . .
Poupon, C. (2011). Quantitative evaluation of 10 tractography algorithms
on a realistic diffusion MR phantom. *Neuroimage, 56*(1), 220–34. http://dx.
doi.org/10.1016/j.neuroimage.2011.01.032

Force, U. (1996). *Guide to clinical preventive services* (2nd ed.). Alexandria, VA:
International Medical Publishing.

Frank, E., Nimgoankar, V.L., Phillips, M.L., & Kupfer, D.J. (2015). All the
world's a (clinical) stage: Rethinking bipolar disorder from a longitudinal
perspective. *Molecular Psychiatry, 20,* 23–31. http://dx.doi.org/10.1038/
mp.2014.71

Frazier, J. A., Breeze, J. L., Papadimitriou, G., Kennedy, D. N., Hodge, S. M.,
Moore, C. M., . . . Makris, N. (2007). White matter abnormalities in
children with and at risk for bipolar disorder. *Bipolar Disorders, 9*(8),
799–809. http://dx.doi.org/10.1111/j.1399-5618.2007.00482.x

Friston, K. (2002). Beyond phrenology: What can neuroimaging tell us about
distributed circuitry? *Annual Review of Neuroscience, 25,* 221–50. http://dx.
doi.org/10.1111/j.1399-5618.2007.00482.x

Gazzaniga, M. S. (2000). Cerebral specialization and interhemispheric
communication: Does the corpus callosum enable the human condition.
Brain, 123, 1293–1326. http://dx.doi.org/10.1093/brain/123.7.1293

Geller, B., Craney, J., Bolhofner, K., Nickelsburg, M., Williams, M., &
Zimerman, B. (2002). Two-year prospective follow-up of children with a
prepubertal and early adolescent bipolar disorder phenotype. *American
Journal of Psychiatry, 159*(6), 927–33. http://dx.doi.org/10.1176/appi.
ajp.159.6.927

Giedd, J. N., Blumenthal, J., Jeffries, N. O., Castellanos, F. X., Liu, H.,
Zijdenbos, A., . . . Rapoport, J. L. (1999). Brain development during

childhood and adolescence: A longitudinal MRI study. *Nature Neuroscience*, *2*(10), 861–3. http://dx.doi.org/10.1038/13158

Giorgio, A., Watkins, K. E., Douaud, G., Behrens, T. E., Matthews, P. M., James, A. C., ... Johansen-Berg, H. (2007). Developmental changes in white matter microstructure in adolescence. *Journal of Neurology, Neurosurgery and Psychiatry*, *78*, 1019–20.

Goodwin, F. K., & Jamison, K. R. (2007). *Manic-depressive illness: Bipolar disorders and recurrent depression* (2nd ed.). New York, NY: Oxford University Press.

Gross, J. J., & Thompson, R. A. (2007). Emotion regulation: Conceptual foundations. In J. J. Gross (Ed.), *Handbook of emotion regulation* (pp. 3–24). New York: Guilford Press.

Guyer, A. E., Monk, C. S., McClure, E. B., Nelson, E. E., Roberson-Nay, R., Adler, A. D., ... Ernst, M. (2008). A developmental examination of amygdala response to facial expressions. *Journal of Cognitive Neuroscience*, *20*, 1565–82. http://dx.doi.org/10.1162/jocn.2008.20114

Hagmann, P. (2005). *From diffusion MRI to brain connectomics*. Doctoral dissertation, Ecole Polytechnique Fédérale de Lausanne (EPFL), Switzerland.

Hajek, T., Carrey, N., & Alda, M. (2005). Neuroanatomical abnormalities as risk factors for bipolar disorder. *Bipolar Disorders*, *7*(5), 393–403. http://dx.doi.org/10.1111/j.1399-5618.2005.00238.x

Hare, T. A., Tottenham, N., Galvan, A., Voss, H. U., Glover, G. H., & Casey, B. J. (2008). Biological substrates of emotional reactivity and regulation in adolescence during an emotional Go-Nogo task. *Biological Psychiatry*, *63*, 927–34. http://dx.doi.org/10.1016/j.biopsych.2008.03.015

Hariri, A. R., Mattay, V. S., Tessitore, A., Fera, F., & Weinberger, D. R. (2003). Neocortical modulation of the amygdala response to fearful stimuli. *Biological Psychiatry*, *53*, 494–501. http://dx.doi.org/10.1016/S0006-3223(02)01786-9

Hariri, A. R., Tessitore, A., Mattay, V. S., Fera, F., & Weinberger, D. R. (2002). The amygdala response to emotional stimuli: A comparison of faces and scenes. *Neuroimage*, *17*, 317–23. http://dx.doi.org/10.1006/nimg.2002.1179

Harrison, P. J. (2002). The neuropathology of primary mood disorder. *Brain*, *125*, 1428–49. http://dx.doi.org/10.1093/brain/awf149

Hasan, K. M. (2006). Diffusion tensor eigenvalues or both mean diffusivity and fractional anisotropy are required in quantitative clinical diffusion tensor MR reports: Fractional anisotropy alone is not sufficient. *Radiology*, *239*, 611–12. http://dx.doi.org/10.1148/radiol.2392051172

Hasan, K. M., & Narayana, P. A. (2006). Retrospective measurement of the diffusion tensor eigenvalues from diffusion anisotropy and mean diffusivity in DTI. *Magnetic Resonance Medicine*, *56*(1), 130–7. http://dx.doi.org/10.1002/mrm.20935

Haznedar, M. M., Roversi, F., Pallanti, S., Baldini-Rossi, N., Schnur, D. B., LiCalzi, E. M., ... Buchsbaum, M. S. (2005). Fronto-thalamo-striatal gray and white matter volumes and anisotropy of their connections in bipolar spectrum illnesses. *Biological Psychiatry*, *57*(7), 733–42. http://dx.doi.org/10.1016/j.biopsych.2005.01.002

Heng, S., Song, A. W., & Sim, K. (2010). White matter abnormalities in bipolar disorder: Insights from diffusion tensor imaging studies. *Journal of Neural Transmission, 117*(5), 639–54. http://dx.doi.org/10.1007/s00702-010-0368-9

Henriques, J. B., & Davidson, R. J. (1990). Regional brain electrical asymmetries discriminate between previously depressed and healthy control subjects. *Journal of Abnormal Psychology, 99*(1), 22–31. http://dx.doi.org/10.1037/0021-843X.99.1.22

Houenou, J., Wessa, M., Douaud, G., Leboyer, M., Chanraud, S., Perrin, M., . . . Paillere-Martinot, M. L. (2007). Increased white matter connectivity in euthymic bipolar patients: Diffusion tensor tractography between the subgenual cingulate and the amygdalo-hippocampal complex. *Molecular Psychiatry, 12*(11), 1001–10. http://dx.doi.org/10.1038/sj.mp.4002010

Immordino-Yang, M. H., & Singh, V. (2013). Hippocampal contributions to the processing of social emotions. *Human Brain Mapping, 34*(4), 945–55. http://dx.doi.org/10.1002/hbm.21485

Jones, D. K., & Cercignani, M. (2010). Twenty-five pitfalls in the analysis of diffusion MRI data. *NMR in Biomedicine, 23*, 803–20. http://dx.doi.org/10.1002/nbm.1543

Kafantaris, V., Kingsley, P., Ardekant, B., Saito, E., Lencz, T., Lim, K., & Szeszko, P. (2009). Lower orbital frontal white matter integrity in adolescents with bipolar I disorder. *Journal of the American Academy of Child and Adolescent Psychiatry, 48*(1), 79–86. http://dx.doi.org/10.1097/CHI.0b013e3181900421

Karpati, A. (2002). Stature and pubertal stage assessment in American boys: The 1988–1994 third national health and nutrition examination survey. *Journal of Adolescent Health, 30*, 205–12. http://dx.doi.org/10.1016/S1054-139X(01)00320-2

Kaufman, J., Birmaher, B., Brent, D., Rao, U., Flynn, C., Moreci, P., . . . Ryan, N. D. (1997). Schedule for Affective Disorders and Schizophrenia for School-Age Children-Present and Lifetime Version (K-SADS-PL): Initial reliability and validity data. *Journal of the American Academy of Child & Adolescent Psychiatry, 36*, 980–8. http://dx.doi.org/10.1097/00004583-199707000-00021

Kessler, R. C. (2011). National Comorbidity Survey: Adolescent Supplement (NCS-A), 2001–2004. ICPSR28581-v4. Ann Arbor, MI: Inter-university Consortium for Political and Social Research [distributor].

Killgore, W. D. S., Oki, M., & Yurgelun-Todd, D. A. (2001). Sex-specific developmental changes in amygdala responses to affective faces. *Neuroreport, 12*(2), 427–33. http://dx.doi.org/10.1097/00001756-200102120-00047

Kupfer, D. J., & Regier, D. A. (2011). Neuroscience, clinical evidence, and the future of psychiatric classification in *DSM-5. American Journal of Psychiatry, 168*, 172–4. http://dx.doi.org/10.1176/appi.ajp.2011.11020219

Ladouceur, C. D. (2012). Neural systems supporting cognitive affective interactions in adolescence: The role of puberty and implications for affective disorders. *Frontiers in Integrative Neuroscience, 6*, 65. http://dx.doi.org/10.3389/fnint.2012.00065

Ladouceur, C. D., Diwadkar, V. A., White, R., Bass, J., Birmaher, B., Axelson, D. A., & Phillips, M. L. (2013). Fronto-limbic function in unaffected offspring at familial risk for bipolar disorder during an emotional working memory paradigm. *Developmental Cognitive Neuroscience, 5*, 185–96. http://dx.doi.org/ 10.1016/j.dcn.2013.03.004

Ladouceur, C. D., Farchione, T., Diwadkar, V., Pruitt, P., Radwan, J., Axelson, D. A., ... Phillips, M. L. (2011). Differential patterns of abnormal activity and functional connectivity in amygdala-prefrontal circuitry in bipolar and bipolar-NOS youth. *Journal of the American Academy of Child and Adolescent Psychiatry, 50*(12), 1275–89. http://dx.doi.org/10.1016/j. jaac.2011.09.023

Ladouceur, C. D., Peper, J. S., & Dahl, R. E. (2012). White matter development in adolescence: The influence of puberty and implications for affective disorders. *Developmental Cognitive Neuroscience, 2*(1), 34–56. http://dx.doi. org/10.1016/j.dcn.2011.06.002

Lebel, C., Walker, L., Leemans, A., Phillips, L., & Beaulieu, C. (2008). Microstructural maturation of the human brain from childhood to adulthood. *Neuroimage, 40*(3), 1044–55. http://dx.doi.org/10.1016/j. neuroimage.2007.12.053

Leibenluft, E., Charney, D., & Pine, D. S. (2003). Researching the pathophysiology of pediatric bipolar disorder. *Biological Psychiatry, 53*, 1009–20. http://dx.doi.org/10.1016/S0006-3223(03)00069-6

Luna, B., Garver, K., Urban, T., Lazar, N., & Sweeney, J. (2004). Maturation of cognitive processes from late childhood to adulthood. *Child Development, 75*, 1357–72. http://dx.doi.org/10.1111/j.1467-8624.2004.00745.x

Luna, B., Padmanabhan, A., & O'Hearn, K. M. (2011). What has fMRI told us about the development of cognitive control through adolescence? *Brain and Cognition, 72*, 101–13. http://dx.doi.org/10.1016/j. bandc.2009.08.005

Macritchie, K. A. N., Lloyd, A. J., Bastin, M. E., Vasudev, K., Gallagher, P., Eyre, R., ... Young, A. H. (2010). White matter microstructural abnormalities in euthymic bipolar disorder. *British Journal of Psychiatry, 196*(1), 52–8. http://dx.doi.org/10.1192/bjp.bp.108.058586

Mahon, K., Burdick, K. E., & Szeszko, P. R. (2010). A role for white matter abnormalities in the pathophysiology of bipolar disorder. *Neuroscience and Biobehavioral Reviews, 34*(4), 533–54. http://dx.doi.org/10.1016/j. neubiorev.2009.10.012

Mahon, K., Wu, J., Malhotra, A. K., Burdick, K. E., Derosse, P., Ardekani, B. A., & Szeszko, P. R. (2009). A voxel-based diffusion tensor imaging study of white matter in bipolar disorder. *Neuropsychopharmacology, 34*, 1590–1600. http://dx.doi.org/10.1038/npp.2008.216

Makris, N., Kennedy, D. N., McInerney, S., Sorensen, A. G., Wang, R., Caviness, J., V. S., & Pandya, D. N. (2005). Segmentation of subcomponents within the superior longitudinal fascicle in humans: A quantitative, in vivo, DT-MRI study. *Cerebral Cortex, 15*, 854–69. http://dx.doi.org/10.1093/cercor/bhh186

Matthews, A., & MacLeod, C. (2002). Induced processing biases have causal effects on anxiety. *Cognition and Emotion, 16*(3), 331–54. http://dx.doi.org/ 10.1080/02699930143000518

McIntosh, A. M., Maniega, S. M., Lymer, G. K. S., McKirdy, J., Hall, J., Sussmann, J. E. D., ... Lawrie, S. M. (2008). White matter tractography in bipolar disorder and schizophrenia. *Biological Psychiatry, 64*(12), 1088–92. http://dx.doi.org/10.1016/j.biopsych.2008.07.026

Merikangas, K. R., Akiskal, H., Angst, J., Greenberg, P. E., Hirschfeld, R. M., Petukhova, M., & Kessler, R. C. (2007). Lifetime and 12-month prevalence of bipolar spectrum disorder in the National Comorbidity Survey replication. *Archives of General Psychiatry, 64*, 543–52. http://dx.doi.org/ 10.1001/archpsyc.64.5.543

Merikangas, K. R., Jin, R., He, J. P., Kessler, R. C., Lee, S., Sampson, N. A., . . . Zarkov, Z. (2011). Prevalence and correlates of bipolar spectrum disorder in the world mental health survey initiative. *Archives of General Psychiatry, 68*(3), 241–51. http://dx.doi.org/10.1001/archgenpsychiatry.2011.12

Monk, C. S., McClure, E. B., Nelson, E. E., Zarahn, E., Bilder, R. M., Leibenluft, E., . . . Pine, D. S. (2003). Adolescent immaturity in attention-related brain engagement to emotional facial expressions. *Neuroimage, 20*, 420–8. http://dx.doi.org/10.1016/S1053-8119(03)00355-0

Mori, S., & Barker, P. B. (1999). Diffusion magnetic resonance imaging: Its principle and applications. *The Anatomical Record, 15*, 102–9.

Mori, S., Crain, B. J., Chacko, V. P., & van Zijl, P. C. (1999). Three-dimensional tracking of axonal projections in the brain by magnetic resonance imaging. *Annals of Neurology, 45*, 265–9.

Morris, J. S., Friston, K. J., Buchel, C., Frith, C. D., Young, A. W., Calder, A. J., & Dolan, R. J. (1998). A neuromodulatory role for the human amygdala in processing emotional facial expressions. *Brain, 121*(Pt. 1), 47–57. http://dx. doi.org/10.1093/brain/121.1.47

Ozer, E. M., Macdonald, T., & Irwin, C. E., Jr. (2002). Adolescent health care in the United States: Implications and projections for the new millennium. In J. T. Mortimer & R. W. Larson (Eds.), *The changing adolescent experience: Societal trends and the transition to adulthood* (pp. 129–74). New York, NY: Cambridge University Press. http://dx.doi.org/10.1017/ CBO9780511613913.006

Paus, T. (2005). Mapping brain maturation and cognitive development during adolescence. *Trends in Cognitive Sciences, 9*(2), 60–8. http://dx.doi.org/ 10.1016/j.tics.2004.12.008

Paus, T. (2010). Growth of white matter in the adolescent brain: Myelin or axon? *Brain and Cognition, 72*, 26–35. http://dx.doi.org/10.1016/j. bandc.2009.06.002

Peake, S. J., Dishion, T. J., Stormshak, E. A., Moore, W. E., & Pfeifer, J. H. (2013). Risk-taking and social exclusion in adolescence: Neural mechanisms underlying peer influences on decision-making. *Neuroimage, 15*, 23–34. http://dx.doi.org/10.1016/j.neuroimage.2013.05.061

Peper, J. S., Pol, H. E. H., Crone, E. A., & Van Honk, J. (2011). Sex steroids and brain structure in pubertal boys and girls: A mini-review of neuroimaging studies. *Neuroscience, 191*, 28–37. http://dx.doi.org/10.1016/j. neuroscience.2011.02.014

Perlis, R., Miyahara, S., Marangell, L. B., Wisniewski, S. R., Ostacher, M., Bowden, C. L., . . . Nierenberg, A. A. (2004). Long-term implications of early onset in bipolar disorder: Data from the first 1000 participants in the systematic treatment enhancement program for bipolar disorder

(STEP-BD). *Biological Psychiatry, 55,* 875–81. http://dx.doi.org/10.1016/j. biopsych.2004.01.022

Perrin, J. S., Herve, P. Y., Leonard, G., Perron, M., Pike, G. B., Pitiot, A., ... Paus, T. (2008). Growth of white matter in the adolescent brain: Role of testosterone and androgen receptor. *Journal of Neuroscience, 28*(38), 9519–24. http://dx.doi.org/10.1523/JNEUROSCI.1212-08.2008

Perrin, J. S., Leonard, G., Perron, M., Pike, G. B., Pitiot, A., Richer, L., ... Paus, T. (2009). Sex differences in the growth of white matter during adolescence. *Neuroimage, 45,* 1055–66. http://dx.doi.org/10.1016/j. neuroimage.2009.01.023

Pfefferbaum, A., Mathalon, D. H., Sullivan, E. V., Rawles, J. M., Zipursky, R. B., & Lim, K. O. (1994). A quantitative magnetic resonance imaging study of changes in brain morphology from infancy to late adulthood. *Archives of Neurology, 51,* 874–87. http://dx.doi.org/10.1001/ archneur.1994.00540210046012

Phillips, M. L. (2003). Understanding the neurobiology of emotion perception: Implications for psychiatry. *British Journal of Psychiatry, 182,* 190–2. http://dx.doi.org/10.1192/bjp.182.3.190

Phillips, M. L., Ladouceur, C. D., & Drevets, W. C. (2008). A neural model of voluntary and automatic emotion regulation: Implications for understanding the pathophysiology and neurodevelopment of bipolar disorder. *Molecular Psychiatry, 13*(9), 833–57. http://dx.doi.org/10.1038/mp.2008.65

Phillips, M. L., & Vieta, E. (2007). Identifying functional neuroimaging biomarkers of bipolar disorder: Toward *DSM-V. Schizophrenia Bulletin, 33,* 893–904. http://dx.doi.org/10.1093/schbul/sbm060

Phillips, M. L., Young, A. W., Senior, C., Brammer, M., Andrew, C., Calder, A. J., ... David, A. S. (1997). A specific neural substrate for perceiving facial expressions of disgust. *Nature, 389*(6650), 495–8. http://dx.doi.org/ 10.1038/39051

Pine, D. S., Cohen, P., Gurley, D., Brook, J., & Ma, Y. (1998). The risk for early-adulthood anxiety and depressive disorders in adolescents with anxiety and depressive disorders. *Archives of General Psychiatry, 55,* 56–64. http://dx. doi.org/10.1001/archpsyc.55.1.56

Post, R. M., Luckenbaugh, D. A., Leverich, G. S., Altshuler, L. L., Frye, M. A., Suppes, T., ... Walden, J. (2008). Incidence of childhood-onset bipolar illness in the USA and Europe. *British Journal of Psychiatry, 192,* 150 1. http://dx.doi.org/10.1192/bjp.bp.107.037820

Price, J., Carmichael, S., & Drevets, W. (1996). Networks related to the orbital and medial prefrontal cortex: A substrate for emotional behavior? In G. Holstege, R. Bandler, & C. B. Saper (Eds.), *Progress in Brain Research* (Vol. 107; pp. 523–36). Amsterdam: Elsevier Science B.V.

Rajkowska, G. (2002). Cell pathology in bipolar disorder. *Bipolar Disorders, 4*(2), 105–16. http://dx.doi.org/10.1034/j.1399-5618.2002.01149.x

Regier, D. A., Narrow, W. E., Kuhl, E. A., & Kupfer, D. J. (2009). Conceptual development of *DSM-V. American Journal of Psychiatry, 166,* 645–50. http://dx.doi.org/10.1176/appi.ajp.2009.09020279

Saxbe, D. E., Yang, X. F., Borofsky, L. A., & Immordino-Yang, M. H. (2012). The embodiment of emotion: Language use during the feeling of social emotions predicts cortical somatosensory activity. *Social Cognitive and Affective Neuroscience, 8*(7), 806–12. http://dx.doi.org/10.1093/scan/nss075

Schmithorst, V. J., & Yuan, W. (2010). White matter development during adolescence as shown by diffusion MRI. *Brain and Cognition, 72,* 16–25. http://dx.doi.org/10.1016/j.bandc.2009.06.005

Seemuller, F., Riedel, M., Dargel, S., Djaja, N., Schennach-Wolff, R., Dittmann, S., … Severus, E. (2010). [Bipolar depression. Spectrum of clinical pictures and differentiation from unipolar depression]. *Nervenarzt, 81*(5), 531–8. http://dx.doi.org/10.1007/s00115-009-2850-x

Silk, J. S., Stroud, L. R., Siegle, G. J., Dahl, R. E., Lee, K. H., & Nelson, E. E. (2012). Peer acceptance and rejection through the eyes of youth: Pupillary, eyetracking and ecological data from the Chatroom Interact Task. *Social Cognitive and Affective Neuroscience, 7*(1), 93–105. http://dx.doi.org/10.1093/scan/nsr044

Song, S. K., Sun, S. W., Ramsbottom, M. J., Chang, C., Russell, J., & Cross, A. H. (2002). Dysmyelination revealed through MRI as increased radial (but unchanged axial) diffusion of water. *Neuroimage, 17*(3), 1429–36. http://dx.doi.org/10.1006/nimg.2002.1267

Sowell, E. R., Petersen, B. S., Thompson, P. M., Welcome, S. E., Henkenius, A. L., & Toga, A. W. (2003). Mapping cortical change across the human life span. *Nature Neuroscience, 6,* 309–15. http://dx.doi.org/10.1038/nn1008

Spear, L. P. (2011). Rewards, aversions and affect in adolescence: Emerging convergences across laboratory animal and human data. *Developmental Cognitive Neuroscience, 1,* 390–403. http://dx.doi.org/10.1016/j.dcn.2011.08.001

Sporns, O., Tononi, G., & Kötter, R. (2005). The human connectome: A structural description of the human brain. *PLoS Computational Biology, 1,* 245–51. http://dx.doi.org/10.1371/journal.pcbi.0010042

Steinberg, L. (2005). Cognitive and affective development in adolescence. *Trends in Cognitive Sciences, 9*(2), 69–74. http://dx.doi.org/10.1016/j.tics.2004.12.005

Steinberg, L. (2007). Risk-taking in adolescence: New perspectives from brain and behavioral science. *Current Directions in Psychological Science, 16,* 55–9. http://dx.doi.org/10.1111/j.1467-8721.2007.00475.x

Surguladze, S. A., Brammer, M. J., Young, A. W., Andrew, C., Travis, M. J., Williams, S. C. R., & Phillips, M. L. (2003). A preferential increase in the extrastriate response to signals of danger. *Neuroimage, 19*(4), 1317–28. http://dx.doi.org/10.1016/S1053-8119(03)00085-5

Sussmann, J. E., Lymer, G. K. S., McKirdy, J., Moorhead, T. W. J., Maniega, S. M., Job, D., … McIntosh, A. M. (2009). White matter abnormalities in bipolar disorder and schizophrenia detected using diffusion tensor magnetic resonance imaging. *Bipolar Disorders, 11*(1), 11–18. http://dx.doi.org/10.1111/j.1399-5618.2008.00646.x

Thapar, A., Collishaw, S., Pine, D. S., & Thapar, A. K. (2012). Depression in adolescence. *Lancet, 379*(9820), 1056–67. http://dx.doi.org/10.1016/S0140-6736(11)60871-4

Thompson, R. A. (1994). Emotion regulation: A theme in search of definition. In N. A. Fox (Ed.), *The development of emotion regulation:*

Biological and behavioral considerations (Vol. 59; Nos. 2–3). Monographs of the Society for Research in Child Development (pp. 25–52).

Tost, H., & Meyer-Lindenberg, A. (2010). I fear for you: A role for serotonin in moral behavior. *Proceedings of the National Academy of Sciences of the United States of America, 107*(40), 17071–2. http://dx.doi.org/10.1073/pnas.1012545107

Tsai, S., Lee, J., & CC, C. (1999). Genetics of bipolar disorder. *Journal of Affective Disorders, 52*, 145–52. http://dx.doi.org/10.1016/S0165-0327(98)00066-4

Tsuang, M., & Faraone, S. (1990). *The genetics of mood disorders.* Baltimore, MD: John Hopkins University Press.

Van der Gucht, E., Morriss, R., Lancaster, G., Kinderman, P., & Bentall, R. P. (2009). Psychological processes in bipolar affective disorder: Negative cognitive style and reward processing. *British Journal of Psychiatry, 194*, 146–51. http://dx.doi.org/10.1192/bjp.bp.107.047894

Vederine, F.-E., Wessa, M., Leboyer, M., & Houenou, J. (2011). A meta-analysis of whole-brain diffusion tensor imaging studies in bipolar disorder. *Progress in Neuro-Psychopharmacology and Biological Psychiatry, 35*(8), 1820–6. http://dx.doi.org/10.1016/j.pnpbp.2011.05.009

Versace, A., Acuff, H., Bertocci, M. A., Bebko, G., Almeida, J. R. C., Perlman, S. B., ... Phillips, M.L. (2015). White matter structure in youth with behavioral and emotional dysregulation disorders: A probabilistic tractographic study. *JAMA Psychiatry, 72*(4), 367–76. http://dx.doi.org/10.1001/jamapsychiatry.2014.2170

Versace, A., Almeida, J. R., Hassel, S., Walsh, N. D., Novelli, M., Klein, C. R., ... Phillips, M. L. (2008). Elevated left and reduced right orbitomedial prefrontal fractional anisotropy in adults with bipolar disorder revealed by tract-based spatial statistics. *Archives of General Psychiatry, 65*(9), 1041–52. http://dx.doi.org/10.1001/archpsyc.65.9.1041

Versace, A., Almeida, J. R., Quevedo, K., Thompson, W. K., Terwilliger, R. A., Hassel, S., ... Phillips, M. L. (2010). Right orbitofrontal corticolimbic and left corticocortical white matter connectivity differentiate bipolar and unipolar depression. *Biological Psychiatry, 68*(6), 560–7. http://dx.doi.org/10.1016/j.biopsych.2010.04.036

Versace, A., Ladouceur, C. D., Romero, S., Birmaher, B., Axelson, D. A., Kupfer, D. J., & Phillips, M. L. (2010). Altered development of white matter in youth at high familial risk for bipolar disorder: A diffusion tensor imaging study. *Journal of the American Academy of Child and Adolescent Psychiatry, 49*, 1249–59.

Versace, A., Thompson, W. K., Zhou, D., Almeida, J. R. C., Hassel, S., Klein, C. R., ... Phillips, M.L. (2010). Abnormal left and right amygdala-orbitofrontal cortical functional connectivity to emotional faces: State versus trait vulnerability markers of depression in bipolar disorder. *Biological Psychiatry, 67*(5), 422–31. http://dx.doi.org/10.1016/j.biopsych.2009.11.025

Wahlstrom, D., White, T., & Luciana, M. (2010). Neurobehavioral evidence for changes in dopamine system activity during adolescence. *Neuroscience and Biobehavioral Reviews, 34*, 631–48. http://dx.doi.org/10.1016/j.neubiorev.2009.12.007

Wakana, S., Caprihan, A., Panzenboeck, M. M., Fallon, J. H., Perry, M., Gollub, R., ... Mori, S. (2007). Reproducibility of quantitative tractography methods applied to cerebral white matter. *Neuroimage, 36*(3), 630–44. http://dx.doi.org/10.1016/j.neuroimage.2007.02.049

Wang, F., Kalmar, J. H., He, Y., Jackowski, M., Chepenik, L. G., Edmiston, E. E., ... Blumberg, H. P. (2009). Functional and structural connectivity between the perigenual anterior cingulate and amygdala in bipolar disorder. *Biological Psychiatry, 66*(5), 516–21. http://dx.doi.org/10.1016/j.biopsych.2009.03.023

Wessa, M., Houenou, J., Leboyer, M., Chanraud, S., Poupon, C., Martinot, J. L., & Paillere-Martinot, M. L. (2009). Microstructural white matter changes in euthymic bipolar patients: A whole-brain diffusion tensor imaging study. *Bipolar Disorders, 11*(5), 504–14. http://dx.doi.org/10.1111/j.1399-5618.2009.00718.x

Whittle, S., Yap, M. B. H., Sheeber, L., Dudgeon, P., Yücel, M., Pantelis, C., ... Allen, N. B. (2011). Hippocampal volume and sensitivity to maternal aggressive behavior: A prospective study of adolescent depressive symptoms. *Development and Psychopathology, 23*, 115–29. http://dx.doi.org/10.1017/S0954579410000684

World Health Organization. (2001). *World health report 2001 – Mental health: New understanding, new hope.* Retrieved from www.who.int/whr/2001/en/

Wu, T., Mendola, P., & Buck, G. (2002). Ethnic differences in the presence of secondary sex characteristics and menarche among US girls: The third national health and nutrition examination survey, 1988–1994. *Pediatrics, 110*, 752–7. http://dx.doi.org/10.1542/peds.110.4.752

Yurgelun-Todd, D. A., Silveri, M. M., Gruber, S. A., Rohan, M. L., & Pimentel, P. J. (2007). White matter abnormalities observed in bipolar disorder: A diffusion tensor imaging study. *Bipolar Disorders, 9*(5), 504–12. http://dx.doi.org/10.1111/j.1399-5618.2007.00395.x

Zanetti, M. V., Jackowski, M. P., Versace, A., Almeida, J. R., Hassel, S., Duran, F. L., ... Phillips, M. L. (2009). State-dependent microstructural white matter changes in bipolar I depression. *European Archives of Psychiatry and Clinical Neuroscience, 259*(6), 316–28. http://dx.doi.org/10.1007/s00406-009-0002-8

11 Paying Attention to a Field in Crisis
Psychiatry, Neuroscience, and Functional Systems of the Brain

Amir Raz and Ethan Macdonald

Introduction

A few short weeks before the long-awaited publication of *DSM-5*, Thomas Insel, director of the National Institute of Mental Health (NIMH), stated that the manual suffers from a "lack of validity" (Insel, 2013). To remedy this problem, he envisaged a new direction for psychiatry whereby clinicians and researchers classify disorders based on underlying neurobiological causes rather than on highly variable symptoms.

The anticipation of *DSM-5* and professional efforts surrounding it generated unprecedented questioning from both consumers and practitioners. The public, advocacy groups, and even senior members of the psychiatric community raised questions, not only regarding decisions to include or exclude specific types of problems from the revised manual but also concerning the scientific foundation of the whole enterprise. Many of these criticisms were based on recognizing the limited advances that have been made in the biological understanding and treatment of mental disorders.

Psychiatry aims to link behavioral science to underlying mechanisms, using the techniques of neuroscience. Yet decades of work on cognitive, molecular, and systems neuroscience have taught most scientists a lesson in humility: despite an enormous investment in research with an emphasis on the neural correlates of typical and atypical behavioral "phenotypes," breakthroughs are sorely lacking. In spite of the global efforts and the accumulation of a large body of findings, the lack of clinical advances has undermined many working assumptions concerning the neurobiological basis of psychiatric distress.

The genetic and neuroimaging revolutions – which seemed poised to elucidate and ultimately explain conditions categorized as psychopathologies and psychiatric disorders – have produced modest results that speak only obliquely to the vast, complex dynamics revealed by behavioral science. Many scholars are disillusioned with imaging studies of the living human brain, and further recognize that genetic

273

polymorphisms putatively appearing to increase risk of schizophrenia in one person may actually predispose another to bipolar disorder (Bilder, 2011). Furthermore, some scientists argue that the therapeutic effects of drugs that comprise the backbone of modern psychiatry – antidepressants and atypical antipsychotics – are largely indistinguishable from placebos in common clinical situations (Raz & Harris, in press). These findings challenge the extent to which the study of pharmaceutical drugs contributes to our understanding of psychological conditions.

Neuroscience and biology have given us neither the hoped for refinement of diagnostic criteria nor the sensitivity and specificity required for effective clinical practice. Psychiatry needs an entirely new approach that would allow us to understand – in a tangible way – the diversity of experience in illness and in health. Whereas older models of the *DSM* represented psychiatric illnesses as categories discontinuous with "normal" functioning, the NIMH strategy with respect to the Research Domain Criteria (RDoC) project emphasizes the potential continuity of psychopathology with normal functioning. For example, RDoC recognizes "attention" as a construct under the "cognitive systems" domain in the belief that examining its underlying mechanisms may account for both everyday behavior and related pathologies, such as ADHD.

Recent neuroimaging studies have clarified some of the neuroanatomical pathways involved in attention networks. Appreciating the challenges cognitive neuroscience faces, as well as the limitations of current techniques, is important in assessing the strength of particular neuroscientific findings and their implications for psychiatry and psychology. Critics have censured cognitive neuroscience for interpreting neuroimaging results in naïve ways that amount to a "new phrenology" (Uttal, 2001). These criticisms are justified in many areas of research, where reverse inferences and unsupported assumptions run rampant, as well as in some unscrupulous clinical applications, but they do not invalidate the field as a whole (Raz, 2012). But imaging the living brain and drawing conclusions from the enormous amount of data collected poses both technical and conceptual challenges.

In that spirit, our chapter sketches a new model for psychiatry that draws on recent work in the cognitive neuroscience of attention. We provide a detailed example of how operationalizing psychological and mental terms – in this case, "attention" – as a functional "organ system" (Posner & Fan, 2008) opens avenues to the integration of biobehavioral science and clinical psychiatry and allows us to transcend the old clinical dichotomy of functional and organic (Raz & Wolfson, 2010).

Why Should Psychiatrists Pay Attention to the Scientific Study of Attention?

Attention is a central theme in cognitive science, linking brain with behavior and advancing psychology with the techniques of neuroscience. Although experimental psychology has probably examined the topic of attention more than any other field (Raz & Buhle, 2006), the cognitive neuroscience of attention involves a larger social context that extends far beyond laboratory experiments, with innovative applications to mental health, education, human performance, and many other domains (Posner, 2012a). By understanding attention in terms of the orchestration of several separate control networks, we can consolidate behavioral, imaging, and genetic findings into a coherent whole. Moreover, we can elucidate individual differences in attention and outline the roles of early experience, upbringing, and environment in the development of attention networks. The scientific study of attention, therefore, provides critical insights into an alternative model that can help reorient psychiatry.

In the following sections, we show how viewing attention as a functional organ system – with its own anatomy, circuitry, and cellular structure – aids in our conceptualization of many psychopathologies. Moreover, we will argue that the pathologies of attention comprise a sizeable domain within the field of psychiatry and provide a way to group problems that transcends traditional diagnostic categories. This approach builds on our knowledge of the evolutionary and developmental bases of a principle brain mechanism of voluntary control, and thus paves the way to a better understanding of how genetics and culture together shape control systems. By studying the unique neurobiological and functional characteristics of brain networks, researchers can systematically search for genetic variations (e.g., polymorphisms) associated with differences in the regulation of cognition, emotion, thought, and action. Identifying this kind of variation can shed considerable light on both typical and atypical behaviors and provide critical insights to psychiatry.

The mapping of the human genome offers the potential to increase understanding of how biology and environment interact to produce individual differences in temperament and other dimensions of human behavior and functioning. Many genes exhibit variations that code for different phenotypes, which, in turn, can alter the efficiency of specific attention networks. The dopamine receptor D4 gene (*DRD4*), for example, has several versions that differ in having two, four, or seven repeats of a portion of the gene, and these variations may correlate with the temperamental trait of sensation-seeking – the tendency to seek out novel, varied, and intense sensory experiences (LaHoste et al., 1996). These genetic variations interact with specific aspects of the social environment. Thus, in the presence of the seven-repeat *DRD4* variant, parenting has a significant effect on an array of temperamental dimensions that correspond to some of the symptoms found in children diagnosed with ADHD (Sheese, Voelker, Rothbart, & Posner, 2007). Children with the seven-repeat allele who had a lower quality of parenting had unusually high levels of sensation-seeking, including impulsivity. By identifying children who are more susceptible to environmental factors, we can determine which children will benefit most from therapies that aim to improve attention. Hence, genetic variation provides a tool for refining our understanding of environmental influences.

A systematic account of the biological substrates of attention and their relation to social processes can clarify the impact that genetic variation has on each network. For example, experimental studies examining spatial orienting suggest that anxious people orient toward negative and positive targets in a similar manner, but highly anxious individuals have trouble disengaging from the negative target when the cue is invalid (Posner, Walker, Friedrich, & Rafal, 1984). These findings complement data from recent studies showing an inverse correlation between negative affect and effortful control (e.g., Rothbart, 2011). Overall, this research suggests that clinicians may use attention training as a strategy to bolster executive attention and help patients disengage from negative ideation.

The three-network model of attention systems described in this chapter provides researchers and practitioners with tools to examine clinical interventions, rehabilitation programs, educational methods, and even parenting styles. By construing attention as a functional organ system, we focus on its functional connectivity, neuroanatomy, network dynamics, cellular structure, and electrochemical mechanisms. This multilevel integrative view shows the way toward interdisciplinary work unifying the social world, life experiences, biological processes, and computational sciences.

Although attention networks occupy a central place in psychological and cognitive science, they have had relatively limited application in mental health theory and practice. Looking into the past and projecting into the future, attention research may be expected to have a much wider impact. Half a century ago, researchers largely focused on demonstrating that attention changes specific operations in the information-processing hierarchy – from input all the way to behavioral outcome. However, since the 1990s, neuroimaging has increasingly elucidated the focal brain areas that subserve attention networks. Investigators now study the brain regions within these networks that operationalize the computations performed by attention and monitor their patterns and rhythmic activations in real time. Present since early childhood, attention networks evolve throughout the life span and into adulthood via changes in connectivity (Posner, Rothbart, Sheese, & Voelker, 2014). Although genetic variations interacting with environment give rise to individual differences in the efficiency of control networks that compose attention, recent findings show that practice can improve the operation of specific attention networks by altering overarching brain states (Rabipour & Raz, 2012). Future studies may lead to new methods to ameliorate deficiencies and enhance performance.

Attention as a Functional Organ System: A Metaphor for a New Psychiatry

The notion of attention is part of our everyday "folk psychology." Titchener (1909) considered attention "the heart of the psychological enterprise"; and William James (1890) contended that, "Everyone knows what attention is. It is the taking possession of the mind in clear and vivid form of one out of what seem several simultaneous objects or trains of thought." This subjective definition, which construes attention intuitively as a unitary process under voluntary control, bears little resemblance to the working models of attention developed by cognitive neuroscientists (Posner, 2012a), who view attention in terms of a variety of networks that coordinate or facilitate much of human experience and consciousness.

We will outline a view of attention as a set of three distinct networks (alerting, orienting, and executive attention). Overall, we consider "attention" to be a "functional organ system." According to the *Oxford English Dictionary*, an organ "system" refers to "a set of organs or parts in an animal body of the same or similar structure, or subserving the same function," as exemplified by the digestive system. The term "functional" organ system serves to bridge an outdated dichotomy between "functional" (i.e., psychological) and "organic" (biological) mental disorders (Beer, 1996) that continues to influence clinical thinking (Miresco & Kirmayer, 2006).

Over the last half-century, the three-network model of attention has been continually refined (Posner, 2012a). Although most of the research has focused on visual attention, this approach generalizes across all sensory modalities (Posner, 2012b). Briefly, *alerting* can be conceptualized as a foundation upon which orienting and executive attention rest. It maintains sensitivity to incoming stimuli. *Orienting* concerns the selection of information from incoming stimuli. Lastly, *executive attention* involves complex higher-order processing, including conflict monitoring and inhibitory control (Posner & Fan, 2008; Posner & Petersen, 1990).

Table 11.1. *Attention Systems Involved in Visual Attention*

Function	Anatomical Structures	Neuromodulator/ Neurotransmitter	Brain Sites	Measures
Orienting	Superior parietal Temporal parietal junction Frontal eye fields Superior colliculus	Acetylcholine	A1, V1, S1 (Primary auditory, visual, and somatosensory cortexes)	Eye-tracking
Alerting	Locus coruleus Right frontal and parietal cortex	Norepinephrine	Orienting system	Autonomic changes, event-related potentials
Executive Attention	Anterior cingulate Lateral ventral Prefrontal Basal ganglia	Dopamine	All over the brain	Stroop, McGurk, Simon, Go/NoGo, Stop task

Brain structures that house the three control networks active in studies of a tripartite broad classification of attention, the corresponding dominant neuromodulators, and the sites of function. Although this illustration focuses on vision, the sources of attention effects appear similar in other modalities (Macaluso, Frith, & Driver, 2000). Adapted from "Attention as an Organ System" by M. J. Posner & J. Fan (2008).

Each network is associated with its own set of physiological activations, neuroanatomical structures, and neuromodulators (see Table 11.1; Posner & Fan, 2008; Rueda, Posner, & Rothbart, 2011).

As neuroimaging studies have shown, a wide variety of cognitive tasks correspond to brain signal changes distributed over a set of neural areas; each of these areas relate to specific mental operations that contribute to the overall cognitive task (Posner & Raichle, 1994, 1998). In the study of attention, the specific neural areas identified have been more consistent than for many other cognitive functions. For example, in order to shift visual attention to a new object, one has to disengage attention from its current focus, move it to the location of the new target, and engage the new object. Many experiments have shown that specific areas of the brain are involved in the operations of *disengage* (i.e., the parietal lobe), *move* (i.e., the superior colliculus), and *engage* (i.e., the pulvinar), and these areas collectively form a functional control system (Posner, 2012b). Together, these loci perform the task of orienting (cf. Losier & Klein,

2001). Because attention involves specialized networks to carry out different functions, damage to any module can produce distinct impairments in achieving and maintaining the alert state, orienting to sensory events, or controlling thoughts and feelings (Raz & Buhle, 2006).

Localizing mental operations in separate, yet connected, brain areas suggests a solution to the old problem of how brain localization could occur when widely diffuse damage is observed to produce the same general behavioral effect (e.g., extinction; Karnath & Rorden, 2012). To perform an integrated task, the brain must orchestrate the activity of a distributed network of functionally related anatomical regions; yet, the computations underlying any single mental operation (for example, engagement during orienting, which is orchestrated by the pulvinar) occurs locally. In this view, brain regions coordinate to perform multiple cognitive functions and are not solely defined by the few mental operations ascribed to them in a particular theoretical model or experimental setting (Macdonald & Raz, 2014).

The following sections present evidence for each attentional network and outline their implications for conceptualizing, diagnosing, and treating psychiatric conditions.

Alerting Attention

Alerting often appears as a foundational form of attention characterized by individual sensitivity to incoming stimuli, be they visual or other sensory types (Posner, 2012a). In laboratory studies, any stimuli presented to a subject will produce brain activity and physiological arousal compared to the resting state. To separate the activity underlying alerting attention from the resting state, alerting responses are generally measured during the interval between a warning signal and a stimulus. During this period, brain physiology reflects activity suppression, and the parasympathetic nervous system engages as an individual prepares for a swift response to the anticipated stimuli. Alerting increases the efficiency of sensory processing, including processing nontarget stimuli, such as distractors, and influencing orienting and attention networks as needed. Unfortunately, research on the alerting network has been relatively limited, compared with the volume of work on executive and orienting attention networks. As a result, despite the alerting network's fundamental role in attention, we know less about it.

Anatomically, alerting involves operations in the right frontal and right parietal regions (Posner, 2012a). Evidence in support of this localization includes lesion studies, wherein damage to the right parietal cortex, but not the left, has been associated with diminished alerting capacities

(Posner, Inhoff, Friedrich, & Cohen, 1987). Recent neuroimaging studies corroborate these findings, showing activity in the parietal and frontal regions during the alert state (Raz & Buhle, 2006). Using a combination of separate modalities, a plausible functional anatomy of the alert state has been posited (Figure 11.1).

The primary neurotransmitter of the alerting network is norepinephrine (NE), which is known to cause widespread effects within the regions that underlie alerting. The source of the brain's NE pathways, the locus coeruleus, appears to be the substrate for the influence of attention on arousal (Posner, 2012a), and warning signals trigger activity in this area (Aston-Jones & Cohen, 2005). Drugs that reduce or inhibit the release of NE can block the effect of warning signals (Marrocco & Davidson, 1998), whereas NE release enhancers may have the opposite effect (Posner, 2012a). The NE pathway originating in the locus coeruleus connects to regions of the frontal and parietal lobe, where it influences other networks. Studies designed to distinguish between orienting and alerting responses suggest that NE is a primary neuromodulator for the alerting system (Beane & Marrocco, 2004).

Pathologies of alerting due to individual differences in NE modulation have not been directly studied, although other influences on the alerting network have been identified. For example, some people with ADHD and learning disorders have a genetic variation in the alpha-2A receptor gene *ADRA2A* (Posner, 2012a), which may reflect alertness functioning. Children with ADHD also have increased difficulty maintaining an alert state without a warning signal (Swanson et al., 1991), as well as poorer performance with stimuli presented to the right hemisphere (Posner, 2012a). Of course, some degree of alerting attention is needed for nearly every experimental task of attention. Understanding the bases of individual differences in alerting may allow for more nuanced conceptualizations of cognitive functioning.

Orienting Attention

The vast majority of studies on attention have involved orienting to sensory – predominantly visual – events. Orienting, which involves either effortful or reflexive directing of awareness to a stimulus, exists in two major forms: overt and covert. This distinction depends on whether overt physical actions (e.g., eye movements) accompany directing awareness to a new stimulus. Of the three types of attention networks, orienting provides the strongest evidence of mental operations, and researchers usually decompose it into a number of subsidiary processes (e.g., engaging, disengaging, moving). Results from studies since the 1980s,

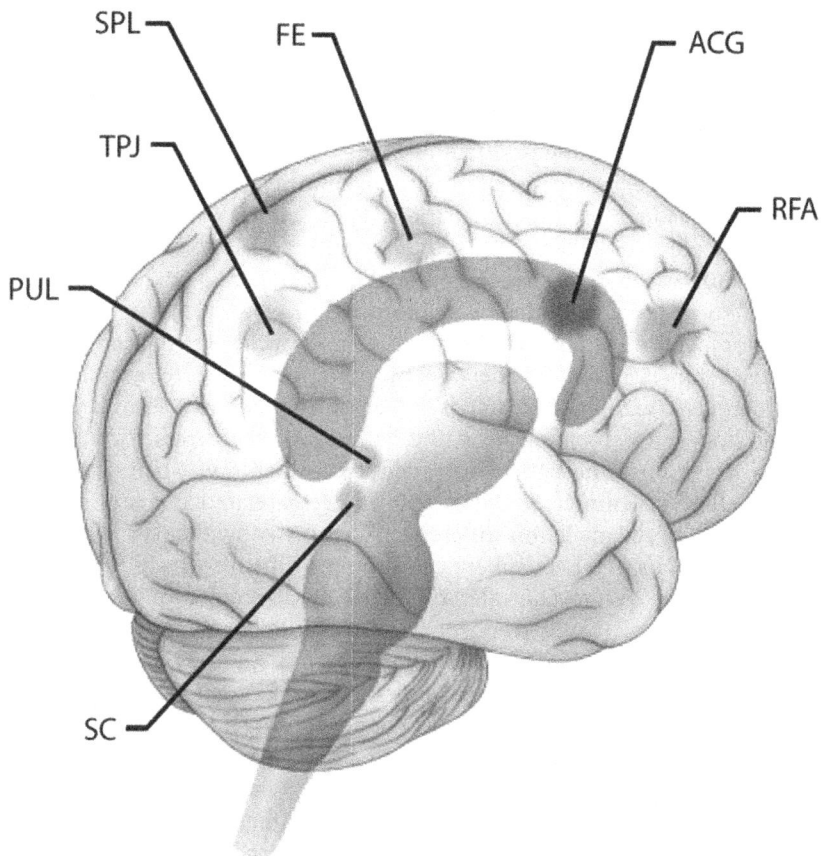

Figure 11.1. A sketch of the functional anatomy of the attention networks. The pulvinar, superior colliculus, superior parietal lobe, and frontal eye fields are often activated in studies of the orienting network. The temporoparietal junction is active when a target occurs at a novel location. The anterior cingulate gyrus is an important part of the executive network. Right frontal and parietal areas are active when people maintain the alert state. PUL: pulvinar; SC: superior colliculus; SPL: superior parietal lobe; FE: frontal eye fields; TPJ: temporoparietal junction; ACG: anterior cingulate gyrus; RFA: right frontal area. Adapted with permission from "Hypnosis and Neuroscience: A Cross Talk Between Clinical and Cognitive Research" by A. Raz & T. Shapiro, 2002, *Archives of General Psychiatry, 59*(1), 88. Copyright © (2002) American Medical Association. All rights reserved. (See Color Plate.)

including clinical, experimental, and imaging studies, support the general approach toward localization but suggest somewhat different decompositions of the operations involved. As new methods of neuroimaging have become available, increasingly sophisticated experiments have been applied to the problem of orienting to sensory input.

Anatomical regions associated with visual orienting include the temporoparietal junction, superior parietal lobe, frontal eye fields, and the superior colliculus (Posner, 2012a). A paradox of lesion studies in the early 1980s was that the superior parietal lobe seemed to be the area most related to producing difficulty in disengaging from a current focus of attention. Yet, most clinical data point to inferior lesions in the temporoparietal junction and/or the superior temporal lobe to account for neurological "extinction"; that is, when simultaneously stimulated on either side of a perceptual field, the patient only perceives stimulus on one side – even if the patient can identify both stimuli when presented separately (Vuilleumier & Rafal, 2000). Event-related imaging studies have served to reconcile this difference. We now know that lesions in two separate regions in a hemisphere can produce difficulty in shifting attention to stimuli in the contralateral visual field, but for quite different reasons. Lesions of the temporoparietal junction or superior temporal lobe are important when a novel or unexpected stimulus occurs. When functioning normally, this area allows disengagement from a current focus of attention in order to shift to the new event. It also plays a critical role in producing the core elements of the hemispatial neglect syndrome (or extinction), in which a person becomes unaware of or inattentive to sensations and events on one side of the body. In addition, considerable clinical evidence suggests that in humans, lateralization in the right-temporal parietal junction may be more important to the deficit than lateralization in corresponding areas of the left hemisphere (Mesulam, 1981; Perry & Zeki, 2000). A different brain region, the superior parietal lobe (SPL), appears critical for voluntary shifts of attention following a cue. Event-related functional magnetic resonance (fMRI) studies have found this region to be active following a cue that informs the person to shift attention covertly (i.e., without eye movement) to the target (Corbetta, Kincade, Ollinger, McAvoy, & Shulman, 2000). The SPL is part of a larger network that includes frontal eye fields and the superior colliculus; this network appears to orchestrate both covert shifts of attention and eye movements toward targets (Corbetta, 1998). During visual search – when people voluntarily move their attention from location to location while searching for a visual target – the SPL is also active. By linking the findings of lesion studies with converging evidence from event-related imaging studies, research on orienting has identified a network of behavioral and anatomical features collectively responsible for the movement of attention in either a covert or overt manner (Figure 11.1 and 11.2).

Further distinctions between covert and overt orienting have been posited at a cellular level (Posner, 2012a). For instance, a specific type of neuron seems to be involved in covert shifts of attention (Schafer & Moore, 2007; Thompson, Biscoe, & Sato, 2005), which also continues to attend to, or hold, the locations of cues during delay intervals (Armstrong, Chang, & Moore, 2009). Thus, cellular differentiation contributes to the distinction between motor systems involved in saccades and circuits involved in covert orienting.

Cholinergic systems play a vital role in orienting attention. Even in cases where NE release, and therefore warning signals, cannot occur, orienting can still take place (Marrocco & Davidson, 1998). Studies in monkeys have utilized the acetylcholine (ACh) blocker, scopolamine (which slows covert orienting), to elucidate the role of ACh in orienting (Davidson & Marrocco, 2000). These findings further point to differences in neurotransmitters between alerting and orienting systems.

Abnormalities in the orienting network may contribute to neuropsychological conditions. For example, Alzheimer's patients with degeneration in the superior parietal lobe have difficulty dealing with cues in the central visual field that are meant to inform them to shift their attention (Parasuraman, Greenwood, Haxby, & Grady, 1992). In addition, of the two main pathways that process visual information in the brain, the ventral information-processing stream represents the "what" stream, which seems to identify objects rather than locate them in space. Patients with lesions of the thalamus (e.g., the pulvinar) show subtle deficits in visual-orienting tasks that are likely related to the ventral information-processing stream. It seems plausible, therefore, that a critical element of orienting would be a vertical network of brain areas related to voluntary eye movements and to processing novel input, but a precise model that includes a role for all visual areas implicated in orienting is still lacking.

The methods of neuroimaging have proven useful in testing the general proposition that mental operations involved in a given task are distributed across multiple brain areas (Posner & Raichle, 1998). Nearly two decades of work have shown many tasks to be associated with the activation of widely spaced networks that are presumed to carry out particular operations. We are still unsure as to the exact operations that occur at each location, even in a relatively simple act such as shifting attention to a novel event. However, imaging data link clinical observations with experimental results to support the general idea of localization of specific operations.

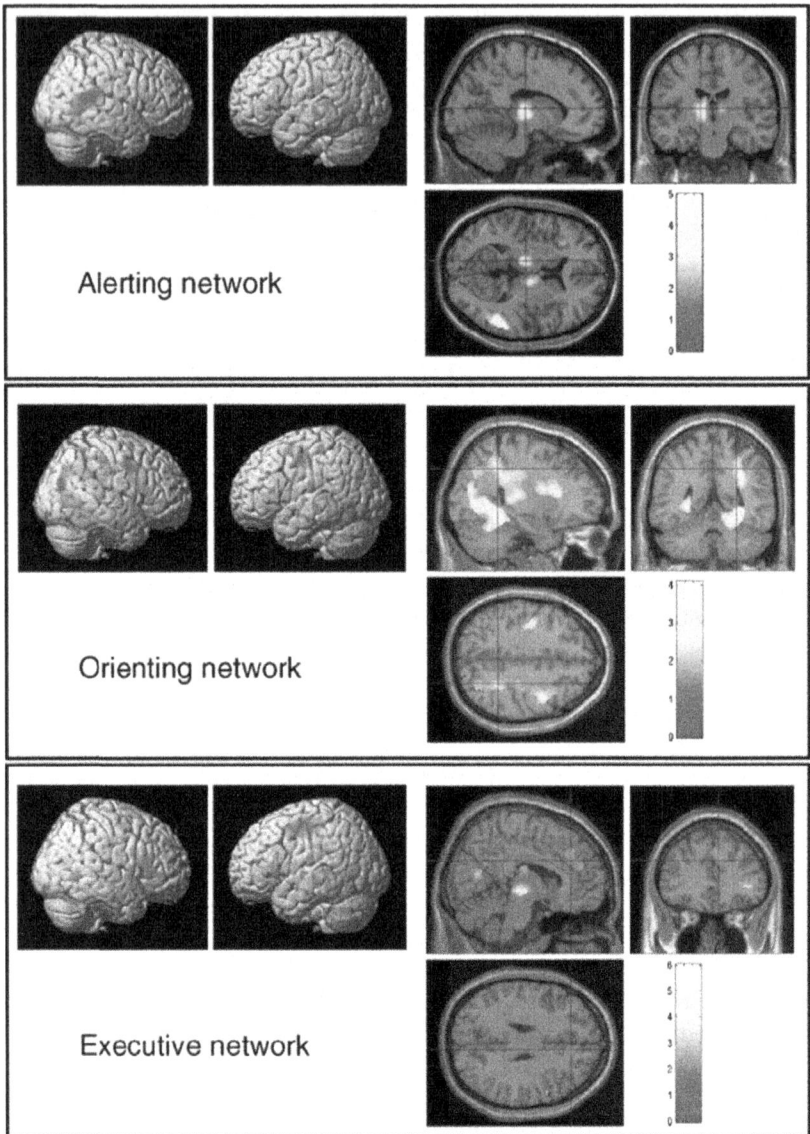

Figure 11.2. Cross-sectional views of the three attention networks. The alerting network shows thalamic activation, the orienting network shows parietal activation, and the conflict network shows anterior cingulate cortex activation. The color bar shows fMRI signal level (Z-scores) above the 0.05 significance threshold. fMRI images collected from 16 healthy adults performing the ANT in a 3 Tesla MRI scanner (Fan et al., 2001). Reprinted from *NeuroImage, 26*, J. Fan, B. D. McCandliss, J. Fossella, J. I. Flombaum, & M. I. Posner, "The Activation of Attentional Networks," p. 476, Copyright 2005, with permission from Elsevier. (See Color Plate.)

Executive Attention

The executive attention network is perhaps the most multifaceted of the functional systems of attention, involving the neural processing required for resolution of conflicts, monitoring, and self-regulation. Common tests of executive attention generally include perceptual conflicts or higher-level brain processing (e.g., Stroop or visual search tasks), and performance on such tasks of executive attention has proven amenable to top-down modulation (Lifshitz, Aubert Bonn, Fischer, Kashem, & Raz, 2013) and cognitive training (Rabipour & Raz, 2012). Moreover, cognitive training programs aimed at strengthening executive attention networks have been found to increase intelligence and self-regulation scores in children (Rueda, Checa, & Santonja, 2008). Although this network has long been associated with the handling of sensory conflicts, recent findings now illuminate the wide-reaching implications of executive attention in self-regulation.

The executive attention network, while interacting with other forms of attention, is anatomically distinct. Exploration of brain activity in the cingulate during tasks of conflict resolution (Pardo, Pardo, Janer, & Raichle, 1990; Posner, 2012a) led to the discovery of the network. In conflict paradigms, including Stroop tasks, the anterior cingulate cortex (ACC) becomes active and contributes to a dynamic process of conflict monitoring and top-down control with the dorsolateral prefrontal cortex (MacDonald, Cohen, Stenger, & Carter, 2000). Utilization of modified Stroop paradigms has further illuminated a distinction between emotional and cognitive areas of the ACC (Bush et al., 1998) – a discovery that has implications for executive control of cognitive and emotional impulses. The major areas of executive attention interface with functionally adjacent brain areas, while maintaining their autonomy as a distinct network (Figure 11.1 and Figure 11.2).

Areas of the executive attention network exhibit particular cell morphologies that provide clues regarding function. Spindle cells are found in areas of the ACC and anterior insula that are unique to great apes and humans (Posner, 2012a). Their presence, as well as the time course of their development, suggest higher cortical functioning concurrent with the development of executive attention. Of course, these cells are not necessarily the same ones that are active during fMRI scans, but further investigation into the function of these cells might provide key insights.

As behavioral genetics advances, novel research paradigms have begun to unravel relationships between genes and executive attention. For example, *DRD4* and *MAOA* polymorphisms, selected for study because of the importance of dopaminergic pathways in executive attention, have been correlated with performance on an attention network test, and alleles have been identified that correlate both with increased ACC activity and enhanced conflict resolution (Fan, Fossella, Sommer, Wu, & Posner, 2003). Studies of such genetic variation, while in their infancy, will lead to better understanding of the complex gene-brain-environment interactions during development that contribute to cognitive functioning.

Critically important in psychiatric disorders, executive attention has been implicated in a wide range of disorders, including borderline personality and schizophrenia (Posner, 2012a). Such transdiagnostic approaches, congruent with the advent of the RDoC, may prove essential to the development of a scientific basis for psychiatry that is grounded in cognitive neuroscience.

The Functional Anatomy and Genetics of Attention Systems

In summary, recent research has mapped the functional anatomy of multiple systems in the brain. Event-related fMRI studies have identified brain areas or networks associated with alerting, orienting, and executive attention (Fan, McCandliss, Fossella, Flombaum, & Posner, 2005). Research on the effects of warning signals (e.g., alerting or expectation of when a target will occur) have shown that, while sustained vigilance involves mainly areas of the right cerebral hemisphere, phasic changes in alertness following warning signals tend to operate through left hemisphere sites (Coull, Nobre, & Frith, 2001). Event-related fMRI studies of orienting (cf. Corbetta & Shulman, 2002) identify a dorsal system that includes the interparietal sulcus and frontal eye fields as key sites triggered by volitional shifts of attention. A more ventral parietal-frontal network serves as a "circuit breaker" leading to shifts of attention, particularly to novel stimuli. The more ventral system has been identified as a major site where cortical lesions produce attentional neglect. There is considerable agreement on which cortical areas orchestrate shifts of attention toward sensory information, but the subcortical areas are still largely unclear (Posner, 2004; Posner, 2012a).

Much effort has been given to determining the exact role of specific areas, including the ACC and lateral prefrontal cortex. Several researchers have argued that the cingulate involves a monitoring function, whereas lateral prefrontal areas act more directly to suppress neural activity in unselected areas (e.g., Cohen, Aston-Jones, & Gilzenrat, 2004). Although consensus on the sites involved in executive attention exists, active debates continue on whether these brain areas operate as a whole or via local, specific operations (Posner, 2004, Posner, 2012a).

Initial work on the molecular genetics of attention provided evidence on the roles that *MAOA, COMT, DRD4,* and *DAT1* genes play in measures of attention control (Fossella et al., 2002), and major studies from a large group at National Institutes of Health (NIH) have confirmed the role of *COMT* in attention (Blasi et al., 2005). In addition, researchers have identified two cholinergic genes that influence individual differences in the orienting network (Parasuraman, Greenwood, Kumar, & Fossella, 2005). Neuroimaging has been used to further explore the anatomy of these genetic differences (Egan et al., 2003; Fan et al., 2003). The area of cognitive genetics has become a large field, allowing the study of individual differences in attention at the molecular level (Goldberg & Weinberger, 2004). As findings from this field accumulate, we may soon have refined biological correlates of psychiatric distress that can guide the development of clinical interventions based on cultivating our attentional capacities.

Neurodevelopment of Attention

The field of developmental cognitive neuroscience has traced the development of the attention systems in some detail (e.g., Posner, 2012a; Posner et al., 2014; Rothbart, Posner, & Kieras, 2006). Not only is this field of particular importance for understanding neurodevelopmental disorders such as ADHD, but it also sheds light on the impact of environmental factors on attention (Posner, 2012a).

In adults, most cognitive and emotional self-regulation involves a network of brain regions drawing on structures such as the ACC, the insula, and areas of the basal ganglia related to executive attention. During infancy and throughout early development, however, control systems depend primarily on a brain network involved in orienting to sensory events that includes areas of the parietal lobe and frontal eye fields (Posner, 2012a).

Over the first few years of life, emotion regulation is a major aspect of development. fMRI studies on newborns and infants up to a year old (Gao et al., 2009), as well as on children and adolescents (Fair et al., 2009; Fair, Dosenbach, Petersen, & Schlaggar, 2012; Fransson et al., 2007), have provided data on two attention networks related to control systems: the frontoparietal network and the cingulo-opercular network. During early development the two networks cooperate closely together, while in adulthood the cingulo-opercular network becomes independent from the frontoparietal network. Drawing on the neural substrates of the orienting network, the frontoparietal network is important for rapid adaptive control on shorter timescales, whereas the cingulo-opercular network draws on the executive network's neural infrastructure to maintain stable attentional sets over longer timescales.

These patterns of connectivity suggest that the control structures involved in executive attention – including structures on the medial aspect of the frontal lobe (e.g., ACC) and parietal lobe (e.g., operculum) – are active during early development, maturing to wield fuller control only later in life. The parallels identified by studies of brain networks of attention in adults (e.g., Posner & Fan, 2008) and developmental studies of resting fMRI connectivity (e.g., Fair et al., 2009; Fair et al., 2012) may help unravel the story of the development of attention in infants and young children.

Researchers, including Posner and others, have pursued the study of changes in control in early life, from orienting to executive attention, showing increased frontoparietal (i.e., orienting) resting network activity and reduced cingulo-cuneus (i.e., executive) activity during infancy (Posner, Rothbart, Sheese, & Voelker, 2012). As children develop, executive functioning increases, as indexed by both behavioral measures and neural correlates.

During infancy, orienting serves as the primary control system; later in childhood, effortful control becomes dominant. Control during infancy may be mainly in relation to emotion and only later related to executive functioning. Parents and caregivers probably propel the development of self-regulation and exercise executive systems by presenting novel stimuli (e.g., new objects or people). Reading to the child may be another form of this type of stimulation. Some cultures make "active watching" (e.g., observation and imitation) the main learning venue of the developing young. "High motivation to learn" among the children of Aka and Bofi foragers in the Congo Basin rainforest "occurs early and often. Infants climb into their parents' laps to watch them cook, play an instrument or make a net" (B. S. Hewlett, Fouts, Boyette, & B. L Hewlett, 2011). Such cultures may prepare the executive attention network of infants by orienting to novel stimuli. The cingulate system appears to function, at least for the detection of errors, as early as seven months of age (Berger, Tzur, & Posner, 2006; Boduroglu et al., 2009; cf. Ketay, Aron, & Hedden, 2009); with epigenetic and environmental interactions shaping the development of the networks in later life (Sheese et al., 2007; Voelker, Sheese, Rothbart, & Posner, 2009), training can increase the efficiency of white matter connections, even in adults (Tang et al., 2010). Therefore, assuming that infants and adults share similar mechanisms with regard to novelty, cingulate activity may forge connections found in later life. Better understanding of the development of attention systems will have implications for child-rearing, pedagogy, and treating attention-related disorders.

Attention Training: Meditation and Hypnosis

Learning shapes attention systems well into adulthood. Attentional capacities are malleable, and attention can be trained in a number of ways. Michael Posner and colleagues, for example, have tried to distinguish attention training (e.g., conflict-related tasks) from attention state training (e.g., meditative practices accompanied by changes in mind/body states; 2009). Furthermore, they have demonstrated alterations in white matter connectivity in critical areas related to the ACC after attention state training (Tang et al., 2010). Attention state training can improve attention performance and response to stress, and measures of attention have been used with individuals as young as four years old.

The potential clinical value of forms of attentional training such as meditation and hypnosis is apparent from research on pain regulation (Holroyd, 1996); modulation of the immune system (Kiecolt-Glaser, Marucha, Atkinson, & Glaser, 2001); and treatment effectiveness (Kirsch, Montgomery, & Sapirstein, 1995).

Clinical hypnosis involves the deliberate use of attentional capacities to manage symptoms, change behaviors, and produce other helpful outcomes (Nash & Barnier, 2012). During a hypnotherapy session, a therapist uses suggestion in the form of hypnotic instruction to bring about such outcomes in a client. Individuals vary widely in their ability to respond to hypnotic instructions and suggestions. We can measure this individual trait, which is known as hypnotizability, via the use of scales; but no biological marker currently exists for indexing either hypnotizability or the hypnotic experience. In other words, neither a brain scan nor a blood test can determine if a person is highly hypnotizable or if someone is currently experiencing hypnotically induced alterations or effects. In fact, most children are highly hypnotizable, with an age peak of about eleven to twelve years, but hypnotizability seems to gradually diminish for many people thereafter; and adult hypnotizability is a relatively stable characteristic that is normally distributed in the population (Kohen & Olness, 2011; Raz, 2012). A few studies, however, have found that individuals can increase their hypnotic responsiveness through training (Gorassini et al., 1999). Although it is controversial, hypnotizability training aims to teach individuals to direct their attention in a specific fashion to achieve a hypnotic experience (cf. Rabipour & Raz, 2012; Spanos et al., 1989). Although critics argue that the observed responses may result from a combination of factors, including training-to-task and a certain measure of theatrics and self-deception, little research has examined hypnotic training in depth. It would be interesting to know, for example, whether people with low hypnotizability who undergo training can achieve the ability of highly hypnotizable but untrained people to override automatic effects such as those measured by executive tasks (Lifshitz et al., 2013). Attention training is a form of cognitive intervention, similar to hypnotic training, that is aimed at exercising specific control networks (Rabipour & Raz, 2012). Behavioral programs, including attention training, have become ubiquitous; proponents claim that they can be valuable adjuncts, if not rivals, to conventional pharmacotherapy for certain disorders (e.g., Tourette syndrome), especially in children (Piacentini et al., 2010; Steeves et al., 2012). Finding nondrug treatments for mental and neurological disorders might help patients avoid or limit the side effects of medication; however, this nascent field is still in its infancy (cf. Rabipour & Raz, 2012).

Tourette Syndrome: Intervening through the Functional System of Attention

Tourette syndrome (TS) is a neuropsychiatric condition marked by compulsive, habitual movements and vocalizations. Individuals with TS frequently report that these tics are preceded by physical sensations or urges to tic. These proceeding sensations and urges, known as premonitory urges, resemble the sensations and desires to blink that one may get when holding their eyes open for too long. Researchers often consider premonitory urges to be "semivoluntary" since, as with blinking, they can be suppressed only with a great deal of effort and discomfort. Moreover, many individuals with TS find that their tics ameliorate during times of deep mental focus.

Because of its close relationship to other diagnoses, we will use TS as an illustration of how to apply findings from attention research to the study and treatment of clinical populations. Although some may construe TS as a neurological condition, a strong psychological component has been noted for well over a century (Kushner, 1999), and the past decade has seen a revival of behavioral interventions that exploit top-down control (Wile & Pringsheim, 2013). Furthermore, TS symptoms overlap with other conditions, including Obsessive Compulsive Disorder (OCD) and Attention Deficit Hyperactivity Disorder (ADHD). "Pure" TS is hard to find and usually occurs alongside multiple co-morbidities of attention and emotional regulation (Freeman et al., 2000). Hence, some researchers have characterized TS as an impulse-control disorder related to ADHD and OCD.

Following the logic of RDoC, models of attention would unite TS with impulse-control disorders on the basis of putatively shared neurobiological substrates, as suggested by studies of individuals who have comorbid TS (Freeman et al., 2000) or experience urges (Blumberg et al., 2003; Bush, 2008; Raz et al., 2009; Shafritz, Collins, & Blumberg, 2006; Sowell et al., 2008). In a large-scale study, Freeman et al. (2000) sampled thousands of individuals with TS from twenty-two countries. ADHD and OCD formed the bulk of TS-comorbid diagnoses, contributing to 60 and 27 percent, respectively, of all TS cases. Impairment of the attention system responsible for emotional and behavioral regulation is likely central to these disorders (Raz & Buhle, 2006; Raz et al., 2009). These results highlight the potential for attention research to elucidate both the neurobiological substrate of psychopathology and the mechanisms underlying the clinical effects of current therapies.

Whereas TS was once thought to result from an oversensitivity to dopamine in the basal ganglia, the neurobiological mechanisms appear to be more complex (Felling & Singer, 2011; Leckman, Bloch, Smith, Larabi, & Hampson, 2010). Therefore, pharmacological dopamine blockers, the standard treatment for TS, have fallen short in successfully ameliorating tics for many patients (Peterson & Cohen, 1998; Phelps, 2008; Pringsheim & Pearce, 2010). These drugs frequently induce intolerable side effects, including sedation, parkinsonism, cognitive dulling, dry mouth, fatigue, dizziness, weight gain, and metabolic syndrome (Swain, Scahill, Lombroso, King, & Leckman, 2007). In light of such challenges with pharmacotherapy, efforts have been redoubled to develop cognitive-behavioral interventions for TS (Piacentini et al., 2010), whereas others have examined TS biology more closely (Leckman et al., 2010).

A shared neural circuitry among TS, ADHD, and OCD is consistent with findings that approximately 90 percent of individuals with TS qualify for multiple diagnoses (Freeman, 2007; Robertson, 2006; Scahill, Bitsko, Visser, & Blumberg, 2009). TS, ADHD, and OCD all involve irregularities in the internal neural circuitry that modulate impulse control and in executive attention (Eddy, Rickards, & Cavanna, 2012; Willcutt, Doyle, Nigg, Faraone, & Pennington, 2005). TS research has focused on cortico-striatal-thalamo-cortical (CSTC) loops involved in habit formation and information transmission between the basal ganglia and the cortex (Alexander, DeLong, & Strick, 1986; Graybiel & Canales, 2000; Leckman et al., 2010). Decreased volume of the caudate nucleus (part of the basal ganglia) in childhood is a predictor of tic severity in adulthood (Bloch, Leckman, Zhu, & Peterson, 2005); and frontostriatal loop activation, particularly in subcortical structures, influences tic symptom severity (Peterson et al., 1998). Cognitive neuroscientists have further elucidated these subcortical structures as key nodes in the attentional system that may contribute to ADHD (Casey et al., 1997). Both OCD and TS involve include dysfunction of CSTC loops (Harrison et al., 2009); and novel findings from deep brain stimulation suggest that direct modulation of basal ganglia activity can improve OCD symptoms (Welter et al., 2011). Taken together, the neurobiology of comorbid TS blur the distinction between "compulsion" and "tic" and implicate attention as a central component of the condition.

Cognitive-behavioral therapies, which train attention, have been found to surpass pharmacological treatments as effective therapies for TS (Piacentini et al., 2010; Steeves et al., 2012). In response to the considerable empirical evidence supporting habit reversal training (Feldman, Storch, & Murphy, 2011) and comprehensive behavioral intervention for tics (CBIT; Piacentini et al., 2010), recent Canadian guidelines for evidence-based treatment of TS identify cognitive-behavioral approaches as first line treatments for TS (Steeves et al., 2012). These therapies employ classic tools of attention training (AT; Rabipour & Raz, 2012) in that they require sustained attention, awareness, and focus.

Attention may play a key role in tic disorders. When tested with the Stroop task, for instance, groups with TS demonstrate poorer inhibitory function compared to control groups (Eddy et al., 2012; Raz et al., 2009). In addition, tic suppression reduces cognitive performance (Conelea & Woods, 2008), and stress induction raises tic frequency (Conelea, Woods, & Brandt, 2011). We have found preliminary evidence that attention training is effective at reducing tic expression, and six-month follow up data suggest long-term efficacy and increased quality of life (Rabipour & Raz, 2012).

Additional research avenues remain to be explored. For example, using combinations of attention training and neuroimaging techniques, it may be possible to probe the relationships between executive attention training, the unusual ACC patterns in OCD (Freeman et al., 2000), and the abnormal ACC anatomy in adults with TS (Müller-Vahl et al., 2009). Moreover, TS is a unique context for studying impulse control because the overt behavioral expression of tics lends itself to quantitative measurement, even during novel experimental paradigms.

There is evidence that hypnotic suggestion can override processes previously believed to be impermeable to top-down influences (Lifshitz et al., 2013; Raz, Kirsch, Pollard, & Nitkin-Kaner, 2006; Raz, Moreno-Íniguez, Martin, & Zhu, 2007; Raz, Shapiro, Fan, & Posner, 2002);

and hypnosis has been shown to modulate tic expression (Kushner, 1999; Raz, Keller, Norman, & Senechal, 2007). Interestingly, like suggestibility, tic severity peaks during childhood development (Leckman et al., 1998). Because of its ability to bridge controlled and seemingly automatic processes, hypnosis may be an effective tool for attention and TS research alike (Raz, Moreno-Íniguez, et al., 2007). For example, hypnosis can be used to empower individuals to exert executive control over an otherwise involuntary tic. Hypnosis can alter the voluntariness of the semivoluntary tics characteristic of TS in ways that may be similar to attention training, CBIT, or habit reversal training (HRT; Feldman et al., 2011). With regard to HRT and CBIT, hypnosis may have potential as a useful adjunct to attention training. In these training programs, individuals with TS engage in behaviors called "competing responses" when they feel the urge to tic. These competing responses are incompatible with the motions and vocalizations of the tic. Because it can help make voluntary behaviors more automatic, hypnosis may simultaneously increase the elements of suggestion in CBIT and HRT and decrease the difficulty of employing competing responses. Furthermore, hypnosis has proven itself a powerful analgesic (Montgomery, DuHamel, & Redd, 2000), and may provide new ways of reducing the sensory discomfort associated with the premonitory urges that individuals with TS often suffer.

Another approach to clinical intervention has proposed using meditation to improve attention, self-regulation, and emotional control (Perlman, Salomons, Davidson, & Lutz, 2010; Tang et al., 2007; Zeidan, Johnson, Diamond, David, & Goolkasian, 2010). Studies have reported that expert meditators show significant alterations in ACC activity and effortless control over previously challenging and effortful modes of attention (Tang, Rothbart, & Posner, 2012). Such approaches have yet to be applied to conditions such as TS, but there is enough evidence to encourage further investigation.

As research on neural functioning in psychiatric disorders moves from biological reductionism to an integration of neurobiology and psychology, with social science clarifying the contexts of functioning and adaptation, the clinical importance of attention as a mediator of tics and other impulse-related problems suggests the utility of transdiagnostic research frameworks, such as RDoC. The history of approaches to TS shows how the psychiatric pendulum has swung from completely psychological to extremely biological explanations, and then, most recently, back to a more balanced perspective, in which neurobiology, psychology, and social interactional processes all contribute to symptom production. This interactional perspective supports the search for cognitive-behavioral interventions (Kirmayer & Crafa, 2014; Raz, Keller, et al., 2007).

Although TS represents a particularly interesting condition for the study of attention, it is but one example of how findings on attention systems might be applied to psychiatry. Similar approaches may be useful to help ADHD patients build sustained attention and to help OCD patients alleviate compulsions.

Conclusion

In this chapter, we have emphasized the importance of development in the study of attention as a functional system. Studies conducted over the last decade have revealed key aspects of the neurodevelopment of attention networks. This research shapes our efforts to understand how experience and genetics interact to produce the executive attention network, with possible consequences for developmental problems of children and adults (Posner, 2012a; Posner & Rothbart, 2005).

Approaching attention as a functional organ system – with specific control networks carrying its basic functions – provides a useful direction for psychiatry (Posner & Fan, 2008). Setting aside diagnostic criteria for discrete disorders (as in the *DSM*), the framework we have presented shows how molecular, neural network, and cognitive studies can be integrated to provide a view of attention that illuminates its role in the development of children and the everyday performance of adults. Disorders of attention comprise an important subset of the problems addressed by modern psychiatry. Attention systems also play a role in adapting to many conditions. Attention training, therefore, can be a powerful tool to influence behavior and modulate cognition, affect, and action in a wide range of problems. As we have shown, linking clinical symptomatology to functional systems through the behavioral and brain sciences breaks down the functional/organic distinction and actually supports the use of psychological and psychosocial interventions for a wide range of putatively "biological" disorders.

REFERENCES

Albin, R. L., & Mink, J. W. (2006). Recent advances in Tourette syndrome research. *Trends in Neurosciences, 29*(3), 175–82. http://dx.doi.org/10.1016/j.tins.2006.01.001

Alexander, G. E., DeLong, M. R., & Strick, P. L. (1986). Parallel organization of functionally segregated circuits linking basal ganglia and cortex. *Annual Review of Neuroscience, 9*(1), 357–81. http://dx.doi.org/10.1146/annurev.ne.09.030186.002041

Armstrong, K. M., Chang, M. H., & Moore, T. (2009). Selection and maintenance of spatial information by frontal eye field neurons. *Journal of Neuroscience, 29*(50), 15621–9. http://dx.doi.org/10.1523/ JNEUROSCI.4465-09.2009

Aston-Jones, G., & Cohen, J. D. (2005). An integrative theory of locus coeruleus-norepinephrine function: Adaptive gain and optimal performance. *Annual Review of Neuroscience, 28*(1), 403–50. http://dx.doi.org/10.1523/ JNEUROSCI.4465-09.2009

Beane, M., & Marrocco, R. T. (2004). Cholinergic and noradrenergic inputs to the posterior parietal cortex modulate the components of exogenous attention. In M. Posner (Ed.), *Cognitive neuroscience of attention* (pp. 313–25). New York, NY: Guilford.

Beer, M. D. (1996). The dichotomies: Psychosis/neurosis and functional/ organic – A historical perspective. *History of Psychiatry, 7*(26), 231–55. http://dx.doi.org/10.1177/0957154X9600702603

Berger, A., Tzur, G., & Posner, M. (2006). Infant brains detect arithmetic errors. *Proceedings of the National Academy of Sciences of the United States of America, 103*(33), 12649–53. http://dx.doi.org/10.1073/ pnas.0605350103

Bilder, R. M. (2011). Neuropsychology 3.0: Evidence-based science and practice. *Journal of the International Neuropsychological Society, 17*(1), 7–13. http://dx.doi.org/10.1017/S1355617710001396

Blasi, G., Mattay, V. S., Bertolino, A., Elvevåg, B., Callicott, J. H., Das, S., ... Weinberger, D. R. (2005). Effect of catechol-O-methyltransferase val158met genotype on attentional control. *Journal of Neuroscience, 25*(20), 5038–45. http://dx.doi.org/10.1523/JNEUROSCI.0476-05.2005

Bloch, M. H., Leckman, J. F., Zhu, H., & Peterson, B. S. (2005). Caudate volumes in childhood predict symptom severity in adults with Tourette syndrome. *Neurology, 65*(8), 1253–8. http://dx.doi.org/10.1212/01. wnl.0000180957.98702.69

Blumberg, H. P., Kaufman, J., Martin, A., Whiteman, R., Zhang, J. H., Gore, J. C., ... Peterson, B. S. (2003). Amygdala and hippocampal volumes in adolescents and adults with bipolar disorder. *Archives of General Psychiatry, 60*(12), 1201–8. http://dx.doi.org/10.1001/ archpsyc.60.12.1201

Boduroglu, A., Shah, P., & Nisbett, R. E. (2009). Cultural differences in allocation of attention in visual information processing. *Journal of Cross-Cultural Psychology, 40*(3), 349–60. http://dx.doi.org/10.1177/ 0022022108331005

Bush, G. (2008). Neuroimaging of attention deficit hyperactivity disorder: Can new imaging findings be integrated in clinical practice? *Child and Adolescent Psychiatric Clinics of North America, 17*(2), 385–404. http://dx.doi. org/10.1016/j.chc.2007.11.002

Bush, G., Whalen, P. J., Rosen, B. R., Jenike, M. A., McInerney, S. C., & Rauch, S. L. (1998). The counting Stroop: An interference task specialized for functional neuroimaging: Validation study with functional MRI. *Human Brain Mapping, 6*(4), 270–82.

Casey, B., Castellanos, F. X., Giedd, J. N., Marsh, W. L., Hamburger, S. D., Schubert, A. B., ... Sarfatti, S. E. (1997). Implication of right frontostriatal circuitry in response inhibition and attention-deficit/hyperactivity disorder. *Journal of the American Academy of Child & Adolescent Psychiatry, 36*(3), 374–83. http://dx.doi.org/10.1097/00004583-199703000-00016

Cohen, J. D., Aston-Jones, G., & Gilzenrat, M. S. (2004). A systems-level perspective on attention and cognitive control: Guided activation, adaptive gating, conflict monitoring, and exploitation versus exploration. In M. Posner (Ed.), *Cognitive neuroscience of attention* (pp. 71–90). New York, NY: Guilford.

Conelea, C. A., & Woods, D. W. (2008). Examining the impact of distraction on tic suppression in children and adolescents with Tourette syndrome. *Behaviour Research and Therapy, 46*(11), 1193–1200. http://dx.doi.org/10.1016/j.brat.2008.07.005

Conelea, C. A., Woods, D. W., & Brandt, B. C. (2011). The impact of a stress induction task on tic frequencies in youth with Tourette syndrome. *Behaviour Research and Therapy, 49*(8), 492–7. http://dx.doi.org/10.1016/j.brat.2011.05.006

Corbetta, M. (1998). Frontoparietal cortical networks for directing attention and the eye to visual locations: Identical, independent, or overlapping neural systems? *Proceedings of the National Academy of Sciences of the United States of America, 95*(3), 831–8. http://dx.doi.org/10.1073/pnas.95.3.831

Corbetta, M., Kincade, J. M., Ollinger, J. M., McAvoy, M. P., & Shulman, G. L. (2000). Voluntary orienting is dissociated from target detection in human posterior parietal cortex. *Nature Neuroscience, 3*(3), 292–7. http://dx.doi.org/10.1038/73009

Corbetta, M., & Shulman, G. L. (2002). Control of goal-directed and stimulus-driven attention in the brain. *Nature Reviews Neuroscience, 3*(3), 201–15. http://dx.doi.org/10.1038/nrn755

Coull, J., Nobre, A., & Frith, C. (2001). The noradrenergic α2 agonist clonidine modulates behavioural and neuroanatomical correlates of human attentional orienting and alerting. *Cerebral Cortex, 11*(1), 73–84. http://dx.doi.org/10.1093/cercor/11.1.73

Davidson, M. C., & Marrocco, R. T. (2000). Local infusion of scopolamine into intraparietal cortex slows covert orienting in rhesus monkeys. *Journal of Neurophysiology, 83*(3), 1536–49.

Eddy, C. M., Rickards, H. E., & Cavanna, A. E. (2012). Executive functions in uncomplicated Tourette syndrome. *Psychiatry Research, 200*(1), 46–8. http://dx.doi.org/10.1016/j.psychres.2012.05.023

Egan, M. F., Kojima, M., Callicott, J. H., Goldberg, T. E., Kolachana, B. S., Bertolino, A., ... Dean, M. (2003). The BDNF val66met polymorphism affects activity-dependent secretion of BDNF and human memory and hippocampal function. *Cell, 112*(2), 257–69. http://dx.doi.org/10.1016/S0092-8674(03)00035-7

Fair, D. A., Cohen, A. L., Power, J. D., Dosenbach, N. U., Church, J. A., Miezin, F. M., ... Petersen, S. E. (2009). Functional brain networks develop from a "local to distributed" organization. *PLOS Computational Biology*, 5(5), e1000381. http://dx.doi.org/10.1371/journal.pcbi.1000381

Fair, D. A., Dosenbach, N. U., Petersen, S. E., & Schlaggar, B. L. (2012). Resting state studies on the development of control systems. In M. Posner (Ed.), *Cognitive neuroscience of attention* (Vol. 2, pp. 291–311). New York, NY: Guilford.

Fan, J., Fossella, J., Sommer, T., Wu, Y., & Posner, M. (2003). Mapping the genetic variation of executive attention onto brain activity. *Proceedings of the National Academy of Sciences of the United States of America*, 100(12), 7406–11. http://dx.doi.org/10.1073/pnas.0732088100

Fan, J., McCandliss, B. D., Fossella, J., Flombaum, J. I., & Posner, M. (2005). The activation of attentional networks. *Neuroimage*, 26(2), 471–9. http://dx. doi.org/10.1016/j.neuroimage.2005.02.004

Feldman, M. A., Storch, E. A., & Murphy, T. K. (2011). Application of habit reversal training for the treatment of tics in early childhood. *Clinical Case Studies*, 10(2), 173–83. http://dx.doi.org/10.1177/1534650111400728

Felling, R. J., & Singer, H. S. (2011). Neurobiology of Tourette syndrome: current status and need for further investigation. *Journal of Neuroscience*, 31(35), 12387–95. http://dx.doi.org/10.1523/JNEUROSCI.0150-11.2011

Fossella, J., Sommer, T., Fan, J., Wu, Y., Swanson, J. M., Pfaff, D. W., & Posner, M. I. (2002). Assessing the molecular genetics of attention networks. *BMC Neuroscience*, 3(1), 14. http://dx.doi.org/10.1186/1471-2202-3-14

Fransson, P., Skiöld, B., Horsch, S., Nordell, A., Blennow, M., Lagercrantz, H., & Åden, U. (2007). Resting-state networks in the infant brain. *Proceedings of the National Academy of Sciences of the United States of America*, 104(39), 15531–6. http://dx.doi.org/10.1073/pnas.0704380104

Freeman, R. D. (2007). Tic disorders and ADHD: Answers from a world-wide clinical dataset on Tourette syndrome. *European Child & Adolescent Psychiatry*, 16(9), 15–23. http://dx.doi.org/10.1007/s00787-007-1003-7

Freeman, R. D., Fast, D. K., Burd, L., Kerbeshian, J., Robertson, M. M., & Sandor, P. (2000). An international perspective on Tourette syndrome: Selected findings from 3500 individuals in 22 countries. *Developmental Medicine & Child Neurology*, 42(7), 436–47. http://dx.doi.org/10.1017/S0012162200000839

Gao, W., Zhu, H., Giovanello, K. S., Smith, J. K., Shen, D., Gilmore, J. H., & Lin, W. (2009). Evidence on the emergence of the brain's default network from 2-week-old to 2-year-old healthy pediatric subjects. *Proceedings of the National Academy of Sciences of the United States of America*, 106(16), 6790–5. http://dx.doi.org/10.1073/pnas.0811221106

Goldberg, T. E., & Weinberger, D. R. (2004). Genes and the parsing of cognitive processes. *Trends in Cognitive Sciences*, 8(7), 325–35. http://dx.doi.org/10.1016/j.tics.2004.05.011

Gorassini, D. R., Spanos, N. P., Kirsch, I., Capafons, A., Carde-a-Buelna, E., & Amigó, S. (1999). The Carleton skill training program for modifying hypnotic suggestibility: Original version and variations. In I. Kirsch, A.

Capafons, E. Carde-a-Buelna, & S. Amigó (Eds.), *Clinical hypnosis and self-regulation* (pp. 141–77). Washington, DC: American Psychological Association.

Graybiel, A. M., & Canales, J. J. (2000). The neurobiology of repetitive behaviors: Clues to the neurobiology of Tourette syndrome. *Advances in Neurology, 85,* 123–31.

Harrison, B. J., Soriano-Mas, C., Pujol, J., Ortiz, H., López-Solà, M., Hernández-Ribas, R., . . . Pantelis, C. (2009). Altered corticostriatal functional connectivity in obsessive-compulsive disorder. *Archives of General Psychiatry, 66*(11), 1189–1200. http://dx.doi.org/10.1001/archgenpsychiatry.2009.152

Hewlett, B. S., Fouts, H. N., Boyette, A. H., & Hewlett, B. L. (2011). Social learning among Congo Basin hunter-gatherers. *Philosophical Transactions of the Royal Society B: Biological Sciences, 366*(1567), 1168–78. http://dx.doi.org/10.1098/rstb.2010.0373

Holroyd, J. (1996). Hypnosis treatment of clinical pain: Understanding why hypnosis is useful. *International Journal of Clinical and Experimental Hypnosis, 44*(1), 33–51. http://dx.doi.org/10.1080/00207149608416066

Insel, T. (2013). Transforming diagnosis [Blog post]. Retrieved from www.nimh.nih.gov/about/director/2013/transforming-diagnosis.shtml

James, W. (1890). *The principles of psychology* (Vol. 1). New York, NY: Henry Holt. http://dx.doi.org/10.1037/10538-000

Karnath, H. O., & Rorden, C. (2012). The anatomy of spatial neglect. *Neuropsychologia, 50*(6), 1010–17. http://dx.doi.org/10.1016/j.neuropsychologia.2011.06.027

Ketay, S., Aron, A., & Hedden, T. (2009). Culture and attention: Evidence from brain and behavior. *Progress in Brain Research, 178,* 79–92. http://dx.doi.org/10.1016/S0079-6123(09)17806-8

Kiecolt-Glaser, J. K., Marucha, P. T., Atkinson, C., & Glaser, R. (2001). Hypnosis as a modulator of cellular immune dysregulation during acute stress. *Journal of Consulting and Clinical Psychology, 69*(4), 674–82. http://dx.doi.org/10.1037/0022-006X.69.4.674

Kirmayer, L. J., & Crafa, D. (2014). What kind of science for psychiatry? *Frontiers in Human Neuroscience, 8,* 435. http://dx.doi.org/10.3389/fnhum.2014.00435

Kirsch, I., Montgomery, G., & Sapirstein, G. (1995). Hypnosis as an adjunct to cognitive-behavioral psychotherapy: A meta-analysis. *Journal of Consulting and Clinical Psychology, 63*(2), 214–20. http://dx.doi.org/10.1037/0022-006X.63.2.214

Kohen, D. P., & Olness, K. (2011). *Hypnosis and hypnotherapy with children.* New York, NY: Routledge

Kushner, H. I. (1999). *A cursing brain? The histories of Tourette syndrome.* Cambridge, MA: Harvard University Press.

LaHoste, G., Swanson, J., Wigal, S., Glabe, C., Wigal, T., King, N., & Kennedy, J. (1996). Dopamine D4 receptor gene polymorphism is associated with attention deficit hyperactivity disorder. *Molecular Psychiatry, 1*(2), 121–4.

Leckman, J. F., Bloch, M. H., Smith, M. E., Larabi, D., & Hampson, M. (2010). Neurobiological substrates of Tourette's disorder. *Journal of Child and*

Adolescent Psychopharmacology, 20(4), 237–47. http://dx.doi.org/10.1089/cap.2009.0118

Leckman, J. F., Zhang, H., Vitale, A., Lahnin, F., Lynch, K., Bondi, C., ... Peterson, B. S. (1998). Course of tic severity in Tourette syndrome: The first two decades. *Pediatrics, 102*(1), 14–19. http://dx.doi.org/10.1542/peds.102.1.14

Lifshitz, M., Aubert Bonn, N., Fischer, A., Kashem, I. F., & Raz, A. (2013). Using suggestion to modulate automatic processes: From Stroop to McGurk and beyond. *Cortex, 49*(2), 463–73. http://dx.doi.org 10.1016/j.cortex.2012.08.007

Losier, B. J., & Klein, R. M. (2001). A review of the evidence for a disengage deficit following parietal lobe damage. *Neuroscience & Biobehavioral Reviews, 25*(1), 1–13. http://dx.doi.org/10.1016/S0149-7634(00)00046-4

Macaluso, E., Frith, C. D., & Driver, J. (2000). Modulation of human visual cortex by crossmodal spatial attention. *Science, 289*(5482), 1206–8. http://dx.doi.org/10.1126/science.289.5482.1206

MacDonald, A. W., Cohen, J. D., Stenger, V. A., & Carter, C. S. (2000). Dissociating the role of the dorsolateral prefrontal and anterior cingulate cortex in cognitive control. *Science, 288*(5472), 1835–8. http://dx.doi.org/10.1126/science.288.5472.1835

Macdonald, E., & Raz, A. (2014). The marginalization of phenomenological consciousness [Book review]. *Frontiers in Human Neuroscience, 8*, 306. http://dx.doi.org/10.3389/fnhum.2014.00306

Marrocco, R. T., & Davidson, M. C. (1998). Neurochemistry of attention. In R. Parasuraman (Ed.), *The attentive brain* (pp. 35–50). Cambridge, MA: MIT Press.

Mesulam, M. (1981). A cortical network for directed attention and unilateral neglect. *Annals of Neurology, 10*(4), 309–25. http://dx.doi.org/10.1002/ana.410100402

Miresco, M., & Kirmayer, L. (2006). The persistence of mind-brain dualism in psychiatric reasoning about clinical scenarios. *American Journal of Psychiatry, 163*(5), 913–18. http://dx.doi.org/10.1176/appi.ajp.163.5.913

Montgomery, G. H., DuHamel, K. N., & Redd, W. H. (2000). A meta-analysis of hypnotically induced analgesia: How effective is hypnosis? *International Journal of Clinical and Experimental Hypnosis, 48*(2), 138–53. http://dx.doi.org/10.1080/00207140008410045

Müller-Vahl, K. R., Kaufmann, J., Grosskreutz, J., Dengler, R., Emrich, H. M., & Peschel, T. (2009). Prefrontal and anterior cingulate cortex abnormalities in Tourette Syndrome: Evidence from voxel-based morphometry and magnetization transfer imaging. *BMC Neuroscience, 10*(1), 47. http://dx.doi.org/10.1186/1471-2202-10-47

Nash, M. R., & Barnier, A. J. (Eds.). (2012). *The Oxford handbook of hypnosis: Theory, research, and practice.* New York, NY: Oxford University Press.

Parasuraman, R., Greenwood, P. M., Haxby, J. V., & Grady, C. L. (1992). Visuospatial attention in dementia of the Alzheimer type. *Brain, 115*(3), 711–33. http://dx.doi.org/10.1093/brain/115.3.711

Parasuraman, R., Greenwood, P. M., Kumar, R., & Fossella, J. (2005). Beyond heritability: Neurotransmitter genes differentially modulate visuospatial

attention and working memory. *Psychological Science, 16*(3), 200–7. http://dx.
doi.org/10.1111/j.0956-7976.2005.00804.x

Pardo, J. V., Pardo, P. J., Janer, K. W., & Raichle, M. E. (1990). The anterior
cingulate cortex mediates processing selection in the Stroop attentional
conflict paradigm. *Proceedings of the National Academy of Sciences of the United
States of America, 87*(1), 256–9. http://dx.doi.org/10.1073/pnas.87.1.256

Perlman, D. M., Salomons, T. V., Davidson, R. J., & Lutz, A. (2010).
Differential effects on pain intensity and unpleasantness of two meditation
practices. *Emotion, 10*(1), 65–71. http://dx.doi.org/10.1037/a0018440

Perry, R., & Zeki, S. (2000). The neurology of saccades and covert shifts in
spatial attention: An event-related fMRI study. *Brain, 123*(11), 2273–88.
http://dx.doi.org/10.1093/brain/123.11.2273

Peterson, B. S., & Cohen, D. J. (1998). The treatment of Tourette's syndrome:
Multimodal, developmental intervention. *Journal of Clinical Psychiatry,
59*(1), 62–72.

Peterson, B. S., Skudlarski, P., Anderson, A. W., Zhang, H., Gatenby, J. C.,
Lacadie, C. M., ... Gore, J. C. (1998). A functional magnetic resonance
imaging study of tic suppression in Tourette syndrome. *Archives of General
Psychiatry, 55*(4), 326–33. http://dx.doi.org/10.1001/archpsyc.55.4.326

Phelps, L. (2008). Tourette's disorder: Genetic update, neurological correlates,
and evidence-based interventions. *School Psychology Quarterly, 23*(2), 282–9.
http://dx.doi.org/10.1037/1045-3830.23.2.282

Piacentini, J., Woods, D. W., Scahill, L., Wilhelm, S., Peterson, A. L.,
Chang, S., ... Levi-Pearl, S. (2010). Behavior therapy for children with
Tourette disorder. *Journal of the American Medical Association, 303*(19),
1929–37. http://dx.doi.org/10.1001/jama.2010.607

Posner, M. (2004). *Cognitive neuroscience of attention* (1st ed.). New York, NY:
Guilford Press.

Posner, M. (2012a). *Attention in a social world.* New York, NY: Oxford University
Press. http://dx.doi.org/10.1093/acprof:oso/9780199791217.001.0001

Posner, M. (2012b). *Cognitive neuroscience of attention* (2nd ed.). New York, NY:
Guilford Press.

Posner, M., & Fan, J. (2008). Attention as an organ system. In J. R. Pomerantz
(Ed.), *Topics in integrative neuroscience* (pp. 31–61). New York, NY:
Cambridge University Press. http://dx.doi.org/10.1017/
CBO9780511541681.005

Posner, M., Inhoff, A. W., Friedrich, F. J., & Cohen, A. (1987). Isolating
attentional systems: A cognitive-anatomical analysis. *Psychobiology, 15*(2),
107–21.

Posner, M., & Petersen, S. E. (1990). The attention system of the human brain.
Annual Review of Neuroscience, 13(1), 25–42. http://dx.doi.org/10.1146/
annurev.ne.13.030190.000325

Posner, M., & Raichle, M. E. (1994). *Images of mind.* New York, NY: Scientific
American Library/Scientific American Books.

Posner, M., & Raichle, M. E. (1998). The neuroimaging of human brain
function. *Proceedings of the National Academy of Sciences of the United States of
America, 95*(3), 763–4. http://dx.doi.org/10.1073/pnas.95.3.763

Posner, M., & Rothbart, M. K. (2005). Influencing brain networks: Implications for education. *Trends in Cognitive Sciences, 9*(3), 99–103. http://dx.doi.org/10.1016/j.tics.2005.01.007

Posner, M., Rothbart, M. K., Sheese, B. E., & Voelker, P. (2012). Control networks and neuromodulators of early development. *Developmental Psychology, 48*(3), 827–35. http://dx.doi.org/10.1037/a0025530

Posner, M. I., Rothbart, M. K., Sheese, B. E., & Voelker, P. (2014). Developing attention: Behavioral and brain mechanisms. *Advances in Neuroscience.* http://dx.doi.org/10.1155/2014/405094

Posner, M. I., Walker, J. A., Friedrich, F. J., & Rafal, R. D. (1984). Effects of parietal injury on covert orienting of attention. *Journal of Neuroscience, 4*(7), 1863–74.

Pringsheim, T., & Pearce, M. (2010). Complications of antipsychotic therapy in children with Tourette syndrome. *Pediatric Neurology, 43*(1), 17–20. http://dx.doi.org/10.1016/j.pediatrneurol.2010.02.012

Rabipour, S., & Raz, A. (2012). Training the brain: Fact and fad in cognitive and behavioral remediation. *Brain and Cognition, 79*(2), 159–79. http://dx.doi.org/10.1016/j.bandc.2012.02.006

Raz, A. & Harris, C. (Eds.). (in press). *Talking placebos: Modern perspectives on placebos in society.* Oxford, England: Oxford University Press.

Raz, A. (2012). Hypnosis as a lens to the development of attention. *Consciousness and Cognition, 21*, 1595–8. http://dx.doi.org/10.1016/j.concog.2012.05.011

Raz, A., & Buhle, J. (2006). Typologies of attentional networks. *Nature Reviews Neuroscience, 7*(5), 367–79. http://dx.doi.org/10.1038/nrn1903

Raz, A., Hongtu, Z., Shan, Y., Bansal, R., Zhishun, W., Alexander, G. M., . . . Peterson, B. S. (2009). Neural substrates of self-regulatory control in children and adults with Tourette syndrome. *Canadian Journal of Psychiatry, 54*(9), 579–88.

Raz, A., Keller, S., Norman, K., & Senechal, D. (2007). Elucidating Tourette's syndrome: Perspectives from hypnosis, attention and self-regulation. *American Journal of Clinical Hypnosis, 49*(4), 289–309. http://dx.doi.org/10.1080/00029157.2007.10524506

Raz, A., Kirsch, I., Pollard, J., & Nitkin-Kaner, Y. (2006). Suggestion reduces the Stroop effect. *Psychological Science, 17*(2), 91–5. http://dx.doi.org/10.1111/j.1467-9280.2006.01669.x

Raz, A., Moreno-Íniguez, M., Martin, L., & Zhu, H. (2007). Suggestion overrides the Stroop effect in highly hypnotizable individuals. *Consciousness and Cognition, 16*(2), 331–8. http://dx.doi.org/10.1016/j.concog.2006.04.004

Raz, A., Shapiro, T., Fan, J., & Posner, M. (2002). Hypnotic suggestion and the modulation of Stroop interference. *Archives of General Psychiatry, 59*(12), 1155. http://dx.doi.org/10.1001/archpsyc.59.12.1155

Raz, A., & Wolfson, J. B. (2010). From dynamic lesions to brain imaging of behavioral lesions: Alloying the gold of psychoanalysis with the copper of suggestion. *Neuropsychoanalysis: An Interdisciplinary Journal for Psychoanalysis and the Neurosciences, 12*(1), 5–18. http://dx.doi.org/10.1080/15294145.2010.10773621

Robertson, M. M. (2006). Mood disorders and Gilles de la Tourette's syndrome: An update on prevalence, etiology, comorbidity, clinical associations, and implications. *Journal of Psychosomatic Research, 61*(3), 349–58. http://dx.doi.org/10.1016/j.jpsychores.2006.07.019

Rothbart, M. K. (2011). *Becoming who we are: Temperament and personality in development.* New York, NY: Guilford Press.

Rothbart, M. K., Posner, M., & Kieras, J. (2006). Temperament, attention, and the development of self-regulation. In K. McCartney & D. Phillips (Eds.), *Blackwell handbook of early childhood development* (pp. 338–57). Malden, MA: Blackwell. http://dx.doi.org/10.1002/9780470757703.ch17

Rueda, M., Checa, P., & Santonja, M. (2008). Training executive attention in preschoolers: Lasting effects and transfer to affective self-regulation. Paper presented at the Annual Meeting of the Cognitive Neuroscience Society, San Francisco, CA, USA.

Rueda, M., Posner, M., & Rothbart, M. (2011). Attention and self regulation. In R. F. Baumeister & K. D. Vohs (Eds.), *Handbook of self-regulation: Research, theory and applications* (2nd ed., pp. 284–99). New York, NY: Guilford Press.

Scahill, L., Bitsko, R., Visser, S., & Blumberg, S. (2009). Prevalence of diagnosed Tourette syndrome in persons aged 6–17 years, United States, 2007. *Morbidity and Mortality Weekly Report, 58*(21), 581–5.

Schafer, R. J., & Moore, T. (2007). Attention governs action in the primate frontal eye field. *Neuron, 56*(3), 541–51. http://dx.doi.org/10.1016/j.neuron.2007.09.029

Shafritz, K. M., Collins, S. H., & Blumberg, H. P. (2006). The interaction of emotional and cognitive neural systems in emotionally guided response inhibition. *Neuroimage, 31*(1), 468–75. http://dx.doi.org/10.1016/j.neuroimage.2005.11.053

Sheese, B. E., Voelker, P. M., Rothbart, M. K., & Posner, M. (2007). Parenting quality interacts with genetic variation in dopamine receptor D4 to influence temperament in early childhood. *Development and Psychopathology, 19*(4), 1039. http://dx.doi.org/10.1017/S0954579407000521

Sowell, E. R., Kan, E., Yoshii, J., Thompson, P. M., Bansal, R., Xu, D., . . . Peterson, B. S. (2008). Thinning of sensorimotor cortices in children with Tourette syndrome. *Nature Neuroscience, 11*(6), 637–9. http://dx.doi.org/10.1038/nn.2121

Spanos, N. P., Lush, N. I., & Gwynn, M. I. (1989). Cognitive skill-training enhancement of hypnotizability: Generalization effects and trance logic responding. *Journal of Personality and Social Psychology, 56*(5), 795–804. http://dx.doi.org/10.1037/0022-3514.56.5.795

Steeves, T., McKinlay, B. D., Gorman, D., Billinghurst, L., Day, L., Carroll, A., . . . Sandor, P. (2012). Canadian guidelines for the evidence-based treatment of tic disorders: Behavioural therapy, deep brain stimulation, and transcranial magnetic stimulation. *Canadian Journal of Psychiatry [Revue Canadienne de Psychiatrie], 57*(3), 144–51.

Swain, J. E., Scahill, L., Lombroso, P. J., King, R. A., & Leckman, J. F. (2007). Tourette syndrome and tic disorders: A decade of progress. *Journal of the American Academy of Child & Adolescent Psychiatry, 46*(8), 947–68. http://dx.doi.org/10.1097/chi.0b013e318068fbcc

Swanson, J. M., Posner, M., Potkin, S., Bonforte, S., Youpa, D., Fiore, C., … Crinella, F. (1991). Activating tasks for the study of visual-spatial attention in ADHD children: A cognitive anatomic approach. *Journal of Child Neurology, 6*(Suppl. 1), S119–27.

Tang, Y.-Y., Lu, Q., Geng, X., Stein, E. A., Yang, Y., & Posner, M. (2010). Short-term meditation induces white matter changes in the anterior cingulate. *Proceedings of the National Academy of Sciences of the United States of America, 107*(35), 15649–52. http://dx.doi.org/10.1073/pnas.1011043107

Tang, Y.-Y., Ma, Y., Wang, J., Fan, Y., Feng, S., Lu, Q., … Fan, M. (2007). Short-term meditation training improves attention and self-regulation. *Proceedings of the National Academy of Science of the United States of America, 104*(43), 17152–6. http://dx.doi.org/10.1073/pnas.0707678104

Tang, Y.-Y., & Posner, M. (2009). Attention training and attention state training. *Trends in Cognitive Sciences, 13*(5), 222–7. http://dx.doi.org/10.1016/j.tics.2009.01.009

Tang, Y.-Y., Rothbart, M. K., & Posner, M. (2012). Neural correlates of establishing, maintaining, and switching brain states. *Trends in Cognitive Sciences, 16*(6), 330–7. http://dx.doi.org/10.1016/j.tics.2012.05.001

Thompson, K. G., Biscoe, K. L., & Sato, T. R. (2005). Neuronal basis of covert spatial attention in the frontal eye field. *Journal of Neuroscience, 25*(41), 9479–87. http://dx.doi.org/10.1523/JNEUROSCI.0741-05.2005

Titchener, E. B. (1909). *The psychology of feeling and attention.* New York, NY: Macmillan.

Uttal, W. R. (2001). *The new phrenology: The limits of localizing cognitive processes in the brain.* Cambridge, MA: MIT Press.

Voelker, P., Sheese, B. E., Rothbart, M. K., & Posner, M. (2009). Variations in catechol-O-methyltransferase gene interact with parenting to influence attention in early development. *Neuroscience, 164*(1), 121–30. http://dx.doi.org/10.1016/j.neuroscience.2009.05.059

Vuilleumier, P. O., & Rafal, R. D. (2000). A systematic study of visual extinction between- and within-field deficits of attention in hemispatial neglect. *Brain, 123*(6), 1263–79. http://dx.doi.org/10.1093/brain/123.6.1263

Welter, M.-L., Burbaud, P., Fernandez-Vidal, S., Bardinet, E., Coste, J., Piallat, B., … Devaux, B. (2011). Basal ganglia dysfunction in OCD: Subthalamic neuronal activity correlates with symptoms severity and predicts high-frequency stimulation efficacy. *Translational Psychiatry, 1*(5), e5. http://dx.doi.org/10.1038/tp.2011.5

Wile, D. J., & Pringsheim, T. M. (2013). Behavior therapy for Tourette syndrome: A systematic review and meta-analysis. *Current Treatment Options in Neurology, 15*(4), 385–95. http://dx.doi.org/10.1007/s11940-013-0238-5

Willcutt, E. G., Doyle, A. E., Nigg, J. T., Faraone, S. V., & Pennington, B. F. (2005). Validity of the executive function theory of attention-deficit/ hyperactivity disorder: A meta-analytic review. *Biological Psychiatry, 57*(11), 1336–46. http://dx.doi.org/10.1016/j.biopsych.2005.02.006

Zeidan, F., Johnson, S. K., Diamond, B. J., David, Z., & Goolkasian, P. (2010). Mindfulness meditation improves cognition: Evidence of brief mental training. *Consciousness and Cognition, 19*(2), 597–605. http://dx.doi.org/10.1016/j.concog.2010.03.014

12 *Reflections*
Hearing Voices – How Social Context Shapes
Psychiatric Symptoms

T. M. Luhrmann

From the first, psychiatry has been torn between understanding serious mental illness as a dramatic expression of the strains of ordinary living and as a disease, as something fundamentally different from the everyday, more like pellagra or diabetes than sadness.

Freud thought that mental illness arose out of emotional conflict. To be human was to live with impulses we could not acknowledge and losses we could not bear. Ordinary life was thus a habituated management of personal pain. "Depression" and "psychosis" were simply names we gave to patterns of self-management which were so woefully inadequate that those who used them could not function. Diagnosis was not particularly important. What mattered to Freud was the clinician's ability to recognize particular patterns of interpreting emotions and responding to them – emotion–motivation–behavior bundles, if you will – and to help the person who enacted these patterns recognize them as patterns, as choices, which could be changed. The psychoanalyst empathized with a patient as a person like himself, struggling with similar burdens of thwarted love and future death, and the psychoanalyst understood that whatever medicine the person might take, what truly mattered in the end was the ability to help that person to recognize why they responded to people as they did.

Kraepelin was born the same year as Freud (1856) in a similar European milieu. But when Kraepelin looked at people with serious mental illness, he saw disease. He set out to identify specific diseases by identifying symptoms that marked people off as different, and distinguishing these diseases from one another by symptom cluster, illness trajectory, and outcome. He paid attention to family history, not because he thought that families might socialize similar responses to life's challenges, but because he thought that these diseases might be heritable. He assumed that our hope of treating them was to distinguish them clearly enough to understand them. The biomedically oriented psychiatrist within the Kraepelinian tradition empathizes with a patient as a person different from himself, struggling with an alien and unchosen burden, like someone who has been diagnosed with cancer. She understands that whatever compassionate care she may offer, her most important intervention is to prescribe the right medication. She puts her faith in science.

Freud's model dominated American psychiatry until the last decades of the twentieth century, when it was replaced more and more by a Kraepelinian one. And because the shift was born out of disappointment and frustration with an approach that, in the end, did not seem to cure serious mental illness, the biomedical psychiatry that emerged in response presented itself as an entirely new beginning. As Nancy Andreasen wrote in one of the manifestos of the period:

> Psychiatry now recognizes that the serious mental illnesses as diseases in the same sense that cancer or high blood pressure are diseases. Mental illnesses are diseases that affect the brain, which is an organ of the body just as the heart or the stomach is. People who suffer from mental illness suffer from a sick or broken brain, not from a weak will, laziness, bad character or a bad upbringing. (Andreasen, 1984, p. 8)

This book, explained one of its blurbs, "chronicles a revolution in psychiatry that has returned this battered specialty to its birthplace in medicine."

It is now clear that the simple biomedical approach to serious psychiatric illness has failed in turn. As Raz and Macdonald point out, "decades of work on cognitive, molecular and systems neuroscience have taught most scientists a lesson in humility. Despite an enormous investment in research with an emphasis on the neural correlates of typical and atypical behavioral "phenotypes," breakthroughs are sorely lacking." At least, the confidence that these illnesses would be understood as brain disorders with clearly identifiable genetic causes and clear, targeted pharmacological interventions – what some researchers call the bio-bio-bio model: brain lesion, genetic cause, pharmacological cure – has faded into mist (Read, 2005). To be sure, it would be too strong to say that we should no longer think of a condition such as schizophrenia as a brain disease. One often has a profound sense, when confronted with a person diagnosed with schizophrenia, that something has gone badly wrong with the brain.

Yet the outcome of two decades of serious psychiatric science is that schizophrenia now appears to be a complex outcome of many unrelated causes – the genes you inherit, but also whether your mom fell ill during her pregnancy, whether you got beaten up as a child or were stressed as an adolescent, even how much sun your skin has seen. It's not just about the brain. It's not just about genes. In fact, in terms of causation, schizophrenia looks more and more like diabetes. A messy array of risk factors predisposes someone to develop diabetes: smoking, being overweight, collecting fat around the middle rather than on the hips, high blood pressure, and family history. These risk factors are not intrinsically connected to one another. Some of them have something to do with genes, but most of them do not. In fact they hang together so loosely that physicians now speak of a metabolic "syndrome," something far looser and vaguer than an "illness," let alone a "disease." Psychiatric researchers increasingly think about schizophrenia and other psychiatric illnesses in similar terms.

And so the NIMH has shifted the scientific emphasis back to the ways in which people with serious mental illness are, in effect, more like the rest of us. The structure of the new approach to research is to search for specific alterations of specific human psychobiological symptoms, and to abandon (at least in the research) specific categories of disease. It is a remarkable experiment for a scientific field defined for decades by nosological categories.

Some see this new orientation as a mistake. Laurence Kirmayer and Daina Crafa, for example, describe it as impoverished and conceptually flawed:

Moving the search for mechanism back several steps in the causal chain to putative endophenotypes may increase the likelihood of finding certain lower-level mechanisms but it will not provide a complete explanation of how most symptoms are produced nor will it adequately address the role in psychopathology of processes of self-understanding, coping, and interpersonal communication or interaction with others. (Kirmayer & Crafa, 2014, p. 4)

This is an understandable response and many people are sympathetic to it – including many psychiatric scientists who have spent their careers focused on specific diseases and now see the scaffolding of their research ripped out from under them. Kirmayer and Crafa are particularly concerned that the emphasis on neuroscience will diminish the attention to cultural variation and social meaning in the study of mental illness.

My take is more optimistic. I think that this may be an opportunity not only for psychiatry, but for anthropology. From my reading, the RDoC criteria take seriously the basic insight of anthropology: that humans are fundamentally social animals and that the social gets under our skins in profound ways. It remains to be seen, of course, whether NIMH funding will acknowledge the contributions anthropology has to offer. Nevertheless, the shift invites us to think carefully about the specific ways in which social context shapes psychiatric illness.

Let me offer three examples of the way that social context may direct specific psychological processes and so shape psychiatric symptoms. The three chapters, other than Bilder's (Chapter 8), which form this section suggest that attention, emotion regulation, and early trauma shape symptom expression. The work that I and my colleagues have done with people with serious psychotic disorder suggests that social context may shape the way people attend to their voices; the inferences they draw about who is speaking to them, and thus, how they experience their voices emotionally; and, in general, the risk that someone will fall ill with psychosis.

When someone becomes psychotic and begins to hear voices, they often experience a wide range of auditory events (Tuttle, 1902). They hear bad voices and good voices, voices that command and voices that comment. They have internal events and external events and events that seem somehow in between. They hear hissing and murmuring and sounds that seem to fall off cars as they pass and resolve into voices. When I and my colleagues interviewed twenty people with serious psychotic disorder in each of Accra (Ghana); Chennai (India); and San Mateo (California), we found that they reported quite different experiences (Luhrman, Padmavati, Tharoor, & Osei, 2014; Luhrmann, Padmavati, Tharoor, & Osei, in press). In general, Americans hated their voices. They experienced their voices as assaults, and they reported that their voices were more violent. None of them reported their voice-hearing experiences to be primarily or exclusively positive. By contrast, many patients in Accra and Chennai described their voice-hearing experience as positive – half the patients in Accra, and over a third of those in Chennai. They more often talked about liking their voices, even when they said that the voices were mean. They did, to be sure, report voices that were caustic and told them to kill themselves – but less often.

Why would people with psychosis experience hallucinated voices differently in different social settings? There is no reason to think that the disease process of psychosis differs in these different settings. We concluded that local expectations shaped the ways that subjects were paying attention to the complex array of auditory events. In particular, we thought that local expectations about the mind – what we could call local theory of mind, the ways people understand thoughts and feelings – might alter the way people attend to sensory or quasi-sensory data. Americans imagine the mind as a separate, private place – as "bounded," to use Charles Taylor's (2007) phrase, walled off from an external material world (D'Andrade, 1987). There are no cultural expectations that there are many supernatural beings who talk frequently. Even

American Christians who embrace a faith in which God speaks back need to learn that God will do so frequently, and they are not taught that God will speak back audibly (Luhrmann, 2012). The only meanings Americans tend to ascribe to their auditory hallucinations is that they are the signs of being "crazy," and so it makes sense that Americans would dislike their voices, and feel them to be intrusions. This may lead them to attend more to their least pleasant experiences.

Ghanaians and South Asians, by contrast, live in social worlds in which spirits are widely understood to be present. It is not the case that the only meaning of hearing a voice is that one is crazy. The large majority of our Ghanaian subjects were Christian. They understood demons to be real, and they took God to be capable of controlling them. Our Chennai subjects were largely Hindu. They live within a social world in which Hindu spirits take command of human bodies and speak to them. There are distinctive class and caste expectations involved, but it is an evident part of this social world that invisible spirits can speak. Some of our Chennai subjects even experienced their voices as having the playfulness associated with some Hindu avatars. For both Accra and Chennai subjects, then, there would be more of a cultural invitation to attend to their most positive voices and to treat those voices as real invisible beings.

It is important to be clear that these differences in voice hearing are differences in emphasis. They are not absolute. There was no question that subjects in Chennai and Accra were ill. They knew they were ill and they would have preferred not to be ill. But they were much less critical of their voices – on average – than the Americans were.

Another striking difference in voice hearing was that in general, our American subjects did not know who was speaking to them. Subjects in Accra and Chennai were far more likely to say that they knew the real humans who spoke to them in this disembodied way. They were also more likely to say that the voices gave them good advice, and that they valued the advice – even if they did not like the voices. They were more likely to treat their voices as sources of comfort and aid during their illness, rather than as the cause of their illness, as the Americans often insisted. We concluded that differences in the culturally varied experience of the self may have shifted the way people incorporated voice hearing into their daily lives.

One of the most robust observations in cultural psychology and psychological anthropology is that Europeans and Americans imagine themselves as individuals – set apart and in contrast to others. The more "independent" emphasis of what we typically call the "West" and the more "interdependent" emphasis of other societies has been demonstrated ethnographically and experimentally many times in many places – among them, India and Africa (Markus, Mullally, & Kitayama, 1997; Nisbett, 2003). This research does not suggest that people experience themselves in the same ways outside of the West; its point is that relationships with others are far more salient to the way non-Westerners (and certainly, South Asians and Africans) interpret their experience than they are to Westerners.

We believe that these social expectations about persons may shape the voice-hearing experience of those with serious psychotic disorder. The Chennai and Accra patients were more comfortable interpreting their voices as relationships, and not as the sign of a violated mind. Although there is robust evidence that emotional dysregulation contributes to the emergence of serious psychotic disorder, these data suggest that to some extent, the tendency to infer that voices are people may mitigate some of the distress. A number of studies have now suggested that psychosis has a more benign course and trajectory outside of the West, with the best data coming from India (Hopper, Harrison, Janca, & Sartorius, 2007). It is possible that these differences in voice hearing contribute to that more benign course and outcome.

It appears from our evidence that auditory hallucinations are not only construed differently in different cultural settings, but that their affective tone actually shifts – an observation in accord with the new cognitive-developmental model of psychotic hallucinations, which argues that cognitive bias – as well as cognitive deficit – shapes the rate, content, and phenomenology of psychotic hallucination. (Bentall, Fernyhough, Morrison, Lewis, & Corcoran, 2007) We suggest that everyday expectations determine (to some extent) the way subjects attend to the messy array of auditory events that occur for most people with serious psychotic disorder and, in consequence, alter those auditory phenomena: that everyday, socially shaped expectations alter not only how what is heard is interpreted, but what is actually heard. And it is possible that these differences have clinical implications (Connor & Birchwood, 2013).

The evidence that early-life adversity increases the risk of developing serious psychotic disorder, as well as suicide, is increasingly robust (Bentall, Wickham, Shevlin, & Varese, 2012). People who are humiliated and abused and bullied are more likely to fall ill with schizophrenia. People who are born poor or live poor are more likely to develop schizophrenia. People with dark skins are more likely to fall ill in white-skinned neighborhoods, probably (scientists think) because they feel their lesser social status more keenly. People who live urban, too, are more likely to fall ill with the condition, perhaps because they are more likely to feel socially threatened. When life beats people up, they are at more risk of developing psychosis, and for the most part both our epidemiology and our ethnography suggest that the best way to understand social causation in schizophrenia is through the experience of social defeat: a social encounter in which one person physically or symbolically loses to another (see Morgan, McKenzie, & Fearon, 2008, for summary; see also McKenzie, & Shah, Chapter 13, *this volume*). And it is striking that back before the biomedical turn in psychiatry, anthropologists had argued that something like the bodily experience of social defeat explained why some societies had higher-than-average rates of schizophrenia. They saw a daily, constant grind of humiliation and rejection that – they thought – made people ill (Desjarlais, 1995, Hopper, 2003, Jenkins & Barrett, 2004; Scheper-Hughes, 1979). My own work on homeless psychotic women on the streets of Chicago makes it abundantly clear that homelessness is not the best way for our society to treat persons who are falling ill with psychosis, although evidence suggests that it is now normative for such people to experience bouts of homelessness in the United States. That work also suggests that the experience of living on the street with psychosis may exacerbate existing illness and heighten the symptoms of those who are already ill (Luhrmann, 2007).

Indeed, in a forthcoming collection of case studies on the experience of psychosis, we suggest that the social patterning of increased risk of schizophrenia for some social worlds and better outcomes for others can be explained by different vulnerabilities to social defeat (Luhrmann & Marrow, n.d.). Schizophrenia is not only more common in some social conditions, but its effects are mitigated in others, most notably in India and probably elsewhere in the developing world, where both its course and outcome are more benign. We argue that for all the pain in madness everywhere, there seems to be more opportunities for social defeat for a person with madness in the West.

The old bio-bio-bio world invited anthropologists to argue about whether diagnostic categories were real. The new RDoC approach invites us to think about psychiatric illness as a complex syndrome, and to ask how specific social patterns change them. That in turn invites us to think differently, not only about biology but about culture – to deessentialize it, just as we are deessentializing psychopathology. It invites us to ask not what is different about Ghanaian culture, but what it is about a specific sense of self that might be found in another culture, or an expectation about how the mind works, or what counts as trauma. It could be a remarkable opportunity to rethink our field.

312   *T. M. Luhrmann*

REFERENCES

Andreasen, N. (1984). *The broken brain.* New York, NY: Harper & Row.
Bentall, R., Fernyhough, C., Morrison, A., Lewis, S., & Corcoran, R. (2007). Prospects for a cognitive-developmental account of psychotic experiences. *British Journal of Clinical Psychology, 46,* 155–73. http://dx.doi.org/10.1348/014466506X123011
Bentall, R. P., Wickham, S., Shevlin, M., & Varese, F. (2012). Do specific early life adversities lead to specific symptoms of psychosis? A study from the 2007 Adult Psychiatric Morbidity Survey. *Schizophrenia Bulletin, 38*(4), 734–40. http://dx.doi.org/ 10.1093/schbul/sbs049
Bilder, R. M. (2015). Dimensional and categorical approaches to mental illness: Let biology decide. In L. J. Kirmayer, R. Lemelson, & C. A. Cummings (Eds.), *Re-visioning psychiatry: Cultural phenomenology, critical neuroscience, and global mental health* (pp. 179–205). New York, NY: Cambridge University Press.
Connor, C., & Birchwood, M. (2013). Power and perceived expressed emotion of voices: Their impact on depression and suicidal thinking in those who hear voices. *Clinical Psychology and Psychotherapy, 20,* 199–205. http://dx.doi.org/10.1002/cpp.798
D'Andrade, R. (1987). A folk model of the mind. In D. Holland & N. Quinn (Eds.), *Cultural models in language and thought* (pp. 113–47). Cambridge, England: Cambridge University Press. http://dx.doi.org/10.1017/CBO9780511607660.006
Desjarlais, R. (1995). *Shelter blues.* Philadelphia: Pennsylvania University Press.
Hopper, K., Harrison, G., Janca, A., & Sartorius, N. (Eds.). (2007). *Recovery from schizophrenia.* New York, NY: Oxford University Press.
Hopper, K. (2003). *Reckoning with homelessness.* Ithaca, NY: Cornell University Press.
Jenkins, J., & Barrett, R. (Eds.). (2004). *Schizophrenia, culture, and subjectivity.* Cambridge, England: Cambridge University Press.
Kirmayer, L., & Crafa, D. (2014). What kind of science for psychiatry? *Frontiers in Human Neuroscience, 8,* 435. http://dx.doi.org/10.3389/fnhum.2014.00435
Luhrmann, T. M. (2007). Social defeat and the culture of chronicity: Or, why schizophrenia does so well over there and so badly here. *Culture, Medicine, and Psychiatry, 31,* 135–72. http://dx.doi.org/10.1007/s11013-007-9049-z
Luhrmann, T. M. (2012). *When God talks back.* New York, NY: Knopf.
Luhrmann, T. M., & Marrow, J. (Eds.). (2015). *Our most troubling madness: Schizophrenia and social condition.* Manuscript in preparation.
Luhrmann, T. M., Padmavati, R., Tharoor, H., & Osei, A. (2015). Differences in hearing voices associated with psychosis in San Mateo, Chennai and Accra. *British Journal of Psychiatry, 206*(1), 41–4. http://dx.doi.org/10.1192/bjp.bp.113.139048
Luhrmann, T. M., Padmavati, R., Tharoor, H., & Osei, A. (in press). Social kindling of voice-hearing in serious psychotic disorder. *Topics in Cognitive Science.*

Markus, H. R., Mullally, P. R., & Kitayama, S. (1997). Selfways: Diversity in modes of cultural participation. In U. Neisser & D. A. Jopling (Eds.), *The conceptual self in context: Culture, experience, self-understanding* (pp. 13–61). Cambridge, England: Cambridge University Press.

McKenzie, K. , & Shah, J. (2015). Understanding the social etiology of psychosis. In L. J. Kirmayer, R. Lemelson, & C. A. Cummings (Eds.), *Re-visioning psychiatry: Cultural phenomenology, critical neuroscience, and global mental health* (pp. 317–42). New York, NY: Cambridge University Press.

Morgan, C., McKenzie, K., & Fearon, P. (Eds.). (2008). *Society and psychosis.* Cambridge, England: Cambridge University Press. http://dx.doi.org/10.1017/CBO9780511544064

Nisbett, R. (2003). *The geography of thought.* New York, NY: Free Press.

Raz, A., & Macdonald, E. (2015). Paying attention to a field in crisis: Psychiatry, neuroscience, and functional systems of the brain. In L. J. Kirmayer, R. Lemelson, & C. A. Cummings (Eds.), *Re-visioning psychiatry: Cultural phenomenology, critical neuroscience, and global mental health* (pp. 273–304). New York, NY: Cambridge University Press.

Read, J. (2005). The bio-bio-bio model of madness. *The Psychologist, 18,* 596–97.

Scheper-Hughes, N. (1979). *Saints, scholars, and schizophrenics.* Berkeley: University of California Press.

Taylor, C. (2007). *A secular age.* Cambridge, MA: Harvard University Press.

Tuttle, G. (1902). Hallucinations and illusions. *American Journal of Psychiatry, 58,* 443–67.

Section Three

Cultural Contexts of Psychopathology

13   Understanding the Social Etiology of Psychosis

Kwame McKenzie and Jai Shah

Introduction

Prevention of mental illness is considered to be a public health priority, and the World Health Organization (WHO) has amassed an impressive array of evidence-based strategies (Hosman, Jane-Llopis, & Saxena, 2005). These strategies demonstrate that effective prevention can reduce the risk of mental disorders. Although the rhetoric surrounding the importance of preventing mental illness from public health and government departments is rarely matched by the level of implementation of actual strategies, it is generally accepted that social risk factors are important in the genesis and maintenance of common mental disorders and affective states. These disorders are considered to be the result of a complex array of individual vulnerability factors (including biological factors) that interact with social factors to produce symptoms.

There is little disagreement that life events such as loss of a job, divorce, being a victim of a crime, or being exposed to organized violence may cause psychological illness. That chronic stressors such as poverty, domestic abuse, and racial discrimination increase risk is also not contentious. Whether members of the scientific community or the lay public, we agree that, for instance, loss of money or social position can make you feel sad, demoralized, and may cause depression. We agree that you can develop psychological symptoms following a traumatic event. And we agree that anxiety disorders may follow exposure to something that makes you frightened or uneasy. However, because of the commonsense nature, or face validity, of these associations, the mechanisms by which they actually occur may not be given as much scrutiny as they deserve.

A significant research effort is now attempting to identify how social experiences get under the skin and alter gene expression, neurochemistry, and neural circuitry (see, for example, Labonté, Farah, & Turecki, Chapter 8, *this volume*). Furthermore, despite the fact that we are not entirely clear about the mechanisms by which the social environment interacts with biology, governments, public health officials, and mental health specialists seem comfortable with the logical extension of the *zeitgeist* – that interventions designed to decrease exposure to, or the action of, harmful social determinants could lessen the risk of developing mental illness. But they are more comfortable with this approach when considering some mental illnesses more than others. Although psychotic disorders are linked to many of the same social determinants as common mental disorders, they have rarely been the target of major prevention efforts.

Schizophrenia and other psychoses are substantial public health problems that impose a profound impact on national economies, health and social systems, affected individuals, and their families and carers. Recent advances in our understanding of the pathophysiology of psychosis have focused on the brain mechanisms that underlie particular symptoms in the search for improved pharmacological treatments. This may have inadvertently supported the perception that psychoses are "brain diseases" and that models of prevention based on a population health approach focusing on the impact of social determinants may not be relevant. However, a growing literature is outlining the associations between a number of social or societal variables and the onset, course, and outcome of psychosis (Cantor-Graae, 2007; Jones & Fernyhough, 2007; Myin-Germeys & van Os, 2008; Selten & Cantor-Graae, 2005; Shevlin, Houston, Dorahy, & Adamson, 2008; Walker, Mittal, & Tessner, 2008; van Os, Kenis, & Rutten, 2010). Unfortunately, unlike common mental disorders where there are clear and easy-to-understand models of causation, there is so far no agreed-on model or framework for how various social factors modulate the risk of psychotic illnesses. Although these processes are complex, there is a need for simplified models that can facilitate the understanding of these issues by policy makers and health planners and guide the development and targeting of intervention strategies and the evaluation of their effectiveness, as well as the identification of areas for further research. A simplified model could also help us better communicate what we think is going on and build the consensus that has allowed progress in prevention of other psychiatric disorders and in mental health promotion.

The social world is hard to investigate. Particular social determinants may have impacts at single or multiple levels. They may affect the individual, family, group, city, or country, or any mixture of these levels. Teasing out which level is affected can be difficult. The impacts that the risk factors have can be proximal to the exposure, or there may be a significant delay – a latency effect – that needs to be taken into account when trying to measure outcomes. Additionally, social factors may trigger a train of events that increase or change risk over the life course.

Different factors can interact to either decrease or amplify each other's effects. A further complication, according to March, Morgan, Bresnahan, and Susser (2008), is the necessity of distinguishing between social conditions (such as being unemployed) and social processes (such as the mechanisms through which the experience of being unemployed is made unpleasant). Both may be related to the development of mental health problems, but different interventions may be required to change their impacts. Thus, although there is a growing understanding of how social factors may increase the risk of developing a psychotic illness (Jones & Fernyhough, 2007; Kirkbride & Jones, 2011; March & Susser, 2006; Miller et al., 2001; Nuechterlein & Dawson, 1984; Susser, St. Clair, & He, 2008), there is little agreement as to how the information should be ordered.

Social Factors and Psychotic Illness

There are a variety of explanatory models for the impact of social factors on psychotic illness. Social factors may change the exposure to or action of biological risk factors or they may have a direct, toxic effect on individuals and their families. Genetic and epigenetic processes interacting with social factors at the individual, group, and societal levels over a life course produce a complex and interconnected web of causation (Kirkbridge & Jones, 2011; March & Susser, 2006; see also Labonté, Farah, & Turecki, Chapter 8, *this volume*).

Understanding how different social factors change the risk of psychosis has been problematic. In part, this reflects the many possible and interconnected mechanisms and multiple levels through which this could occur (Kirkbridge & Jones, 2011; March & Susser, 2006; Susser et al., 2008). An example would be the reported association between prenatal malnutrition and an increased risk of schizophrenia during adolescence. This association could reflect the impact of nutritional stress on the hypothalamic-pituitary-adrenal (HPA) axis or the direct effects of low levels of nutrients on DNA stability or expression (to name just two theories). At a different level, others have reported that urban or rural residence during famine may change the risk of exposure to malnutrition by determining access to supplementary food, which may be more plentiful in rural areas (Susser et al., 2008). In addition, the reactivity of the HPA axis to nonnutritional forms of stress may be linked to rural or urban residence, as may the number of adverse life events, which may be subsequently important in triggering a psychotic breakdown.

A further problem in trying to understand etiology may derive from the fact that until recently a dichotomy has existed between those who focus on the brain and those who focus on the environment. This produces conceptual difficulties because mental illness straddles both. From a biological perspective, the brain helps us adapt to the environment, but it also develops in response to the environment. Some environmental factors promote healthy brain development and some impede it, but many have a variable impact depending on context. Whether environmental events contribute to individual vulnerability or resiliency depends on many factors, including the previous history of environmental exposures (Daskalakis, Bagot, Parker, Vinkers, & Kloet, 2013). Individuals who have been exposed to more positive environmental influences, that is, fewer social risk factors, tend to be more resilient. For these individuals, exposure to indeterminate social factors leads to the development of a more resilient coping style and they are more likely to be able to meet new challenges. However, if a person has been exposed to more social risk factors for mental illness, some environmental factors are more likely to be experienced as burdensome, and this may further undermine the development of resilience.

These processes have neurodevelopmental parallels: Both the structure and function of the brain are linked to environmental influences. Van Os and colleagues (2010) have detailed the development of brain architecture, as well as neurocognition, affect regulation, and social cognition throughout childhood. They reviewed the associations between specific factors in the social environment and neurocognitive development and linked problems in neurocognitive development during childhood to a later increased risk of schizophrenia (van Os et al., 2010). The best evidence to date associates increased risk of psychosis with growing up in an urban environment, early life adversity, minority group position, and cannabis use.

The mechanisms by which these experiences influence individual biologies are discussed in the next section, but the environment has further impact on mental illness. Mental illness is diagnosed when particular thoughts, behaviors, or functions are considered aberrant. The diagnosis of psychopathology reflects a judgment that a person has not responded properly or adapted adequately to the environment. However, what constitutes a proper response is socially and culturally determined. Consequently, mental illnesses can be viewed as not simply an individual's difficulties in responding or adapting to their environment, but as others' subjective assessments of the adequacy of the way in which that individual responds or adapts. Whether we label an adaptation as aberrant or not is socially mediated, but this normative judgment cannot be circumvented by defining mental disorders in terms of brain dysfunction. If mental illnesses are disorders of adaptation, and the way the brain adapts is in part a response to social and environmental contexts, then mental illness lies in the interaction between brain and environment.

The brain is married to the environment, and it is in that relationship that we view mental illnesses. Trying to understand the marriage by looking at only one partner is unlikely to give an accurate picture. Investigating one without the other resembles attempts to understand and repair a marriage without both parties present. It may give a distorted view of what is happening and may not offer the best basis for treatment. The movement away from research that focuses entirely on the brain or the environment toward investigations that focus on the interactions between the two, as well as the mechanisms underlying those interactions, is a crucial development in the field (van Os et al., 2010).

How Does the Environment Get under the Skin?

There are a number of possible mechanisms through which the environment may have an impact on psychosis risk. In order to clarify the complex nature of the inquiry, in this chapter we will consider just one of the explanatory models for the impact of social factors on psychotic illness: the "vulnerability-stress model" (Myin-Germeys & van Os, 2008; Nuechterlein & Dawson, 1984). This model posits that genetic or developmental vulnerabilities interact with social adversity to influence a common pathway leading to stress-related effects that may culminate in psychosis (Mason et al., 2004; Miller et al., 2001).

Genetic, biochemical, and neurological evidence support the link between stress and psychosis (Jones & Fernyhough, 2007; Walker & Diforio, 1997; Walker, Mittal, & Tessner, 2008). Stress involves some of the best-studied pathways through which environment affects both short- and long-term physiological functioning in social species. Stress activates the HPA axis, which plays a pivotal role in governing physiological responses to threats. This hormonal cascade begins with the hypothalamic release of corticotropin-releasing hormone (CRH), which stimulates the secretion of adrenocorticotropic hormone (ACTH) from the pituitary gland into the bloodstream. ACTH in turn stimulates the production and release of glucocorticoids (GC), or stress hormones (cortisol in humans), from the adrenal cortex, which migrate to several brain areas, including the hippocampus, where they bind to receptors. GC receptor binding exerts an inhibitory or negative feedback loop on the system. Receptor binding in the brain and other organ systems allows GCs to affect neural function, immune responses, and cardiovascular function, as well as other processes important in the stress response (Walker, Mittal, & Tessner, 2008).

However, acquired vulnerabilities such as prenatal exposures, perinatal complications, drug and child abuse, or neglect can dysregulate this response to stress. Links between the physiology of stress and that of psychosis have been reported. For example, the hippocampus, which plays a key role in returning HPA activity to baseline levels, is reduced in volume in psychotic disorders (Geuze, Vermetten, & Bremner, 2005; Fusar-Poli et al., 2007; Lieberman et al., 2001; Steen, Mull, McClure, Hamer, & Lieberman, 2006). Comparisons of monozygotic twins suggest that this reduction is at least partially environmentally caused because the hippocampal volume of the twin with schizophrenia is significantly smaller than that of the healthy twin, presumably reflecting differences in their environmental exposures and life experiences (van Erp et al., 2004).

In a related series of processes, stress also alters the activity of mesolimbic and mesocortical pathways in the brain, which are involved in the transmission of dopamine (a neurotransmitter that may mediate psychotic symptoms) to the limbic system and the prefrontal cortex, respectively (Kapur, 2003; Seeman & Kapur, 2000; Soares & Innis, 1999). Experimental support for this is found, for example, in studies in which psychotic symptoms are associated with increased dopamine release in the mesolimbic pathway after amphetamine challenge (Laruelle & Abi-Dargham, 1999). Over time, in at-risk individuals, exposure to moderate levels of stress can lead to sensitization, leading to an enhanced and persistent dopamine response. Building on this theory, those with higher rates of life stressors may be at particular risk of developing a psychotic illness.

Epidemiologic studies support the impact of life stressors at multiple levels. Cumulative exposure to traumatic life events, or the number of life events experienced, is associated with an increased risk for psychosis (Cantor-Graae, 2007; Selten & Cantor-Graae, 2005, 2007; Shevlin et al., 2008), and the British National Psychiatric Morbidity Survey has reported that adverse life events are associated with subsequent psychotic experiences in the general population (Johns et al., 2004; Wiles et al., 2006). In addition to traumatic major life events, the accumulation of minor events or "daily hassles" has also been linked to psychotic illness (Myin-Germeys & van Os, 2007).

However, it is not just the accumulation of life events that is important. Life events may trigger a train of other events. For instance, loss of a parent as a child (which has been associated with increased risk of later psychosis) could increase the chance of living in poverty and thus exposure to other stress-inducing environmental risk factors associated with psychosis. At the level of gene-environment interaction, it has been suggested that even minor life events and daily hassles interact with polymorphisms known to be involved in dopamine neurotransmission to cause differential stress reactivity and psychotic experiences (van Winkel et al., 2008). Of note, the same polymorphism has been shown to correlate with differential risk for psychosis in individuals who use cannabis (Caspi et al., 2005), further highlighting the complex interplay between multiple biological and environmental risk factors.

Literature outlining the association between childhood trauma and psychosis describes in further detail the psychological, as well as neuro-biological mechanisms, linking adverse experiences to psychosis (van Winkel, van Nierop, Myin-Germeys, & van Os, 2013). These mechanisms include the psychological concepts of social defeat – that is, "the negative experience of being excluded from the majority group" (Selten, van der Ven, Rutten, & Cantor-Graae, 2013) – and negative self-esteem. These processes have neural correlates: sensitization of the mesolimbic dopamine system, which produces a heightened response to low-level stressors; changes in the immune system; and concomitant changes in the size and function of stress-related brain structures, such as the hippo-campus and the amygdala. These mechanisms also interact, as exemplified by the hypothesis that chronic exposure to social defeat may lead to sensi-tization of the mesolimbic dopaminergic system and increased risk of schizophrenia (Selten et al., 2013). According to the hypothesis, social defeat is "the common denominator" for several environmental risk factors, including childhood trauma, urban upbringing, migration, and drug use.

Despite the identification of putative neural mechanisms, it appears that the genes under consideration in much of the current research are not specifically involved in the genesis of psychosis, but more generally in regulating mood (e.g., the serotonin transporter gene), neuroplasticity (brain-derived neurotrophic factor; BDNF), and the stress-response system (the *FKBP5* gene). Moreover, researchers studying families with a strong genetic predisposition for schizophrenia have found that a cumulative adversity index – which includes childhood illness, family instability, and cannabis use – is significantly associated with the risk of schizophrenia and that this is independent of genetic risk (Husted, Ahmed, Chow, Brzustowicz, & Bassett, 2012). Genetic variants and environmental exposures can also interact in ways that are protective and not just harmful. Instead of focusing on "vulnerability genes" that confer increased risk in the presence of certain environments, Belsky and colleagues call for an appreciation of "plasticity genes" that confer a nuanced *differential* susceptibility: increased risk in some environments and decreased risk in others (Belsky et al., 2009).

Physiologically and cognitively, exposure to early developmental stres-sors (such as childhood trauma) may act by sensitizing people to later adverse events, major or minor. Such exposures may increase the likelihood of adverse events, for instance, by shaping the capacity of individuals to form relationships (Myin-Germeys & van Os, 2008; Wright, Turkington, Kingdon, & Ramirez Basco, 2009). Alternately, they may interface with a person's attributional style – potentially making them more prone to psychotic thinking (Bentall, Kinderman, & Kaney, 1994).

The Importance of Place

Moving from the individual to the ecological, there is a wealth of evidence about the impact of the physical environment on health, as well as a growing literature on its impact on mental health. There is evidence that the level of noise, light, and the quality of the fabric of the built environment are all important determinants of health (Cooper, Boyko, & Codinhoto, 2008). In addition, seeing nature, having access to green space, and taking part in activities such as community gardens are generally beneficial for mental health across all age groups. Thus, planting trees in urban areas, making sure that there are parks, and maintaining lawns all have the potential to improve mental well-being, decrease stress, and increase effective management of major life issues. Studies report that children exposed to nature and green space have improved ability to learn, better memory, and better attention (Cooper et al., 2008). At a community level, green space is associated with higher levels of perceived social connectedness to the community and decreased levels of violence (Cooper et al., 2008)

Although there may be beneficial effects from contact with nature, on a global basis people are increasingly moving to cities. According to the most recent version of the United Nation's World Urbanization Prospects study, "over half of the world's population (54 percent) lives in urban areas." This figure is expected to increase to 67 percent in 2050, based on an estimated increase in world population to 9.3 billion (rev.; United Nations, 2014). Because of this trend, work on psychosis has focused mainly on the impact of urban living rather than on the possible benefit of exposure to green spaces.

A major branch of investigation into the social etiology of psychotic illness began in 1939 with Faris and Dunham's work on the urban environment (Faris & Dunham, 1939). Since then, research has focused on better defining urbanicity as a risk factor for psychosis. Studies have demonstrated that the higher risk of psychotic illness for those living in cities is not due to social drift but is associated with being born in or growing up in an urban environment. Moreover, the larger the city, the greater the risk for psychosis (Allardyce et al., 2005; Boydell &

McKenzie, 2008; Kelly et al., 2010; van Os, Hanssen, Bijl, & Vollebergh, 2001). Of course, living in an urban environment is associated with a number of different types of exposures, including the fragmentation of community bonds and economic disparities. Allardyce and colleagues found that, after adjusting for social fragmentation and deprivation, there was only a nonsignificant trend toward an association between urbanicity and schizophrenia (Allardyce et al., 2005).

Other factors may be important for the association between place and psychosis. For instance, Silver and colleagues documented that the proportion of people moving in and out of an area is associated with higher rates of schizophrenia (Silver, Mulvey, & Swanson, 2002). Another pilot study reported that increased social cohesion and social efficacy in areas in London were associated with a reduced incidence of psychosis (Boydell et al., 2001); and after controlling for individual deprivation, Boydell and colleagues found the rate of schizophrenia correlated with increasing neighborhood inequality, but only in more deprived areas (Boydell, van Os, McKenzie, & Murray, 2004).

Many of the benefits of social bonds and community relations have been captured in the notion of "social capital," which is associated with better mental health (McKenzie & Harpham, 2006). In a study with data from the United Kingdom, Kirkbride, Morgan, and colleagues (2007) used multilevel Poisson regression to model the simultaneous effects of individual- and neighborhood-level factors. They found that 23 percent of the incidence of schizophrenia could be attributed to neighborhood-level social risk factors, including socioeconomic deprivation, voter turnout (a proxy for social capital), ethnic fragmentation (proxy for segregation), and ethnic density (95 percent confidence interval 9.9–42.2). One percent increases in voter turnout and ethnic segregation were both independently associated with a reduced incidence of schizophrenia of 5 percent, independent of age, sex, ethnicity, deprivation, and population density (Kirkbride, Morgan, et al., 2007). Of course, there are a number of different mechanisms through which such social ecological factors could have their impact on psychosis. Stress may be just one of a number of mediators (Susser et al., 2008).

The neural processes that could mediate the association between urban environments and mental illness have only recently begun to be documented. Increased levels of stress linked to urban residence are considered important, as are models of psychological appraisal and neurocognitive development. There is some evidence that urban upbringing and city living change social evaluative stress processing in humans. Those who live in a city have increased amygdala activity, and being brought up in a city affects the perigenual anterior cingulate cortex, a key region for regulation of negative affect and stress. Because different parts of the social brain may have different critical developmental periods and social impacts may exert their effects at different times, research findings indicate that brain regions differ in their vulnerability and reactions to city living across the lifespan (Lederbogen et al., 2011; Meyer-Lindenberg, 2010).

The urban environment is not the only ecological factor involved in the risk of psychosis, but it is one of the better researched. Our aim here is not to document all the risk factors for psychosis, but to demonstrate that, taken as a whole, the literature reports that social factors are associated with psychosis risk at both individual and ecological levels. There is evidence for an increased risk of schizophrenia with greater exposure to some individual risk factors and with a greater number of risk factors, generally. This involves multiple mechanisms and an interplay between genetic, epigenetic and environmental factors.

An Integrative Conceptual Framework

A framework for categorizing or organizing different associations of psychotic illnesses with social factors may be helpful for developing prevention or mental health promotion initiatives, as well as for further research in the field. Although we have highlighted the "stress hypotheses," this umbrella conceptual framework allows for inclusion of different perspectives on causation and mechanisms. A simplified conceptual model would build on the literature and posit four dimensions of interest: (1) exposure to individual-level social factors linked to psychosis, (2) exposure to ecological-level social or environmental factors linked to psychosis, (3) interaction between individual and ecological social factors, and (4) time.

Individual-Level Social Factors

At the individual level, the model would be similar to heart disease: There is an inherited risk, but whether one develops a heart attack or not depends on other risk, protective, and health promotion factors that one encounters. Accordingly, the risk of developing a psychosis for any individual depends in part on inherited vulnerabilities, but in addition rests on the balance of exposures to factors that either increase risk for illness or enhance mental health. In addition to genetic and other biological risk factors, the list of social risk factors could include the use of certain drugs (especially cannabis), racial discrimination, and childhood experiences influencing development, such as bullying and psychological trauma, separation from parents, and other adversities (Boydell et al., 2004). The number and severity of exposures as well as their interactions may all contribute to the risk of developing a psychotic illness.

Previous work has shown that the greater the number of risk factors, the higher the risk of psychosis (Cantor-Graae, 2007; Johns et al., 2004; Selten & Cantor-Graae, 2005, 2007; Shevlin et al., 2008; Wiles et al., 2006). However, further complexity is introduced by work on child brain development. This work has shown that the same exposure may have negative or positive impacts on the developing brain, depending on the individual's previous history of exposure to social determinants. If the balance of exposures has been negative, then an otherwise neutral factor may be experienced as negative. Alternatively, if the balance of exposures has been positive, some challenges may actually enhance brain development (Knudsen, Heckman, Cameron, & Shonkoff, 2006).

Ecological-Level Social Factors

At the ecological level, social factors may change the environmental exposures and consequent risk for a whole population or increase the vulnerability of specific socially demarcated groups. The model here is similar to that of diabetes, where changes in the availability and quality of certain types of food and cultural changes in activity with increasingly sedentary lifestyles have led to markedly increased rates of the illness. Groups with similar individual-level risk factors may have different rates of illness dependent on the social-ecological environment. In addition to factors like diet and exposure to infectious diseases which influence early neurodevelopment, environmental risk factors that may contribute to the risk of psychosis include city birth and city living, social cohesion, social fragmentation, being a member of a minority group living in areas with low population densities of one's group, and migrants from countries that are predominantly black living in countries that are predominantly white (Allardyce et al., 2005; Cooper et al., 2008; Bentall, Kinderman, & Kaney, 1994; Boydell et al., 2001; Boydell et al., 2004; Boydell & McKenzie, 2008; Faris & Dunham, 1939; Kelly et al., 2010; Silver, Mulvey, & Swanson, 2002; Spauwen & van Os, 2006; Wright et al., 2009; van Os et al., 2001).

Interactions Between Individual and Ecological-Level Social Factors

But in the real world individual and ecological risks interact. Some ecological factors may decrease the rates of illness, either by decreasing the impact of individual risk factors or by reducing the possibility of exposure to individual social risks. The social safety net, for instance, may mitigate the impact of life events. Some ecological factors could interact with individual-level factors to change risk. For example, urbanization may decrease the capacity to cope with social risk factors such as marital problems or unemployment. The impact of minority-group membership on psychosis risk may be linked to the density of that minority group in a geographic region or neighborhood (Shaw et al., 2012).

Individual and ecological factors may not simply be independent variables acting in concert, but may interact in ways that amplify or dampen each other's effects. For example, at an individual level, use of cannabis may increase a person's risk of developing a psychotic illness. At an ecological level, the availability of cannabis in the community could increase the risk of cannabis use in the first place. Moreover, depending on social context, regular cannabis use may offer access to a subculture, or a different environment, characterized by an increase in daily hassles and life events, which increases the risk of exposure to other social factors associated with psychosis. Exposure to more life events and daily hassles may lead to higher levels of perceived stress and so increase cannabis use, thus further increasing the risk of psychosis. The link between individual and ecological processes in this example may trigger a chain of events resulting in further interactions among social risk factors. Social factors also may alter biological risk in multiple ways. For example, socio-cultural factors at an ecological level, such as the trend toward older paternal age at conception, may change psychosis risk in offspring at a population level by increasing the rate of children with genetic vulnerability (March & Susser, 2006).

New evidence is rapidly emerging in this field. Binbay and colleagues, for instance, have reported that the association between familial liability to severe mental illness and the expression of illnesses within the psychotic spectrum is stronger in more deprived neighborhoods, in high-unemployment neighborhoods, and in neighborhoods high in social control (Binbay et al., 2012).

Time

The final dimension in the model of psychopathology is time, which is important in several ways. First, sufficient exposure to an individual-level or ecological risk factor may only occur over time. Second, time may be needed for the interaction between individual and ecological risk factors to amplify. Third, there are sensitive periods in brain development during which exposure to certain risk factors may be more important.

For instance, being born and brought up in a city is etiologically more significant in schizophrenia than living in a city per se (Lederbogen, Haddad, & Meyer-Lindenberg, 2013; Marcelis, Takei, & van Os, 1999; Pedersen & Mortensen, 2001). Other risk factors such as separation from parents may be more important in childhood than adult life. Fourth, there may be a delay in time between the exposure to a risk factor and the development of psychosis. For instance, the impact of maternal mal-nutrition on psychosis risk may only be evident when offspring reach early adulthood (Susser et al., 2008). Lastly, the impact that a social factor has on an individual may be determined in part by the cumulative or profound effect of previous life experiences. These include the history of prior exposures linked to sensitization or resilience and the way that history may change our perception of our environment. A ten-year follow-up study on a population sample of 3,021 people in Germany recently reported that early adversity may impact later expression of psychosis by increasing exposure to later adversity and/or by rendering individuals more sensitive to later adversity if these early experiences are severe. (Lataster, Myin-Germeys, Lieb, Wittchen, & van Os, 2012)

Case Study

In order to clarify the utility of this four-dimensional approach, we will apply the conceptual model to understanding the increased incidence of psychosis among people of African and Caribbean origin in the United Kingdom. A difference in rates of illness between two groups in the same country suggests that social risk may be, at least partially, the cause of the difference and is an appropriate target for prevention (Kirkbride & Jones, 2011).

The incidence rate of schizophrenia varies across the globe and for different populations within a country. There are consistent reports of elevated rates of schizophrenia and psychosis in various migrant and ethnic minority groups in Europe (Cantor-Graae & Selten, 2005) and the United States (Bresnahan et al., 2007). In a meta-analysis, the vast majority of studies reported that migrants are at increased risk of psychosis (Bourque, van der Ven, & Malla, 2011). Migrants are nearly three times more likely to develop schizophrenia than nonmigrants, but not all migrants are equal. When moving to high-income countries, migrants from countries where the population is predominantly black skinned are nearly twice as likely to develop schizophrenia as migrants from countries where the populations are predominantly white skinned. Similarly, migrants from low-income countries are more likely to be diagnosed with schizophrenia when they move to high-income countries compared to migrants who move from one high-income country to another (Cantor-Graac & Selten, 2005).

The best-studied and most consistent findings in this area involve people from Africa and the Caribbean who live in the United Kingdom (Fearon & Morgan, 2006; Fearon et al., 2006). Their risk of schizophrenia is between two and six times that of other people in the United Kingdom (Cantor-Graae & Selten, 2005; Fearon & Morgan, 2006; Fearon et al., 2006). The African-origin and Caribbean-origin populations are quite different. The African-origin population has been in the United Kingdom since the Roman era. The next significant migrations were in the 16th century and then post-1980. They comprise a mixture of economic migrants from Commonwealth countries and refugees fleeing persecution in their countries of origin. The Caribbean-origin population was invited to come to the United Kingdom from colonies to help fill post–World War II labor shortages. Subsequently, migration was severely restricted by changes in immigration laws from 1968 onwards. The largest proportion of Caribbean immigrants is from Jamaica, but there are people from most of the English-speaking Caribbean. Caribbean-origin communities are found throughout the United Kingdom, although by far the largest concentrations are in London and Birmingham.

There are approximately 1.5 million people of African or Caribbean origin in the United Kingdom, split roughly equally between the two groups. Although there is significant diversity within and between these groups, they have often been considered together in research. This conflation is partially due to the underlying belief that racial discrimination or the process of racialization experienced by both groups are important factors in the increased incidence of mental health problems, but also due to co-location of African and Caribbean origin populations, similarities in current socioeconomic position, and the increased use of "Black British" as an identity for second and third generations of both groups. Indeed, as of the 2011 census, the majority of people of both African and Caribbean origin in the United Kingdom were born there. Nonetheless, the conflation of people of African and Caribbean origin has also been cemented by literature historically comparing "black" populations to "white" populations.

Altough the veracity of reported high rates of schizophrenia has at times been questioned, and more rigorous studies have decreased the size of the increased risk, the weight of evidence suggests that the findings are not simply an artifact of misdiagnosis (Morgan & Hutchinson, 2009). People of both African and Caribbean origin in the United Kingdom are at increased risk of being diagnosed with schizophrenia (Fearon et al.,

2006). The possible reasons for the increased risk are many and varied. Using the proposed conceptual framework, they can be organized along the following four dimensions.

Individual-Level Risk Factors

There is no evidence of an increased rate of genetic markers for psychosis in people of Caribbean origin. With regard to biological risks, neither obstetric complications nor other neurodevelopmental risk factors show greater frequency in the African or Caribbean population (Dean et al., 2007; Hutchinson et al., 1997).

Cannabis use is an important risk factor for psychosis that is linked to genetic susceptibility (van Os et al., 2010). The greatest risk occurs with cannabis use during adolescence. The stereotype of cannabis use being prevalent in the Caribbean has led to questions as to whether this is a particularly important risk factor in the African-Caribbean population. However, studies have failed to demonstrate increased rates of cannabis use or misuse in young African Caribbeans (Sharpley, Hutchinson, McKenzie, & Murray, 2001).

The Caribbean-origin group in the United Kingdom are disadvantaged materially; they have some of the highest unemployment rates in the country and are more likely than most other ethnic minority groups to be members of lower socioeconomic groups and to live in substandard housing. People of Caribbean and African origin are more likely than the host population to have been separated from at least one of their parents for a year before the age of sixteen. Evidence also implicates the role of life events and daily hassles linked to discrimination. Although Gilvarry and colleagues (1999) reported no difference in the number of major life events experienced by patients with psychosis across ethnic groups, African Caribbeans were more likely to attribute life events to racism. In turn, life events due to racism have been associated with increased risks of physical and mental health problems (Karlsen & Nazroo, 2002). A recent meta-analysis reported that being the victim of perceived racism has a direct impact on stress reactivity and may increase the risk of illness, but perceptions of victimization may also trigger a train of events that leads to unhealthy behaviors, such as smoking and eating high-calorie foods (Pascoe & Richmand, 2009). Thus, those who experience perceived racism also tend to have more unhealthy lifestyles.

The association between perceived discrimination and psychosis has been demonstrated in cross-sectional and longitudinal studies (Janssen et al., 2003; Karlsen, Nazroo, McKenzie, Bhui, & Weich, 2005). Research also demonstrates that you do not have to be a direct victim of racial discrimination for this factor to affect psychosis risk. Those who were not victims of direct racial abuse or attack but who believed that employers discriminate against ethnic minorities were more likely to suffer from a psychosis (Karlsen & Nazroo, 2002). This may be because the belief that employers discriminate influences everyday perceptions and inter-actions at work, and over time, this belief may become a chronic stressor, or daily hassle.

In summary, although there is little evidence for biological factors, the risk of being exposed to a number of individual-level risk factors for psychosis is increased in both the African and Caribbean population of the United Kingdom.

Ecological Level Risk Factors

Migrants have an increased risk of psychosis, but those from countries that are predominantly black migrating to countries that are predomi-nantly white have a higher risk still (Cantor-Graae & Selten, 2005), with the most conclusive evidence coming from the United Kingdom and the Netherlands. The same is true for migrants from low-income countries (Selten, Cantor-Graae, & Kahn, 2007). This contrasts with the incidence of schizophrenia and psychosis in the Caribbean and in the African sites included in the WHO incidence studies, which were not significantly different from those of the white British population in the United Kingdom (Bhugra et al., 1996; Hickling & Rodgers-Johnson, 1995; Mahy, Mallett, Leff, & Bhugra, 1999). These findings argue for the importance of place in the incidence of psychosis in these groups.

Place can be considered on a societal level – for instance, the overall reception of migrants may be an important contextual factor. But there are more prosaic social factors, such as the greater likelihood that people of African and Caribbean origin in the United Kingdom will live in cities. Being born and brought up in a city is one of the most important risk factors for the development of psychosis, as discussed earlier. There have not been many ecological analyses undertaken in these communities. However, in the United Kingdom, people of both African and Caribbean origin are more likely to live in inner city areas, which have high rates of poverty, social fragmentation, and low levels of social capital. In addition, Boydell and colleagues (2001) and Kirkbride and colleagues (Kirkbride, Fearon, et al., 2007) have shown that the relative risk of schizophrenia in black Caribbeans living in the United Kingdom rises significantly (and in a dose-response fashion) as the proportionate size of that minority group in the local population falls. This could be because in such a setting social networks, supports, and resources become less available and more exclusionary to minorities (Whitley & McKenzie, 2005).

Interaction of Individual and Ecological Factors

The study by Hutchinson and colleagues (1996) of the rates of schizophrenia in first-degree relatives of people with schizophrenia demonstrated the interaction between individual and ecological factors. Individual risk of schizophrenia was increased in first-degree relatives of people with schizophrenia. Hutchinson compared the risk of developing schizophrenia in first-degree relatives of people of Caribbean origin in the Caribbean and people of Caribbean origin in the United Kingdom. His group found that the first-degree relatives who lived in the United Kingdom had a higher incidence rate of schizophrenia than those who lived in the Caribbean. They concluded that the environment in the United Kingdom amplified the effect of familial risk (Hutchinson et al., 1996).

There are potentially similar models for the interaction of substance use and social environment, in which substance use could lead to involvement with a different social environment with more frequent exposure to adverse life events. In addition, although individuals of African and Caribbean origin are more likely to encounter financial difficulties and social disadvantage such as unemployment, limited social networks, and separation from or loss of a parent before age sixteen (Morgan et al., 2007; Morgan et al., 2008), they are also more likely to live in environments that further increase the rates of adverse life events due to social fragmentation and the associated lack of social safety-nets and access to social support. The impact of life events may be increased by decreased ability at a community level to provide effective restitution. In support of this theory, Boydell and colleagues (2004) demonstrated that the association between low levels of social capital and the incidence of psychosis is only seen in lower socioeconomic groups.

Time

Etiological theories of psychosis often focus on childhood and adolescence. This is partly because of neurodevelopmental hypotheses of schizophrenia which suggest that early childhood incidents are important in producing vulnerability, but also because of the apparently slow development of psychosis over time. During sensitive periods of functional and structural brain development, such as adolescence (Blakemore & Mills, 2014), people of African and Caribbean origin are more likely to be living in cities, separated from a parent, and living in poverty. Therefore, they are more likely to be exposed to individual and ecological insults, thus increasing their risk of developing psychosis.

Time can also be considered across generations. The second generation of people of African and Caribbean origin are reported to be at higher risk of psychosis than the first generation. This may in part be because more second-generation children than first-generation children will have grown up in families with a psychotic parent or sibling. It may also reflect the fact that first-generation immigrants tend to stick together geographically, while second-generation immigrants are more likely to disperse. The risk of psychosis is increased in those who move from areas with higher proportions of immigrant groups because of the density effect reported above (Shaw et al., 2012). Lastly, the generation effect could reflect differences in expectations between first and second generations. First-generation immigrants often make a calculated choice to move countries. They expect there will be difficulties, but they compare the problems in the new country to the difficulties they left behind in the old country. Members of the second generation are born and brought up in the new country. They rightly expect equity of opportunity, but evidence shows that, like their parents, they do not get it. Thwarted aspirations then may play out differently in the first generation and the second generation. The first generation may downplay or discount their problems because they feel they have made the right decision to move and they are better off than they were, whereas the second generation cannot make such a calculation and may feel a more intense sense of injustice and disqualification.

Developing Interventions

This simplified four-dimensional model may be useful in considering potential prevention initiatives, as each dimension can be linked to specific types of strategies. Prevention at an individual level will aim to decrease amount of exposure or limit the number of different social factors to which an individual is exposed. This could be allied with health-promotion efforts to enhance behaviors, and expose individuals to social factors known to strengthen mental health. The aim is to decrease risk factors, increase protective factors, and build resilience.

At an ecological level, the aim would be to develop healthy environments. Cross-government approaches, including the targeting of improved accessibility to nursery and preschool education for lower income children, as well as better schools for adolescents, and job creation for young adults, have all been considered important. Community development coupled with social renewal and decreased income inequality are also part of a group of actions that may decrease social fragmentation.

Where interactions between individual and ecological factors lead to an amplification or spiraling of risk, targeting such interactions may be important. If neither individual risk factors nor environmental risk factors can be reduced, then remedial strategies aimed at uncoupling the links between factors could be effective. This is essentially a harm reduction or minimization approach. For instance, if it is not possible to decrease the amount of cannabis that is in the community or individual use of it, then trying to decrease the secondary impacts through decriminalization may decrease the number of people who move to a more noxious social environment because of substance misuse.

Of course, considerations of time and temporal trajectories of development are essential. Understanding the stages of development at which particular risk factors act is important for targeting age-specific prevention strategies for maximal effect. Understanding the longer-term impacts of particular risk factors may give an indication of how long preventive strategies should last, and understanding the time-scales over which social factors exert their effects helps evaluators pick the right time frame to assess the effectiveness of interventions. In the case of migration-related psychosis, a temporal perspective points to the transgenerational processes that may increase risk and raises the possibility that different prevention strategies may be needed in first and second-generation groups.

Conclusion

In this chapter, we have outlined a framework for considering how a range of social factors, acting over time and through stressful life events or daily hassles, could contribute, independently or through ongoing interactions, to the development of psychotic illness. The importance of such models for conceptualizing the social etiology of psychosis lies in demonstrating the complex and multifaceted interplay between individual and ecological dimensions, their interactions, and temporal trajectories. The framework also throws into relief the gaps in current knowledge. Our hope is that this framework can directly assist in the design of future research, the planning of interventions aimed at particular risk and protective factors, the training of health and mental health professionals, and the construction and implementation of health and social systems that can more effectively respond to the needs of at-risk populations.

REFERENCES

Allardyce, J., Gilmour, H., Atkinson, J., Rapson, T., Bishop, J., & McCreadie, R. G. (2005). Social fragmentation, deprivation and urbanicity: Relation to first-admission rates for psychoses. *British Journal of Psychiatry, 187*, 401–6. http://dx.doi.org/10.1192/bjp.187.5.401

Belsky, J., Jonassaint, C., Pluess, M., Stanton, M., Brummett, B., & Williams, R. (2009). Vulnerability genes or plasticity genes? *Molecular Psychiatry, 14*, 746–54. http://dx.doi.org/10.1038/mp.2009.44

Bentall, R. P., Kinderman, P., & Kaney, S. (1994). The self, attributional processes and abnormal beliefs: Towards a model of persecutory delusions. *Behaviour Research Therapy, 32*(3), 331–41. http://dx.doi.org/10.1016/0005-7967(94)90131-7

Bhugra, D., Hilwig, M., Hossein, B., Marceau, H., Neehall, J., Leff, J., ... Der, G. (1996). First-contact incidence rates of schizophrenia in Trinidad and one-year follow-up. *British Journal of Psychiatry, 169*(5), 587–92. http://dx.doi.org/10.1192/bjp.169.5.587

Binbay, T., Drukker, J., Alptekin, K., Elbi, H., Aksu Tanik, F., Özkinay, F., ... van Os, J. (2012). Evidence that the wider social environment moderates the association between familial liability and psychosis spectrum outcome. *Psychological Medicine, 42*, 2499–2510. http://dx.doi.org/10.1017/S0033291712000700

Blakemore, S.-J., & Mills, K. L. (2014). Is adolescence a sensitive period for sociocultural processing? *Annual Review of Psychology, 65*, 187–205. http://dx.doi.org/10.1146/annurev-psych-010213-115202

Bourque, F., van der Ven, E., & Malla, A. (2011). A meta-analysis of the risk for psychotic disorders among first- and second-generation immigrants. *Psychological Medicine, 41*(5), 897–910. http://dx.doi.org/10.1017/S0033291710001406

Boydell, J., & McKenzie, K. (2008). Society, place and space. In C. Morgan, K. McKenzie, & P. Fearon (Eds.), *Society and psychosis* (pp. 77–94). Cambridge, England: Cambridge University Press.

Boydell, J., van Os, J., McKenzie, K., Allardyce, J., Goel, R., McCreadie, R. G., & Murray, R. M. (2001). Incidence of schizophrenia in ethnic minorities in London: Ecological study into interactions with environment. *British Medical Journal, 323*(7325), 1336–8. http://dx.doi.org/10.1136/bmj.323.7325.1336

Boydell, J., van Os, J., McKenzie, K., & Murray, R. M. (2004). The association of inequality with the incidence of schizophrenia: An ecological study. *Social Psychiatry & Psychiatric Epidemiology, 39*(8), 597–9. http://dx.doi.org/10.1007/s00127-004-0789-6

Bresnahan, M., Begg, M. D., Brown, A., Schaefer, C., Sohler, N., Insel, B., ... Susser, E. (2007). Race and risk of schizophrenia in a US birth cohort: Another example of health disparity? *International Journal of Epidemiology, 36*(4), 751–8. http://dx.doi.org/10.1093/ije/dym041

Cantor-Graae, E. (2007). The contribution of social factors to the development of schizophrenia: A review of recent findings. *Canadian Journal of Psychiatry, 52*(5), 277–86. http://dx.doi.org/10.3410/f.1116901.572995

Cantor-Graae, E., & Selten, J. P. (2005). Schizophrenia and migration: A meta-analysis and review. *American Journal of Psychiatry, 162*(1), 12–24. http://dx.doi.org/10.1176/appi.ajp.162.1.12

Caspi, A., Moffitt, T., Cannon, M., McClay, J., Murray, R., Harrington, H., … Craig, I. (2005). Moderation of the effect of adolescent-onset cannabis use on adult psychosis by a functional polymorphism in the catechol-O-methyltransferase gene: Longitudinal evidence of a gene X environment interaction. *Biological Psychiatry, 57*(10), 1117–27. http://dx.doi.org/10.1016/j.biopsych.2005.01.026

Cooper, R., Boyko, C., & Codinhoto, R. (2008). The effect of the physical environment on mental and capital wellbeing. In D. Flynn (Ed.), *Mental capital and wellbeing: Making the most of ourselves in the 21st century.* Retrieved from www.gov.uk/government/collections/mental-capital-and-wellbeing

Daskalakis, N. P., Bagot, R. C., Parker, K. J., Vinkers, C H., & de Kloet, E. R. (2013). The three-hit concept of vulnerability and resilience: Toward understanding adaptation to early-life adversity outcome. *Psychoneuroendocrinology, 38*(9), 1858–73. http://dx.doi.org/10.1016/j.psyneuen.2013.06.008

Dean, K., Dazzan, P., Lloyd, T., Morgan, C., Morgan, K., Doody, G. A., … Fearon, P. (2007). Minor physical anomalies across ethnic groups in a first episode psychosis sample. *Schizophrenia Research, 89*(1–3), 86–90. http://dx.doi.org/10.1016/j.schres.2006.08.019

Faris, R., & Dunham, H. (1939). *Mental disorders in urban areas.* Chicago, IL: University of Chicago Press.

Fearon, P., Kirkbride, J. B., Morgan, C., Dazzan, P., Morgan, K., Lloyd, T., … Murray, R. M. (2006). Incidence of schizophrenia and other psychoses in ethnic minority groups: Results from the MRC AESOP Study. *Psychological Medicine, 36*(11), 1541–50. http://dx.doi.org/10.1017/S0033291706008774

Fearon, P., & Morgan, C. (2006). Environmental factors in schizophrenia: The role of migrant studies. *Schizophrenia Bulletin, 32*(3), 405–8. http://dx.doi.org/10.1093/schbul/sbj076

Fusar-Poli, P., Perez, J., Broome, M., Borgwardt, S., Placentino, A., Caverzasi, E., … McGuire, P. (2007). Neurofunctional correlates of vulnerability to psychosis: A systematic review and meta-analysis. *Neuroscience & Biobehavioral Reviews, 31*(4), 465–84. http://dx.doi.org/10.1016/j.neubiorev.2006.11.006

Geuze, E., Vermetten, E., & Bremner, J. D. (2005). MR-based in vivo hippocampal volumetrics: 2. Findings in neuropsychiatric disorders. *Molecular Psychiatry, 10*(2), 160–84. http://dx.doi.org/10.1038/sj.mp.4001579

Gilvarry, C. M., Walsh, E., Samele, C., Hutchinson, G., Mallett, R., Rabe-Hesketh, S., … Murray, R. M. (1999). Life events, ethnicity and perceptions of discrimination in patients with severe mental illness. *Social Psychiatry and Psychiatric Epidemiology, 34*(11), 600–8. http://dx.doi.org/10.1007/s001270050181

Hickling, F. W., & Rodgers-Johnson, P. (1995). The incidence of first contact schizophrenia in Jamaica. *British Journal of Psychiatry, 167*(2), 193–6. http://dx.doi.org/10.1192/bjp.167.2.193

Hosman, C., Jane-Llopis, E., & Saxena, S. (2005). *Prevention of mental disorders: Effective interventions and policy options.* Oxford, England: Oxford University Press.

Husted, J. A., Ahmed, R., Chow, E. W., Brzustowicz, L. M., & Bassett, A. S. (2012). Early environmental exposures influence schizophrenia expression even in the presence of strong genetic predisposition. *Schizophrenia Research, 137*(1–3), 166–8. http://dx.doi.org/10.1016/j.schres.2012.02.009

Hutchinson, G., Takei, N., Bhugra, D., Fahy, T. A., Gilvarry, C., Mallett, R., ... Murray, R. M. (1997). Increased rate of psychosis among African-Caribbeans in Britain is not due to an excess of pregnancy and birth complications. *British Journal of Psychiatry, 171*, 145–7. http://dx.doi.org/10.1192/bjp.171.2.145

Hutchinson, G., Takei, N., Fahy, T. A., Bhugra, D., Gilvarry, C., Moran, P., ... Murray, R. M. (1996). Morbid risk of schizophrenia in first-degree relatives of white and African-Caribbean patients with psychosis. *British Journal of Psychiatry, 169*, 776–80. http://dx.doi.org/10.1192/bjp.169.6.776

Janssen, I., Hanssen, M., Bak, M., Bijl, R. V., de Graaf, R., Vollebergh, W., ... van Os, J. (2003). Discrimination and delusional ideation. *British Journal of Psychiatry, 182*, 71–6. http://dx.doi.org/10.1192/bjp.182.1.71

Johns, L. C., Cannon, M., Singleton, N., Murray, R. M., Farrell, M., Brugha, T., ... Meltzer, H. (2004). Prevalence and correlates of self-reported psychotic symptoms in the British population. *British Journal of Psychiatry, 185*, 298–305. http://dx.doi.org/10.1192/bjp.185.4.298

Jones, S. R., & Fernyhough, C. (2007). A new look at the neural diathesis–stress model of schizophrenia: The primacy of social-evaluative and uncontrollable situations. *Schizophrenia Bulletin, 33*(5), 1171–7. http://dx.doi.org/10.1093/schbul/sbl058

Kapur, S. (2003). Psychosis as a state of aberrant salience: A framework linking biology, phenomenology, and pharmacology in schizophrenia. *American Journal of Psychiatry, 160*(1), 13–23. http://dx.doi.org/10.1176/appi.ajp.160.1.13

Karlsen, S., & Nazroo, J. Y. (2002). Relation between racial discrimination, social class, and health among ethnic minority groups. *American Journal of Public Health, 92*(4), 624–31. http://dx.doi.org/10.2105/AJPH.92.4.624

Karlsen, S., Nazroo, J. Y., McKenzie, K., Bhui, K., & Weich, S. (2005). Racism, psychosis and common mental disorder among ethnic minority groups in England. *Psychological Medicine, 35*(12), 1795–1803. http://dx.doi.org/10.1017/S0033291705005830

Kelly, B. D., O'Callaghan, E., Waddington, J. L., Feeney, L., Browne, S., Scully, P. J., ... Larkin, C.(2010). Schizophrenia and the city: A review of literature and prospective study of psychosis and urbanicity in Ireland. *Schizophrenia Research, 116*(1), 75–89. http://dx.doi.org/10.1016/j.schres.2009.10.015

Kirkbride, J. B., Fearon, P., Morgan, C., Dazzan, P., Morgan, K., Murray, R. M., & Jones, P. B. (2007). Neighbourhood variation in the incidence of psychotic disorders in Southeast London. *Social Psychiatry and Psychiatric Epidemiology, 42*(6), 438–45. http://dx.doi.org/10.1007/s00127-007-0193-0

Kirkbride, J. B., & Jones, P. B. (2011). The prevention of schizophrenia: What can we learn from eco-epidemiology? *Schizophrenia Bulletin, 37*(2), 262–71. http://dx.doi.org/10.1093/schbul/sbq120

Kirkbride, J. B., Morgan, C., Fearon, P., Dazzan, P., Murray, R. M., & Jones, P. B. (2007). Neighbourhood-level effects on psychoses: Re-examining the role of context. *Psychological Medicine, 37*(10), 1413–25. http://dx.doi.org/10.1017/S0033291707000499

Knudsen, E. I., Heckman, J. J., Cameron, J. L., & Shonkoff, J. P. (2006). Economic, neurobiological and behavioral perspectives on building America's future workforce. *Proceedings of the National Academy of Sciences of the United States of America, 27*, 10155–62. http://dx.doi.org/10.1073/pnas.0600888103

Labonté, B., Farah , A., & Turecki, G. (2015). Early-life adversity and epigenetic changes: Implications for understanding suicide. In L. J. Kirmayer, R. Lemelson, & C. A. Cummings (Eds.), *Re-visioning psychiatry: Cultural phenomenology, critical neuroscience, and global mental health* (pp. 206–35). New York, NY: Cambridge University Press.

Laruelle, M., & Abi-Dargham, A. (1999). Dopamine as the wind of the psychotic fire: New evidence from brain imaging studies. *Journal of Psychopharmacology, 13*(4), 358–71. http://dx.doi.org/10.1177/026988119901300405

Lataster, J., Myin-Germeys, I., Lieb, R., Wittchen, H.-U., & van Os, J. (2012). Adversity and psychosis: A 10-year prospective study investigating synergism between early and recent adversity in psychosis. *Acta Psychiatrica Scandinavica, 125*(5), 388–99. http://dx.doi.org/10.1111/j.1600-0447.2011.01805.x

Lederbogen, F., Haddad, L., & Meyer-Lindenberg, A. (2013) Urban social stress – Risk factor for mental disorders. The case of schizophrenia. *Environmental Pollution, 183*, 2–6. http://dx.doi.org/10.1016/j.envpol.2013.05.046

Lederbogen F., Kirsch, P., Haddad, L., Streit, F., Tost, H., Schuch, P., . . . Meyer-Lindenberg, A. (2011). City living and urban upbringing affect neural social stress processing in humans. *Nature, 474*(7352), 498–501. http://dx.doi.org/10.1038/nature10190

Lieberman, J., Chakos, M., Wu, H., Alvir, J., Hoffman, E., Robinson, D., & Bilder, R. (2001). Longitudinal study of brain morphology in first episode schizophrenia. *Biological Psychiatry, 49*(6), 487–99. http://dx.doi.org/10.1016/S0006-3223(01)01067-8

Mahy, G. E., Mallett, R., Leff, J., & Bhugra, D. (1999). First-contact incidence rate of schizophrenia on Barbados. *British Journal of Psychiatry, 175*, 28–33. http://dx.doi.org/10.1192/bjp.175.1.28

Marcelis, M., Takei, N., & van Os, J. (1999). Urbanization and risk for schizophrenia: Does the effect operate before or around the time of illness onset? *Psychological Medicine, 29*, 1197–1203. http://dx.doi.org/10.1017/S0033291799008983

March, D., Morgan, C., Bresnahan, M., & Susser, E. (2008). Conceptualising the social world. In C. Morgan, K. McKenzie, & P. Fearon (Eds.), *Society and psychosis* (pp. 41–57). Cambridge, England: Cambridge University Press.

March, D., & Susser, E. (2006). Taking the search for causes of schizophrenia to a different level [Invited commentary]. *American Journal of Epidemiology, 163*(11), 979–81. http://dx.doi.org/10.1093/aje/kwj170

Mason, O., Startup, M., Halpin, S., Schall, U., Conrad, A., & Carr, V. (2004). Risk factors for transition to first episode psychosis among individuals with "at-risk mental states." *Schizophrenia Research, 71*(2–3), 227–37. http://dx.doi.org/10.1016/j.schres.2004.04.006

McKenzie, K., & Harpham, T. (2006). *Social capital and mental health.* London, England: Jessica Kingsley.

Meyer-Lindenberg A. (2010). From maps to mechanisms through neuroimaging of schizophrenia. *Nature, 468*(7321), 194–202. http://dx.doi.org/10.1038/nature09569

Miller, P., Lawrie, S. M., Hodges, A., Clafferty, R., Cosway, R., & Johnstone, E. C. (2001). Genetic liability, illicit drug use, life stress and psychotic symptoms: Preliminary findings from the Edinburgh study of people at high risk for schizophrenia. *Social Psychiatry and Psychiatric Epidemiology, 36*(7), 338–42. http://dx.doi.org/10.1007/s001270170038

Morgan, C., & Hutchinson, G. (2009). The social determinants of psychosis in migrant and ethnic minority populations: A public health tragedy. *Psychological Medicine, 40,*(5), 705–9. http://dx.doi.org/10.1017/S0033291709005546

Morgan, C., Kirkbride, J., Hutchinson, G., Craig, T., Morgan, K., Dazzan, P., . . . Fearon, P. (2008). Cumulative social disadvantage, ethnicity and first-episode psychosis: A case-control study. *Psychological Medicine, 38*(12), 1701–15. http://dx.doi.org/10.1017/S0033291708004534

Morgan, C., Kirkbride, J., Leff, J. Craig, T., Hutchinson, G., Mckenzie, K., . . . Fearon, P. (2007). Parental separation, loss and psychosis in different ethnic groups: A case-control study. *Psychological Medicine, 37*(4), 495–503. http://dx.doi.org/10.1017/S0033291706009330

Myin-Germeys, I., & van Os, J. (2007). Stress-reactivity in psychosis: Evidence for an affective pathway to psychosis. *Clinical Psychology Review, 27*(4), 409–24. http://dx.doi.org/10.1016/j.cpr.2006.09.005

Myin-Germeys, I., & van Os, J. (2008). Adult adversity: Do early environment and genotype create lasting vulnerabilities for adult social adversity in psychosis? In C. Morgan, K. McKenzie, & P. Fearon (Eds.), *Society and psychosis* (pp. 127–42). Cambridge, England: Cambridge University Press.

Nuechterlein, K. H., & Dawson, M. E. (1984). A heuristic vulnerability/stress model of schizophrenic episodes. *Schizophrenia Bulletin, 10*(2), 300–12. http://dx.doi.org/10.1093/schbul/10.2.300

Pascoe, E. A., Richmand, L. S. (2009). Perceived discrimination and health: A meta-analytic review. *Psychology Bulletin, 135*(4), 531–54.

Pedersen, C. B., & Mortensen, P. B. (2001). Evidence of a dose-response relationship between urbanicity during upbringing and schizophrenia risk. *Archives of General Psychiatry, 58,* 1039–46.

Seeman, P., & Kapur, S. (2000). Schizophrenia: More dopamine, more D2 receptors. *Proceedings of the National Academy of Sciences of the United States of America, 97*(14), 7673–5. http://dx.doi.org/10.1073/pnas.97.14.7673

Selten, J. P., & Cantor-Graae, E. (2005). Social defeat: Risk factor for schizophrenia? *British Journal of Psychiatry, 187,* 101–2. http://dx.doi.org/10.1192/bjp.187.2.101

Selten, J. P., & Cantor-Graae, E. (2007). Hypothesis: Social defeat is a risk factor for schizophrenia? *British Journal of Psychiatry, 51*(Suppl.), s9–12. http://dx.doi.org/10.1192/bjp.191.51.s9

Selten, J. P., Cantor-Graae, E., & Kahn, R. S. (2007). Migration and schizophrenia. *Current Opinion in Psychiatry, 20*(2), 111–15. http://dx.doi.org/10.1097/YCO.0b013e328017f68e

Selten, J. P., van der Ven, E., Rutten, B. P. F., & Cantor-Graae, E. (2013). The social defeat hypothesis of schizophrenia: An update. *Schizophrenia Bulletin, 39*(6), 1180–6. http://dx.doi.org/10.1093/schbul/sbt134

Sharpley, M. S., Hutchinson, G., McKenzie, K., & Murray, R. M. (2001). Understanding the excess of psychosis among the African-Caribbean population in England: Review of current hypotheses. *British Journal of Psychiatry, 178*(Suppl. 40), s60–8.

Shaw, R. J., Atkin, K., Bécares, L., Albor, C. B., Stafford, M., Kiernan, K. E., ... Pickett, K. E. (2012). Impact of ethnic density on adult mental disorders: Narrative review. *British Journal of Psychiatry, 201*(1), 11–19. http://dx.doi.org/10.1192/bjp.bp.110.083675

Shevlin, M., Houston, J. E., Dorahy, M. J., & Adamson, G. (2008). Cumulative traumas and psychosis: An analysis of the National Comorbidity Survey and the British Psychiatric Morbidity Survey. *Schizophrenia Bulletin, 34*(1), 193–9. http://dx.doi.org/10.1093/schbul/sbm069

Silver, E., Mulvey, E., & Swanson, J. (2002). Neighbourhood structural characteristics and mental disorder: Faris and Dunham revisited. *Social Science and Medicine, 55*(8), 1457–70. http://dx.doi.org/10.1016/S0277-9536(01)00266-0

Soares, J. C., & Innis, R. B. (1999). Neurochemical brain imaging investigations of schizophrenia. *Biological Psychiatry, 46*(5), 600–15. http://dx.doi.org/10.1016/S0006-3223(99)00015-3

Spauwen, J., & van Os, J. (2006). The psychosis proneness: Psychosis persistence model as an explanation for the association between urbanicity and psychosis. *Epidemiologia e Psichiatria Sociale, 15*(4), 252–7. http://dx.doi.org/10.1017/S1121189X00002128

Steen, R. G., Mull, C., McClure, R., Hamer, R. M., & Lieberman, J. A. (2006). Brain volume in first-episode schizophrenia: Systematic review and meta-analysis of magnetic resonance imaging studies. *British Journal of Psychiatry, 188*, 510–18. http://dx.doi.org/10.1192/bjp.188.6.510

Susser, E., St. Clair, D., & He, L. (2008). Latent effects of prenatal malnutrition on adult health: The example of schizophrenia. *Annals of the New York Academy of Sciences, 1136*, 185–92. http://dx.doi.org/10.1196/annals.1425.024

United Nations (2014). *World urbanization prospects* (rev. ed.). Retrieved from http://esa.un.org/unpd/wup/

van Erp, T. G. M., Saleh, P. A., Huttunen, M., Lönnqvist, J., Kaprio, J., Salonen, O., ... Cannon, T. D. (2004). Hippocampal volumes in schizophrenic twins. *Archives of General Psychiatry, 61*, 346–53. http://dx.doi.org/10.1001/archpsyc.61.4.346

van Os, J., Hanssen, M., Bijl, R. V., & Vollebergh, W. (2001). Prevalence of psychotic disorder and community level of psychotic symptoms: An urban-rural comparison. *Archives of General Psychiatry, 58*(7), 663–8. http://dx.doi.org/10.1001/archpsyc.58.7.663

van Os, J., Kenis, G., & Rutten, B. P. (2010). The environment and schizophrenia. *Nature*, *468*(7321), 203–12. http://dx.doi.org/1038/nature09563

van Winkel, R., Henquet, C., Rosa, A., Papiol, S., Fananas, L., De Hert, M., . . . Myin-Germeys, I. (2008). Evidence that the COMT(Val158Met) polymorphism moderates sensitivity to stress in psychosis: An experience-sampling study. *American Journal of Medical Genetics Part B: Neuropsychiatric Genetics*, *147B*(1), 10–17. http://dx.doi.org/10.1002/ajmg.b.30559

van Winkel, R., van Nierop, M., Myin-Germeys, I., & van Os, J. (2013). Chiildhood trauma as a cause of psychosis: Linking genes, psychology, and biology. *Canadian Journal of Psychiatry*, *58*(1), 44–51.

Walker, E., Mittal, V., & Tessner, K. (2008). Stress and the hypothalamic pituitary adrenal axis in the developmental course of schizophrenia. *Annual Reviews of Clinical Psychology*, *4*, 189–216. http://dx.doi.org/10.1146/annurev.clinpsy.4.022007.141248

Walker, E. F., & Diforio, D. (1997). Schizophrenia: A neural diathesis-stress model. *Psychological Review*, *104*(4), 667–85. http://dx.doi.org/10.1037/0033-295X.104.4.667

Whitley, R., & McKenzie, K. (2005). Social capital and psychiatry: Review of the literature. *Harvard Review of Psychiatry*, *13*(2), 71–84. http://dx.doi.org/10.1080/10673220590956474

Wiles, N. J., Zammit, S., Bebbington, P., Singleton, N., Meltzer, H., & Lewis, G. (2006). Self-reported psychotic symptoms in the general population: Results from the longitudinal study of the British National Psychiatric Morbidity Survey. *British Journal of Psychiatry*, *188*, 519–26. http://dx.doi.org/10.1192/bjp.bp.105.012179

Wright, J., Turkington, D., Kingdon, D., & Ramirez Basco, M. (2009). *Cognitive-behavior therapy for severe mental illness: An illustrated guide*. Washington, DC: American Psychiatric Publishing.

14   Toward a Cultural Neuroscience of Anxiety Disorders
The Multiplex Model

Devon E. Hinton and Naomi M. Simon

Introduction

In this chapter, we propose a model to describe the various ways in which biological mechanisms of anxiety and their psychological correlates are embedded in, shape, and are shaped by particular cultural contexts. Our approach focuses on a set of processes, including attentional looping, catastrophic cognitions, and interpretive biases, and uses several versions of our "multiplex model" in order to illustrate the profound effects of culture on panic attacks, panic disorder, worry/generalized anxiety disorder (GAD), posttraumatic stress disorder (PTSD), anxiety symptoms, and somatization more generally. In doing so, we illustrate how local conceptualizations of the body alter the experience of somatic and panic-related symptoms. Our illustrations come mainly from research and clinical work with traumatized Cambodian refugees.

The multiplex models illustrate the importance of a dimensional approach to psychopathology – such as catastrophic cognitions, panic, somatic sensations, trauma associations, biology of trauma (e.g., amygdala reactivity) – in line with NIMH's RDoC initiative (Morris & Cuthbert, 2012; Sanislow et al., 2010; see also Kirmayer & Crafa, 2014, for critique); the models also provide insights into how a biocultural phenomenology of mental disorders may be advanced. More specifically, the multiplex models demonstrate how certain somatic symptoms may be subject to "bioattentional" looping, a positive feedback effect whereby interpretation of the symptoms in terms of the local ethnophysiology, ethnopsychology, and ethnospirituality may "loop back" and amplify their physiological effects, creating a vicious circle (for a review, see Hinton & Good, 2009; Hinton & Hinton, 2002; Hinton, Hinton, Eng, & Choung, 2012; Hinton & Kirmayer, 2013; Kirmayer & Blake, 2009; Kirmayer & Sartorius, 2007). As conceptualized in the multiplex models, trauma associations and metaphor associations also may play a role in the generation and escalation of the somatic symptoms and general distress. Furthermore, the multiplex models are nested in that they involve core processes embedded within the matrices of other processes, including coping, treatment, and interpersonal contexts (e.g., Kleinman & Becker, 1998), what we refer here to as sociocultural pragmatics. Altogether, the models demonstrate how anxiety ontologies can vary greatly across cultures, with important implications for assessment and treatment.

We begin by describing the trauma background of Cambodian and Vietnamese refugees and their high rates of PTSD, as well as the different types of panic attacks and multiple somatic complaints they experience. We then present the multiplex model, building on Clark's (1986, 1988) model of panic attack, to explain the high rate of panic-related disorders (and somatization) among the Cambodian population and discuss how our model applies to trauma-related disorders. Because catastrophic cognitions play a key role in generating panic among Cambodian refugees (and in shaping anxiety-related experiencing), we describe the contents of these cognitions in detail, focusing on the cultural syndrome of "*khyâl* attack" ("wind attack"). We next describe how bioattentional looping and catastrophic cognitions underlie anxiety episodes that Cambodians label as a "wind attack." We illustrate our discussion with a case study on orthostatic panic, a form of panic attack common among Cambodian refugees and also discuss treatment implications. In our concluding remarks, we introduce a more generalized version of the multiplex model, the anxiety multiplex model, which incorporates a biological dimension and can be used to evaluate and treat anxiety disorder episodes in cultural context.

Trauma-Related Anxiety Disorders Among Southeast Asian Refugees

Southeast Asian refugees in the United States have experienced many traumatic events that may increase their risk of anxiety disorders. Before arriving in the United States, Cambodian refugees passed through periods of extreme adversity (Kiernan, 1996). Several years of bloody civil war preceded the Khmer Rouge rule from 1975 to 1979. During the Khmer Rouge period, a quarter of Cambodia's population of eight million people died from starvation, illness, and execution – most commonly by means of a blow to the back of the neck, after which the body was dumped into a large burial pit. In 1979, during the Vietnamese invasion, many Cambodians were caught in cross-fire, while others died of starvation after being driven into the jungle by the Khmer Rouge. Many also fled to the Thai border. Getting to the border camps along paths mined and patrolled by marauders was risky, and once in these camps, Cambodians often lived for months or even years under local warlords, often besieged by Khmer Rouge,

Vietnamese, and Thai soldiers. This was followed by a stay in inner Thailand's chaotic and often dangerous refugee camps while awaiting permission to emigrate to the United States (Kiernan, 1996). On arrival in the United States, Cambodians had to adjust to a completely new culture and language, often living in urban settings where they faced poverty and contexts of endemic violence.

Likewise, Vietnamese refugees passed through years of civil war (Mollica et al., 1998) before communists gained control of the country in 1975. Many refugees were former Southern Vietnamese soldiers and officials whom the communists had imprisoned, often for over ten years. In prison, these political detainees were subjected to illness, torture, slave labor, and starvation. The detainees' property was seized, and their spouses and children sent to jungle areas to face harassment, illness, overwork, and starvation. On attempting escape by boat to the United States, many Vietnamese confronted dehydration, starvation, and seasickness, and many were raped, beaten, and/or robbed by pirates. Most Vietnamese attempted to escape in small boats, which posed multiple risks: becoming lost at sea, capsizing in a storm, or running out of fuel and then floating on the waves until either death or rescue occurred. If they survived, Vietnamese refugees stayed in refugee camps that were often dangerous, and on arriving in the United States most had to adapt to difficult urban circumstances.

As would be expected given these levels of trauma, Cambodian and Vietnamese refugees have very high levels of trauma and high rates of PTSD. In a community survey of adult Cambodians in Long Beach, CA, 62 percent were found to have PTSD (Marshall, Schell, Elliott, Berthold, & Chun, 2005; Mollica, et al., 1998). These two refugee groups also have elevated rates of panic disorder (PD), as evaluated in psychiatric clinic populations: among Cambodian refugees, a rate of 60 percent (Hinton, Ba, Peou, & Um, 2000) and among Vietnamese refugees, a rate of 50 percent (Hinton, Chau, et al., 2001). In addition, Southeast Asian refugees have extremely high rates of certain subtypes of panic attacks, some culturally specific, which include "orthostatic panic" (panic triggered by dizziness and other sensations experienced on rising to standing from a sitting or lying position); "gastrointestinal panic" (panic with prominent gastrointestinal distress, much more common among Cambodian refugees); "sore neck panic" (panic focusing on neck sensations – this subtype is also much more common among Cambodian refugees); and "headache panic" (panic focused on head pain, which often is migraine in type) (Hinton et al., 2000; Hinton, Chau, et al., 2001). More generally, distressed Southeast Asian patients often have somatic complaints, such as dizziness, as a central part of their clinical presentation (Hinton, Hinton, et al., 2012).

The Multiplex Model of Somatic Symptoms and Panic Attacks

Panic attacks are a central aspect of both panic disorder and PTSD (Ehlers & Clark, 2000; Jones & Barlow, 1990). PTSD-type panic attacks are classifiable by their triggers: a sudden noise, anger, a flashback, or exposure to a trauma-related stimulus, such as meeting someone who resembles a perpetrator. By contrast, PD-related panic attacks are characterized by catastrophic cognitions that give rise to impending death or insanity. PD-related panic attacks may be classified in several ways: by what provokes the attack (e.g., an odor, standing up, exertion, traveling in a car, going to a shopping mall); by the sensation of most concern to the person (e.g., chest pain); or by the specific catastrophic cognition the person has during the attack. For example, among Westernized, English speakers, common fears are that dizziness indicates an imminent stroke, that shortness of breath indicates asphyxia, and that palpitations or chest tightness indicate a heart attack.

Why do traumatized Southeast Asian refugees have such a high rate of somatic complaints, panic attack, and panic disorder? What mechanisms produce the culture-related somatic symptoms and panic attack subtypes? In this section, we will try to answer these questions by introducing the multiplex model of somatic symptoms, panic attacks, and panic disorder.

Clark's Model of Panic

According to Clark's (1986) model of panic attack, a bodily sensation – such as shortness of breath or palpitations – triggers a catastrophic cognition, that is, fear that the sensation signifies a dangerous physiological event. This surge of fright can intensify the sensation by two "looping mechanisms" (cf. Hinton & Good, 2009; Hinton & Hinton, 2002; Kirmayer & Blake, 2009; Kirmayer & Sartorius, 2007; see also Ryder & Chentsova-Dutton, Chapter 16, *this volume*):

- *Attentional amplification,* in which fear causes the person to focus on the symptoms, thus amplifying them; and
- *Biological amplification,* in which fear affects the autonomic nervous system and other biological systems that, in turn, worsen certain symptoms; for example, fear causes palpitations from sympathetic nervous system (SNS) activation, cold hands and feet caused by vasoconstriction from SNS activation, and rapid, shallow breathing through central nervous system effects.

TRIGGER STIMULUS
(internal or external)

Perceived
threat

Interpretation of
sensations as catastrophic

Apprehension

Body
sensations

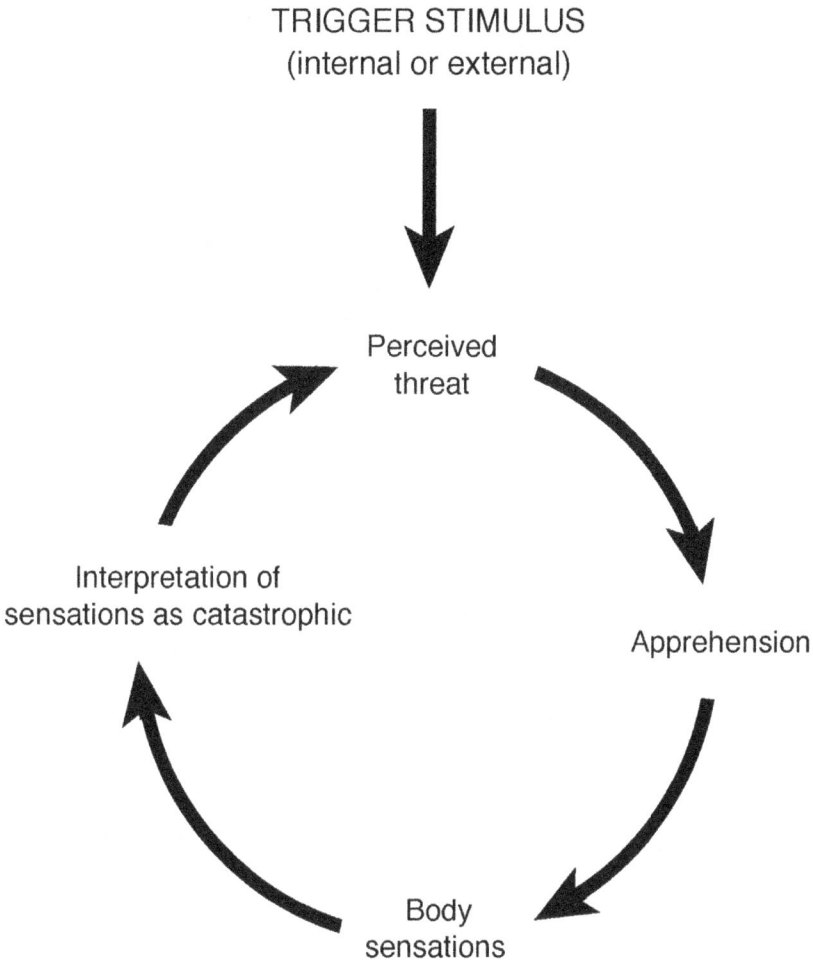

Figure 14.1. The generation of a panic attack according to Clark's cognitive model. Reprinted from *Behaviour Research and Therapy, 24*(4), D. M. Clark, "A Cognitive Approach to Panic," p. 463, Copyright 1986, with permission from Elsevier.

The subsequent attentional and biological amplification of symptoms will cause the person to be even more frightened that there is a dangerous disturbance of the body. This increased fear further worsens the somatic symptoms (Clark & Wells, 1997). In this way, the person becomes increasingly caught up in an escalating spiral of fear (see Figures 14.1 and 14.2). (This model equally applies to mental symptoms of anxiety, such as racing thoughts, poor concentration, and forgetfulness.)

SITUATION:
Walking my dog in the park

Slightly breathless, tightness in my chest

"Maybe there is something wrong"

Anxious

THOUGHT
"I'm having a heart attack"
&
IMAGE
See myself collapsed and
my dog looking lost

More breathless
Chest pain
Racing heart
Dizzy

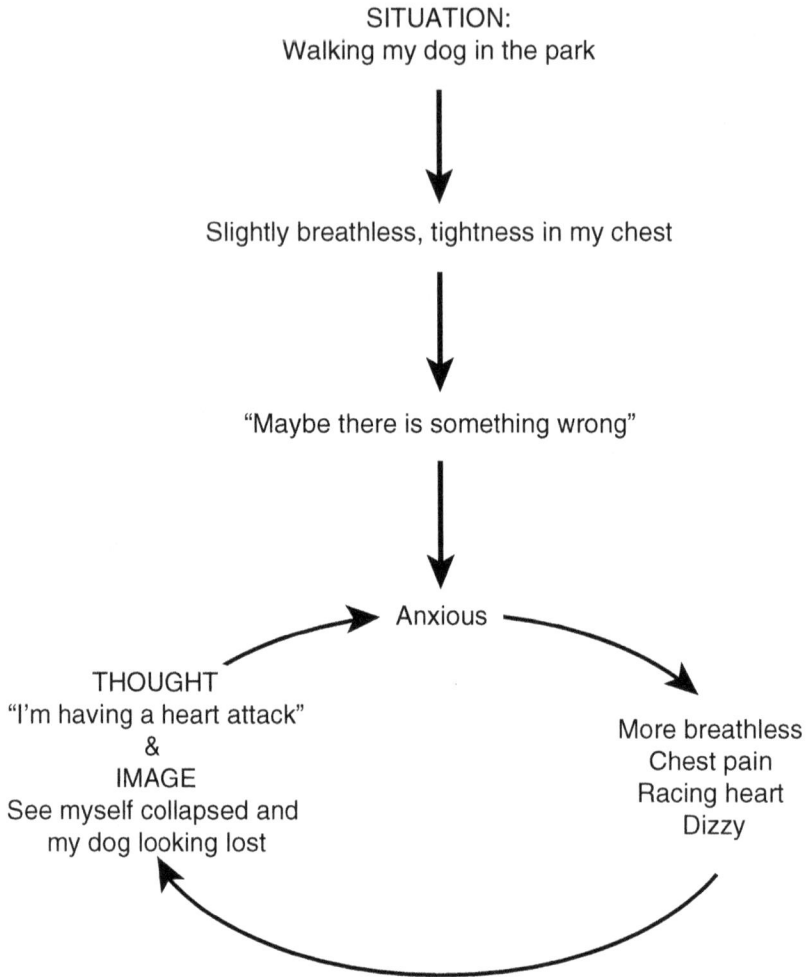

Figure 14.2. An example of the generation of a panic attack according to Clark's cognitive model. Reprinted from "Cognitive Therapy for Anxiety Disorders," by D. M. Clark & A. Wells, in L. J. Dickstein, M. B. Riba, & J. M. Oldham (Eds.), *Review of Psychiatry*, p. I-22. Copyright 1997 by the American Psychiatric Publishing.

The importance of attention and interpretation of symptom meaning in Clark's model suggests that cultural influences will play a key role in what we refer to as bioattentional looping and associated psychological distress as it plays out in a specific context. In particular, Clark's model suggests that panic attacks and PD (characterized by repeated, disabling panic attacks) – and other disorders involving panic attacks and PD, like somatization, GAD, and PTSD – will vary across cultures in several ways. The frequency of panic attacks and panic disorder may vary because a culture may provide many potential catastrophic interpretations of common somatic symptoms, for example, that certain somatic symptoms signal an imminent stroke (Hinton, Chong, Pollack, Barlow, & McNally, 2008; Hinton, Pich, Safren, Pollack, & McNally, 2006). Certain panic triggers may be unique to a culture or may be much more frequent in one culture than in another owing to specific ideas about what may cause physiological dysregulation. Among Vietnamese refugees, for example, being hit by a cold wind may cause panic, and among Cambodian refugees, standing up from a sitting or lying position as well as encountering certain smells often does (D. E. Hinton, Hinton, Pham, Chau, & Tran, 2003; Hinton, Pich, Chhean, Pollack, & Barlow, 2004). The catastrophic cognitions that are prominent in a panic attack may reflect differences in the cultural syndromes to which the panic attack symptoms are attributed and the physiological disturbance that it is feared the panic attack symptoms indicate (Hinton, Pich, Marques, Nickerson, & Pollack, 2010).

Clark's model would also suggest great variation in panic symptoms. The *DSM-5* (APA, 2013) lists certain somatic symptoms in the panic attack criteria (see Table 14.1), but the symptoms that are most salient for patients or emphasized during panic attacks may vary because particular somatic sensations are expected or are the focus of particular concern. For example, dizziness appears to be prominent in the panic attacks of Cambodian and Vietnamese refugees (Hinton, Hinton, et al., 2012). Other symptoms related to autonomic arousal that are not included in the *DSM-5* panic attack description may give rise to catastrophic cognitions in certain cultural contexts. Among Cambodian refugees, tinnitus and neck soreness are common in panic attacks because those symptoms are thought to be produced by the ethnophysiological disturbances in which the windlike substance *khyâl*, along with blood, are thought to surge upward in the body to cause various disastrous forms of *khyâl* attack (Hinton, Pich, et al., 2010).

The Clark model would also indicate that the ways in which panic disorder and panic attacks are treated in a culture will vary radically. How panic is treated will depend on the cultural syndrome or physiological disturbance to which the somatic symptoms and associated affect are attributed. Moreover, according to the Clark model, the interpersonal consequences of having panic attacks and panic disorder will vary greatly across culture: it will depend on their causal attributions in that culture, as seen, for example, in the responses to *khyâl* attacks among Cambodian

Table 14.1 *Panic Attack Specifier*

An abrupt surge of intense fear or intense discomfort that reaches a peak within minutes, and during which time four (or more) of the following symptoms occur:

Note: The abrupt surge can occur from a calm state or an anxious state.
1.   Palpitations, pounding heart, or accelerated heart rate.
2.   Sweating.
3.   Trembling or shaking.
4.   Sensations of shortness of breath or smothering.
5.   Feelings of choking.
6.   Chest pain or discomfort.
7.   Nausea or abdominal distress.
8.   Feeling dizzy, unsteady, light-headed, or faint.
9.   Chills or heat sensations.
10. Paresthesias (numbness or tingling sensations).
11. Derealization (feelings of unreality) or depersonalization (being detached from oneself).
12. Fear of losing control or "going crazy."
13. Fear of dying.

Source. Reprinted with permission from the *Diagnostic and Statistical Manual of Mental Disorders* (5th ed.), p. 214 (Copyright @2013). American Psychiatric Association.

refugees or *ataque de nervios* in Latino populations (see Lewis-Fernández & Aggarwal, Chapter 18, *this volume*).

A Hybrid Model of Panic and Somatization: The Multiplex Model of Panic Attacks and Somatization

Clark's model can be extended to a broader model of the generation of somatic symptoms and anxiety episodes that applies across cultures (Figure 14.3), which we have called the "multiplex model of somatic symptom and panic attack generation" (Hinton et al., 2000; Hinton, Chau, et al., 2001; Hinton, Hofmann, et al., 2008). This model explains how high rates of somatic symptoms, panic attacks, and unique panic subtypes are generated among trauma-exposed Cambodian and Vietnamese refugees. In addition to the psychological theory of panic-attack generation (Barlow, 2002; Clark, 1986), the multiplex model incorporates aspects of fear network theory (Foa & Kozak, 1998), the biology of fear, and anthropological models of somatization (Good, 1977; Kirmayer & Young, 1998; Kleinman & Kleinman, 1994).

According to the multiplex model, a trigger – anger, exertion, a worry episode, orthostatic hypotension (i.e., a drop in blood pressure on standing up), head rotation, hyperventilation, or thinking about a traumatic

SOCIO-CULTURAL PRAGMATICS
• Attempts at self-cure (e.g.,"coining") •
• Role of the somatic symptoms or panic attack-associated cultural syndrome as an idiom of distress •
• Economic, identity, and interpersonal effects of having the symptom or panic attack
(e.g., as a result of labeling the symptoms or panic attack as indicating a certain cultural syndrome) •

Trauma associations to the sensation

Catastrophic cognitions about the sensation
(e.g., attribution of the sensation to a cultural syndrome:
among Cambodian refugees, attribution of the sensation to the onset of a *khyâl* attack)

A sensation
(e.g., dizziness or palpitations)

Escalating distress and arousal

Trigger of sensations
(e.g., worry, stress, or anger)

Metaphoric resonances
of the sensation

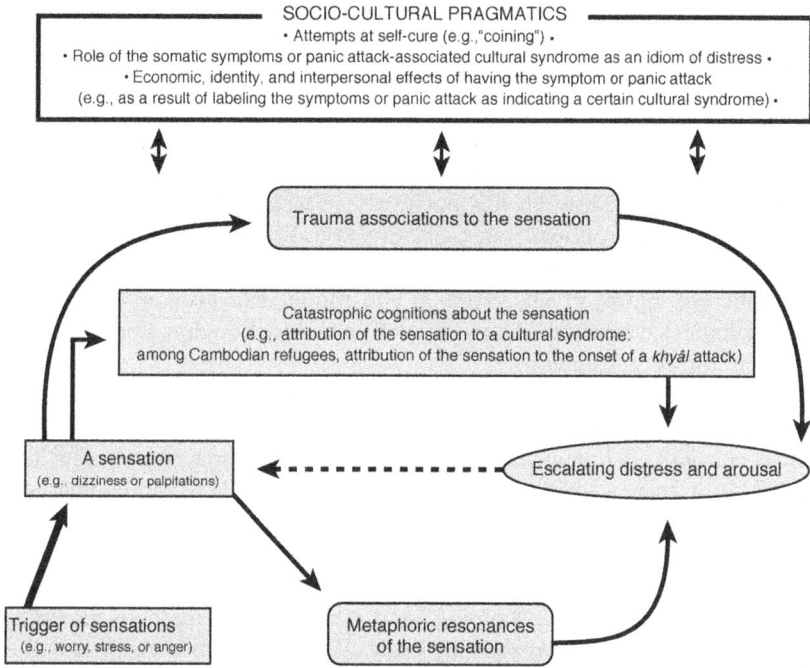

Figure 14.3. The generation of a somatic complaint and/or a panic attack according to the multiplex model. There are many possible triggers of the initial sensation: worry, stress, fear, anger, exertion (e.g., climbing stairs), metaphor-guided somatization, smells, trauma recall, startle, motion sickness. The sensation may also result from hypervigilant surveying of the body for symptoms (1) when in a self-perceived weak state or (2) when engaging in an activity, like standing up, that is feared to induce sensations and trigger a dangerous physiological disturbance. Once induced, the sensation may activate dysphoric networks such as catastrophic cognitions about the sensation. As indicated in the figure, all levels of the model may be influenced by sociocultural pragmatics: attempts at cure, the role of the symptom or syndrome as a culturally sanctioned idiom of distress, and the economic, identity, and interpersonal effects of having a somatic symptom or panic attack and its associated syndrome.

event – causes the individual to experience a bodily sensation such as dizziness. The sensation then activates one or more types of dysphoria networks: catastrophic cognitions, trauma associations, and/or metaphoric resonances. Activation of these dysphoria networks increases anxiety, and this heightened anxiety further increases the bodily sensation by such means as attentional amplification (e.g., greater scrutiny of the body in search of feared symptoms such as, among Cambodian refugees, symptoms thought to be part of a *khyâl* attack: dizziness and neck soreness) and biological amplification (e.g., an increase in SNS activity). When the sensation that initially triggered panic is intensified, and other sensations possibly induced, the dysphoria networks become further activated by those new and intensified sensations and the accompanying distress. Through this positive feedback or bioattentional loop, the person may experience an escalating spiral of arousal that leads to a panic attack, as depicted in Figure 14.3 (Hinton, Chau, et al., 2001; Hinton, Hofmann, et al., 2010). (The model can also be applied to psychological symptoms of anxiety such as racing thoughts, poor concentration, and forgetfulness.)

As the model shows, certain other variables will play a key part in the experiencing of panic attacks and the course of panic disorder, what we call socio-cultural pragmatics. For example, the person may try to treat the episodes or to prevent them in certain ways. Methods of self-coping and help-seeking depend on how panic attack symptoms are labeled and understood. Self-coping may consist simply of running outside for air when feeling short of breath; taking a pill such as an anxiolytic medication; or, in the case of a Cambodian refugee, "coining" and other physical methods aimed at regulating the flow of *khyâl* in the body. If the problem is recurrent, the person may seek treatment between episodes with religious leaders, traditional healers, or biomedical experts. Others in the sufferer's social world may respond to somatic complaints and panic attacks in ways that may range from solicitous concern to irritation, stigmatization, and rejection.

A somatic complaint or panic episode also may be understood and interpreted by others as an "idiom of distress," that is, as a culturally sanctioned way of expressing distress. These idioms may also shape illness experience. Thus, a person who feels extreme distress might embody and enact the panic attack form in that culture – for example, *ataque*-type panic attacks in the Latino context or *khyâl*-type panic attacks in the Cambodian context – for lack of other ways of expressing extremely negative affect and desperation. Somatic symptoms and panic attacks might then become a sort of psychological "safety-valve," or alternative pathway to express and work through extreme distress (Carr & Vitaliano, 1985; Lewis-Fernández & Aggarwal, Chapter 18, *this volume*).

In addition to individual physiological and psychological dynamics, therefore, the course of panic attacks and panic disorder will be influenced by the ways that the particular form and interpretation of the disorder, affects the afflicted person's social networks, identity, position and status. This will depend in large part on the attribution or labeling of the distress as a certain type of syndrome or other kind of "disturbance."

Cultural Syndromes and the Multiplex Model: The Example of *Khyâl* Attacks among Cambodian Refugees

Cambodians and Vietnamese often consider anxiety symptoms to be generated by dangerous physiological dysregulations. This interpretation of physiological arousal leads to frequent panic attacks driven by catastrophic cognitions. To illustrate this phenomenon, we address below the Cambodian ethnophysiology of *khyâl* (for a discussion of these same processes among Vietnamese patients, see Hinton et al., 2003; Hinton, Chau, et al., 2001). For the multiplex model of cultural syndromes, see Figure 14.4. This figure unpacks the processes involving catastrophic cognitions that are present but are only partially depicted in the panic attack multiplex model (Figure 14.3).

A person asks certain types of questions on first noticing a bodily symptom. "Why am I having this sensation? What is causing it? Does this sensation indicate a serious medical problem?" Cambodians interpret somatic sensations in terms of *khyâl*, as detailed in Figure 14.5 and Table 14.2 (Hinton, Pich, et al., 2010). *Khyâl* refers to external "wind" and to a key element of bodily physiology: an air that courses through the inner conduits of the body alongside blood (Figure 14.5, Table 14.2). Cambodians refer to almost any anxiety episode, especially a panic attack, as a *kaeut khyâl* ("wind attack"), one of nine cultural concepts of distress recognized by *DSM-5* (APA, 2013).

According to the Cambodian conceptualization, the healthy person's blood and *khyâl* ("inner air") run unimpeded through conduits in the body (Hinton, Pich, et al., 2010). But if the flow of blood and *khyâl* is blocked, joint discomfort or cold hands and feet result, with the knee and elbow being considered the most frequent locations of blockage. If not corrected, this blockage is thought to lead to the "death" of the limb distal to the blockage as a result of insufficient blood perfusion. Moreover, if blood and *khyâl* cannot flow outward along the limb, they ascend upward in the body, bringing about various disturbances (see Figure 14.5): Blood and *khyâl* surge upward and enter *the thorax*, causing palpitations and shortness of breath, as well as possibly cardiac arrest and fatal asphyxia; *the neck vessels*, causing neck soreness and possibly neck-vessel rupture; and *the head*, causing dizziness, tinnitus (*khyâl* exiting from the ears), blurry vision (*khyâl* exiting the eyes), and possibly syncope, deafness, and blindness.

In Figure 14.5 and Table 14.2, we show how a Cambodian refugee might interpret each somatic anxiety symptoms in terms of *khyâl* and how this interpretation leads to catastrophic cognitions about those symptoms. The Cambodian's conceptualization of the physiology of somatic anxiety symptoms, according to which the symptoms are

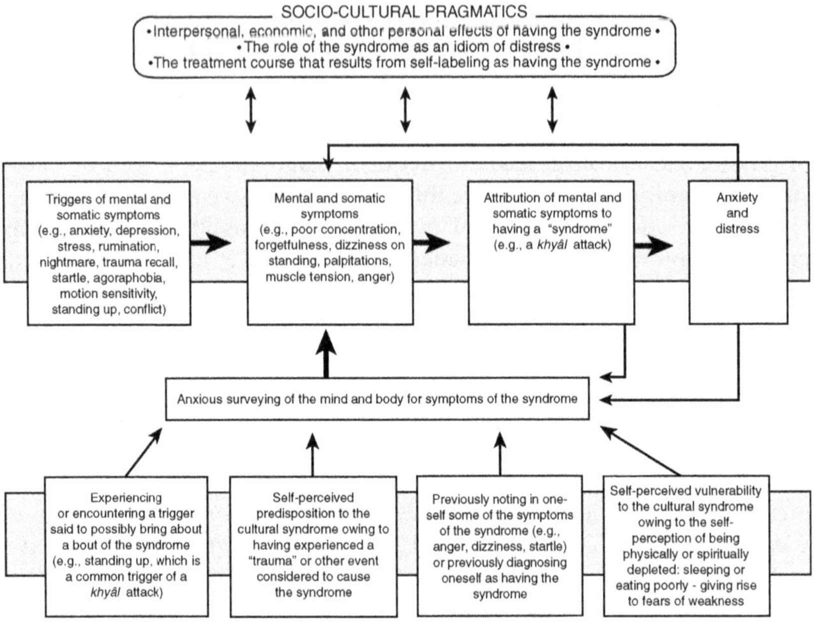

Figure 14.4. A multiplex model of the generation of a cultural syndrome. A trigger such as anxiety, standing up, or a conflict brings about an initial symptom. If the symptom is attributed to a syndrome, this will bring about more scrutinizing of the mind and body in search of syndrome-associated symptoms. This attribution also may give rise to catastrophic cognitions about syndrome-related disasters, and those catastrophic cognitions then result in anxiety and distress. That anxiety and distress may lead to more mental and somatic symptoms, thus creating more fear of having the syndrome. As indicated, hypervigilant surveying of the mind and body for symptoms results from several processes, such as experiencing a trigger that is known to cause a bout of the syndrome. This multiplex model is nested in that it takes into account sociocultural pragmatics: It shows the importance of the reaction of the social network to the person having the syndrome and its symptoms, as well as the economic effects and the effects of treatments that are self-administered, sought out, and received owing to labeling symptoms as a certain kind of disorder. (In some cases, a syndrome may not lead to anxiety and distress, but rather may just serve as an explanatory frame for behaviors such as anger, even a justificatory frame, that is, a frame that excuses behaviors. But the rest of the model still applies.)

produced by the flow of blood and *khyâl*, profoundly influences the interpretation of anxiety states and gives rise to fears of dire physical outcomes caused by a pathomechanics of blood and *khyâl*. Although *khyâl* may be a culture-specific concern, these thoughts fit the same form

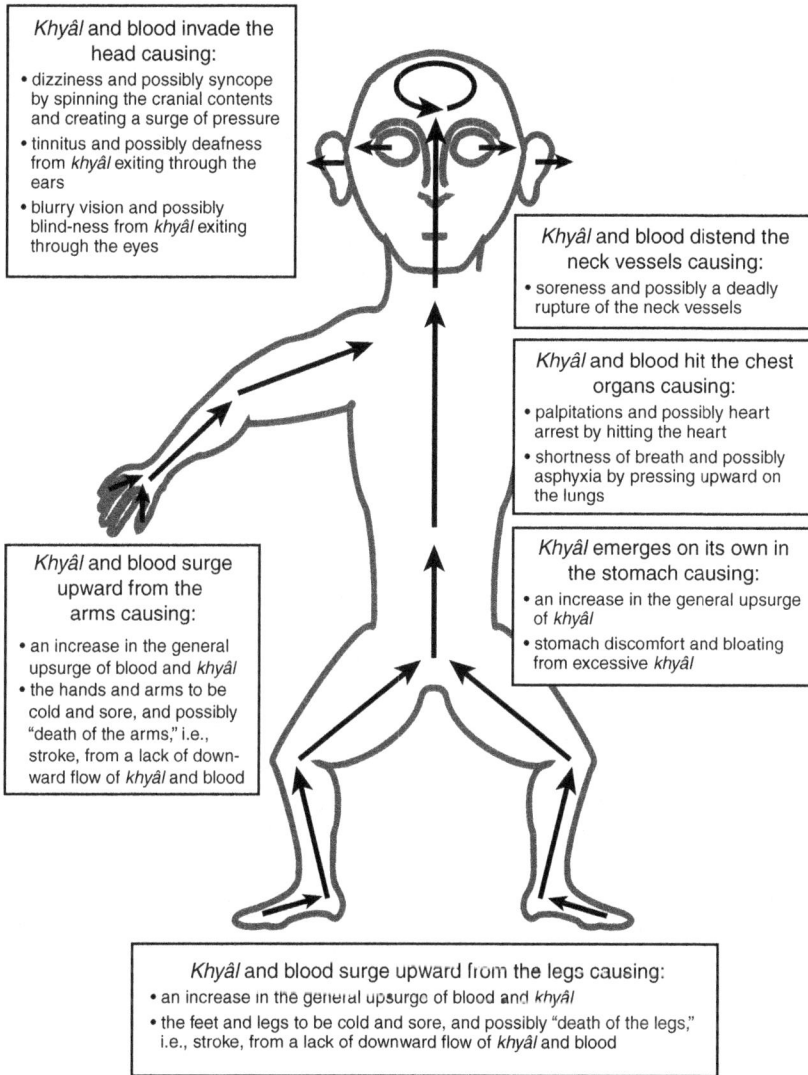

Khyâl and blood invade the head causing:
• dizziness and possibly syncope by spinning the cranial contents and creating a surge of pressure
• tinnitus and possibly deafness from khyâl exiting through the ears
• blurry vision and possibly blind-ness from khyâl exiting through the eyes

Khyâl and blood distend the neck vessels causing:
• soreness and possibly a deadly rupture of the neck vessels

Khyâl and blood hit the chest organs causing:
• palpitations and possibly heart arrest by hitting the heart
• shortness of breath and possibly asphyxia by pressing upward on the lungs

Khyâl and blood surge upward from the arms causing:
• an increase in the general upsurge of blood and khyâl
• the hands and arms to be cold and sore, and possibly "death of the arms," i.e., stroke, from a lack of down-ward flow of khyâl and blood

Khyâl emerges on its own in the stomach causing:
• an increase in the general upsurge of khyâl
• stomach discomfort and bloating from excessive khyâl

Khyâl and blood surge upward from the legs causing:
• an increase in the general upsurge of blood and khyâl
• the feet and legs to be cold and sore, and possibly "death of the legs," i.e., stroke, from a lack of downward flow of khyâl and blood

Figure 14.5. A *khyâl* attack: ethnophysiology, symptoms, and associated disasters. The arrows represent the flow of *khyâl* and blood upward in the body during a *khyâl* attack. During the healthy state, *khyâl* and blood flow downward in the direction opposite to the arrows, with *khyâl* exiting the body through the hands and feet, through bodily pores, and down through the gastrointestinal tract, but during a *khyâl* attack, *khyâl* and blood surge upward in the body to cause the disasters outlined above.

Table 14.2 *The Interpretation of Somatic Symptoms in Terms of a Khyâl Attack: Correlated Physiological State and Feared Consequence*

Symptom	Correlated Physiological State	Feared Consequence
Dizziness	A surge of *khyâl* and blood into the head	Syncope, "*khyâl* attack," and "*khyâl* overload" (*khyâl koeu*)
Tinnitus	A pressure-like escape of *khyâl* from the ears, with tinnitus being called "*khyâl* exits from the ears" (*khyâl ceuny taam treujieu*)	Deafness, *khyâl* attack, and *khyâl* overload
Blurry vision	A pressurelike escape of *khyâl* from the eyes	Blindness, *khyâl* attack, and *khyâl* overload
Headache	A rush of *khyâl* and blood into the head and its vessels	Syncope, *khyâl* attack, and *khyâl* overload
Neck soreness	A surge of *khyâl* and blood into the neck vessels	Bursting of the neck vessels, *khyâl* attack, and *khyâl* overload
Nausea	An accumulation of excessive *khyâl* in the stomach and abdomen, with the *khyâl* threatening to rise upward in the body	*Khyâl* rising upward from the abdomen into the body to cause asphyxia, cardiac arrest, and various cerebral catastrophes, to cause a *khyâl* attack and *khyâl* overload
Palpitations	An upward surge of *khyâl* and blood from the limbs or stomach that presses on the heart, interfering with its pumping; and the heart overexerts itself trying to pump blood and *khyâl* through blocked vessels	Cardiac arrest and all disasters associated with a weakened heart, such as poor circulation in the limbs resulting in coagulation in the limbs, with the limb blockage then causing a surge of *khyâl* and blood upward in the body
Shortness of breath	An upward surge of *khyâl* from the limbs or stomach to press on the lungs and cause shortness of breath	Asphyxia, *khyâl* attack, and *khyâl* overload
Soreness in the legs or arms	A blocking of the flow of *khyâl* and blood at the arm and leg joints, with sore joints being called "plugged vessels" (*cok sosai*) or "blocked *khyâl*" (*sla khyâl*)	"Death" of the limbs from a lack of outward flow along the limbs as well as a surge of *khyâl* and blood upward in the body to cause various disasters: asphyxia, heart arrest, neck-vessel rupture, and syncope
Cold hands or feet	A blocking of the outward flow of *khyâl* and blood at the limb joints, preventing the perfusion of the hands or feet	"Death" of the limbs from a lack of outward flow along the limbs as well as a surge of *khyâl* and blood upward in the body to cause various disasters: asphyxia, heart arrest, neck-vessel rupture, and syncope

Table 14.2 (*cont.*)

Symptom	Correlated Physiological State	Feared Consequence
Poor appetite	A direct effect of excessive bodily *khyâl*	Weakness from poor food intake, which in turn may cause various physiological consequences: dizziness on standing, palpitations on exposure to stimuli, and a predisposition to *khyâl* attacks.
Energy depletion	A direct effect of excessive bodily *khyâl* that worsens the energy depletion that initially produced the *khyâl* attack (e.g., the depletion that was caused by overexertion, poor sleep, or poor appetite)	A weakened heart that may result in dizziness on standing, heart arrest on slight provocation, and *khyâl* attacks, with *khyâl* attacks being caused by a weakened heart that does not adequately pump the *khyâl* and blood through the body, thereby resulting in coagulation-caused plugs in the limbs and thus an upward surge of *khyâl* and blood into the trunk, that is, a *khyâl* attack

as the catastrophic cognitions in Western cultures that often increase anxiety symptoms to the point of panic (Clark, 1996; Harvey, Richards, Dziadosz, & Swindell, 1993). In the West, these cognitions include fear of death and disability ("Am I having a stroke?" "Is this a heart attack?") and fear of insanity ("Am I having a nervous breakdown?"). The natural result of such catastrophic thinking – about *khyâl* concerns or other catastrophic explanations of symptoms – is increased anxiety, as indicated by several studies, one of which correlates panic intensity with the severity of associated catastrophic cognitions (Hedley, Hoffart, Dammen, Eckeberg, & Friis, 2000). The Cambodian refugee's complex explanatory models for anxiety symptoms, the *khyâl* ethnophysiology, provide one source of catastrophic fears that may drive panic responses.

Cambodian Self-Treatment of Khyâl-Related Panic Attacks

Because Cambodians consider anxiety attacks to be generated by *khyâl*, they self-treat anxiety attacks through *khyâl*-extraction techniques, most frequently "coining" and "cupping" (Hinton, Pich, et al., 2010). Coining is performed on the arms, chest, back, and neck. To coin, a Cambodian dips the edge of a coin in "*khyâl* oil," a menthol substance that purportedly promotes *khyâl*'s escape from the body. The coin edge is then dragged across the skin in a proximal-to-distal direction, producing a linear mark (for film footage of "coining" and other ways Cambodians treat *khyâl*, see www.khyalattack.com). Cambodians worriedly assess the color of the streaks: Red denotes minimal *khyâl* accumulation, whereas a darker hue, especially purple, indicates excessive *khyâl*. A dark hue like purple causes great concern and leads to more coining and, if indicated owing to severity, another "*khyâl*-removal" technique, which is often cupping. In cupping, the rim of a warmed glass is placed against the skin, usually on the back or on the forehead. When the glass cools the contained air contracts, and the resulting vacuum is considered to pull the *khyâl* upward through skin pores into the glass.

Ideally, coining and other methods are performed by a family member or friend – it is impossible to coin or cup one's own back, for example – so a *khyâl* attack is often a highly interpersonal event. Also, because these attacks are often thought to be caused by "worry" or depressive thoughts, which are believed to weaken the body and predispose a person to attacks, anyone in the family who may have contributed to worry or sadness is aware of this possible causation. This can result in a process of interpersonal looping (Kirmayer & Sartorius, 2007). For example, blame might fall on a husband who has been suspected of infidelity or a child who is not going to school. *Khyâl* attacks are read by others as an idiom of distress, part of the Cambodian conceptualization of sociosomatics (Kleinman & Becker, 1998).

Somatic Symptoms and the Multiplex Model: Four Dimensions of Somatic Sensations

As specified in the multiplex model (Figure 14.3), the sensation that initiates distress and possibly panic may be produced by many different triggers, including worry, an exacerbation of chronic anxiety, acute fear, or simply standing up. Once the sensation is triggered, the individual reacts according to specific cultural meanings and personal associations.

As suggested earlier in this chapter, a somatic symptom can be conceived of as having four dimensions (the process of biological causation might be considered a fifth dimension):

1. Associated local interpretive schemas, which include ethnophysiology, ethnopsychology, and ethnospirituality as well as related syndromes (i.e., the symptom may be interpreted in terms of local ideas about the workings of the mind, the physiology of the body, and the nature of the spirit world, such as an attack by a "ghost");
2. Associated trauma-related emotions, meanings, and memories;

3. Associated metaphoric resonances (i.e., the symptom may be present in key metaphors to express distress in the culture); and
4. Role as a cultural idiom of distress (i.e., as a culturally recognized indicator of distress).

These networks of meaning can explain the prominence of certain somatic symptoms in somatization and the anxiety disorders of individuals and cultural groups.

Let us see how this model (Figure 14.3) applies to dizziness among Cambodian refugees, a very common distress presentation in that group, as well as among Vietnamese refugees (for a review, see Hinton & Hinton, 2002; Hinton, Hinton, et al., 2012). Generally speaking, dizziness may be induced in multiple ways: by activation of the autonomic nervous system owing to stress, anxiety, or fear; hyperventilation during emotional upset; motion sickness from riding in a car or from simply walking through a crowd. Among Cambodians, all these are common causes, and so too standing up (i.e., orthostasis). And among Cambodian refugees, worry is a particularly common trigger of dizziness, with worry themes ranging from financial issues to concerns about health. Worry appears to induce dizziness through metaphor-guided somatization, rapid induction of arousal, and, perhaps, a biological predisposition for this group to experience dizziness during states of dysphoria (Hinton et al., 2000, Hinton, Um, & Ba, 2001a, 2001b; Hinton, Chau, et al., 2001; Hinton, Pich, et al., 2010).

Cambodians consider dizziness to be the key indicator of a sudden upward movement of blood and *khyâl* all the way to the head, a severe state called a "*khyâl* attack" (or "wind attack," *kaeut khyâl*). On experiencing dizziness, a Cambodian may search the body for other signs of excessive inner *khyâl* and a dysregulation of blood and *khyâl* flow – cold hands and feet, shortness of breath, palpitations, sore neck, tinnitus – and will fear the various catastrophes associated with excessive inner *khyâl* (Figure 14.5, Table 14.2): stroke, asphyxia, heart arrest, deafness, vision loss, syncope, and rupture of neck vessels.

During the Pol Pot period, many physical and psychological traumas were associated with experiences of dizziness. Starvation combined with overwork in rice fields or construction often caused Cambodians to feel dizzy on standing up. Malaria was widespread during the Pol Pot period. Many died from the disease, while those who recovered endured months of recurrent attacks, which, typically began with chills followed by intense fever, accompanied by nausea, anxiety, palpitations, shortness of breath, and severe dizziness. Malaria may predispose individuals to panic disorder by forming trauma associations with symptoms of autonomic arousal such as chills, dizziness, and palpitations. Dizziness was also experienced by many during the Pol Pot period on seeing bloodied, injured or decaying bodies, a frequent event, and on witnessing executions, also common. (Exposure to the sight of blood and injury can cause fear along with a drop in blood pressure related to a vaso-vagal fainting response.) More generally, any trauma marked by dizziness that resulted from a surge of fear that occurred at that time may be encoded in memory in association with dizziness and may be recalled later on experiencing dizziness for any reason, setting up a potential vicious circle between bodily distress and trauma memory.

Cambodians frequently describe distress with dizziness images; if a child acts out and causes distress, a Cambodian may say, "my son shakes me" (*goun greulok knyom*). "Being busy" is "to be spinning rapidly" (*rewuel*). Worry itself is described as a kind of spinning of the mind, a turning of the head from one problem to another, as in "I think here and then I think there" (*kut anjeh anjoh*) or "I think up and then I think down" (*kut nih, kut nuh*). Traumatized Cambodian patients at our psychiatric clinic often string together such expressions when explaining why they feel dizzy, another common expression being, "My son shakes me. He makes me dizzy" (*goun greulok khyom, wul muk*). Sometimes dizziness brings existential and social issues to mind, such as confronting life's meaning or experiencing confused anger with circling thoughts about a personal dilemma; that is, a sensation like dizziness may evoke its related networks of metaphoric meaning and associated distress. Owing to these various distress idioms cast in dizziness images, patients tend to somaticize dizziness during distress through metaphor-guided somatization, and additionally others in their social network may well read "dizziness" as an idiom of distress because the link of dizziness to worry is well known. For these reasons, dizziness serves as an idiom of distress that may be embodied as an expression of distress, a sort cry for help.

Now let us see how this model (Figure 14.3) applies to neck soreness among Cambodian refugees, a very common distress presentation in this group (Hinton, Chhean, et al., 2006; Hinton, Um, & Ba, 2001c). Neck complaints also are extremely common among Cambodian refugee patients and often give rise to panic. Anxiety states – from worry to panic – increase tension in shoulder and neck musculature, primarily the trapezius muscle, which may cause pain (Arena, Bruno, Hannah, & Meador, 1995; Hazlett, Mcleod, & Hoehn-Saric, 1994; Noyes & Hoehn-Saric, 1998). Anxiety and panic also increase the tension of the frontalis muscle, producing a feeling of pressure in the head (Hoehn-Saric, Mcleod, & Zimmerli, 1991).

Cambodians may attribute neck tension to excessive *khyâl*, and imagine a pressurized rise of blood and *khyâl* into the neck and possibly upward into the confines of the cranium. So neck soreness may trigger panic attacks as the sufferer visualizes the rising blood and *khyâl* bursting the neck vessels and spinning the cranial contents to cause dizziness and possibly syncope, and imagines the *khyâl* shooting forth from the ears to cause tinnitus and shooting from the eyes to cause blurry vision (Hinton, Chhean, et al., 2006; Hinton, Um, et al., 2001c). Thus, neck soreness leads to a hypervigilant surveying of the body for all the somatic signs of a *khyâl* attack, further causing bioattentional looping, symptom amplification, and possibly panic.

Many Cambodian refugees survived brutal beatings to the body and head; the most common form of execution was a blow to the back of the head, and some survived this assault. These events may by recalled by neck tension. In addition, Cambodians worked as many as fifteen hours a day during the Pol Pot period. Dam building was one of the most difficult tasks, and involved carrying buckets of dirt balanced at either end of a rod placed across the shoulders. Some Cambodian refugees in the United States who develop a sore neck may experience vivid flashbacks of this labor, and commonly cite it as the origin of their pain (Hinton, Chhean, et al., 2006; Hinton, Um, et al., 2001c).

The English language has many metaphors concerning posture and weight-carrying that associate upright posture with health and moral rectitude, while slouching is a sign of being weighed-down, overburdened, or "unable to bear any more." Similarly, in Khmer, many distress expressions are based on the neck. For example, to describe a state of being overwhelmed by financial or other problems, one may say *tnguen go*, meaning "heavy in the neck." A Cambodian may tell someone, "Don't carry that pole at your neck, with its heavy load, all by yourself" (*gom reek khluen aeng*), meaning "let me help with your burden." Or, if one gives a little money to someone in financial distress, one "helps to carry the pole at the neck, with its heavy load" (*juey reek*). (Neck soreness will also serve as an idiom of distress for the reasons described above for dizziness.)

The Multiplex Model of Panic: The Example of Orthostatic Panic Among Cambodian Refugees

Many Cambodian patients experience anticipatory anxiety in certain situations that may contribute to the risk of panic attacks. On arising from bed in the morning, for example, if a traumatized Cambodian slept poorly and is worrying about some problem – with worry and poor sleep

both considered processes that weaken the body – he or she may anticipate feeling dizzy on standing (Hinton, Hofmann, et al., 2010; Hinton,
Um, et al., 2001a). The expectation of having dizziness and a *khyâl*
attack on standing may lead to both increased bodily attention and
physiological arousal (Clark, 1986). Sensations of dizziness, along with
other autonomic arousal symptoms, may then activate trauma associations, metaphoric resonances, and catastrophic cognitions. This activation of fear networks produces yet greater anxiety. Because dizziness
and other autonomic sensations may be increased by autonomic arousal,
a vicious cycle results and may culminate in panic (see Figure 14.3). The
processes of symptom generation and amplification are illustrated in the
following case vignette.

A Case Example of Orthostatic Panic

On initial presentation to the psychiatric clinic, fifty-nine-year-old Chan
was having orthostatic panic attacks three times a week. On standing, he
experienced severe dizziness, along with cold hands, palpitations, and
neck soreness. He would immediately sit down, fearing "*khyâl* overload,"
cardiac arrest, neck-vessel rupture, and "death of the hands and legs"
(*ngoeup day ngoeup ceung*). Chan's panic attack would last about an hour.
During about a third of these attacks, Chan had visual flashbacks of
either the brutal execution of his two brothers or the butchered bodies
of two villagers killed by Pol Pot's soldiers for having tried to escape.
Chan's dizziness, neck tension, and palpitations were particularly severe.
To relieve these symptoms, he would immediately begin to "coin" his
neck and limbs in an attempt to remove excessive inner *khyâl*.

In the Khmer Rouge period, Chan had worked twelve-hour days; twice
a day he was fed a watery broth that contained only a few grains of rice.
The work was mainly rice transplantation and dam building, the latter
entailing digging up and carrying dirt in a bucket to help construct a
dam. During those tasks – with his misery compounded by a scorching
sun, a gnawing hunger, and chronic malaria – he often felt dizzy, especially after bending over. Many people collapsed while working, some
never standing up again.

In the Pol Pot period, Chan, like most Cambodians, suffered from
severe malaria. Chan had malarial attacks every day for six months, with
each episode lasting forty-five minutes, marked by rigors and palpitations. Even after a malarial attack commenced, he was forced to continue working. He would struggle to accomplish his task, but when the
attack intensified, he experienced extreme dizziness and collapsed; lying
vertiginous and helpless, he would be dragged to the side of the field.

During these episodes, Chan was accused by his captors of feigning illness and was threatened with execution.

One of Chan's flashbacks on standing up replayed the following. In the Khmer Rouge period, just before the Vietnamese invasion of his village, Chan and his two brothers were transplanting rice about an hour's walk from the village. Suddenly, Khmer Rouge solders arrived and arrested all three. The soldiers had learned that Chan's two brothers had been government soldiers prior to the invasion. The Khmer Rouge routinely hunted down and executed all former soldiers. Although Chan had worked as a rice farmer his entire life, he was also arrested and charged with two crimes: being related to a soldier and not revealing his brothers' identities to the authorities. Three Khmer Rouge soldiers escorted Chan's brothers about fifty yards away while another three soldiers guarded Chan. One of the soldiers lit a cigarette, and while blowing smoke into Chan's face, told him that they intended to kill and eviscerate his brothers, consume their livers, and drink their gall bladder bile. (In this way, according to the Khmer Rouge reasoning, they would assimilate the brothers' vital essence and power, thought to reside in those body parts.) Chan's heart pounded, his chest tightened, and his face flushed with blood; in his head he felt a whirling spiral of fear and rage, made worse by the cigarette fumes. He watched as the Khmer Rouge bound his brothers' hands behind their backs and then killed them with a rifle shot into the chest. The soldiers escorted Chan to view his brothers' bodies and forced him to watch as they cut abdomens open, removed the livers – the gall bladder still attached – and placed the organs on a banana leaf. Overcome with panic, nausea, dizziness, and leg weakness, Chan thought himself about to collapse. The soldiers released him, loudly announcing that he would experience a similar fate if he committed any errors.

The other flashback that Chan had on standing up involved an event that occurred a few weeks after the execution of his brothers. The Khmer Rouge commanded the villagers to assemble before their leader's house. Chan and his fellow villagers were forced to view the butchered corpses of two people who had tried to escape. Their body parts were in orderly heaps arranged by type: eight limbs (four legs and four arms); two heads, severed at the neck; and two eviscerated trunks, the flaps of skin draping like small open doors, revealing an abdominal cavity from which the liver had been extricated in order to be eaten. Weak-kneed, dizzy, and nauseated, Chan stared at the horrifying image of his own likely fate. Luckily, a month later the Vietnamese invaded his village, and he seized the moment to escape and managed to reach the Thai border.

Years later, in the United States, other events had caused Chan to become more anxious, which he recounted on his presentation for psychiatric care at a clinic in Lowell, Massachusetts. His eighteen-year-old son had stopped attending school, stayed out late, and acted very disrespectfully toward him, often using rude language. Thinking about his son made Chan angry, anxious, and dizzy. When he stood up and felt dizzy, thoughts about this son entered his mind, increasing his distress and dysphoria. For Chan, dizziness brought back specific traumas that occurred in Cambodia, and if he became distressed for any reason, for example by worrying that standing up could cause him to collapse, the resulting dizziness activated those memory networks. Also, when he thought about a current social or financial problem, such as his son's behavior, dizziness and other symptoms occurred that predisposed him to panic on standing. Sometimes, if he thought about his conflict with his son just before standing, severe dizziness and panic occurred on rising. Chan was concerned that worry about his son "weakened" him (both directly and by affecting sleep and appetite), predisposing him to dizziness on standing. In addition, he and his wife were having conflicts, many centering on how to deal with the son.

Figure 14.6 summarizes key features of Chan's case from the perspective of the multiplex model. This can guide treatment interventions (for a discussion of how treatment follows from the Multiplex Model,

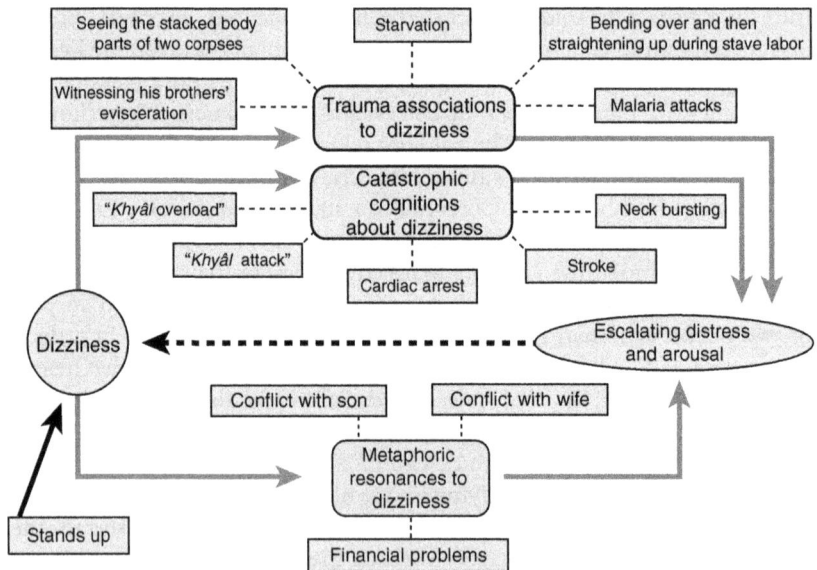

Figure 14.6. The generation of an orthostatic panic attack according to the multiplex model: The case of Chan.

see Hinton, Rivera, Hofmann, Barlow, & Otto, 2012). For example, Chan's catastrophic cognitions about standing up were addressed. We educated him about how the panic attacks were generated, and how his fear drove the symptoms, how the dizziness triggered his trauma memories. His memory associations were explored, in part as a way of investigating the link to past trauma. He was taught through interoceptive exposure to fear dizziness less and to reassociate positive memories to dizziness (e.g., traditional Cambodian games that induced dizziness). His current life situation was discussed and suggestions provided. He was taught applied muscle relaxation, which helped to reduce the physiological mechanisms that generate orthostatic dizziness. He used this and other techniques when he was distressed, such as when standing up seemed to be escalating to panic. He was educated about panic, such as teaching about the role of breathing in generating panic, and was taught how to use controlled breathing to reduce distress.

Conclusion

In this chapter, we have used Cambodian examples to illustrate how multiplex models (Figure 14.3, 14.4, and 14.7) explain the generation of somatic symptoms, panic attacks, and panic disorder, and how the episodes of distress occur, such as those triggered by worry. These episodes of distress are a key aspect of trauma-related disorder (Hinton, Hofmann, Pitman, Pollack, & Barlow, 2008). The panic and somatization multiplex model reveals how particular bodily symptoms may be induced and amplified, in some cases bringing about panic and in other cases illness worry or anxiety. The cultural syndrome multiplex model demonstrates how arousal, somatic symptoms, and cultural interpretation of symptoms interact through bioattentional looping to create a certain anxiety experience and presentation, a certain anxiety reality, centered on a cultural syndrome (Figure 14.4).

The multiplex model (and versions thereof) illustrates how the experiencing of somatic symptoms of anxiety and panic varies across cultures. There are cross-cultural differences in the initial triggers of somatic sensations, and in the catastrophic cognitions, metaphoric resonances, and trauma associations activated by the sensation. There are differences in the cultural syndromes to which sensations and panic may be attributed. There are differences in sociocultural pragmatics: treatments used for somatic symptoms and panic attacks, the use of somatic symptoms and panic attacks as idioms of distress, and the interpersonal, identity, and economic consequences of somatic symptoms and panic attacks. Clinical implications of the multiplex model were also discussed.

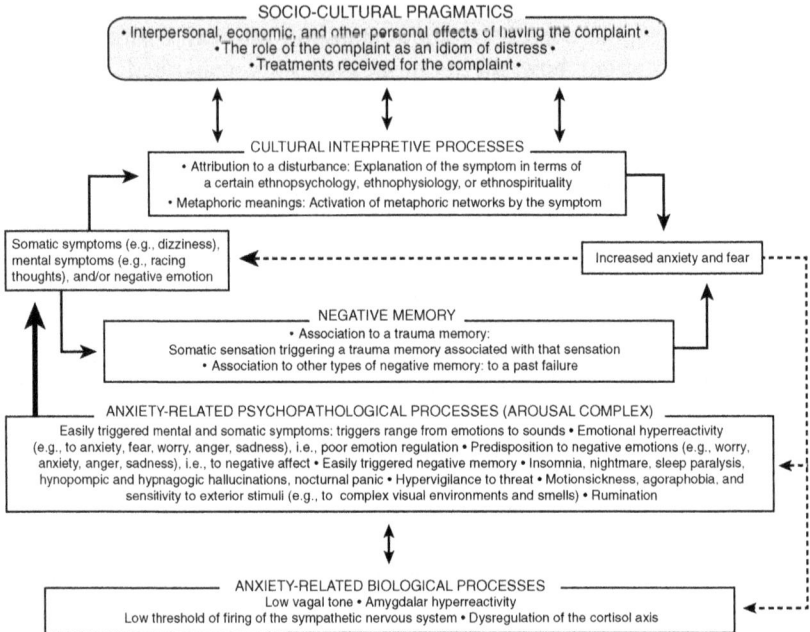

Figure 14.7. The multiplex anxiety model: a biocultural model of cultural influences on anxiety-related disorders. Feedback loops occur when cultural interpretive processes and negative memories increase arousal and distress, and when cultural interpretive processes lead to bioattentional looping, such as surveying the body for feared symptoms (see Figure 14.4).

(Please note the model works equally well for mental symptoms of anxiety such as poor concentration, racing thoughts, and forgetfulness.)

A broader version of the multiplex model, the "multiplex anxiety model" (Figure 14.7), depicts the role of anxiety-related biological processes in producing anxiety episodes. The biology of anxiety, stress, and trauma feeds into all aspects of the model: the biology leads to a predisposition to worry and to other negative emotions and to somatic and emotional hyperreactivity to sounds, smells, and even to emotional states such as worry. For example, poor vagal control may result in poor emotion regulation (and orthostatic dizziness), whereas amygdala hyperreactivity may produce startle and the recall of negative memories (Heim et al., 2000; Hinton, Hofmann, Pollack, & Otto, 2009). In all, three partially overlapping biological processes have been associated with fear or anxiety-related disorders (panic, phobias, PTSD): (1) hyperreactivity of the amygdala, a highly conserved and interconnected almond-shaped collection of nuclei in the medial temporal lobe that is particularly sensitive to potential threat; (2) dysregulation of the HPA axis, which orchestrates the synthesis and release of stress hormones (see Labonté, Farah, & Turecki, Chapter 8, *this volume*); and (3) low cardiac vagal tone (heart rate variability), which impairs the "self-regulatory capacity to adjust rapidly to stressful stimuli" (Porges, 2011), by, for example, inhibiting the SNS fight-or-flight mechanism activated by the amygdala or dampening the HPA axis response. Biological contributions to hyperreactivity and impaired self-regulation in the face of stress may be an initiating factor in the deleterious, bioattentional looping effects captured by the multiplex model.

The anxiety multiplex model is biocultural in that it not only takes into consideration the biological generation of symptoms but also posits that symptoms are generated by culturally shaped psychological processes operating in parallel with biology. For example, if the person learns to control worry by distancing from that affect, by engaging in loving-kindness meditation practices, or by learning to shift attention from rumination to mindful awareness of breath, then this will have biological effects, such as altering vagal tone, which will reduce many of the other symptoms of arousal (Hinton et al., 2009). Here we have looping effects between psychological and biological processes based on their parallelism (Cromwell & Panksepp, 2011).

The anxiety multiplex model posits that anxiety-related biological processes generate a potential "anxiety symptom pool," the symptoms of the arousal complex (Shorter, 1992). And as indicated in Figure 14.7, we hypothesize that the symptoms of the anxiety symptom pool, that is, the arousal complex, will be interpreted in terms of the local ethnopsychology, ethnophysiology, and ethnospirituality (e.g., nightmares may be attributed to a spirit assault or anxiety states to possession), and that this will lead to concern about having a culturally specified problem. This concern will lead to an increase of the very feared symptoms, to a kind of vicious loop we have called bioattentional looping. This is because the concern about having a culturally salient disorder may lead to increased arousal and to arousal symptoms (biological amplification) and to increased scanning of the body and mind for symptoms associated with the feared disorder of body, mind, or spiritual state (attentional amplification). These attentional and biological mechanisms worsen the symptoms and create spirals that result in ever greater autonomic arousal and self-scanning and to a progressive worsening of all the symptoms. At the same time, the symptoms in the anxiety pool – such as somatic symptoms and emotions like fear – will tend to activate trauma recall, which will in turn increase the anxiety symptoms and unleash another type of looping (i.e., trauma-association looping) that contributes to worsening, as trauma associations lead to more fear and somatic sensations that lead to more trauma associations.

These processes are nested within other processes, as illustrated in Figure 14.7, what we call sociocultural pragmatics. The person will tend to engage in self-help processes and traditional types of healing, and may be treated by biomedical or psychological therapies, which will influence the course of particular episodes of the illness and the general disorder. Being labeled as having a certain syndrome will also lead to certain interpersonal consequences, which may include the recognition and legitimation of one's suffering and opportunities for help and compensation, but also may result in an altered social identity and stigmatization. These are further types of looping as the effects of attempted treatments, interpersonal process, and economic effects feedback on other processes, such as influence current levels of arousal and hence the anxiety symptom pool. These loopings might be called treatment looping, interpersonal looping, and economic looping (cf. Kirmayer & Sartorius, 2007; McNally & Frueh, 2012), processes represented by the directional arrows in Figure 14.7.

The multiplex model emphasizes the central role of bioattentional looping, the importance of cultural interpretive processes (e.g., attribution of symptoms to cultural syndromes and the interpretation of symptoms in terms of a certain ethnopsychology, ethnophysiology and ethnospirituality), and the activation of negative memory. These processes are nested so that events at one level may have repercussions at other levels. The model highlights the importance of examining how self-help and other interventions alter the unfolding of acute episodes of distress and the course of the disorder over time. The multiplex model suggests the need for detailed analysis of episodes to understand the links between individual phenomenology and networks of personal and cultural meaning.

The multiplex model illustrates how particular cultural systems may interact with biological vulnerability and attentional processes, but also emphasizes individual difference. Personal history and experiences shape biological risk: There will be a certain genetic predisposition to the arousal complex that may be modified by epigenetic mechanisms (Bohacek, Gapp, Saab, & Mansuy, 2013; see also Labonté, Farah, & Turecki, Chapter 8, *this volume*). Individuals may have certain vagal and other biological states; insecurity and social conflict that gives rise to stress and worry; trauma histories; certain cultural interpretations of anxiety symptoms; and the use of particular therapeutic practices.

According to the multiplex model of arousal-related processes, bioattentional looping between these different experiential zones plays a key role in producing the anxiety reality. This model reveals the importance of the analysis of psychiatric symptoms and syndromes along multiple dimensions of meaning, and it provides insights into how to advance a biocultural phenomenology of anxiety and mental disorders on the individual and cultural levels. The model shows how anxiety will vary across individuals and local and global contexts, and has important treatment implications by pointing toward ways to develop culturally consonant therapeutic interventions.

We would argue that the multiplex model, which is a model of how acute episodes are generated, is best conceived as situated in a more general arousal complex (Figure 14.8). Individuals from a group with extreme trauma, such as Cambodians, will tend to present with all aspects of psychopathology depicted in the complex, an example of extreme trauma disorder. Moreover, we would argue that all aspects of this more general arousal complex will be give rise to cultural interpretation and interpersonal and personal consequences (Figure 14.9). The nested aspect of multiplex models within the arousal complex should always be considered. The nested models (Figures 14.7–14.9) are a more general model of the local biocultural ontologies of trauma and anxiety (see also Hinton & Good, 2015; Hinton & Hinton, 2015). More generally, multiplex models show a more dynamic view of biocultural ontologies that takes into account explanatory models and illness schemas, that focus on episode analysis, and that take into account multiple levels of looping.

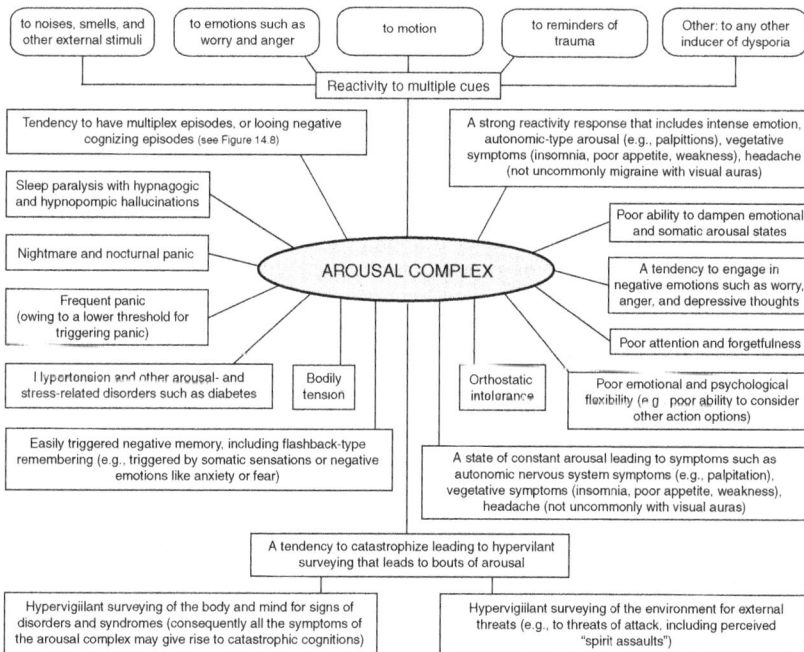

Figure 14.8. The arousal complex. Activation of any node will tend to activate all other nodes of the network. Trauma survivors, such as Cambodian refugees, will tend to have all these symptoms. This is a form of complex trauma that seemingly generates this extreme trauma complex.

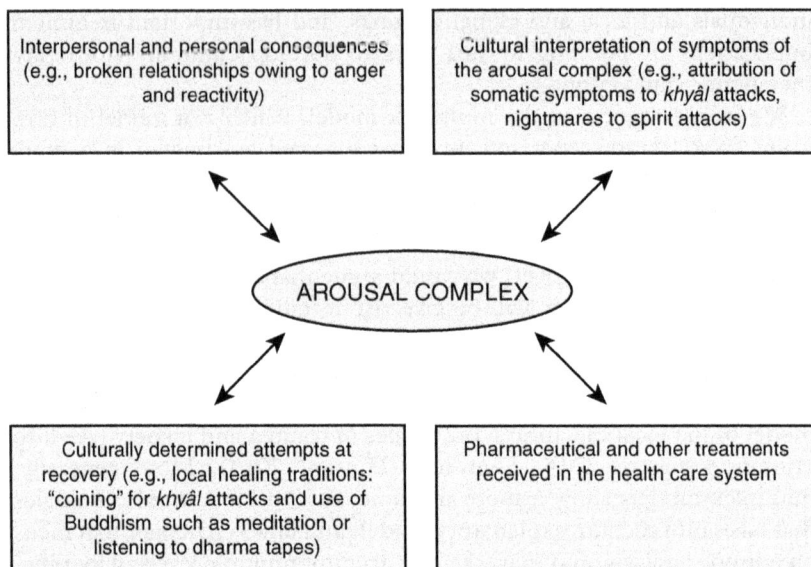

Figure 14.9. The social and cultural course of symptoms of the arousal complex.

REFERENCES

American Psychiatric Association (2013). *Diagnostic and statistical manual of mental disorders* (5th ed.). Washington, DC: Author.

Arena, J., Bruno, G., Hannah, S., & Meador, K. (1995). A comparison of frontal electromyographic biofeedback training, trapezius electromyographic biofeedback training, and progressive muscle relaxation therapy in the treatment of tension headache. *Headache, 35,* 411–19. http://dx.doi.org/10.1111%2Fj.1526-4610.1995.hed3507411.x

Barlow, D. H. (2002). *Anxiety and its disorders: The nature and treatment of anxiety and panic* (2nd ed.). New York, NY: Guilford Press.

Bohacek, J., Gapp, K., Saab, B. J., & Mansuy, I. M. (2013). Transgenerational epigenetic effects on brain functions. *Biological Psychiatry, 73*(4), 313–20. http://dx.doi.org/10.1016%2Fj.biopsych.2012.08.019

Carr, J. E., & Vitaliano, P. P. (1985). The theoretical implications of converging research on depression and the culture-bound syndromes. In A. Kleinman & B. J. Good (Eds.), *Culture and depression: Studies in anthropology and cross-cultural psychiatry of affect and disorder* (pp. 244–67). Berkeley: University of California Press.

Clark, D. M. (1986). A cognitive approach to panic. *Behaviour Research and Therapy, 24,* 461–470. http://dx.doi.org/10.1016%2F0005-7967%2886%2990011-2

Clark, D. M. (1988). A cognitive model of panic. In S. J. Rachman & J. Maser (Eds.), *Panic: Psychological perspectives.* Hillsdale, NJ: Lawrence Erlbaum.

Clark, D. M. (1996). Panic disorder: From theory to therapy. In P. M. Salkovskis (Ed.), *Frontiers of cognitive therapy* (pp. 318–44). New York, NY: Guilford Press.

Clark, D. M., & Wells, A. (1997). Cognitive therapy for anxiety disorders. In L. Dickstein, M. Riba, & J. Oldham (Eds.), *Review of psychiatry*. Washington, DC: American Psychiatric Association.

Cromwell, H. C., & Panksepp, J. (2011). Rethinking the cognitive revolution from a neural perspective: How overuse/misuse of the term "cognition" and the neglect of affective controls in behavioral neuroscience could be delaying progress in understanding the BrainMind. *Neuroscience and Biobehavioral Reviews, 35*(9), 2026–35. http://dx.doi.org/10.1016%2Fj.neubiorev.2011.02.008

Ehlers, A., & Clark, D. (2000). A cognitive model of posttraumatic stress disorder. *Behaviour Research and Therapy, 38*, 319–45. http://dx.doi.org/10.1016%2FS0005-7967%2899%2900123-0

Foa, E. B., & Kozak, M. J. (1998). Clinical applications of bioinformational theory: Understanding anxiety and its treatment. *Behavior Therapy, 29*, 675–90. http://dx.doi.org/10.1016%2FS0005-7894%2898%2980025-7

Good, B. J. (1977). The heart of what's the matter: The semantics of illness in Iran *Culture, Medicine, and Psychiatry, 1*, 25–58.

Harvey, J. M., Richards, J. C., Dziadosz, T., & Swindell, A. (1993). Misinterpretation of ambiguous stimuli in panic disorder. *Cognitive Therapy and Research, 17*, 235–48. http://dx.doi.org/10.1007%2FBF01172948

Hazlett, R., Mcleod, R., & Hoehn-Saric, R. (1994). Muscle tension in generalized anxiety disorder: Elevated muscle tonus or agitated movement. *Psychophysiology, 31*, 189–95. http://dx.doi.org/10.1111%2Fj.1469-8986.1994.tb01039.x

Hedley, L., Hoffart, A., Dammen, T., Ekeberg, O., & Friis, S. (2000). The relationship between cognitions and panic attack intensity. *Acta Psychiatrica Scandinavica, 102*, 300–2. http://dx.doi.org/10.1034%2Fj.1600-0447.2000.102004300.x

Heim, C., Newport, D. J., Heit, S., Graham, Y. P., Wilcox, M., Bonsall, R., … Nemeroff, C. B. (2000). Pituitary-adrenal and autonomic responses to stress in women after sexual and physical abuse in childhood. *JAMA, 284*(5), 592–7. http://dx.doi.org/10.1001%2Fjama.284.5.592

Hinton, D. E., Ba, P., Peou, S., & Um, K. (2000). Panic disorder among Cambodian refugees attending a psychiatric clinic: Prevalence and subtypes. *General Hospital Psychiatry, 22*, 437–44. http://dx.doi.org/10.1016%2FS0163-8343%2800%2900102-X

Hinton, D. E., Chau, H., Nguyen, L., Nguyen, M., Pham, T., Quinn, S., & Tran, M. (2001). Panic disorder among Vietnamese refugees attending a psychiatric clinic: Prevalence and subtypes. *General Hospital Psychiatry, 23*, 337–44. http://dx.doi.org/10.1016%2FS0163-8343%2801%2900163-3

Hinton, D. E., Chhean, D., Pich, V., Um, K., Fama, J. M., & Pollack, M. H. (2006). Neck-focused panic attacks among Cambodian refugees; A logistic and linear regression analysis. *Journal of Anxiety Disorders, 20*, 119–38. http://dx.doi.org/10.1016%2Fj.janxdis.2005.02.001

Hinton, D. E., Chong, R., Pollack, M. H., Barlow, D. H., & McNally, R. J. (2008). *Ataque de nervios:* Relationship to anxiety sensitivity and dissociation predisposition. *Depression and Anxiety*, 25, 489–95. http://dx doi.org/10.1002%2Fda.20309

Hinton, D. E., & Good, B. J. (2009). *Culture and panic disorder*. Palo Alto, CA: Stanford University Press.

Hinton, D. E., & Good, B. J. (Eds.). (2015). *Culture and PTSD: Trauma in historical and global perspective*. Philadelphia: University of Pennsylvania Press.

Hinton, D. E., & Hinton, A. L. (Eds.). (2015). *Genocide and mass violence: Memory, symptom, and recovery*. Cambridge, England: Cambridge University Press.

Hinton, D. E., Hinton, A. L., Eng, K.-T., & Choung, S. (2012). PTSD and key somatic complaints and cultural syndromes among rural Cambodians: The results of a needs assessment survey. *Medical Anthropology Quarterly*, 29, 147–54. http://dx.doi.org/10.1111%2Fj.1548-1387.2012.01224.x

Hinton, D. E., & Hinton, S. D. (2002). Panic disorder, somatization, and the new cross-cultural psychiatry: The seven bodies of a medical anthropology of panic. *Culture, Medicine, and Psychiatry*, 26, 155–78.

Hinton, D. E., Hinton, S. D., Pham, T., Chau, H., & Tran, M. (2003). "Hit by the wind" and temperature-shift panic among Vietnamese refugees. *Transcultural Psychiatry*, 40, 342–76. http://dx.doi.org/10.1177% 2F13634615030403003

Hinton, D. E., Hofmann, S. G., Orr, S. P., Pitman, R. K., Pollack, M. H., & Pole, N. (2010). A psychobiocultural model of orthostatic panic among Cambodian refugees: Flashbacks, catastrophic cognitions, and reduced orthostatic blood-pressure response. *Psychological Trauma: Theory, Research, Practice, and Policy*, 2, 63–70. http://dx.doi.org/10.1037%2Fa0018978

Hinton, D. E., Hofmann, S. G., Pitman, R. K., Pollack, M. H., & Barlow, D. H. (2008). The panic attack–PTSD model: Applicability to orthostatic panic among Cambodian refugee. *Cognitive Behaviour Therapy*, 27, 101–16.

Hinton, D. E., Hofmann, S. G., Pollack, M. H., & Otto, M. W. (2009). Mechanisms of efficacy of CBT for Cambodian refugees with PTSD: Improvement in emotion regulation and orthostatic blood pressure response. *CNS Neuroscience and Therapeutics*, 15(3), 255–63. http://dx.doi. org/10.1111%2Fj.1755-5949.2009.00100.x

Hinton, D. E., & Kirmayer, L. J. (2013). Local responses to trauma: Symptom, affect, and healing. *Transcultural Psychiatry*, 50, 607–21.

Hinton, D. E., Pich, V., Chhean, D., Pollack, M. H., & Barlow, D. H. (2004). Olfactory-triggered panic attacks among Cambodian refugees attending a psychiatric clinic. *General Hospital Psychiatry*, 26, 390–7. http://dx.doi.org/ 10.1016%2Fj.genhosppsych.2004.04.007

Hinton, D. E., Pich, V., Marques, L., Nickerson, A., & Pollack, M. H. (2010). Khyâl attacks: A key idiom of distress among traumatized Cambodia refugees. *Culture, Medicine, and Psychiatry*, 34, 244–78. http://dx.doi.org/ 10.1007%2Fs11013-010-9174-y

Hinton, D. E., Pich, V., Safren, S. A., Pollack, M. H., & McNally, R. J. (2006). Anxiety sensitivity among Cambodian refugees with panic disorder: A factor analytic investigation. *Journal of Anxiety Disorders*, 20(3), 281–95. http://dx.doi.org/10.1016%2Fj.janxdis.2005.02.006

Hinton, D. E., Rivera, E., Hofmann, S. G., Barlow, D. H., & Otto, M. W. (2012). Adapting CBT for traumatized refugees and ethnic minority patients: Examples from culturally adapted CBT (CA-CBT). *Transcultural Psychiatry, 49*, 340–65. http://dx.doi.org/10.1177%2F1363461512441595

Hinton, D. E., Um, K., & Ba, P. (2001a). Kyol goeu ("wind overload") part I: A cultural syndrome of orthostatic panic among Khmer refugees. *Transcultural Psychiatry, 38*, 403–32. http://dx.doi.org/10.1177% 2F136346150103800401

Hinton, D. E., Um, K., & Ba, P. (2001b). Kyol goeu ("wind overload") part II: Prevalence, characteristics and mechanisms of kyol goeu and near-kyol goeu episodes of Khmer patients attending a psychiatric clinic. *Transcultural Psychiatry, 38*, 433–60. http://dx.doi.org/10.1177%2F136346150103800402

Hinton, D. E., Um, K., & Ba, P. (2001c). A unique panic-disorder presentation among Khmer refugees: The sore-neck syndrome. *Culture, Medicine, and Psychiatry, 25*(3), 297–316.

Hoehn-Saric, R., Mcleod, D., & Zimmerli, W. (1991). Psychophysiological response patterns in panic disorder. *Acta Psychiatrica Scandinavica, 83*, 4–11. http://dx.doi.org/10.1111%2Fj.1600-0447.1991.tb05503.x

Jones, J. C., & Barlow, D. (1990). The etiology of posttraumatic stress disorder. *Clinical Psychology Review, 10*, 299–328. http://dx.doi.org/ 10.1016%2F0272-7358%2890%2990064-H

Kiernan, B. (1996). *The Pol Pot regime: Race, power, and genocide in Cambodia under the Khmer Rouge, 1975–79.* New Haven, CT: Yale University Press.

Kirmayer, L. J., & Blake. (2009). Theoretical perspectives on the cross-cutural study of panic disorder. In D. Hinton & B. Good (Eds.), *Culture and panic disorder* (pp. 31–56). Stanford, CA: Stanford University Press.

Kirmayer, L. J., & Crafa, D. (2014). What kind of science for psychiatry? *Frontiers in Human Neuroscience, 8*(435), 1–12. http://dx.doi.org/10.3389/ fnhum.2014.00435

Kirmayer, L. J., & Sartorius, N. (2007). Cultural models and somatic syndromes. *Psychosomatic Medicine, 69*, 832–40. http://dx.doi.org/10.1097% 2FPSY.0b013e31815b002c

Kirmayer, L. J., & Young, A. (1998). Culture and somatization: Clinical, epidemiological, and ethnographic perspectives. *Psychosomatic Medicine, 60*(4), 420–30.

Kleinman, A., & Becker, A. E. (1998). "Sociosomatics": The contributions of anthropology to psychosomatic medicine. *Psychosomatic Medicine, 60*(4), 389–93.

Kleinman, A., & Kleinman, J. (1994). How bodies remember: Social memory and bodily experience of criticism, resistance, and deligitimation following China's cultural revolution. *New Literary History, 25*, 707–23. http://dx.doi. org/10.2307%2F469474

Labonté, B., Farah, A., & Turecki, G. (2015). Early-life adversity and epigenetic changes: Implications for understanding suicide. In L. J. Kirmayer, R. Lemelson, & C. A. Cummings (Eds.), *Re-visioning psychiatry: Cultural phenomenology, critical neuroscience, and global mental health* (pp. 206–35). New York, NY: Cambridge University Press.

Lewis-Fernández, R., & Aggarwal, N. K. (2015). Psychiatric classification beyond the *DSM*: An interdisciplinary approach. In L. J. Kirmayer, R. Lemelson, & C. A. Cummings (Eds.), *Re-visioning psychiatry: Cultural phenomenology, critical neuroscience, and global mental health* (pp. 434–68). New York, NY: Cambridge University Press.

Marshall, G. N., Schell, T. L., Elliott, M. N., Berthold, S. M., & Chun, C. A. (2005). Mental health of Cambodian refugees 2 decades after resettlement in the United States. *JAMA, 294,* 571–9. http://dx.doi.org/10.1001% 2Fjama.294.5.571

McNally, R. J., & Frueh, B. C. (2013). Why are Iraq and Afghanistan War veterans seeking PTSD disability compensation at unprecedented rates? *Journal of Anxiety Disorders, 27*(5), 520–6.

Mollica, R. F., McInnes, K., Pham, T., Smith, F. M. C., Murphy, E., & Lin, L. (1998). The dose-effect relationships between torture and psychiatric symptoms in Vietnamese ex-political detainees and a comparison group. *Journal of Nervous and Mental Disease, 186,* 543–53. http://dx.doi.org/ 10.1097%2F00005053-199809000-00005

Morris, S. E., & Cuthbert, B. N. (2012). Research Domain Criteria: Cognitive systems, neural circuits, and dimensions of behavior. *Dialogues Clinical Neuroscience, 14*(1), 29–37. http://dx.doi.org/10.1177/1462474511424681

Noyes, R., & Hoehn-Saric, R. (1998). *The anxiety disorders.* Cambridge, England: Cambridge University Press.

Porges, S. W. (2011). *The polyvagal theory: Neurophysiological foundations of emotions, attachment, communication, and self-regulation.* New York, NY: Norton.

Ryder, A. G., & Chentsova-Dutton, Y. E. (2015). Cultural clinical psychology: From cultural scripts to contextualized treatments. In L. J. Kirmayer, R. Lemelson, & C. A. Cummings (Eds.), *Re-visioning psychiatry: Cultural phenomenology, critical neuroscience, and global mental health* (pp. 400–33). New York, NY: Cambridge University Press.

Sanislow, C. A., Pine, D. S., Quinn, K. J., Kozak, M. J., Garvey, M. A., Heinssen, R. K., . . . Cuthbert, B. N. (2010). Developing constructs for psychopathology research: Research domain criteria. *Journal of Abnormal Psychology, 119*(4), 631–9. http://dx.doi.org/10.1037%2Fa0020909

Shorter, E. (1992). *From paralysis to fatigue: A history of psychosomatic illness in the modern era.* Toronto, Canada: Maxwell Macmillan Canada.

15 From the Brain Disease Model to Ecologies of Addiction

Eugene Raikhel

The historian of medicine Charles Rosenberg wrote a few years ago that "[w]e have never been more aware of the arbitrary and constructed qualities of psychiatric diagnoses, yet we have never been more dependent on them than now" (2007, p. 50). This argument could be easily extrapolated from diagnoses to cover psychiatry's categories and concepts more generally, and it would aptly describe the way in which the notion of addiction as a "brain disease" is simultaneously ubiquitous and highly contested today. In North America and elsewhere, the idea of addiction as a "chronic, relapsing brain disease" serves as a guideline for prioritizing funding for basic research on addiction and substance use and has been adopted as an official definition by influential professional organizations such as the American Society of Addiction Medicine (ASAM, 2011). Closely linked to this concept are claims that addiction is not limited to "substance abuse" or "substance use disorders," but encompasses pathological, harmful, or distressing patterns of gambling, eating, sex, technology use, and other behaviors.

Yet one doesn't have to look far to find criticisms of these brain-centered accounts or expansive definitions as reductionist, biomedicalizing, or focused on the wrong factors. As mainstream, a publication as the *New York Times* could in 2014 ask six experts the basic question, "What is Addiction?" and receive six substantially different answers – each emphasizing factors as wide-ranging as poverty, personal choice, genetics, and spirituality ("What is Addiction," 2014). The specifics of distinct definitions, and their attendant critiques of the brain disease model, vary widely. Psychiatrists, psychologists, behavioral economists, and philosophers argue that the brain disease model obscures the role of choice, agency, and social environment in producing the destructive behavioral patterns we associate with addiction (Foddy & Savulescu, 2010; Heyman, 2009; Levy, 2012; Satel & Lilienfeld, 2013). These critics point to the often forgotten finding that many people who use opiates and other addictive drugs habitually for a period of time either "mature out" of heavy use or are able to stop without any therapeutic intervention (Robins, 1993). Other observers argue that designating addiction as a "disease" or "disorder" medicalizes conditions that are more properly understood as "problems of living," social deviance, or simply the contingent (and sometimes harmful) outcomes of people interacting with particular environments (Keane, 2002, p. 568; Peele, 1985; Reinarman, 2005, p. 308). For many critics, this biomedicalization of addiction obscures patterns of structural violence, particularly in light of the overwhelming associations between addiction-related harm and social inequalities, poverty, and incarceration (Bourgois, 2003; Singer, 2007). Anthropologists, historians, and sociologists have played an important role in this critical discourse, drawing attention to the ways in which framing addiction as a brain disease elides psychological, familial, social, economic, institutional, and global systemic factors.[1]

Until recently, most social scientists working in these traditions have treated the brain disease model of addiction and its forerunners, along with other biological knowledge, either as a "black-box" to leave untouched or as rhetoric, ideology, or social construction to be critiqued. However, over the past several years, a growing number of social scientists studying addiction have begun paying attention to materiality, embodiment, and biology in potentially novel ways. We have seen a growing number of calls for a robust and thoughtful engagement between the social and biological sciences of addiction, or at least for an approach that, as Scott Vrecko has put it, "maintains critical ambivalence toward the reality of addiction as a disease, but nevertheless commits to thinking seriously about the physiological" (Campbell, 2010, 2011; Courtwright, 2005; Fraser, Moore, & Keane, 2014; Hansen & Skinner, 2012; Kaye, 2012; Kushner, 2010; Lende, 2005, 2012; Saris, 2013; Singer, 2001; Weinberg, 2011; Vrecko, 2010a, p. 38). These calls are part of a broader shift among many social scientists toward various modes of engagement with the biosciences, many of which aim to contribute to biosocial or ecological accounts of health, illness, and disease (Downey & Lende, 2012; Fitzgerald & Callard, 2014; Lock & Nguyen, 2010; Rose, 2013; Slaby & Choudhury, 2012). This reorientation is often linked to an understanding of biological

---

[1] Throughout the chapter, I draw on the work of social scientists in order to illustrate broader arguments, *not* in an effort to comprehensively review current research. For useful mappings of the social science literatures on addiction see: Weinberg (2011) on sociology; Kushner (2010) on the history of addiction; and Marshall, Ames, and Bennett (2001) and Singer (2012) on the anthropology of alcohol and drugs. Nichter and colleagues (2004) examine a somewhat wider set of qualitative literatures, with a particular focus on methods and applied or engaged social science, as do Page and Singer (2010).

processes as "porous to social and even cultural signals to an unprecedented extent" (Meloni, 2014, p. 2). And indeed, when we look beyond the headlines highlighting addiction as first and foremost a brain disease, we find many researchers in neuroscience and psychiatry seeking to move beyond potentially reductionist interpretations to investigate the multiple links between biological mechanisms, environmental effects, and developmental histories (Volkow, Wang, Fowler, & Tomasi, 2012).

But what does it mean, concretely, for social scientists to think seriously about materiality and biology while maintaining a "critical ambivalence" toward prevailing notions of addiction as brain disease? Or, to put the question in another way, how might the social sciences of addiction advance a critically productive engagement with neuroscience and psychiatry without either treating biology as only a discursive product or making it the foundation of an ontological hierarchy? Moreover, how might we do so in a way that builds upon the decades of important ethnographic and historical research on addiction?

In thinking about these questions, I have found it particularly useful to return to Gregory Bateson's theory of alcoholism as a problem of epistemology (1972). In his influential article "The Cybernetics of 'Self,'" Bateson argues that alcoholics are often unable to maintain sobriety because they identify the "will" or the "self" with conscious mental processes, a misrecognition that is ultimately just an "unusually disastrous variant of Cartesian dualism, the division between Mind and Matter" (1972, p. 313). In conceptualizing their "will" as distinct from and opposed to the "unconscious processes," which they experience as "urges" and "forces," alcoholics commit themselves to a struggle with a reified disease entity that can only escalate as their social relationships deteriorate. Indeed, the reason Alcoholics Anonymous (AA) worked, according to Bateson, was that in declaring their "powerless[ness] over alcohol," its participants were effecting "a change in epistemology, a change in how to know about personality-in-the world" – turning away from a fatal dualism to a way of knowing and acting with a distinctly different set of assumptions about "mind," "self," and "volition" (1972, p. 313).

Some forty years later, Bateson's argument remains radically suggestive. As I read him (perhaps somewhat idiosyncratically), Bateson urges us to think of alcoholism not only in ecological terms (as a system that encompasses the person and her milieu), but also in a way that recognizes that "ontology and epistemology cannot be separated" in the study of human beings (1972, p. 314). In other words, the ways in which we act in the world (including those experienced as distressful or deemed pathological) cannot be meaningfully disentangled from our knowledge of the world – or more specifically, our categories and their attendant logics. This basic premise has, of course, been echoed by much of the literature in science studies and the social sciences of knowledge, particularly in the work of Ian Hacking – who, like Bateson, has often turned to ecological metaphors and emphasized the centrality of epistemology in his efforts to reconceptualize relationships between processes traditionally demarcated as "biological" and "social" (cf. Hacking, 2002).

Working from the idea that a biosocial or ecological account of addiction should start with examining "addiction" as a problem of knowledge, I devote the first part of this chapter to a discussion of the brain disease model of addiction as an epistemic object, tracing its emergence from a particular scientific style of reasoning and examining some of its key social effects. In the remainder of the chapter, I briefly review the social science of addiction literature associated with four conceptual frameworks, which I suggest highlight domains and mechanisms of biosocial entanglement – and are thus particularly fruitful as potential sites of conversation between social scientists and bioscientists. These frameworks are: (1) embodied sensations, (2) will and habit, (3) social and material milieu, and (4) trajectories.

A final caveat regarding the conceptual framing of this chapter: while I use the term "addiction" throughout, I do not restrict myself to its "core" behavioral symptoms, as defined by the current psychiatric literature (e.g., compulsive drug-seeking despite severe consequences); rather, I examine the broader terrain within which substances and practices may or may not be understood or experienced as distressful. Although this approach makes for a somewhat more unwieldy examination of the literature, it is necessary in order to understand distressful or harmful patterns and experiences involving psychoactive drugs, if one accepts that any definition of pathology inherently requires some normative claim or stance.

Addiction as Brain Disease: The NIDA Model

As historians of science and medicine have shown, today's "chronic, relapsing brain disease" model is just the most recent of a long series of attempts to conceptualize addiction to alcohol, opiates, or other drugs as a disease (Acker, 2002; Campbell, 2007; Valverde, 1998). Although these models share certain characteristics, they invoke distinct loci and mechanisms of addictiveness and privilege different forms of intervention and lines of scientific research; in addition, all have been shaped both by their contemporary political and social milieu and by the styles of thought prevailing in contemporaneous scientific communities (Berridge, 2013;

Courtwright, 2005; Gusfield, 1996; Vrecko, 2010b). For example, one of the earliest articulations of the disease concept is often attributed to an eighteenth-century Philadelphia physician, Benjamin Rush (Levine, 1978). Rush understood the habitual drunkard's desire to consume alcohol as a chronic, progressive compulsion that eventually and inevitably led to a loss of control. As with later disease or medical models of addiction, the key point often emphasized about Rush's framing of alcoholism as disease was its distinction from understanding drunkenness either in moral terms (as "bad behavior," laziness, etc.) or in terms of individual choice. The historical moment at which this concept emerged was, of course, no accident. During the early industrial period – and increasingly during the nineteenth century (when disease concepts of addiction became much more widespread) – drinking practices were problematized for their perceived incompatibility with the behavioral strictures then valorized, particularly those of self-reliance, independence, and productivity (Levine, 1978; Room, 2003).

Yet, despite echoes of these predecessors, recent claims that addiction is a brain disease are the product of a distinct style of thought, one that emerged from the expansion of basic research on neurochemistry under the auspices of Richard Nixon's War on Drugs during the early 1970s. Key to this stream of research was the isolation of opiate receptors in nervous tissue in 1973, which helped to consolidate a biomolecular model of addiction by demonstrating a specific mechanism through which drugs could have biological effects (Vrecko, 2010b). During the 1980s and 1990s such basic research on the neurochemical under-pinnings of craving and pleasure gained strength from the widespread availability of new imaging technologies that permitted noninvasive study of brain structure and function (Campbell, 2007; Fraser et al., 2014; Vrecko, 2010b).

All of these conceptual, technical, and political developments made possible the consolidation and public articulation during the 1990s of the idea that addiction is a "chronic, relapsing brain disease" linked to the neurobiology of reward, attention, motivation, and decision making (Kalivas & Volkow, 2005; Leshner, 1997). Because the U.S. National Institute on Drug Abuse (NIDA) has been central to research behind its development and recent NIDA directors Alan Leshner and Nora Volkow have been instrumental in its articulation both within professional circles and among the lay public, the brain disease approach has also been referred to as "the NIDA model" (Courtwright, 2010).[2]

---

[2] In this chapter I use the terms "NIDA model" and "brain disease model" interchangeably.

Perhaps most significantly, this model argues that chronic use of addict-ive substances results in certain neuroadaptations of brain systems involved in reward, attention, and motivation, with enduring effects.

There is an important distinction to make here. The brain disease (or NIDA) model of addiction represents a particular interpretation of experimental findings in neuroscience, and many researchers have used neuroscience to critique the model and propose alternatives (e.g., Levy, 2014). Indeed, as sociologists Suzanne Fraser, David Moore, and Helen Keane have argued, it may be more useful to think of this "model" as a relatively simple narrative, "distilled from the complex neuroscience of drugs and reward" and "strengthened by the appeal of evolutionary logic" (2014, p. 52). Here is a version of the narrative drawn from a review article by Charles Dackis and Charles O'Brien, two leading neuroscientists of addiction:

> Addiction is best conceptualized as a disease of brain reward centers that ensure the survival of organisms and species... Given their function, reward centers have evolved the ability to grip attention, dominate motivation and compel behavior directed toward survival goals, even in the presence of danger and despite our belief that we are generally rational beings. By activating and dysregulating endogenous reward centers, addictive drugs essentially hijack brain circuits that exert considerable dominance over rational thought, leading to progressive loss of control over drug intake in the face of medical, interpersonal, occupational, and legal hazards. (2005, p. 1431)

At the center of most versions of this narrative is the neurotransmitter dopamine, understood to modulate circuits in the midbrain associated with desire, pleasure, and reward. However, there is considerable debate among neuroscientists about the specific causal role played by dopamine in reward – and particularly, whether it mediates the pleasurable effects of reward (glossed in the literature as "liking"); the prediction of future reward ("learning"); or "incentive salience," that is, "the ascription of attractiveness to 'intrinsically neutral' stimuli" (Berridge & Valenstein, 1991, p. 9), also described as "wanting" or "desiring" (Berridge, 2007; Berridge, Robinson, & Aldridge, 2009). As this third "incentive salience" theory argues, organisms come to experience desire ("wanting") in response to stimuli that were initially associated with pleasurable experi-ences ("liking") through processes of conditioning (Berridge, 2007). As certain drugs "plug ... directly into the neurobiological mechanism that ordinarily adjusts learned incentive salience in accordance with physiological states" (Berridge, 2007, p. 413), "wanting" becomes "craving," a response that can be triggered and amplified by the environ-mental stimuli or cues that have become associated with particular drugs, as well as by stress (Dackis & O'Brien, 2005, p. 1432). Such "cue-induced craving" is widely understood in this literature as a central cause of relapse after long periods of abstinence, both because the neuroadaptations resulting from chronic drug use are considered long-standing and because the entire process may take place outside the conscious awareness of potential users (Campbell, 2013; Childress et al., 2008).[3]

A key aspect of the "incentive salience" hypothesis is that it frames addiction as less a problem of pleasure than one of anticipation or desire. For Robinson and Berridge, "incentive salience" or "wanting" is distinct from the experience of pleasure itself – "liking" – which represents a separate process associated with a different set of brain circuits. Daniel Lende suggests that "incentive salience" may be semantically closer to "passion" than "wanting" (Berridge et al., 2009, as cited in Lende, 2012), adding that this view of addiction has implications for the way addiction fits into a broader interpretation of contemporary consumer capitalism (Lende, 2012, p. 350). That is, a theory of addiction as a pathology of anticipation and desire (rather than pleasure) suggests that addictive experiences may have particularly strong affinities with the central logics and affective textures of consumer capitalism (cf. Saris, 2013; Schüll, 2006, 2012).

One of the most significant effects of the NIDA model has been to fuel the expansion of "addiction" as a cultural idiom for understanding multiple pathologies and forms of distress. For many addiction researchers (as well as laypeople), the model's emphasis on the interaction between drugs and basic neurobiological pathways has validated the idea that "various drug dependencies should be conceptualized as a single disorder" (Dackis & O'Brien, 2005, p. 1433). Not only has the model fostered the grouping of alcohol, tobacco, opiates, and many other intoxicants under a single conceptual rubric, but it has brought them together with pleasurable activities such as gambling, video gaming, sex, and eating (Petry, 2006; Volkow & O'Brien, 2007). This idea is based on the finding that such activities activate the same brain circuits as drugs of addiction and that they may do so intensely enough to be subject to the same processes of dysregulation, leading to "compulsive drug-seeking" (Dackis & O'Brien, 2005). Although some scholars have interpreted the

---

[3] There is, of course, much more to this model. Drug reward is understood as associated with other neurotransmitters, in addition to dopamine (Volkow et al., 2012). Many neurobiologists also argue that addiction is associated with reductions in metabolism in the prefrontal cortex and, in the case of certain drugs, "reductions in frontal gray matter density" leading to disruptions in the decision-making and risk assessment capacities often glossed as "executive function" (Dackis & O'Brien, 2005, p. 1432; Volkow et al., 2012).

expansion of addiction-logics as another instance of biomedicalization, others have argued that in broader cultural terms, it may not only normalize pathology (by emphasizing its foundation in basic biological processes rather than ascribing it to characteristics of particular individuals or kinds of people) but also render everyone potentially pathological (Rose, 2003; Schüll, 2006). Despite the continued debates and marked skepticism of many researchers, the idea of behavioral addictions received institutional legitimation with the recategorization of compulsive gambling as an addiction in *DSM-5* (APA, 2013).[4]

However, the relationship between the NIDA model and addiction diagnostics and therapeutics remains profoundly ambivalent. The description and categorization of addictions in the *DSM-5* reflect both the ambition of its developers to bring nosology closer to neurobiology (through the use of diagnostic biomarkers) and its ultimate failure to achieve this goal. On the one hand, the newly formed category of "Substance-Related and Addictive Disorders" consists of brain disorders; this overall framing echoes the idea of addiction as a disorder independent of substances (Fraser et al., 2014). On the other hand, the most significant change between *DSM-IV* (APA, 1994) and *DSM-5* – the erasure of the distinction between substance abuse and dependence, and the replacement of both categories by the heterogeneous category, "substance use disorder" – was justified as much on the basis of the categories' social effects as it was on their neurobiological validity (Fraser et al., 2014, pp. 37–45).

The brain disease model's relationship to addiction therapeutics is similarly equivocal. The rise of the brain disease model been accompanied by a growing enthusiasm for new pharmaceutical treatments for addiction, as well as for interventions involving neurological modulation (such as deep brain stimulation and transcranial magnetic stimulation). Unlike older pharmacological treatments such as disulfiram, which was used as a tool in an essentially behavioral intervention for alcoholism, newer drugs such as naltrexone and acamprosate are understood to directly modulate the neurochemical effects of substances or to reduce sensations of craving (O'Brien, 2005). Similarly, buprenorphine, used in the treatment of opiate dependence since the mid-1990s in a number of countries, was specifically developed as a opiate–substitution therapy

---

[4] Such debates over the validity of behavioral addictions point to another important effect of the "chronic, relapsing brain disease" model of addiction: whereas earlier models emphasized a distinction between "physiological" and "psychological" addiction, or attempted to encompass the two, the NIDA model arguably blurs any clear distinction between these categories.

because its biochemical properties were understood to reduce its potential for dependency, abuse, and "diversion" – problems that had become evident with methadone maintenance therapy since the beginning of its widespread use in the 1970s (Campbell & Lovell, 2012; Meyers, 2013). Simultaneously, many therapeutic and recovery fields throughout the world that are dedicated to addiction employ a dizzying range of psychosocial, talk, and behavioral therapies, which may encode models of personhood and enactments of agency that differ radically from those associated with pharmaceutical interventions. For example, although treatment modalities in North America are legion, none have had the cultural impact nor attained the prevalence of the Twelve Step program and numerous related modes of talk-based therapy, which, as Summerson Carr has argued, share a conception of addiction as a "disease of denial" (Carr, 2013).

In focusing on the effects, consequences, and receptions of the brain disease model, I have perhaps reified it unfairly, paying less attention to instances of profound disagreement, internal critique, and acknowledgment of uncertainty by neuroscientists of addiction. And yet, as Nancy Campbell has pointed out, while most researchers are quite frank about the enormous gaps that remain in explaining mechanisms linking neurobiology to social behavior in compulsive drug use, "there is a persistent gap between what scientists humbly admit to one another and what the public understands them to be saying" (2011, p. 207). Arguably, this gap is at least partly the product of prominent neuroscientists' assumptions that public acceptance of a neurobiological model of addiction will promote rehabilitative and therapeutic (rather than penal and coercive) approaches to intervention and will lead to reduced stigma and, ultimately, to fewer harmful health outcomes for patients (Campbell, 2013). Of course, these aspirational claims sit quite uneasily next to empirical findings of deeply ambivalent social effects of framing addiction in neurobiological terms (Buchman, Illes, & Reiner, 2011; Pescosolido et. al., 2010; Satel & Lilienfeld, 2013), not to mention the prevailing modes of regulating narcotic drugs in many countries, where criminalization and mass incarceration seem to go hand-in-hand with the acceptance of addiction disease models by criminal justice professionals (Courtwright, 2010; Garriott, 2011; Kaye, 2012).

Biosocial Entanglement and Ecologies of Addiction

Even if we set aside the usefulness of such "strategic reductionism," the more vexing question remains of how to link knowledge about neural processes to our explanations of the actions and experiences associated with addiction, and how (if at all) these explanations should guide our interventions. It is sometimes pointed out that even Alan Leshner, while famously arguing that "addiction is a brain disease, and it matters," explained that, in fact, it is "a brain disease for which the social contexts in which it has both developed and is expressed are critically important" (1997). Indeed, researchers building on this model increasingly take into account other internal and external factors shaping addictive behavior, including genes, development, stress, early trauma, social and physical environmental cues, and comorbidity with other psychiatric disorders (Volkow et al., 2012).

However, there is a significant difference between (1) conceptualizing a set of "core" biological processes or "single biological essences" (Kendler, 2012, p. 11) that "develop" and are "expressed" in particular social contexts and (2) thinking about the social and biological as fundamentally inextricable. Even the NIMH's Research Domain Criteria (RDoC) system of classification, which begins not with a category of "addiction" or "substance abuse," but at the level of "positive and negative valence systems," such as reward learning and habit, has been criticized for its inadequate attention to social processes in their own right (as opposed to neural correlates or preconditions for social processes) (Kirmayer & Crafa, 2014). If we understand "addiction" to be a name we give to a set of affects, experiences, and patterned actions that are "emergent" in interactions taking place across different levels of complexity between brain circuits, substances, self-systems, social networks, and markets (to name a few), then we need to pay closer attention to the specific mechanisms through which these interactions take place (Kirmayer & Gold, 2012; Lock & Nguyen, 2010, p. 90). To rephrase it as a question: If we think of addiction not as a brain disease, but as a phenomenon that emerges under a particular set of biosocial and institutional conditions, what do we need to pay attention to?

In the remainder of this chapter, I briefly review the social science of addiction literature associated with four conceptual frameworks or problem spaces, all of which highlight the domains and mechanisms of biosocial entanglement: (1) embodied sensations, (2) will and habit, (3) social and material milieu, and (4) trajectories. These may seem to unlikely categories. Where are the substances? Where are individual psychologies? Where are structural inequalities? As will become clear, I have chosen these categories precisely because they cut across some of the other frameworks, hopefully putting them into conversation with one another. Rather than a systematic review of social science research or an overarching model of addiction, these categories represent conceptual and discursive spaces where social scientists and bioscientists (and particularly neuroscientists) working on addiction might product-ively communicate and engage.

Embodied Sensations

The embodied sensations and states of consciousness associated with both the habitual use of psychoactive substances and what some researchers understand to be the "core" behavioral components of addiction (such as "cue-induced craving") are an important domain where the social sciences can both speak directly to and potentially develop arguments emerging from the neuroscience of addiction. Anthropologists and sociologists have emphasized that the phenomenology of drug use and addiction is not determined solely by the psychochemistry of ingested substances or (in the case of gambling and gaming) by the characteristics of immersive technologies. Rather, a range of perspectives suggests that embodied sensations and states of consciousness are coproduced or mediated by the interaction of these material properties and expectancies, conceptual models of the body, somatic modes of attention, and bodily memories, which are themselves the instantiations of social values, cultural scripts, and patterns of experience (Csordas, 1993; Hinton, Howes, & Kirmayer, 2008). In part, this complexity occurs because many psychoactive substances simultaneously affect multiple circuits in the nervous system, so users must learn to interpret their drug-related sensations and experiences in particular ways. Howard Becker made such a claim years ago when he argued that one becomes a marijuana user by learning to pay attention to certain sensations and subjective experiences (1953).

In an important early study along these lines, Craig MacAndrew and Robert Edgerton (1969) drew on ethnographic evidence of societies in which heavy drinking did not result in disinhibition or negatively valorized behavior to make a strong claim for the cultural specificity of such effects and more generally to argue that "drunken comportment" is determined culturally, rather than pharmacologically. Much of the subsequent discussion in anthropology and sociology focused on the question of whether this argument romanticized indigenous drinking, or at least failed to account for the potential transformation of valorized and socially constructive practices of heavy drinking into more disruptive and painful patterns with the advent of markets and wage labor (Heath, 2004; Marshall, 1982; Room, 1984). However, other work – primarily in experimental psychology – focused on the effects of expectancies related to intoxicated behavior and aggression, with somewhat mixed results (Marlatt & Rohsenow, 1980; Room, 2001; Testa et al., 2006). In general, however, experimental, qualitative, and ethnographic work asking such questions remains wanting.

Close attention to the phenomenology of gambling, gaming, and other activities and practices that are increasingly framed as potentially addictive is especially important, given that these claims are justified primarily on the basis of neurobiological correlates with certain kinds of experience. In her ethnography of video machine gambling in Las Vegas, anthropologist Natasha Dow Schüll pays close attention to the accounts of players – particularly their descriptions of being "in the zone," the "world-dissolving state of subjective suspension and affective calm" that some machine gamblers seek to attain again and again, despite experiencing extremely painful consequences in many domains of their lives (2012, p. 19). Similarly, Jeffrey Snodgrass and his colleagues have argued for an interpretation of World of Warcraft and similar online games as "technologies of absorption," which facilitate states of dissociation and serve to relieve stress, resulting in positive experiences of achievement, competition, or sociality among some players and distressful or problematic patterns among others (Snodgrass, Lacy, Dengah II, Fagan, & Most, 2011).

Setting and meaning deeply shape both the embodied sensations associated with psychoactive drug use or the experience of immersive technologies and the experiences of "cue-induced craving" associated with the brain disease model of addiction. For example, Daniel Lende has argued that the experiences of "wanting more and more" reported by the young drug users in Colombia with whom he worked resonate with the theory of addiction as "incentive sensitization," but in a way that depends on particular social and experiential settings – in this case, the concrete settings of these adolescents' everyday lives (Lende, 2005, 2012; Robinson & Berridge, 1993). Other studies have not only found significant differences in kinds of craving, but also made clear that processes involved in amplifying feelings of wanting, or their resurgence after periods of abstinence, can only take place within specific social and material environments and are mediated by individually or culturally specific meanings, sensations, and expectancies, where multiple kinds of cues may work synergistically to initiate sensations of craving (Bruehl, Lende, Schwartz, Sterk, & Elifson, 2006). Rather than occasioning drug use in some direct or unambiguous way, these experiences of craving may lead potential users to employ various strategies to control drug use – with differing degrees of success and with expectancies or beliefs about craving itself potentially playing an important role (Bruehl et al., 2006; Lee, Pohlman, Baker, Ferris, & Kay-Lambkin, 2010). Finally, as Allison Schlosser and Lee Hoffer have shown in their research with heroin users with co-occurring mental illness, the effects of various psychoactive substances (heroin "highs", the "side" effects of psychiatric medications) and their absence (withdrawal, craving) have complex interactions, which are often managed in relation to one another (2012).

Will and Habit

Much of the conceptual difficulty surrounding ideas of addiction has to do with the way in which the affects, behaviors, and experiences associated with it run counter to widely held Euro-American assumptions about volition, self-control, choice, agency, and autonomy – assumptions that are often reflected in scientific thinking (in both social sciences and biosciences), as much as they are in lay ideas. Thus, during the nineteenth century, alcoholism and other addictions were often framed as "diseases of the will," and it has been argued that this concept arose as a kind of shadow to the normative ideal of the freely choosing subject, in much the same way as Michel Foucault and others have argued that the concept of madness emerged in a mutually constitutive relationship to reason (Foucault, 1965; Valverde, 1998). To put it in very rough terms, the addict was seen as one who was unable to align his actions with his intentions because of a weakness or failure of the will, which was conceptualized as a human capacity alongside reason and emotion. Recent definitions of addiction translate these problems of the will into a language of "self-control" – the loss of which is understood as a core diagnostic criterion (Baler & Volkow, 2006; Weinberg, 2013). Parallel to ideas about the will, a long-running tension has persisted between theories emphasizing the addictiveness of psychoactive substances (or technologies or practices) and those focusing on the vulnerabilities (whether understood in genetic, psychosocial, or cultural terms) of particular individuals or populations (Campbell, 2007; Valverde, 1998).

Significantly, scholars of addiction in the social sciences increasingly discuss it in ways that avoid the binaries of free will and determinism, conceptualizing volition, control, or agency as partial, fragmented, emergent, or distributed across individuals, social networks, or assemblages comprising humans and nonhuman actors (Duff, 2011; Gomart, 2004; Weinberg, 2013). Such work is particularly suggestive because its conceptualizations of volition seem to dovetail with those arising from the neuroscience of addiction. As Jamie Saris has argued, "theorizing in both psychopharmacology and [the neuroscience of] addiction increasingly has given us a sense of the will as an uncertain achievement, less of an essence and more an epiphenomenon of discrete processes that are subject to both degradation and enhancement" (2013, p. 273).

The idea of habit has emerged as particuarly useful in this regard. Mined by both Eve Kosofsky Sedgewick and Mariana Valverde in respective writings on addiction, as a concept that sidesteps the "metaphysical absolutes" of free will and determinism, the notion of habit has recently reemerged as an object of more general interest among social theorists (Bennett, Dodsworth, Noble, Poovey, & Watkins, 2013; Fraser et al., 2014, pp. 22–23; Sedgwick, 1993, p. 137; Valverde, 1998, pp. 36–41). In his neuroanthropological account of addiction, Lende also refers to habit to explain a mode of learning that begins to dominate if and when drug use becomes repetitive, patterned, and compulsive. For Lende, the key point is that from both a neurobiological and a cognitive perspective, such habit learning seems to take place through the same processes associated with the internalization of "cultural models" or practices "through training, skill acquisition, and other forms of patterned practice" (2012, p. 258). Although these uses of the term "habit" are clearly distinct in many ways, each use can be seen as an attempt to displace tensions between free will and determinacy with accounts of human action as embedded in or emerging from individual particularity.

Social and Material Milieu

Social scientists have long emphasized the significance to addiction and substance use of what is variously referred to as milieu, environment, or setting, and more recent work has expanded these arguments, suggesting the literal interpenetration of bodies and environments, both material and social, complicated by the articulation between milieu and the global circuits through which substances and technologies move. For many researchers in the health sciences, the key question regarding environments or settings concerns the availability and accessibility of substances (or technologies). Thus, epidemiological studies have shown that risk of alcohol dependence is substantially affected by the spatial and temporal availability and pricing of alcohol in a given setting (Wagenaar, Salois, & Komro, 2009). Research from neuroscience and psychiatry has transformed this perspective on environments, emphasizing that it is not simply the availability of substances or devices that defines the "riskiness" of an environment in this sense, but the degree to which it is saturated with cues that have become associated with use for the addict (Childress et al., 2008; this idea was, of course, recognized and institutionalized somewhat earlier in AA as an injunction to avoid the "people, places, and things" associated with drug use).

However, for other researchers, the notion of milieu suggests an even more fundamental starting point: the idea that drug use (or any other activities associated with addiction) always takes place in a social setting, which, at least in part, provides actors with a meaningful frame or reference point and shapes motivations. Clearly, the consumption of psychoactive substances is often constructive in that such practices are a means of producing and maintaining social relationships, even when it occurs through disagreement and negotiation, rather than ritual and consensus (Douglas, 1987; Colson & Scudder, 1988; Moore, 2004). The social settings of use are equally important in shaping the ways in which the uses or potential benefits of psychotropic effects are understood (McKenna, 2013).

Moreover, milieu can be conceptualized in relation to the broader circuits of production, exchange, and consumption – through which psychoactive substances flow as commodities. Anthropologists and historians have documented the key roles played by the trade and use of various psychoactive substances (particularly alcohol, tobacco, and opium) and certain foods in extending the reach of capitalism and colonialism over the past three hundred years (Mintz, 1985; Mills & Barton 2007). David Courtwright (2005) calls this "limbic capitalism," arguing that the prevalence of such substances is directly linked to what neurobiology tells us about their inherent addictiveness for humans. Although such a claim perhaps begs for closer attention to the particularities of substance use and meaning, it is clear that embodied desires are often linked to the circuits of consumer capitalism, and that this linkage is facilitated and amplified by numerous entities seeking to profit from it (ranging from narcotrafficking operations to the alcohol, tobacco, gaming, and – as Kalman Applbaum (Chapter 21, *this volume*) reminds us – pharmaceutical industries).

Moreover, social scientists have emphasized that material and social environments not only shape patterns of substance use and behavior but that environments – as well as the capacity of individuals to move between them – are in turn deeply structured by broader political, economic, and social factors in ways that concentrate the incidence of drug-related harm and infectious diseases (particularly HIV) among particular populations (Bourgois, 2003; Page, 1997; Rhodes, 2002; Singer, 2007). State and social policy is extremely significant in this regard, as it often sets the overall framework for understanding particular substances, behaviors, or environments as problems of a specific kind, often with far-reaching unintended consequences. Thus, criminalizing certain drugs has often had the effect of shaping social and material milieu in ways that arguably increase the risk of harm to those with less capacity (in the form of economic or social capital) to move outside of those often marginalized environments (cf. Lende, 2012, p. 349).

The importance of accounting for milieu extends to our understanding of addiction interventions and therapeutics as well. My own ethnographic work has examined the largely behavioral and suggestion-based techniques for managing sobriety that have been popular in Russia for the past thirty years. While these methods are often criticized as paternalistic and for fostering the dependence of patients on physicians, I argue that particular arrangements of authority in the clinical relationship have less to do with particular therapeutics than they do with the broader institutional and social settings in which these therapies are enacted (Raikhel, 2010). The work of anthropologists Anne Lovell and Todd Meyers on the configurations of pharmaceutical therapy for opiate addiction in Marseille, France, and Baltimore, Maryland, respectively, similarly highlights the mutual shaping of therapeutics and social and institutional milieu (Lovell, 2013; Meyers, 2013).

Trajectories

A range of perspectives in the social sciences have emphasized a temporal perspective on illness and health, on individuals undergoing changes, and the relationship between experiences, life-course events, and environmental processes, which William Garriott and I have referred to collectively as "trajectories" (2013).[5] Such a focus on trajectories draws our attention to the key temporal aspect of addiction, framed by philosopher Gilles Deleuze in the question: "Why and how is this experience [of drug use], even when self-destructive, but still vital, transformed into a deadly enterprise of generalized, unilinear dependence? Is it inevitable? If there is a precise point, that is where therapy should intervene" (Deleuze, 2007, p. 254). Almost all attempts to conceptualize addiction address the temporal aspect in some way, whether framed as a shift from use to abuse, from incentive salience to habit, or any other number of distinctions.[6] Significantly, a focus on trajectories also allows for potential conversations between the increasingly neurodevelopmental approaches of neurobiologists and psychiatrists to mental illness, on the one hand, and the emphasis given by social scientists to structural inequities in material resources and power, on the other (with such inequities often intertwined with class and ethnic distinctions). Highlighting the effects of stress and trauma on selves and bodies, as well as the ways in which these effects can create path-dependent outcomes, a trajectories framework permits us to

---

[5] See Raikhel and Garriott (2013) for a more detailed discussion of several social science traditions using the concept of trajectories.

[6] Thanks to Jeffrey Snodgrass for emphasizing this point.

think closely about epidemiological findings such as the association between risk for alcohol dependence and the experience of early childhood adversity (Kessler et al., 2010).

However, work in the social sciences also emphasizes contingency, differentiation, and singularity in the study of addiction trajectories. Anthropologically informed literature on illness and drug-use trajectories emphasizes that norms, role expectations, and understandings of pathology are culturally determined, and that they are differentiated across local conceptualizations of the life course (Nichter, Quintero, Nichter, Mock, & Shakib, 2004). Other research suggests the ways in which institutionalized, enacted, and materialized ideas about specific life trajectories may work to perpetuate themselves, creating a kind of looping effect. For example, in her study of heroin addiction in New Mexico's Española Valley (the area of the United States with the highest per capita rates of heroin overdose), Angela Garcia argues that for some users, the clinical concept of chronicity they encounter in recovery programs dovetails with local Hispano tropes of loss and endlessness (themselves shaped by many decades of land loss and expropriation) and reinforces a sense of hopelessness and "no exit" from addiction (2010). Finally, a very important aspect of this idea is that it draws our attention not to the trajectories of disease entities, but of particular people, highlighting the contingency and irreducibility of individual human lives.[7]

Conclusion: Steps to an Ecology of Addiction

In 1997, the same year that then NIMH director Alan Leshner urged his readers to attend to addiction as a brain disease, Howard Shaffer, a leading researcher on compulsive gambling, described the field of addiction research as beset by "conceptual chaos," (Shaffer, 1997; Leshner, 1997). The subsequent years have seen many researchers, clinicians, policy makers, and patients turn to the brain disease model, at least partly, as a solution to the profound uncertainty and disagreement which has historically characterized knowledge about addiction. Yet, perhaps instead of seeing "chaos" in the multiple conceptual frameworks which inhabit addiction studies, we might see at least the potential for a vibrant "epistemic pluralism," encompassing not only different research styles in neurobiology and the biosciences but also distinct approaches to psychoactive substances and addiction in the social sciences. In other words,

---

[7] Indeed, it is precisely an emphasis on the potential of open-endedness and contingency that distinguishes the notion of trajectory from that of the "career" – an idea that has been widely used in the ethnography of drug and alcohol use (e.g., Waldorf, 1973).

maybe the first "step to an ecology" of addiction is not a unified "model," but a greater engagement between research agendas that approach the question in fundamentally distinct ways. In this chapter, I have described four problem areas which are especially promising for such vital engagement, but there are certainly others as well.

What relevance does this "epistemic pluralism" have for the psychiatry of addiction? Setting aside the potential of more longitudinal approaches in clinical psychiatry, as well as the important arguments for more attention to social, cultural, and political-economic factors in the clinic, such an epistemologically engaged approach draws our attention to whether and how our conceptual categories shape the very behaviors they seek to describe. Depending on which definitions we adopt, our sense of the problem's scale changes dramatically, as do any implications concerning the ontological status of addiction and which interventions are best suited to address the problems. Rather than asking which interpretive framework more closely "carves nature at its joints," perhaps the place to start is to ask which is best suited for the particular purpose at hand, both for psychiatrists and for the patients they care for and serve.

Acknowledgments

Thanks to Laurence Kirmayer, Rob Lemelson, and Connie Cummings for inviting me to contribute to this volume; to Nancy Campbell, William Garriott, Daniel Lende, and Jeff Snodgrass for their comments on earlier versions of this chapter; and to Elle Nurmi for her editorial work.

REFERENCES

Acker, C. J. (2002). *Creating the American junkie: Addiction research in the classic era of narcotic control*. Baltimore, MD: Johns Hopkins University Press.

American Psychiatric Association. (1994). *Diagnostic and statistical manual of mental disorders* (4th ed.). Washington, DC: Author.

American Psychiatric Association. (2013). *Diagnostic and statistical manual of mental disorders* (5th ed.). Washington, DC: Author.

American Society of Addiction Medicine. (2011). Definition of addiction. Adopted April 19, 2011. Retrieved from www.asam.org/research-treatment/definition-of-addiction

Applbaum, K. (2015). Solving global mental health as a delivery problem: Toward a critical epistemology of the solution. In L. J. Kirmayer, R. Lemelson, & C. A. Cummings (Eds.), *Re-visioning psychiatry: Cultural phenomenology, critical neuroscience, and global mental health* (pp. 544–74). New York, NY: Cambridge University Press.

Baler, R. D., & Volkow, N. D. (2006). Drug addiction: The neurobiology of disrupted self-control. *Trends in Molecular Medicine, 12*(12), 559–66. http://dx.doi.org/10.1016/j.molmed.2006.10.005

Bateson, G. (1972). The cybernetics of self: A theory of alcoholism. In *Steps to an ecology of mind*. Northvale, NJ: Jason Aronson.

Becker, Howard S. (1953). Becoming a marihuana user. *American Journal of Sociology, 59*, 235–42. http://dx.doi.org/10.1086/221326

Bennett, T., Dodsworth, F., Noble, G., Poovey, M., & Watkins, M. (2013). Habit and habituation governance and the social. *Body & Society, 19*(2–3), 3–29. http://dx.doi.org/10.1177/1357034X13485881

Berridge, K. C. (2007). The debate over dopamine's role in reward: The case for incentive salience. *Psychopharmacology, 191*(3), 391–431. http://dx.doi.org/10.1007/s00213-006-0578-x

Berridge, K. C., Robinson, T. E., & Aldridge, J. W. (2009). Dissecting components of reward: 'Liking', 'wanting', and learning. *Current Opinion in Pharmacology, 9*(1), 65–73. http://dx.doi.org/10.1016/j.coph.2008.12.014

Berridge, K. C., & Valenstein, E. S. (1991). What psychological process mediates feeding evoked by electrical stimulation of the lateral hypothalamus? *Behavioral Neuroscience, 105*(1), 3–14. http://dx.doi.org/10.1037/0735-7044.105.1.3

Berridge, V. (2013). *Demons: Our changing attitudes to alcohol, tobacco, and drugs.* Oxford, England: Oxford University Press.

Bourgois, P. (2003). Crack and the political economy of social suffering. *Addiction Research & Theory, 11*, 31–7.

Bruehl, A. M., Lende, D. H., Schwartz, M., Sterk, C. E., & Elifson, K. (2006). Craving and control: Methamphetamine users' narratives. *Journal of Psychoactive Drugs, 38*(Suppl. 3), 385–92. http://dx.doi.org/10.1080/02791072.2006.10400602

Buchman, D. Z., Illes, J., & Reiner, P. B. (2011). The paradox of addiction neuroscience. *Neuroethics, 4*(2), 65–77. http://dx.doi.org/10.1007/s12152-010-9079-z

Campbell, N. D. (2007). *Discovering addiction: The science and politics of substance abuse research.* Ann Arbor, MI: University of Michigan Press.

Campbell, N. D. (2010). Toward a critical neuroscience of 'addiction'. *BioSocieties, 5*(1), 89–104. http://dx.doi.org/10.1057/biosoc.2009.2

Campbell, N. D. (2011). The metapharmacology of the "addicted brain." *History of the Present, 1*(2), 194–218. http://dx.doi.org/10.5406/historypresent.1.2.0194

Campbell, N. D. (2013). "Why can't they stop?" A highly public misunderstanding of science. In E. Raikhel & W. Garriott (Eds.), *Addiction trajectories* (pp. 238–63). Durham, NC: Duke University Press. http://dx.doi.org/10.1215/9780822395874-010

Campbell, N. D., & Lovell, A. M. (2012). The history of the development of buprenorphine as an addiction therapeutic. *Annals of the New York Academy of Sciences, 1248*(1), 124–39. http://dx.doi.org/10.1111/j.1749-6632.2011.06352.x

Carr, E. S. (2013). Signs of sobriety: Rescripting American addiction counseling. In E. Raikhel & W. Garriott (Eds.), *Addiction trajectories* (pp. 160–87). Durham, NC: Duke University Press. http://dx.doi.org/10.1215/9780822395874-007

Childress, A. R., Ehrman, R. N., Wang, Z., Li, Y., Sciortino, N., Hakun, J., … O'Brien, C. P. (2008). Prelude to passion: Limbic activation by "unseen" drug and sexual cues. *PLOS One, 3*(1), e1506. http://dx.doi.org/10.1371/journal.pone.0001506

Colson, E., & Scudder, T. (1988). *For prayer and profit: The ritual, economic, and social importance of beer in Gwembe District, Zambia, 1950–1982.* Stanford, CA: Stanford University Press.

Courtwright, D. T. (2005). Mr. ATOD's wild ride: What do alcohol, tobacco, and other drugs have in common? *Social History of Alcohol and Drugs, 20*(1), 105–40.

Courtwright, D. T. (2010). The NIDA brain disease paradigm: History, resistance and spinoffs. *BioSocieties, 5,* 137–47. http://dx.doi.org/10.1057/biosoc.2009.3

Csordas, T. J. (1993). Somatic modes of attention. *Cultural Anthropology, 8*(2), 135–56. http://dx.doi.org/10.1525/can.1993.8.2.02a00010

Dackis, C., & C. O'Brien. (2005). Neurobiology of addiction: Treatment and public policy ramifications. *Nature Neuroscience, 8,* 1431–6. http://dx.doi.org/10.1038/nn1105-1431

Deleuze, G. (2007). Two questions on drugs. In D. Lapoujade (Ed.), *Two regimes of madness: Texts and interviews 1975–1995* (A. Hodges & M. Taaormina, Trans., rev. ed., pp. 151–5). Cambridge, MA: MIT Press.

Douglas, M. (1987). *Constructive drinking: Perspectives on drink from anthropology.* Cambridge, England: Cambridge University Press.

Downey, G. & Lende, D. H. (2012). Neuroanthropology and the encultured brain. In D. H. Lende & G. Downey, *The encultured brain: An introduction to neuroanthropology* (pp. 23–66). Cambridge, MA: MIT Press.

Duff, C. (2011). Reassembling (social) contexts: New directions for a sociology of drugs. *International Journal of Drug Policy, 22*(6), 404–6. http://dx.doi.org/10.1016/j.drugpo.2011.09.005

Fitzgerald, D., & Callard, F. (2015). Social science and neuroscience beyond interdisciplinarity: Experimental entanglements. *Theory, Culture & Society, 32*(1), 3–32. http://dx.doi.org/10.1177/0263276414537319

Foddy, B., & Savulescu, J. (2010). A liberal account of addiction. *Philosophy, Psychiatry, & Psychology, 17*(1), 1–22. http://dx.doi.org/10.1353/ppp.0.0282

Foucault, M. (1965). *Madness and civilization* (R. Howard, Trans.). New York, NY: Pantheon.

Fraser, S., Moore, D., & Keane, H. (2014). *Habits: Remaking addiction.* New York, NY: Palgrave Macmillan.

Garcia, A. (2010). *The pastoral clinic: addiction and dispossession along the Rio Grande.* Berkeley: University of California Press.

Garriott, W. C. (2011). *Policing methamphetamine: Narcopolitics in rural America.* New York, NY: New York University Press.

Gomart, E. (2004). Surprised by methadone: In praise of drug substitution treatment in a French clinic. *Body & Society, 10*(2–3), 85–110. http://dx.doi.org/10.1177/1357034X04042937

Gusfield, J. R. (1996). *Contested meanings: The construction of alcohol problems.* Madison, WI: University of Wisconsin Press.

Hacking, I. (2002). *Historical ontology.* Cambridge, MA: Harvard University Press.

Hansen, H., & Skinner, M. E. (2012). From white bullets to black markets and greened medicine: The neuroeconomics and neuroracial politics of opioid pharmaceuticals. *Annals of Anthropological Practice, 36*(1), 167–82. http://dx.doi.org/10.1111/j.2153-9588.2012.01098.x

Heath, D. (2004). Camba (Bolivia) drinking patterns: Changes in alcohol use, anthropology, and research perspectives. In R. Coomber & N. South (Eds.), *Drug use and cultural contexts "beyond the west": Tradition, change, and post-colonialism* (pp. 119–36). London, England: Free Association Books.

Heyman, G. M. (2009). *Addiction: A disorder of choice.* Cambridge, MA: Harvard University Press.

Hinton, D. E., Howes, D., & Kirmayer, L. J. (2008). Toward a medical anthropology of sensations: Definitions and research agenda. *Transcultural Psychiatry, 45*(2), 142–62. http://dx.doi.org/10.1177/1363461508089763

Hser, Y-I., Longshore, D., & Anglin, M. D. (2007). The life course perspective on drug use: A conceptual framework for understanding drug use trajectories. *Evaluation Review, 31*(6), 515–47. http://dx.doi.org/10.1177/0193841X07307316

Kalivas, P. W., & Volkow, N. D. (2005). The neural basis of addiction: A pathology of motivation and choice. *American Journal of Psychiatry, 162*(8), 1403–13. http://dx.doi.org/10.1176/appi.ajp.162.8.1403

Kaye, K. (2012). De-medicalizing addiction: Toward biocultural understandings. *Advances in Medical Sociology, 14*, 27–51. http://dx.doi.org/10.1108/S1057-6290(2012)0000014006

Keane, H. (2002). *What's wrong with addiction?* Melbourne, Australia: Melbourne University Publishing.

Kendler, K. S. (2012). Levels of explanation in psychiatric and substance use disorders: Implications for the development of an etiologically based nosology. *Molecular Psychiatry, 17*(1), 11–21. http://dx.doi.org/10.1038/mp.2011.70

Kessler, R. C., McLaughlin, K. A., Green, J. G., Gruber, M. J., Sampson, N. A., Zaslavsky, A. M., ... Williams, D. R. (2010). Childhood adversities and adult psychopathology in the WHO World Mental Health Surveys. *The British Journal of Psychiatry, 197*(5), 378–85.

Kirmayer, L. J., & Crafa, D. (2014). What kind of science for psychiatry? *Frontiers in Human Neuroscience, 8*, 435. http://dx.doi.org/10.3389/fnhum.2014.00435

Kirmayer, L. J., & Gold, I. (2012). Re-socializing psychiatry: Critical neuroscience and the limits of reductionism. In S. Choudhury & J. Slaby (Eds.), *Critical neuroscience: A handbook of the social and cultural contexts of neuroscience* (pp. 307–30). Chichester, England: Wiley-Blackwell. http://dx.doi.org/10.1002/9781444343359.ch15

Kushner, H. I. (2010). Toward a cultural biology of addiction. *BioSocieties, 5*(1), 8–24. http://dx.doi.org/10.1057/biosoc.2009.6

Lee, N. K., Pohlman, S., Baker, A., Ferris, J., & Kay-Lambkin, F. (2010). It's the thought that counts: Craving metacognitions and their role in abstinence from methamphetamine use. *Journal of Substance Abuse Treatment, 38*(3), 245–50.

Lende, D. H. (2005). Wanting and drug use: A biocultural approach to the analysis of addiction. *Ethos, 33*(1), 100–24.

Lende, D. H. (2012). Addiction and neuroanthropology. In D. H. Lende & G. Downey (Eds.), *The encultured brain*, (pp. 339–62). Cambridge, MA: MIT Press.

Leshner, A. I. (1997). Addiction is a brain disease, and it matters. *Science, 278*(5335), 45. http://dx.doi.org/10.1126/science.278.5335.45

Levine, H. G. (1978). The discovery of addiction. Changing conceptions of habitual drunkenness in America. *Journal of Studies on Alcohol, 39*(1), 143–74.

Levy, N. (2012). Addiction is not a brain disease (and it matters). *Frontiers in Psychiatry, 4*, 24. http://dx.doi.org/10.3389/fpsyt.2013.00024

Levy, N. (2014). Addiction as a disorder of belief. *Biology & Philosophy, 29*, 337–55. http://dx.doi.org/10.1007/s10539-014-9434-2

Lock, M., & Nguyen, V-K. (2010). *An anthropology of biomedicine.* Chichester, England: Wiley-Blackwell.

Lovell, A.M. (2013). Elusive travelers: Russian narcology, transnational toxicomanias, and the great French ecological experiment. In E. Raikhel & W. Garriott (Eds.), *Addiction trajectories* (pp. 126–59). Durham, NC: Duke University Press.

MacAndrew, C., & Edgerton, R. B. (1969). *Drunken comportment: A social explanation.* Boston, MA: Walter De Gruyter.

Marlatt, G. A., & Rohsenow, D. J. (1980). Cognitive processes in alcohol use: Expectancy and the balanced placebo design. In N. K. Mello (Ed.), *Advances in substance abuse: Behavioral and biological research* (pp. 159–99). Greenwich, CT: JAI.

Marshall, M. (1982). *Through a glass darkly: Beer and modernization in Papua New Guinea.* Boroko, Papua New Guinea: Institute of Applied Social and Economic Research.

Marshall, M., Ames, G. M., & Bennett, L. A. (2001). Anthropological perspectives on alcohol and drugs at the turn of the new millennium. *Social Science & Medicine, 53*(2), 153–64. http://dx.doi.org/10.1016/S0277-9536(00)00328-2

McKenna, S. A. (2013). "We're Supposed to Be Asleep?": Vigilance, paranoia, and the alert methamphetamine user. *Anthropology of Consciousness, 24*(2), 172–90.

Meloni, M. (2014). How biology became social, and what it means for social theory. *The Sociological Review, 62*(3), 593–614. http://dx.doi.org/10.1111/1467-954X.12151

Meyers, T. (2013). *The clinic and elsewhere: Addiction, adolescents, and the afterlife of therapy.* Seattle, WA: University of Washington Press.

Mills, J. H., & Barton, P., Eds. (2007). *Drugs and empires: Essays in modern imperialism and intoxication, c. 1500–c. 1930.* New York, NY: Palgrave Macmillan.

Mintz, S. W. (1985). *Sweetness and power: The place of sugar in modern history.* New York, NY: Viking.

Moore, D. (2004). Beyond subculture in the ethnography of illicit drug use. *Contemporary Drug Problems, 31*(2), 181–212.

Nichter, M., Quintero, G., Nichter, M., Mock, J., & Shakib, S. (2004). Qualitative research: Contributions to the study of drug use, drug abuse, and drug use (r)-related interventions. *Substance Use & Misuse, 39*(10–12), 1907–69. http://dx.doi.org/10.1081/JA-200033233

O'Brien, C. P. (2005). Anticraving medications for relapse prevention: A possible new class of psychoactive medications. *American Journal of Psychiatry, 162*(8), 1423–31. http://dx.doi.org/10.1176/appi.ajp.162.8.1423

Page, J. B. (1997). Needle exchange and reduction of harm: An anthropological view. *Medical Anthropology, 18*(1), 13–33. http://dx.doi.org/10.1080/01459740.1997.9966148

Page, J. B., & Singer, M. (2010). *Comprehending drug use: Ethnographic research at the social margins.* New Brunswick, NJ: Rutgers University Press.

Peele, S. (1985). *The meaning of addiction: Compulsive experience and its interpretation.* Lexington, MA: Lexington Books.

Pescosolido, B. A., Martin, J. K., Long, J. S., Medina, T. R., Phelan, J. C., & Link, B. G. (2010). "A disease like any other"? A decade of change in public reactions to schizophrenia, depression, and alcohol dependence. *American Journal of Psychiatry, 167*(11), 1321–30. http://dx.doi.org/10.1176/appi.ajp.2010.09121743

Petry, N. M. (2006). Should the scope of addictive behaviors be broadened to include pathological gambling? *Addiction, 101*(Suppl. s1), 152–60. http://dx.doi.org/10.1111/j.1360-0443.2006.01593.x

Raikhel, E. (2010). Post-Soviet placebos: Epistemology and authority in Russian treatments for alcoholism. *Culture, Medicine, and Psychiatry, 34*(1), 132–68. http://dx.doi.org/10.1007/s11013-009-9163-1

Raikhel, E., & Garriott, G. (2013). Tracing new paths in the anthropology of addiction. In E. Raikhel & W. Garrett (Eds.), *Addiction trajectories* (pp. 1–35). Durham, NC: Duke University Press. http://dx.doi.org/10.1215/9780822395874-001

Reinarman, C. (2005). Addiction as accomplishment: The discursive construction of disease. *Addiction Research & Theory, 13*, 307–20. http://dx.doi.org/10.1080/16066350500077728

Rhodes, T. (2002). The 'risk environment': A framework for understanding and reducing drug-related harm. *International Journal of Drug Policy, 13*(2), 85–94. http://dx.doi.org/10.1016/S0955-3959(02)00007-5

Robins, L. N. (1993). Vietnam veterans' rapid recovery from heroin addiction: A fluke or normal expectation? *Addiction, 88*(8), 1041–54. http://dx.doi.org/10.1111/j.1360-0443.1993.tb02123.x

Robinson, T. E., & Berridge, K. C. (1993). The neural basis of drug craving: an incentive-sensitization theory of addiction. *Brain Research Reviews, 18*(3), 247–91. http://dx.doi.org/10.1016/0165-0173(93)90013-P

Room, R. (1984). Alcohol and ethnography: A case of problem deflation? *Current Anthropology, 25*(2), 169–78. http://dx.doi.org/10.1086/203107

Room, R. (2001). Intoxication and bad behaviour: Understanding cultural differences in the link. *Social Science & Medicine, 53*(2), 189–98. http://dx.doi.org/10.1016/S0277-9536(00)00330-0

Room, R. (2003). The cultural framing of addiction. *Janus Head, 6*(2), 221–34.

Rose, N. (2003). The neurochemical self and its anomalies. In R. V. Ericson & A. Doyle (Eds.), *Risk and morality* (pp. 407–37). Toronto: University of Toronto Press.

Rose, N. (2013). The human sciences in a biological age. *Theory, Culture & Society, 30*(1), 3–34. http://dx.doi.org/10.1177/0263276412456569

Rosenberg, C. E. (2007). *Our present complaint: American medicine, then and now.* Baltimore, MD: Johns Hopkins University Press.

Saris, A. J. (2013). Committed to will: What's at stake for anthropology in addiction. In E. Raikhel & W. Garriott (Eds.), *Addiction trajectories* (pp. 263–83). Durham, NC: Duke University Press. http://dx.doi.org/10.1215/9780822395874-011

Satel, S., & Lilienfeld, S. O. (2013). Addiction and the brain-disease fallacy. *Frontiers in Psychiatry, 4*, 141. http://dx.doi.org/10.3389/fpsyt.2013.00141

Schlosser, A. V., & Hoffer, L. D. (2012). The psychotropic self/imaginary: Subjectivity and psychopharmaceutical use among heroin users with co-occurring mental illness. *Culture, Medicine, and Psychiatry, 36*(1), 26–50. http://dx.doi.org/10.1007/s11013-011-9244-9

Schüll, N. D. (2006). Machines, medication, modulation: Circuits of dependency and self-care in Las Vegas. *Culture, Medicine, and Psychiatry, 30*(2), 223–47. http://dx.doi.org/10.1007/s11013-006-9018-y

Schüll, N. D. (2012). *Addiction by design: Machine gambling in Las Vegas.* Princeton, NJ: Princeton University Press.

Sedgwick, E. K. (1993). Epidemics of the will. In *Tendencies* (pp. 130–42). Durham, NC: Duke University Press. http://dx.doi.org/10.1215/9780822381860-007

Shaffer, H. J. (1997). The most important unresolved issue in the addictions: Conceptual chaos. *Substance Use & Misuse, 32*(11), 1573–80.

Singer, M. (2001). Toward a bio-cultural and political economic integration of alcohol, tobacco and drug studies in the coming century. *Social Science & Medicine, 53*(2), 199–213. http://dx.doi.org/10.1016/S0277-9536(00)00331-2

Singer, M. (2007). *Drugging the poor: Legal and illegal drugs and social inequality.* Long Grove, IL: Waveland Press.

Singer, M. (2012). Anthropology and addiction: An historical review. *Addiction, 107*(10), 1747–55. http://dx.doi.org/10.1111/j.1360-0443.2012.03879.x

Slaby, J., & Choudhury, S. (2012). Proposal for a critical neuroscience. In S. Choudhury & J. Slaby (Eds.), *Critical neuroscience: A handbook of the social and cultural contexts of neuroscience* (pp. 29–51). Chichester, England: Wiley-Blackwell.

Snodgrass, J. G., Lacy, M. G., Dengah II, H. F., Fagan, J., & Most, D. E. (2011). Magical flight and monstrous stress: technologies of absorption and mental wellness in Azeroth. *Culture, Medicine, and Psychiatry, 35*(1), 26–62. http://dx.doi.org/10.1007/s11013-010-9197-4

Testa, M., Fillmore, M. T., Norris, J., Abbey, A., Curtin, J. J., Leonard, K. E., ... Hayman, L. W. (2006). Understanding alcohol expectancy effects: Revisiting the placebo condition. *Alcoholism: Clinical and Experimental Research, 30*(2), 339–48. http://dx.doi.org/10.1111/j.1530-0277.2006.00039.x

Valverde, M. (1998). *Diseases of the will: Alcohol and the dilemmas of freedom.* Cambridge, England: Cambridge University Press.

Volkow, N. D., & O'Brien, C. P. (2007). Issues for *DSM-V*: Should obesity be included as a brain disorder? *American Journal of Psychiatry, 164*(5), 708–10.

Volkow, N. D., Wang, G. J., Fowler, J. S., & Tomasi, D. (2012). Addiction circuitry in the human brain. *Annual Review of Pharmacology and Toxicology, 52*, 321–36. http://dx.doi.org/10.1146/annurev-pharmtox-010611-134625

Vrecko, S. (2010a). Civilizing technologies' and the control of deviance. *BioSocieties, 5*(1), 36–51. http://dx.doi.org/10.1057/biosoc.2009.8

Vrecko, S. (2010b). Birth of a brain disease: Science, the state and addiction neuropolitics. *History of the Human Sciences, 23*(4), 52–67. http://dx.doi.org/10.1177/0952695110371598

Wagenaar, A. C., Salois, M. J., & Komro, K. A. (2009). Effects of beverage alcohol price and tax levels on drinking: A meta-analysis of 1003 estimates from 112 studies. *Addiction, 104*(2), 179–90. http://dx.doi.org/10.1111/j.1360-0443.2008.02438.x

Waldorf, D. (1973). *Careers in dope.* Englewood Cliffs, NJ: Prentice Hall.

Weinberg, D. (2011). Sociological perspectives on addiction. *Sociology Compass, 5*(4), 298–310. http://dx.doi.org/10.1111/j.1751-9020.2011.00363.x

Weinberg, D. (2013). Post-humanism, addiction and the loss of self-control: Reflections on the missing core in addiction science. *International Journal of Drug Policy, 24*(3), 173–81. http://dx.doi.org/10.1016/j.drugpo.2013.01.009

What is Addiction? (2014, February 10). [Opinion]. *The New York Times.* Retrieved from www.nytimes.com/roomfordebate/2014/02/10/what-is-addiction

16 Cultural-Clinical Psychology
From Cultural Scripts to Contextualized Treatments

Andrew G. Ryder and Yulia E. Chentsova-Dutton

There is a long history of collaboration between psychiatry and psychology. Clinical psychology, in particular, serves as a link between the interdisciplinary study of mental health problems and basic research on mind and behavior carried out by other branches of psychology. Psychology contributes to the basic sciences of normal and abnormal behavior from which clinicians can draw theories of psychopathology and evidence-based interventions. Compared to psychiatry, the standard training model in clinical psychology places a relatively greater emphasis on research production, nondiagnostic clinical assessment, and psychological interventions. For example, clinical psychologists have been quick to embrace dimensional models of personality and psychopathology, driven by research evidence rather than subscribing to the medical tendency to see all disorders as necessarily categorical (see Bilder, Chapter 8, *this volume*).

Yet clinical psychology faces many of the same dilemmas as psychiatry. In addition to similar pressures toward reinvention as a strictly neurobiological discipline, there are familiar tendencies toward overinvestment in favored concepts, models, and interventions. Like psychiatry, clinical psychology tends to locate mental health problems within the individual person; like psychiatry, clinical psychology tends to assume that the most important aspects of the person are universal. There may be acknowledgment that a person's social context can exacerbate symptoms or that upbringing confering different values impacts willingness to talk about these symptoms, but the core illness and the bounded individualized self that suffers from it is fundamentally the same everywhere. Clinical psychology needs its own revisioning parallel to, and in exchange with, psychiatry. In this chapter, we will outline one such revisioned clinical psychology, which we have called "cultural-clinical psychology" (Ryder, Ban, & Chentsova-Dutton, 2011), and discuss how this approach might contribute to new approaches in psychiatry. Although the methods of cultural-clinical psychology are recognizable to mainstream psychologists, a thoroughgoing engagement with cultural variation will require these psychologists to rethink several core assumptions.

400

Levels of Explanation: A Case Example

To anchor and illustrate our discussion we begin with the case of a young immigrant student. Although focusing on a university student would seem to minimize cultural difference, this example serves as a salutary reminder that one does not have to travel far to find very different cultural contexts. Even a young, well-educated, relatively well-to-do person, living in a globalized world and pursuing her studies in English, can nonetheless inhabit a cultural space that differs in many ways from that of her European American counterparts.

Ms. Kim is a twenty-one-year-old woman from South Korea and is currently a second-year undergraduate at an American university. She presents to the university mental health clinic with complaints of headaches and poor sleep. During the initial assessment, she describes wide fluctuations in appetite and weight, including an eight-pound gain in the past two weeks, and sleep dysregulation. On most nights, she spends two to three hours in bed, tossing and turning and "thinking too much" before falling asleep for no more than three to four hours in total. By day, she is exhausted, listless, and dysphoric, with fatigue-induced headaches. She also has trouble maintaining focus and struggles to make even small decisions.

Ms. Kim reports that her troubles began five years ago when her father, an assistant factory manager, was criticized harshly in the media after a persistent toxic leak was reported. She firmly believes her father was innocent of any wrongdoing and was singled out to cover up a serious violation by the plant manager. The whole family was affected by this event. She describes how her father became silent and withdrawn, and how her mother coped by focusing on Ms. Kim and her younger brother. Ms. Kim recalls this attention made her more distressed, in part due to feelings of anger about the injustice and shame that her mother described to her. In turn, this distress ensured her mother attended to her even more closely.

Now that Ms. Kim is a student in the United States, she has little contact with her parents but thinks about them and their situation "nearly constantly." She dwells on the sense that her father was treated unfairly, making her feel hot and irritable, like her "chest will explode"; she reports episodes of "freaking out," crying, and shaking. Moreover, she is increasingly concerned that other people will be uncomfortable around her and offended by her behavior such that even simple gestures might inappropriately reveal her distress to others. To avoid these reactions she has greatly reduced contact with her parents, but feels guilty about doing so and about not performing well enough to justify their sacrifices in providing for her international education.[1]

How best to understand Ms. Kim's situation? In keeping with the biological turn of recent years, we could tell a story about genetic

---

[1] This is a composite case with details altered to protect anonymity.

vulnerability combined with neurobiological disturbances in response to chronic stress. In response to calls for more attention to sociocultural context, we might prefer a story emphasizing Korean social hierarchies, the interpersonal experience of shame, and beliefs about the value and importance of education. Trained as psychologists, we also incline toward stories told at a level between the biological and the social. We believe stories of the mind are worth preserving in the face of both neurobiological determinism and sociocultural accounts of the context of suffering, not least because effective assessment and psychological treatment often require us to work at this level. In this regard, we note several examples of self-perpetuating cycles: Guilt brings about dysphoria, leading to poor school performance, leading to more guilt and thoughts of failure; thoughts of failure interrupt sleep patterns, leading to exhaustion, leading to failure experiences and shame; shame encourages avoidance, leading to poor grades, leading to more shame and guilt about failure; and so on.

In this chapter, we will argue that these biological, psychological, and sociocultural stories are potentially, and simultaneously, "true." Each story is partial, and identifying the "best story" depends on what we want to accomplish (Kirmayer & Young, 1998). Following our own research, we focus in this chapter on the set of interrelated problems characterized by a mixture of dysphoria and anxiety. In *DSM-5* diagnostic terms, these problems include nonpsychotic Major Depressive Disorder, Persistent Depressive Disorder (Dysthymia), Generalized Anxiety Disorder, Social Anxiety Disorder (Social Phobia), and several related personality disorders (e.g., Avoidant Personality Disorder) (American Psychiatric Association, 2013). Numerous local cultural categories that fit in this general conceptual space and that might overlap conceptually and empirically in various degrees with these "Western" categories are also included.

In general, we believe it useful to be "lumpers" of syndromes and "splitters" of symptoms, especially when making cross-cultural comparisons. Kleinman (1988) has noted that overreliance on formal diagnoses can minimize important group variations. When categorizing people for ease of description, study inclusion, or treatment initiation, we therefore prefer broader groupings rather than formal diagnostic labels. For example, recent research on somatization among Chinese was conducted with patients meeting criteria for any depressive disorder as defined by American, Chinese, and International diagnostic systems rather than only with the criteria for major depression in *DSM-IV* (Ryder et al., 2008). At the same time, in order to investigate cultural variations in symptom experience and expression, the same research program draws on a pool of items drawn from all three diagnostic systems, at times further subdividing these symptoms to capture salient cultural differences. For example, distinctions between insomnia and hypersomnia have led to more nuanced descriptions of what somatization among Chinese actually involves (Dere et al., 2013).

For these reasons, we will focus on "serious distress" as the set of clinically significant problems characterized by dysphoria and anxiety rather than on specific diagnostic categories such as major depression, social anxiety disorder, and so on, except when describing previous research on these categories. The specific syndromes in this broad category are hard to separate, whether through presentation, underlying personality traits, or familial heritability, and it is not clear that doing so provides much clinical information (Tyrer, Seivewright, & Johnson, 2003). Moreover, the best evidence currently available supports the same general approach to treatment for these types of conditions, regardless of the specific diagnosis: Cognitive-behavior therapy (CBT), supplemented by SSRIs or their descendants if needed, with maintenance of a strong therapeutic alliance (Nathan & Gorman, 2007). Attention to specific symptoms, meanwhile, is important in order to characterize the culturally shaped experience of seriously distressed people in a more nuanced way. Clinically, attention to specific symptoms allows us to talk more effectively to patients about their particular experiences, assess them in ways more likely to capture these experiences, identify targets for treatment, and track progress over time.

We begin with a brief presentation of our general perspective, which is that culture, mind, and brain are best understood as a single multilevel system. The three following sections then elaborate how, in light of this perspective, we might approach the mechanisms of psychopathology, clinical diagnosis and assessment, and the treatment of serious distress. We conclude by returning to the story of Ms. Kim, to imagine the application of a successfully revisioned psychiatry – undergirded by the basic science of cultural-clinical psychology.

Culture-Mind-Brain: A Systemic View

Cultural-clinical psychology contributes its parent discipline's focus on mind and behavior to the interdisciplinary study of mental health. Mental processes can neither be reduced to some product or process of the brain, nor entirely explained in terms of the sociocultural context. Rather, mind is best understood as an emergent aggregate or ensemble of processes that depend on both neurobiology and social interaction but that require their own language of description and explanatory constructs (e.g., Bassett & Gazzaniga, 2011). Mind involves cognitive processes that are both embodied in a biological organism and embedded in a social world.

A view of the mind as extended beyond the brain in important ways has emerged in recent philosophy and cognitive science (Clark & Chalmers, 1998; Hutchins, 1995; Valsiner & Van der Veer, 2000; Vygotsky, 1978). Studies on embodied cognition demonstrate how the mind depends on inputs from the body and physical environment (Richardson, Marsh, & Schmidt, 2010; Warren, 2006; Wilson & Golonka, 2013). When bodily actions or aspects of the physical environment are habitually used as cognitive tools – whether counting on one's fingers, using an abacus, or pulling out an Internet-connected smartphone – we can talk about an "extended mind" incorporating these tools. Moreover, just as a map and compass can become part of the mind's direction-finding system, so too can a dependable friend become part of the mind's emotion regulation system (Coman & Hirst, 2011; Rimé, 2007). Psychopathology can include problems in the extended mind: For example, depression often includes excessive reassurance seeking, which can serve to alienate people who might ordinarily be supportive (Joiner, Alfano, & Metalsky, 1992; Joiner, Metalsky, Katz, & Beach, 1999).

The idea that mind includes external tools and the social world, along with cognitive processes and subjective experiences, provides a route to understanding how thoroughly mind is shaped by culture, and culture by mind. Cultural psychology is increasingly moving toward the anthropological view that individual people are uniquely situated within their cultural contexts. Work on distributed cognition demonstrates that "cultural knowledge" does not have to be accessible to everyone equally, or at all (Atran, 2001; Sperber & Hirschfeld, 2004). Meanings and practices are socially distributed so that different people within a context can think and act in different, even contradictory, ways that are equally meaningful. Rather than seeking to catalogue what cultural groups "believe" or "do," therefore, we should instead ask questions about how specific aspects of culture shape specific people in specific ways. As we shall see later on, this idea has important clinical implications.

This view of extended mind and its interrelation with culture is consistent with the core claim of cultural-clinical psychology: that culture, mind, and the human brain are *mutually constitutive* – they must be understood as part of a single, multilevel, system (Ryder et al., 2011; see also Kitayama & Park, 2010; Shweder, 1990). No level can be understood without reference to the others, nor can any level be reduced to the others. A particular story might be easier to tell at a certain level; nonetheless, "disorder," "vulnerability," "protective factor," and so on, are emergent properties of the entire system, shaped by all three levels and their complex interactions. Within the research tradition of psychology, there are several lines of inquiry that can help us develop a more systemic model of the emergence and maintenance of serious distress in cultural context. It is to this work that we now turn.

Serious Distress

Humans are socialized into cultural contexts that profoundly shape our goals and the ways in which they can be pursued. Cultural representations guide attention, allowing the person to construct something personally and consensually meaningful out of the vast range of possibilities (Norenzayan, Choi, & Peng, 2007). Specific cognitive schemas emerge in culture-mind-brain as simultaneous products of how the brain stores and retrieves information, how culture directs attention to what is important, and the individual mind and its experiential history. Once well established, schemas powerfully guide the ways in which old information is remembered and how new information is received; schemas require substantial amounts of important information in order to change (Brewer & Treyens, 1981; Rumelhart, 1984; Rumelhart & Ortony, 1977).

The onset of serious distress is confusing and begs for explanation. Episodes are characterized by a plethora of changes in one's sense of self, motivation, view of the future, relationship with God, spirits, or ancestors, ability to self-regulate, experienced and expressed emotions, attention and concentration, thinking, energy levels, bodily sensations, and more. For example, seriously distressed Korean and Japanese students experience not only the symptoms of lack of energy and loss of appetite familiar from *DSM*, but also a multitude of other somatic symptoms, including heartburn, abdominal cramps, dizziness, hot flashes, stiff joints, and palpitations (Saint Arnault & Kim, 2008). These changes are difficult to explain to oneself, let alone to others. Ambiguous events, such as unexpected and unfamiliar "symptom" experiences, are most easily interpreted in light of available schemas, which may be based on recollection of one's own past experiences or stories of other people who had similar events. New information is seen in light of these schemas and also serves to modify or reinforce them.

Whereas schemas are primarily described as mental structures, scripts involve sequences of action that can be enacted and observed by others in the world. For cognitive psychologists, scripts refer to declarative knowledge structures that organize stereotypical events, such as visiting a clinician (Schank & Abelson, 1977). Once activated, scripts provide a structure or scaffold for meaning-making and memory. As with schemas more generally, people tend to expect script-consistent information and will remember events in accordance with it, overlooking instances of minor script-violation but remembering major violations well (Bower, Black, & Turner, 1979). The notion of scripts has been adopted and broadened by psycholinguists, cultural psychologists, and other social scientists interested in cultural models of behavior and cognition (e.g., D'Andrade, 1981; DiMaggio, 1997; Wierzbicka, 1994). In this literature, scripts refer to broader interpretive rules for behaviors and social encounters. As well, whereas the cognitive approach requires scripts to be conscious, explicit, and reportable to others, scripts in this broader social science tradition can include implicit knowledge. Both views inform our understanding of cultural scripts, and we argue these constructs can be particularly useful in understanding models of serious distress (Chentsova-Dutton, Ryder, & Tsai, 2014).

A Multiplicity of Cultural Scripts

Most cultural contexts offer multiple sets of competing scripts that can help direct attention to particular experiences. For example, Iranian adolescents interpreting Western depression symptoms may recruit culturally familiar scripts of how one falls in love, gets physically ill, or goes through puberty, along with concepts of "depression" and "anxiety" (Essau, Olaya, Pasha, Pauli, & Bray, 2013). Sets of competing scripts can emerge during periods of rapid cultural change. In China, for example, psychological representations of "depression" have emerged in recent years, but somatically focused representations of "neurasthenia" are also available (Ryder, Sun, Zhu, Yao, & Chentsova-Dutton, 2012). The specific script that is used depends on a person's learning history combined with situational demands (Pritzker, 2007; Wittink, Dahlberg, Biruk, & Barg, 2008). In our case example, Ms. Kim accesses Korean cultural scripts for *hwa byung*, a somatic syndrome of idiom of distress that links burning sensations in the epigastrium, anger or indignation, and situations of social injustice (Min, 2008; Min, Suh, & Song, 2009).

Like most cultural representations, scripts of distress differ in their stability, popularity, and ability to spread in a given cultural-historical marketplace of ideas. Successful propagation of an idea depends on the credibility and prestige of the source (e.g., a respected healer) and the psychological "susceptibility" of the people who learn these ideas and pass them on. Representations tend to be favored if they feature moderate levels of novelty, if they fit well with other available representations, if they are easy to communicate, and if they have an emotional appeal (see Chentsova-Dutton & Heath, 2009, for a review). Some ideas spread due to well-developed sets of cultural cues that evoke the idea (Berger & Heath, 2005), others because they map onto concerns salient within the cultural contexts (Bangerter & Heath, 2004). For example, the script of *hikikomori*, or social withdrawal seen among youth, may have rapidly spread in Japan due to the salience of concerns about the effects of economic recession and shifting cultural norms (Norasakkunkit, Uchida, & Toivonen, 2012). Finally, cultural contact and globalization powerfully shape local dynamics of idea propagation by ensuring a supply of novel scripts for serious distress. After the fall of the Berlin Wall, for example, the cultural scripts readily available to East Germans for depression as an understandable response to life crises were replaced by scripts grounded in biomedicine and psychoanalysis that were available to West Germans (Angermeyer & Matschinger, 1999; Beck, Matschinger, & Angermeyer, 2003).

Potentially Symptomatizable Experiences

Put aside this book and pay attention to your body and your mind for a moment. Do you notice bodily sensations, perhaps a stiff neck or difficulty swallowing? What about emotions and thoughts, perhaps a vague feeling of anxiety, an intrusive thought, or a sense that it is hard to focus? Kirmayer and colleagues (Kirmayer, 1984; Kirmayer & Sartorius, 2007; Kirmayer & Taillefer, 1997; Robbins & Kirmayer, 1986) argue that ordinary daily life is characterized by a "background noise" of physical sensations. The majority of these sensations pass by unnoticed, others are noticed momentarily but not flagged for sustained attention, others still may be flagged as strange or annoying without being unduly alarming. These are not symptoms, but rather "symptomatizable" experiences. The background noise fluctuates for all kinds of reasons, which become part of the proximate cause of a particular symptom (Broadbent & Petrie, 2007). Different circumstances elicit different emotional reactions, which come with various sets of physiological sensations, subjective experiences, and behavioral responses – not to mention, their own associated cultural scripts. Diurnal rhythms, caffeine intake, hunger, thirst, and fatigue levels, physical activity, and so on, can all play a moment-to-moment role in helping to determine which symptomatizable experiences are more or less likely to be perceived (see also Hinton & Simon, Chapter 14, *this volume*; Kolk, Hanewald, Schagen, & Gijsbers van Wijk, 2003).

Indeed, there is considerable evidence that most healthy people have experiences that, under certain circumstances, we might call symptoms. Even healthy bodies continuously register twinges, aches, pains, and discomforts (Skelton & Pennebaker, 1982). There is good evidence to support extending this idea beyond physical sensations, to encompass a wide range of symptomatizable experiences. Our mood states fluctuate, not always in ways immediately attributable to the situation (Bowen, Clark, & Baetz, 2004; Katerndahl, Ferrer, Best, & Wang, 2007). We have transient impulses, intrusive thoughts, daydreams, and strange ideas (Purdon & Clark, 1993). The interpersonal world is replete with ambiguous and potentially negative occurrences (Chen, Matthews, & Zhou, 2007). Even occasional and nondisruptive dissociative or psychotic experiences turn out to be rather common in the general population (Johns & van Os, 2001; Posey & Losch, 1983).

The quantity and quality of these experiences show substantial individual differences. Some people are more likely to experience notable or potentially worrisome sensations, emotions, and thoughts. Kirmayer and Sartorius (2007) note that the background noise of physical sensations increases with age. Although we believe claims for the contribution of personality traits become exaggerated when cultural context, especially social role, is not considered, we maintain that dispositional characteristics still contribute to understanding and predicting behavior (Ryder, Dere, Sun, & Chentsova-Dutton, 2014). In particular, the broad domain of neuroticism, and its genetic, neurobiological, affective, and interpersonal correlates (Côté & Moskowitz, 1998; Schinka, Busch, & Robichaux-Keene, 2004; Sen, Burmeister, & Ghosh, 2004), has been implicated in the generation of symptomatizable experiences. Neuroticsm and its correlates, moreover, are associated with increased likelihood that a symptomatizable experience will be elaborated into a full-blown symptom (Lahey, 2009; Malouff, Thorsteinsson, & Schutte, 2005).

Notably, neuroticism is also implicated in studies that examine forms of distress that are known to be primarily driven by interpersonal and cultural factors; for example, unexplained medical symptoms or mass psychogenic syndromes (Colligan & Murphy, 1979; Deary, Chalder, & Sharpe, 2007; De Gucht, Fischler, & Heiser, 2004). This research suggests that exposure to particular representations may combine with neuroticism to promote the emergence of symptoms consistent with those representations. Individual differences in the characteristics of sensory, emotional, and cognitive experiences also emerge through variations in personal biography. The vigilance with which one attends to a somatic symptoms or a drop in mood as a potential source of concern is affected not only by neuroticism, but also by past history of somatoaffective experiences (Wiens, 2005). There is evidence that people learn to associate sad mood with particularly negative thoughts during a first depressive episode and that, once the person has recovered, these thoughts can be reactivated by ordinary sadness (Segal & Ingram, 1994; Teasdale, 1988). Thinking about one's sadness can in turn trigger depressive relapse (Abela & Hankin, 2011; Michalak, Hölz, & Teismann, 2011; Nolen-Hoeksema, Wisco, & Lyubomirsky, 2008).

In sum, most people experience a large number of symptomatizable experiences, particularly those who are temperamentally vulnerable or who have been reinforced for paying attention to particular bodily sensations, emotions, thoughts, or other experiences (Whitehead et al., 1994). Not all of these experiences will be registered, attended to, and interpreted. Beyond momentary fluctuations and individual differences, some experiences within this chaotic and shifting background are identified as worthy of sustained attention in a given cultural context. Cultural scripts for serious distress, set against a backdrop of local models of self, emotion, and the body, are implicated in this process by foregrounding certain symptom constituents and coloring them with significance.

Cultural Representations Shape Serious Distress

Symptomatizable experiences interact with cultural scripts, shaping the emergence and maintenance of symptoms. By *symptoms*, we mean specific experiences, suffered by a specific person, in a specific context that construes these experiences as problematic. We understand symptoms as both somatically embodied and contextually embedded (Ryder & Chentsova-Dutton, 2012). These experiences are identified as potentially pathological changes that can be thought about, talked about, worried about, sought help for, and so on. How do experiences become foregrounded as symptoms? Following Kirmayer (1984; Kirmayer & Sartorius, 2007), we argue that the key processes involved in emergence of symptoms from their constituents are selective attention and cognitive-perceptual looping, guided by locally relevant cultural scripts. As noted earlier, we extend this idea beyond the somatic to include thoughts, emotions, perceptions, actions, and interpersonal events.

Recent work in psychology suggests that cognitive representations do not exist purely as mental structures. Instead, they are simulations of lived and embodied experiences, capable of triggering cascades of sensory and behavioral changes, along with responses to these cascades (Barsalou, 2008; Feldman Barrett, 2009). Attending to representations of psychological processes, such as serious distress, cannot be fully separated from the lived experience of these processes. This means that attending to one's symptomatizable experiences through the filter of a cultural script partly constitutes the emerging symptom.

Not only do cultural scripts guide people to selectively attend to particular experiences when they occur, attentional processes can actually contribute to their emergence as symptoms. By leading people to devote more attentional resources to scanning for particular events, scripts increase the likelihood of detecting an instance of whatever one is looking for. We attend to sensations that are considered to be remarkable or threatening in the framework of relevant cultural scripts (Broadbent & Petrie, 2007). For example, Ms. Kim's first experience of "freaking out" may have had its origins in a particular combination of exhaustion, increased emotional lability, an unexpected phone call from her distressed mother, tearfulness combined with social concerns about crying in public, the desire to escape a crowded bus, and a cultural framework in which losing control in public is a shameful failure to bear suffering quietly. Indeed, this cultural framework may have led her to be particularly likely to notice these experiences and to be concerned about them.

Yet this is not all: Attention and concern may have *promoted* the emergence of particular symptoms. Once Ms. Kim had her first few experiences of "freaking out," she would be more likely to scan for signals that a new episode might be imminent, which in turn could increase the likelihood of future episodes. Recent research illustrates that directing attention to representations of past events, emotions, actions, and somatic sensations can lead to cognitive, emotional, behavioral, and physiological changes consistent with these representations (Gonsalves et al., 2004; Lindquist & Barrett, 2008; Price, Finniss, & Benedetti, 2008; Pulvermüller, 2005; Tucker & Ellis, 2004).

Sometimes this effect is fairly general, observable when people attend to thoughts with particular meaning in a given cultural context. For example, in a series of studies European Americans and Asian Americans were randomized to either think about themselves or think about a family member. While watching emotionally valenced film clips, reactivity was higher in European Americans directed to think about themselves, and in Asian Americans directed to think about a family member. This effect emerged not only for self-report, but also for facial behavior and psychophysiological response (Chentsova-Dutton & Tsai, 2010). This effect can also be specific to particular emotions. In a series of studies, researchers used semantic priming and semantic satiation to manipulate the accessibility of particular emotion words. Then, when presented with faces depicting particular emotional states, participants were quicker or slower to perceive these emotions depending on the accessibility of the appropriate word (Lindquist, Barrett, Bliss-Moreau, & Russell, 2006).

A third example demonstrates how symptoms themselves can be generated by expectations. For instance, some people believe that exposure to electromagnetic fields can lead to illness. Content analysis of media reports in the United Kingdom shows that newspaper articles tend to reinforce this view and rarely note the lack of scientific evidence (Eldridge-Thomas & Rubin, 2013). Moreover, an experimental study has demonstrated that exposure to a television report on the symptoms that can result from exposure to electromagnetic fields, combined with a sham exposure, can elicit physical (e.g., tingling) and psychological (e.g., concentration problems) complaints consistent with these cultural representations (Witthöft & Rubin, 2012). Attention to cultural scripts for serious distress is likely to not only increase detection of preexisting symptoms, but to foreground, foster, and constitute these symptoms.

Cultural scripts relevant to serious distress can also affect the course of symptoms. The attention-directing effects of symptom-relevant cultural scripts do not stop with the emergence of a symptom or a set of symptoms. Once symptoms are detected and interpreted, cultural scripts may suggest meaningful action, such as increased vigilance, communication with healers, or self-administered treatment. These steps may trigger additional reactions from the person and his or her social network. Depression is not only a response to particular stressors, but also a trigger of behaviors that generate stressors (Ryder et al., 2012; Starrs et al., 2010). Social rejection might increase the risk of depression, but the interpersonal behaviors that accompany depression can also increase the risk of social rejection. The result is a loop that plays out over months or years and can help turn an acute episode into a chronic problem.

In sum, we can describe two kinds of loops. The first is implicated in the emergence of symptoms from the background noise of symptomatizable experiences. In the language of control systems theory, these are "positive feedback loops" in which the outcome of a process further increases the likelihood of that outcome. Thus, Ms. Kim anxiously monitors her thoughts to make sure she does not think about her parents in public, which increases the likelihood that she will have those very thoughts, which increases her anxiety, which increases her self-monitoring. These loops are inherently unstable, tending to operate over relatively short time periods and eventually resolving either by "burning out" or by shifting the system to a new stable state (Carver & Scheier, 2001).

The second kind of loop is implicated in the maintenance of symptoms once they have emerged, pushing systems toward stability, or homeostasis. For control systems theorists in psychology, stable states are defined by goals and such "negative feedback loops" function by reducing discrepancies between the current state of affairs and these goals (Carver & Scheier, 2001). Ms. Kim wants to avoid anxiety and believes she is likely to have an embarrassing episode if she is in front of other people, so she avoids public places. Each time she successfully avoids a social situation, her anxiety returns to an acceptable baseline. Unfortunately, doing so reduces her contact with other people, reinforces the benefits of avoidance, and denies her the opportunity to learn to cope with her anxiety. These loops promote stability, and as such there are no temporal limits.

Following Kirmayer and Sartorius (2007), we contend that many forms of psychopathology exist in large part because of such loops, and systems of loops. Indeed, the potential for looping effects may be central to why transient symptoms can become more chronic syndromes, rather than just isolated (albeit unpleasant) incidents. Symptoms that frequently get pulled into these kinds of negative feedback loops within a given cultural context are increasingly likely to be labeled. People who are seen, or who see themselves, as fitting these consensually understood categories are more likely to think and act in accordance with them (Link & Phelan, 1999). The consequence might be further suffering, or more effective treatment seeking, but either way the category is reinforced. These looping processes contribute to the maintenance of privileged explanatory categories, such as diagnoses, within a given cultural context.

Diagnosis and Assessment

Symptoms and their configurations in syndromes or disorders vary for all kinds of reasons, many of them shaped by the context in which they are experienced and expressed. Psychopathology emerges from looping processes that bring together many different constituents to generate suffering for the person, and they are maintained by another set of looping processes that perpetuate suffering. In consequence, psychiatric categories are not fixed – indeed, they are often not even categorical (see Bilder, Chapter 8, *this volume*). Nonetheless, if well designed and well suited to a given context, psychiatric diagnoses may have important clinical utility, but clinicians must remember that these categories are provisional and can only be understood in context.

A sufficiently thorough diagnostic assessment should involve a comprehensive integration of the patient's current situation, life history, symptom presentation, and health status to arrive at a description that provides useful information about the underlying pathology and the preferred options for treatment. Although cultural assumptions are embedded in the diagnostic and assessment process, this may be less obvious if both clinician and patient share the same unspoken assumptions. However, the power and influence of Western science means these unspoken assumptions get packaged and exported around the world, both in the research literature and in models of treatment, often to places where people operate under very different assumptions (Kirmayer, 2006).

Assessment of Symptom Scripts

The alternative to proceeding with implicit assumptions about categories of serious distress is to find some way of making explicit the relevant assumptions of the cultural worlds in which a given patient lives. Unfortunately, the sheer range of possibilities that a clinician might encounter makes case-by-case cultural knowledge unrealistic. We therefore return to the central idea of the cultural script. Scripts have particular properties, they work in particular ways, and these ways can be recruited for research and assessment. In the case of Ms. Kim, if the clinician is not familiar with the Korean cultural context, the relevant cultural scripts must be drawn out. First, *normative cultural scripts* characterize shared understandings of how people generally behave. For example, Korean contexts have accessible cultural scripts for suppression of anger, valorizing people – particularly women – who remain calm and bear suffering through difficult times (Kim & Choi, 1995). Second, *deviant cultural scripts* characterize deviations from the norm that are nonetheless comprehensible within the cultural context (Chentsova-Dutton et al., 2014). The cultural script for *hwa byung* supports the normative value of anger suppression while acknowledging that for some people doing so leads to certain symptoms, both somatic (e.g., feeling like her chest will explode) and psychological (e.g., brooding on injustice; Min, 2008; Min et al., 2009).

Knowledge of how cultural scripts work in general may help us to develop and improve assessment techniques to identify and elaborate on underlying cultural scripts. For example, "behavioral functional analysis" is used in CBT to unpack examples of problematic behavioral sequences (Dobson & Dobson, 2009). When Ms. Kim reports frequent episodes of "freaking out," she might be asked to walk through a specific example in considerable detail, beginning with (1) the immediate antecedents, then (2) the sequence of behaviors itself with associated physical sensations, thoughts, and emotional reactions, and finally (3) the intra- and interpersonal consequences. Importantly, and beyond the standard practice in CBT, she might also be asked to share her sense of how other Koreans might typically understand these episodes, in order to situate her unique narrative within an intersubjectively understood cultural script. Done properly, this approach takes an idiosyncratic self-report of "freaking out" – where the therapist might be tempted to "read in" cultural assumptions about what this term means – and converts it into a descriptively rich account of a patient's problem.

Standardized Assessment Tools

The emphasis on cultural scripts does not mean that individual experience is reducible to abstract constructs. Indeed, one implication of understanding culture-mind-brain as a single multilevel system is that people experiencing serious distress in similar ways need not have arrived there via the same path. The initial trigger may have been an acutely stressful event, a difficult conversation, a negative thought, or decreased synthesis of a certain neurotransmitter. Once the system is disturbed, available cultural scripts pull the resulting cascade toward particular symptom configurations. We therefore need an assessment approach that captures the individual narrative *and* the cultural frames in which it is best understood.

One tool for exploring the interplay of personal and cultural frames is the McGill Illness Narrative Interview (MINI; Groleau, Young, & Kirmayer, 2006). The MINI is a multi-stage semi-structured research interview, which first guides respondents through a detailed chronological recounting of their particular illness experience, and then explores salient prototypes and causal models. The Cultural Formulation Interview (CFI) included in *DSM-5* provides a briefer approach designed for regular clinical use (APA, 2013; see Lewis-Fernández & Aggarwal, Chapter 17, *this volume*). The CFI addresses several domains, contextualizing responses by including questions about the perceived perspective of others in the patient's local social world on the meaning and implications of the illness. Had Ms. Kim been administered such a tool, the clinician would have had much more access to how the patient understood her own symptom presentation, and how this understanding related to that of her Korean family or her American classmates.

Despite the benefit of such anthropologically informed instruments, there are many clinical situations where psychological measurement will also be necessary. There is increasing evidence to support the psychometric advantages of using well-constructed assessment instruments designed to reflect culturally relevant symptoms (e.g., Dere et al., 2013; Hinton, Kredlow, Pich, Bui, & Hofmann, 2013). The challenge for researchers conducting comparative studies is to find or develop instruments that capture symptoms that might be endorsed in more than one cultural context. Ryder and colleagues (2008), for example, pooled items from several Western and Chinese measures to create composite measures of somatic and psychological symptom reporting.

One drawback is that researchers and clinicians still do not know how these questions are actually understood in different cultural contexts. Cognitive interviewing techniques show promise in helping researchers understand how respondents arrive at particular answers (Beatty, Cosenza, & Fowler, 2006; Willis, 2005). The results can highlight areas where respondents provide answers for reasons very different than those assumed by the test designers and could prove invaluable for cross-cultural test construction (Pasick, Stewart, Bird, & D'Onofrio, 2001; Willis & Zahnd, 2007). This approach could help develop an instrument broad enough to capture some of the specifics of Ms. Kim's experience of depressive, social anxiety, and *hwa byung* symptoms that could help assess her progress over the course of treatment.

Treatment as a Positive System Intervention

Understanding culture-mind-brain as a single multilevel system has implications for how we think about treatment. We cannot simply line up disorders within culture, mind, and brain categories and then choose treatments that fit these same categories. Depression researchers once searched for the distinction between endogenous (i.e., brain) and reactive (i.e., mind) syndromes (Kendell, 1976; Mendels & Cochrane, 1968). The underlying assumption was that "brain depression" would respond to biological intervention and "mind depression" to psychological intervention. There is now considerable evidence that pharmacological intervention affects self-concept, personality, relationships with others, and so on, and that psychotherapy changes the brain (Knutson et al., 1998; Linden, 2006). At the same time, the effects – and beliefs about the effects – of treatment help to shape culture by shifting norms about options in the face of mental disorder (Pescosolido et al., 2010).

Successful interventions for serious distress can be considered as deliberate perturbations of the culture-mind-brain system, and the point of entry can take place at any level. Moreover, the effectiveness of these interventions is not context-free; there is considerable evidence demonstrating that treatments believable to the client, delivered confidently by the clinician, are more effective (Luborsky, McLellan, Diguer, Woody, & Seligman, 1997; Meyer et al., 2002; Wampold, 2001; Westra, Dozois, & Marcus, 2007). Indeed, both the idea of "the clinician" and the actual clinician herself are woven into the patient's culture-mind-brain (e.g., Benedetti, 2010). Placebo effects can be understood as psychophysiological responses based on patients' expectations and confidence

(Benedetti, 2008), in which the anticipated benefits derive from a cultural system where rituals of the clinic visit, the prescription pad, the pharmacy, the opening of the childproof bottle, and the ingestion of the pill are part of the script for healing (Kirmayer, 2011; McQueen, Cohen, St. John-Smith, & Rampes, 2013; Moerman & Jonas, 2002). Indeed, some patients experience anticipated negative side effects when receiving a placebo – the so-called nocebo effect (Barsky, Saintfort, Rogers, & Borus, 2002).

Cognitive Behavior Therapy: Vicious and Virtuous Loops in Context

Earlier in this chapter, we noted that a common feature of the *DSM* categories lumped into "serious distress" was generally good evidence for their responsiveness to CBT. Although not the only evidence-based treatment approach for these problems, CBT has a robust and growing literature, including studies conducted in non-Western cultural contexts (Horrell, 2008; Wong, 2008). Moreover, we believe the theory of CBT offers a way of thinking about disorder and intervention that fits well with the idea of dysfunctional loops presented here. Hinton and colleagues, in their work on panic attacks in Cambodian cultural contexts, have made pioneering and sustained efforts in this direction (Hinton & Simon, Chapter 14, *this volume*). In Clark's (1986, 1988) model of a panic attack, a physical sensation such as chest tightness creates anxiety about possible heart trouble, and the anxiety leads to more chest tightness, creating a loop that spirals into a panic attack. In Cambodian contexts, the same general structure of a panic attack holds, but a different set of specific cultural beliefs about the body means that neck pain and stiffness, dizziness, and other particular symptoms are catastrophized (Hinton et al., 2006).

This approach could be applied to many other disorders. Figure 16.1 illustrates how the Clark and Wells (1995) model of social anxiety might be adapted to capture the influence of culture and context. Note the several interlocking loops, each contributing to overall dysfunction by worsening how the person experiences the social situation – and possibly worsening the situation for others. Imagine a patient with social anxiety at a party. He is concerned that he will look unappealing if his hands shake, so he clutches his wine glass tightly to steady himself. His tight grip on the wine glass causes his hands to shake more, leading him to imagine that other people are judging him negatively, thereby increasing the sense of social danger and exacerbating safety behaviors and specific symptoms. This much is already recognized in models of emotional symptom exacerbation (Storms & McCaul, 1976).

However, the structure of the self is taken for granted in the original Clark and Wells (1995) model, which assumes an independently

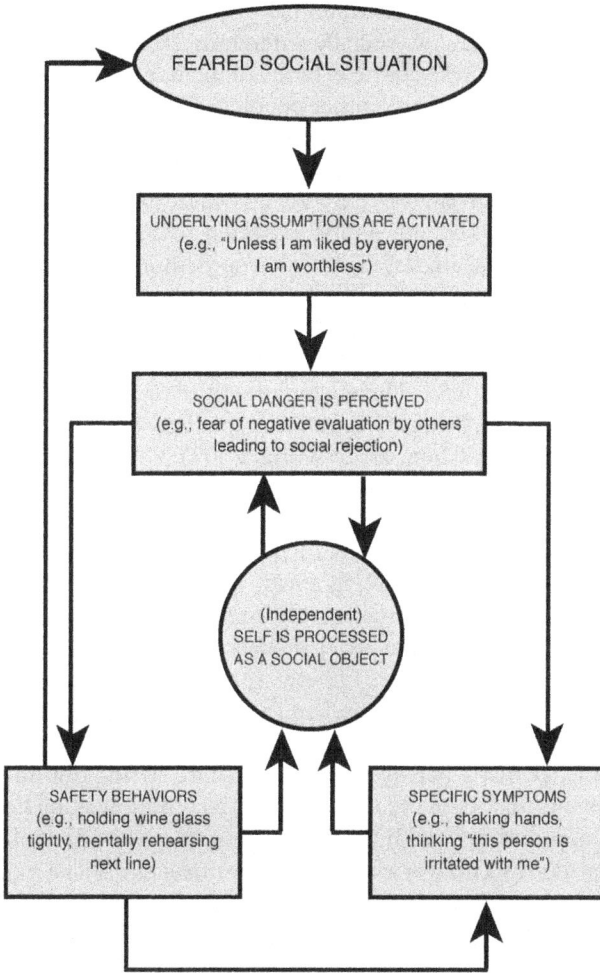

Figure 16.1. Clark and Wells (1995) model of social anxiety (with Western examples). Adapted with permission of Guilford Press, from "A Cognitive Model of Social Phobia," by D. M. Clark & A. Wells, 1995, in R. Heimberg, M. Liebowitz, D. A. Hope, & F. R. Schneier (Eds.), *Social phobia: Diagnosis, assessment and treatment* (p. 71).

construed self-motivated to imagine itself in the eyes of other independent selves. As a major task of the healthy independent self is to promote oneself to others, even moderate social anxiety is detrimental to good functioning (Zhou et al., 2011; Zhu et al., 2014). By contrast, in East Asian cultural contexts (Kim, Kasser, & Lee, 2003; Markus & Kitayama,

1991; Oyserman, Coon, & Kemmelmeier, 2002), the self may be construed interdependently, as socially interconnected. There is evidence that social anxiety in these contexts tends to include prominent concerns about giving offence or making other people feel uncomfortable, with the feared consequence of undermining interpersonal or group harmony (Norasakkunkit, Kitayama, & Uchida, 2012; Zhu et al., 2014).

Indeed, mild social anxiety may be less harmful, and perhaps even beneficial, in contexts where one is expected to monitor for threats to group harmony, as the anxiety signals that something is going wrong and requires smoothing over (Zhu et al., 2014). Shy children in Western cultural contexts tend to be viewed negatively by others, but the reverse appears to be true in Chinese contexts (Chen, DeSouza, Chen, & Wang, 2006; Chen & Tse, 2008). The advantages of shyness may be greater in traditional rural areas, however, and much smaller – and possibly fading – in urban areas (Chen, Chen, Li, & Wang, 2009). Compared to respondents in China, Japan, and Korea, respondents in Australia, Canada, Germany, Netherlands, and the United States reported (a) lower levels of social anxiety, (b) higher levels of perceived life interference due to social anxiety across a series of vignettes, with (c) a stronger correlation between social anxiety and perceived life interference (Rapee et al., 2011).

Let us now "revision" the social anxiety model with examples from Ms. Kim's social avoidance. These speculations are presented in Figure 16.2. Ms. Kim says she prefers to avoid social interactions, trying to escape them as quickly as she can. Because she looks for ways out of conversations, perhaps her eyes frequently dart about. She might then become anxious that these eye movements are communicating her anxiety to others inappropriately, with the feared consequence of disrupting interpersonal harmony. The ways in which these negative social experiences might be perpetuated are depicted in Figure 16.3 as a loop that plays out over a longer time period, incorporating Figure 16.2's shorter-term looping pattern whenever a social interaction is endured. When Ms. Kim exits these interactions, she continues to feel anxious due to the belief that she has made other people feel uncomfortable; when she successfully avoids social interactions, she leaves feeling relieved that she escaped that experience, while assuming that she *would have* made others feel uncomfortable. Either way, the preference for avoidance is reinforced, as are her core beliefs.

If confirmed by research in East Asian cultural contexts, this model could be applied clinically with patients like Ms. Kim to develop a treatment program. Such treatment would be simultaneously evidence-based, grounded in the patient's concerns, and tied to her cultural context. In any competent CBT, the treatment is tailored to the specific feared situations, underlying assumptions, perceived social dangers,

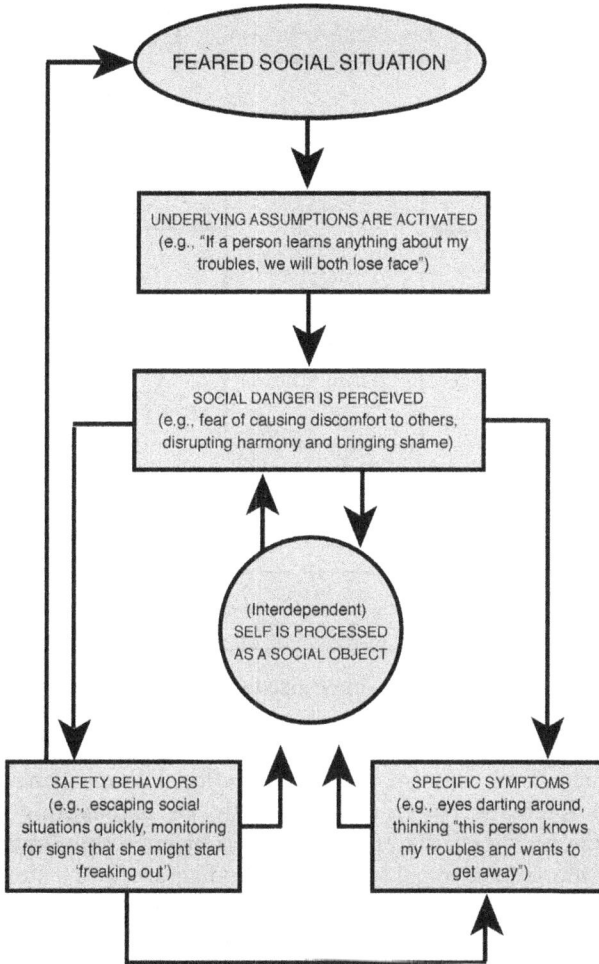

Figure 16.2. Clark and Wells (1995) model of social anxiety (with East Asian examples). Adapted with permission of Guilford Press, from "A Cognitive Model of Social Phobia," by D. M. Clark & A. Wells, 1995, in R. Heimberg, M. Liebowitz, D. A. Hope, & F. R. Schneier (Eds.), *Social phobia: Diagnosis, assessment and treatment* (p. 71).

safety behaviors, and symptoms of each patient, while maintaining this overall structure. Specific therapeutic interventions are designed in a way that blends the general model with the specific patient. Treatment is at once structured and tailored (Dobson & Dobson, 2009).

This approach to treatment bridges the culture-mind-brain view of how serious distress can emerge through looping effects with a

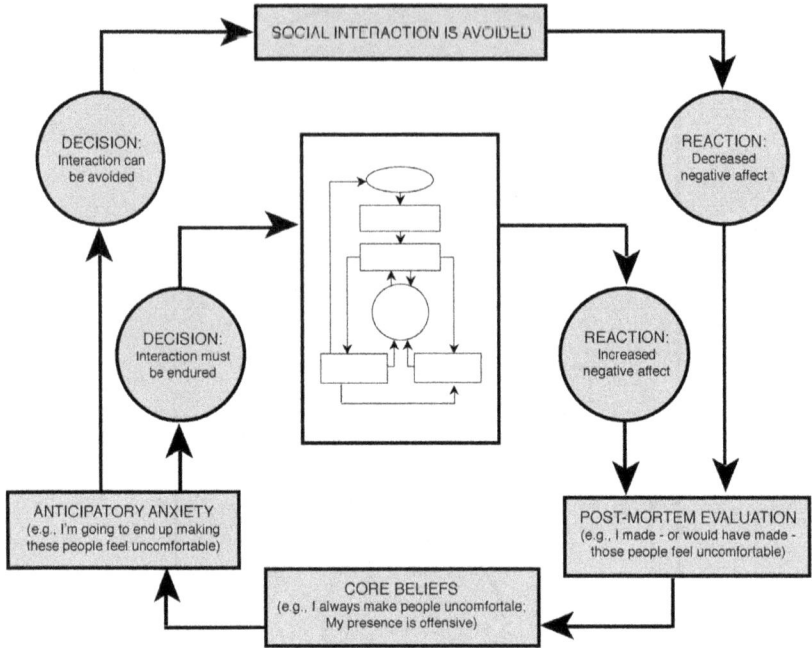

Figure 16.3. Proposed maintenance loop for social anxiety (with East Asian examples).

cognitive-behavioral view of how dysfunctional loops generate and maintain problematic patterns. Importantly, by highlighting loops at the level of mind – the sufferer's thoughts, subjective emotional experiences, and immediate social world – these diagrams tell a story useful to clinicians who are also primarily working at this level. They guide the therapist to consider specific interventions, and help the therapist present these interventions to the patient in a way that fits their particular experience. Such a treatment would work by encouraging positive disturbances in a system that is otherwise looped to generate and maintain distress. A successful treatment involves its own virtuous loops. The hope is that the patient is able to build on these changes and use the skills learned in treatment to encourage more compensatory loops to emerge.

What the clinician must remember – and what can often be forgotten when applying psychological theories that usually are framed as universal – is that mind is shaped by culture, so that all of this work is taking place within a cultural (or intercultural) context. The structure of these diagrams may help guide treatment, but it is in understanding their *content* and their *context* that successful treatment becomes possible. One danger is that content and structure get confused, so that the clinician winds up smuggling in culturally based assumptions that differ from those held by the patient. For example, it is not self-evident that feelings of chest tightness, dizziness, or neck pain might trigger catastrophic thoughts (Hinton & Simon, Chapter 14, *this volume*). Fear of negative evaluation by others is not necessarily the universal root of all social anxieties, and disrupting interpersonal harmony may be a core concern in its own right, not merely one way of being negatively evaluated (Rector, Kocovski, & Ryder, 2006a, 2006b). Awareness of such distinctions, openness to discovering new distinctions, and the ability to explore the patient's life context with both confidence and humility are among the challenges of intercultural work.

Cultural Competence and Its Limits

Successful treatment, no matter how systematized and grounded in evidence, depends on practitioners who are both clinically competent and "culturally competent" (Whitley, 2007). A meta-analysis of fifty-three treatment studies showed no benefit to ethnically matching clinician and patient (Cabral & Smith, 2011), but another meta-analysis of seventy–six treatment studies did show robust benefits for matching clients to *treatments* that have been adapted for specific cultural groups (Griner & Smith, 2006). In any case, it is impractical to assume that clinicians will acquire group-by-group "competence" given the vast range that might be represented in their practice. The number of cultural groups and their internal diversity preclude acquiring knowledge of each one (Ryder & Dere, 2010).

Moreover, cultural and contextual factors are relevant to every case, not just those recognized by the clinician as culturally different. Indeed, if we are going to train clinicians in the cultural features of a specific group, we might start with their own cultural group – no longer taken for granted, but understood as particular way of being in the world (Ryder & Chentsova-Dutton, 2012). Such training should include consideration of the possibility that many of the assumptions of the mental health professions reflect a particularly influential cultural worldview.

People are deeply embedded in their local sociocultural worlds, precluding a cookbook approach no matter how structured the treatment. Rather, the clinician must attend to each patient's available and activated scripts – what they believe, what they believe about others' beliefs, how this frames their action in the world, and how others respond. Clinicians must remember, moreover, that clinical settings themselves affect the scripts that are activated. Instead of attempting to acquire specific knowledge about the whole range of cultural groups likely to be seen in practice, it is far better to appreciate the diversity of cultural experience, and inquire into the specific scripts relevant for a given patient with an attitude of clinical humility about the limits of our knowledge (Kirmayer, 2012). The foundation of "cultural competence," therefore, is not knowledge of cultural probabilities leading to definite answers, but knowledge of cultural possibilities leading to better questions.

A Clinical Case, Revisioned

We began this chapter with the case of Ms. Kim – a fictionalized amalgamation of two real cases. In neither case was there opportunity to follow the treatment, so we conclude with a hopeful fiction: imagining a possible future for the patient, and for a revisioned psychiatry grounded in the science of a revisioned psychology:

The clinical psychologist assigned to Ms. Kim took a detailed history, combining a symptom-based phenomenological interview and an extensive illness narrative. She then administered a comprehensive measure of personality and psychopathology, in a validated Korean translation, plus several specific measures including one to assess *hwa byung*. The next several sessions were spent developing a cognitive-behavioral model based on her particular pattern of serious distress. Due to initial difficulties with building rapport, the psychologist obtained a cultural consultation over video link. They discussed clinical strategies for dealing with Ms Kim's withdrawn interpersonal style, and also helped the psychologist refine her CBT model.

Treatment progressed with regular brief assessments to track progress. Most sessions took place in the psychologist's office, but some social exposure exercises were carried out in the local community. These sessions also allowed the psychologist to observe Ms. Kim in her daily life context. Ms. Kim made steady progress with social anxiety, but continued to struggle with episodes of dysphoria – although these grew somewhat milder with time. In late spring, Ms. Kim decided that she would return to Korea for the summer. Remaining sessions were spent teaching her skills to manage anticipated interactions with her parents, and to help her detect the onset of symptoms so as to counteract the reemergence of dysfunctional loops.

The story we imagine extrapolates from our current state of knowledge to envision a future for clinical care in mental health to be shared by a revisioned psychology and a revisioned psychiatry. This approach would integrate phenomenology with physiological, psychological, and social models of psychopathology to develop assessment and treatment approaches appropriate to the individual client or patient in sociocultural context. In this imagined future, it might not even be necessary to refer specifically to *cultural*-clinical psychology or to *cultural* psychiatry: The fundamental importance of context will be central to our understanding of the person and the patient, and not only for ethnic minorities or international comparisons. Rather, the emphasis on context would be grounded in the recognition of the fundamentally inseparable contributions of culture, mind, and brain to health, illness, and healing.

REFERENCES

Abela, J. R. Z., & Hankin, B. L. (2011). Rumination as a vulnerability factor to depression during the transition from early to middle adolescence: A multiwave longitudinal study. *Journal of Abnormal Psychology, 120*(2), 259–71. http://dx.doi.org/10.1037/a0022796

American Psychiatric Association. (2013). *Diagnostic and statistical manual of mental disorders* (5th ed.). Washington, DC: Author.

Angermeyer, M. C., & Matschinger, H. (1999). Lay beliefs about mental disorders: A comparison between the western and the eastern parts of Germany. *Social Psychiatry and Psychiatric Epidemiology, 34*(5), 275–81. http://dx.doi.org/10.1007/s001270050144

Atran, S. (2001). The trouble with memes. *Human Nature, 12*(4), 351–81. http://dx.doi.org/10.1007/s12110-001-1003-0

Bangerter, A., & Heath, C. (2004). The Mozart effect: Tracking the evolution of a scientific legend. *British Journal of Social Psychology, 43*(4), 605–23. http://dx.doi.org/10.1348/0144666042565353

Barsalou, L. W. (2008). Grounded cognition. *Annual Review of Psychology, 59*, 617–45. http://dx.doi.org/10.1146/annurev.psych.59.103006.093639

Barsky, A. J., Saintfort, R., Rogers, M. P., & Borus, J. F. (2002). Nonspecific medication side effects and the nocebo phenomenon. *Journal of the American Medical Association, 287*(5), 622–7. http://dx.doi.org/10.1001/jama.287.5.622.

Bassett, D. S., & Gazzaniga, M. S. (2011). Understanding complexity in the human brain. *Trends in Cognitive Sciences, 15*(5), 200–9. http://dx.doi.org/10.1016/j.tics.2011.03.006

Beatty, P. C., Cosenza, C., & Fowler, F. J. (2006). Experiments on the structure and specificity of complex survey questions. In *Proceedings of the Survey Research Methods Section of American Statistical Association Conference*, Alexandria, VA. Retrieved from www.amstat.org/sections/srms/proceedings/y2006/Files/JSM2006-000146.pdf

Beck, M., Matschinger, H., & Angermeyer, M. C. (2003). Social representations of major depression in West and East Germany. *Social Psychiatry and Psychiatric Epidemiology, 38*(9), 520–5. http://dx.doi.org/10.1007/s00127-003-0675-7

Benedetti, F. (2008). *Placebo effects: Understanding the mechanisms in health and disease.* Oxford, England: Oxford University Press.

Benedetti, F. (2010). *The patient's brain: The neuroscience behind the doctor-patient relationship.* Oxford, England: Oxford University Press.

Berger, J. A., & Heath, C. (2005). Idea habitats: How the prevalence of environmental cues influences the success of ideas. *Cognitive Science, 29*(2), 195–221. http://dx.doi.org/10.1207/s15516709cog0000_10

Bilder, R. M. (2015). Dimensional and categorical approaches to mental illness: Let biology decide. In L. J. Kirmayer, R. Lemelson, & C. A. Cummings (Eds.), *Re-visioning psychiatry: Cultural phenomenology, critical neuroscience, and global mental health* (pp. 179–205). New York, NY: Cambridge University Press.

Bowen, R., Clark, M., & Baetz, M. (2004). Mood swings in patients with anxiety disorders compared with normal controls. *Journal of Affective Disorders, 78* (3), 185–92. http://dx.doi.org/10.1016/S0165-0327(02)00304-X

Bower, G. H., Black, J. B., & Turner, T. J. (1979). Scripts in memory for text. *Cognitive Psychology, 11*(2), 177–220. http://dx.doi.org/10.1016/0010-0285 (79)90009-4

Brewer, W. F., & Treyens, J. C. (1981). Role of schemata in memory for places. *Cognitive Psychology, 13*(2), 207–30. http://dx.doi.org/10.1016/0010-0285 (81)90008-6

Broadbent, E., & Petrie, K. J. (2007). Symptom perception. In: S. Ayers, A. Baum, C. McManus, S. Newman, K. Wallston, J. Weinman, & R. West (Eds.), *Cambridge handbook of psychology, health and medicine* (2nd ed; pp. 219–23). Cambridge, England: Cambridge University Press.

Cabral, R. R., & Smith, T. B. (2011). Racial/ethnic matching of clients and therapists in mental health services: A meta-analytic review of perceptions, preferences, and outcomes. *Journal of Counseling Psychology, 58*(4), 537–54. http://dx.doi.org/10.1037/a0025266

Carver, C. S., & Scheier, M. (2001). *On the self-regulation of behavior.* Cambridge, England: Cambridge University Press.

Chen, E., Matthews, K. A., & Zhou, F. (2007). Interpretations of ambiguous social situations and cardiovascular responses in adolescents. *Annals of Behavioral Medicine, 34*(1), 26–36. http://dx.doi.org/10.1007/BF02879918

Chen, X., Chen, H., Li, D., & Wang, L. (2009). Early childhood behavioral inhibition and social and school adjustment in Chinese children: A 5-year longitudinal study. *Child Development, 80*, 1692–1704. http://dx.doi.org/10.1111/j.1467-8624.2009.01362.x

Chen, X., DeSouza, A. T., Chen, H., & Wang, L. (2006). Reticent behavior and experiences in peer interactions in Chinese and Canadian children. *Developmental Psychology, 42*, 656–65. http://dx.doi.org/10.1037/0012-1649.42.4.656

Chen, X., & Tse, H. C. H. (2008). Social functioning and adjustment in Canadian-born children with Chinese and European backgrounds. *Developmental Psychology, 44*, 1184–9. http://dx.doi.org/10.1037/0012-1649.44.4.1184

Chentsova-Dutton, Y. E., & Heath, C. (2009). Cultural evolution: Why are some cultural variants more successful than others? In M. Schaller, A. Norenzayan, S. J. Heine, T. Yamagishi, & T. Kameda (Eds.), *Evolution, culture, and the human mind* (pp. 49–70). New York, NY: Taylor & Francis.

Chentsova-Dutton, Y. E., & Ryder, A. G. (2013). Vulnerability to depression in culture, mind, and brain. In M. Power (Ed.), *The Wiley-Blackwell handbook of mood disorders* (2nd ed.; pp. 433–50). Chichester, England: John Wiley & Sons.

Chentsova-Dutton, Y. E., Ryder, A. G., & Tsai, J. L. (2014). Understanding depression across cultural contexts. In I. H. Gotlib & C. L. Hammen (Eds.), *Handbook of depression* (3rd ed.). New York, NY: Guilford.

Chentsova-Dutton, Y. E., & Tsai, J. L. (2010). Self-focused attention and emotional reactivity: The role of culture. *Journal of Personality and Social Psychology, 98*, 507–19.

Clark, A., & Chalmers, D. (1998). The extended mind. *Analysis, 58*(1), 7–19. http://dx.doi.org/10.1093/analys/58.1.7

Clark, D. M. (1986). A cognitive approach to panic. *Behaviour Research and Therapy, 24*(4), 461–70. http://dx.doi.org/10.1016/0005-7967(86)90011-2

(1988). A cognitive model of panic. In S. J. Rachman & J. Maser (Eds.), *Panic: Psychological perspectives.* Hillsdale, NJ: Lawrence Erlbaum.

Clark, D. M., & Wells, A. (1995). A cognitive model of social phobia. In R. Heimberg, M. Liebowitz, D. A. Hope, & F. R. Schneier (Eds.), *Social phobia: Diagnosis, assessment and treatment* (pp. 69–93). New York, NY: Guilford.

Colligan, M. J., & Murphy, L. R. (1979). Mass psychogenic illness in organizations: An overview. *Journal of Occupational Psychology, 52*(2), 77–90. http://dx.doi.org/10.1111/j.2044-8325.1979.tb00444.x

Coman, A., & Hirst, W. (2011). Cognition through social networks: The propagation of induced forgetting and practice effects. *Journal of Experimental Psychology: General, 140*(4), 1–16. http://dx.doi.org/10.1037/a0025247

Côté, S., & Moskowitz, D. S. (1998). On the dynamic covariation between interpersonal behavior and affect: Prediction from neuroticism, extraversion, and agreeableness. *Journal of Personality and Social Psychology, 75*(4), 1032–46. http://dx.doi.org/10.1037/0022-3514.75.4.1032

D'Andrade, R. G. (1981). The cultural part of cognition. *Cognitive Science, 5*(3), 179–95. http://dx.doi.org/10.1207/s15516709cog0503_1

De Gucht, V., Fischler, B., & Heiser, W. (2004). Neuroticism, alexithymia, negative affect, and positive affect as determinants of medically unexplained symptoms. *Personality and Individual Differences, 36*(7), 1655–67. http://dx.doi.org/10.1016/j.paid.2003.06.012

Deary, V., Chalder, T., & Sharpe, M. (2007). The cognitive behavioural model of medically unexplained symptoms: A theoretical and empirical review. *Clinical Psychology Review, 27*(7), 781–97. http://dx.doi.org/10.1016/j.cpr.2007.07.002

Dere, J., Sun, J., Zhao, Y., Persson, T. J., Zhu, X., Yao, S., Bagby, R. M., & Ryder, A. G. (2013). Beyond "somatization" and "psychologization": Symptom-level variation in depressed Han Chinese and Euro-Canadian outpatients. *Frontiers in Psychology, 4*(377), 1–13. http://dx.doi.org/10.3389/fpsyg.2013.00377

DiMaggio, P. (1997). Culture and cognition. *Annual Review of Sociology, 23*, 263–87. http://dx.doi.org/10.1146/annurev.soc.23.1.263

Dobson, D., & Dobson, K. S. (2009). *Evidence-based practice of cognitive behavioral therapy.* New York, NY: Guilford.

Eldridge-Thomas, B., & Rubin, G. J. (2013). Idiopathic environmental intolerance attributed to electromagnetic fields: A content analysis of British newspaper reports. *Plos One, 8*(6), e65713. http://dx.doi.org/10.1371/journal.pone.0065713

Essau, C. A., Olaya, B., Pasha, G., Pauli, R., & Bray, D. (2013). Iranian adolescents' ability to recognize depression and beliefs about preventative strategies, treatments and causes of depression. *Journal of Affective Disorders, 149*(1–3), 152–9. http://dx.doi.org/10.1016/j.jad.2013.01.016

Feldman Barrett, L. (2009). The future of psychology: Connecting mind to brain. *Perspectives on Psychological Science, 4*(4), 326–39. http://dx.doi.org/10.1111/j.1745-6924.2009.01134.x

Fischer, R., & Boer, D. (2011). What is more important for national well-being: Money or autonomy? A meta-analysis of well-being, burnout, and anxiety across 63 societies. *Journal of Personality and Social Psychology, 101*(1), 164–84. http://dx.doi.org/10.1037/a0023663.

Gonsalves, B., Reber, P. J., Gitelman, D. R., Parrish, T. B., Mesulam, M., & Paller, K. A. (2004). Neural evidence that vivid imagining can lead to false remembering. *Psychological Science, 15*(10), 655–60. http://dx.doi.org/10.1111/j.0956-7976.2004.00736.x

Griner, D., & Smith, T. B. (2006). Culturally adapted mental health intervention: A meta-analytic review. *Psychotherapy: Theory, Research, Practice, Training, 43*(4), 531–48. http://dx.doi.org/10.1037/0033-3204.43.4.531

Groleau, D., Young, A., & Kirmayer, L. J. (2006). The McGill Illness Narrative Interview (MINI): An interview schedule to elicit meanings and modes of reasoning related to illness experience. *Transcultural Psychiatry, 43*(4), 671–91. http://dx.doi.org/10.1177/1363461506070796

Hinton, D. E., Chhean, D., Pich, V., Um, K., Fama, J. M., & Pollack, M. H. (2006). Neck-focused panic attacks among Cambodian refugees; a logistic and linear regression analysis. *Journal of Anxiety Disorders, 20*(2), 119–38. http://dx.doi.org/10.1016/j.janxdis.2005.02.001

Hinton, D. E., Kredlow, M. A., Pich, V., Bui, E., & Hofmann, S. G. (2013). The relationship of PTSD to key somatic complaints and cultural syndromes among Cambodian refugees attending a psychiatric clinic: The Cambodian somatic symptom and syndrome inventory (CSSI). *Transcultural Psychiatry, 50*(3), 347–70. http://dx.doi.org/10.1177/1363461513481187

Hinton, D. E., & Simon, N. M. (2015). Toward a cultural neuroscience of anxiety disorders: The multiplex model. In L. J. Kirmayer, R. Lemelson, & C. A. Cummings (Eds.), *Re-visioning psychiatry: Cultural phenomenology, critical neuroscience, and global mental health* (pp. 343–74). New York, NY: Cambridge University Press.

Horrell, S. C. V. (2008). Effectiveness of cognitive-behavioral therapy with adult ethnic minority clients: A review. *Professional Psychology: Research and Practice, 39*(2), 160–8. http://dx.doi.org/10.1037/0735-7028.39.2.160

Hutchins, E. (1995). *Cognition in the wild.* Cambridge, MA: MIT Press.

Johns, L. C., & van Os, J. (2001). The continuity of psychotic experiences in the general population. *Clinical Psychology Review, 21*(8), 1125–41. http://dx.doi.org/10.1016/S0272-7358(01)00103-9

Joiner, T. E., Alfano, M. S., & Metalsky, G. I. (1992). When depression breeds contempt: Reassurance seeking, self-esteem, and rejection of depressed college students by their roommates. *Journal of Abnormal Psychology, 101*(1), 165–73. http://dx.doi.org/10.1016/S0272-7358(01)00103-9

Joiner, T. E., Metalsky, G. I., Katz, J., & Beach, S. R. (1999). Depression and excessive reassurance-seeking. *Psychological Inquiry, 10*(3), 269–78. http://dx.doi.org/10.1207/S15327965PLI1004_1

Katerndahl, D., Ferrer, R., Best, R., & Wang, C. (2007). Dynamic patterns in mood among newly diagnosed patients with major depressive episode or panic disorder and normal controls. *Primary Care Companion to the Journal of Clinical Psychiatry, 9*(3), 183–7. http://dx.doi.org/10.4088/PCC.v09n0303

Kendell, R. E. (1976). The classification of depressions: A review of contemporary confusion. *British Journal of Psychiatry, 129*, 15–28. http://dx.doi.org/10.1192/bjp.129.1.15

Kim, U., & Choi, S.-C. (1995). Indigenous form of lamentation in Korea (Han): Conceptual and philosophical analysis. In Kwon, H.-Y. (Ed.), *Korean cultural roots* (pp. 245–66). Chicago, IL: Integrated Technical Resources.

Kim, Y., Kasser, T., & Lee, H. (2003). Self-concept, aspirations, and well-being in South Korea and the United States. *Journal of Social Psychology, 143*(3), 277–90. http://dx.doi.org/10.1080/00224540309598445

Kirmayer, L. J. (1984). Culture, affect and somatization. *Transcultural Psychiatric Research Review, 21*, 159–88. http://dx.doi.org/10.1177/136346158402100301

Kirmayer, L. J. (2006). Beyond the "new cross-cultural psychiatry": Cultural biology, discursive psychology and the ironies of globalization. *Transcultural Psychiatry, 43*(1), 126–44. http://dx.doi.org/10.1177/1363461506061761

Kirmayer, L. J. (2011). Unpacking the placebo response: Insights from ethnographic studies of healing. *Journal of Mind–Body Regulation, 1*(3), 112–24.

Kirmayer, L. J. (2012). Rethinking cultural competence. *Transcultural Psychiatry, 49*, 149–64. http://dx.doi.org/10.1177/1363461512444673

Kirmayer, L. J., & Sartorius, N. (2007). Cultural models and somatic syndromes. *Psychosomatic Medicine, 69*(9), 832–40. http://dx.doi.org/10.1097/PSY.0b013e31815b002c

Kirmayer, L. J., & Taillefer, S. (1997). Somatoform disorders. In S. Turner & M. Hersen (Eds.), *Adult psychopathology* (3rd ed.; pp. 333–83). New York, NY: John Wiley & Sons.

Kirmayer, L. J., & Young, A. (1998). Culture and somatization: Clinical, epidemiological, and ethnographic perspectives. *Psychosomatic Medicine, 60*(4), 420–30.

Kitayama, S., & Park, J. (2010). Cultural neuroscience of the self: Understanding the social grounding of the brain. *Social Cognitive and Affective Neuroscience, 5*(2–3), 111–29. http://dx.doi.org/10.1093/scan/nsq052

Kleinman, A. (1988). *The illness narratives: Suffering, healing, and the human condition.* New York, NY: Basic Books.

Knutson, B., Wolkowitz, O. M., Cole, S. W., Chan, T., Moore, E. A., Johnson, R. C. ... Reus, V. I. (1998). Selective alteration of personality and social behavior by serotonergic intervention. *American Journal of Psychiatry, 155*(3), 373–9,

Kolk, A. M., Hanewald, G. J., Schagen, S., & Gijsbers van Wijk (2003). A symptom perception approach to common physical symptoms. *Social Science & Medicine, 57*(12), 2343–54. http://dx.doi.org/10.1016/s0277-9536 (02)00451-3

Lahey, B. B. (2009). Public health significance of neuroticism. *American Psychologist, 64*(4), 241–56. http://dx.doi.org/10.1037/a0015309.

Lewis-Fernández, R., & Aggarwal, N. K. (2015). Psychiatric classification beyond the *DSM*: An interdisciplinary approach. In L. J. Kirmayer, R. Lemelson, & C. A. Cummings (Eds.), *Re-visioning psychiatry: Cultural phenomenology, critical neuroscience, and global mental health* (pp. 434–68). New York, NY: Cambridge University Press.

Linden, D. E. J. (2006). How psychotherapy changes the brain – the contribution of functional neuroimaging. *Molecular Psychiatry, 11*, 528–38. http://dx.doi.org/10.1038/sj.mp.4001816

Lindquist, K. A., & Barrett, L. F. (2008). Constructing emotion: The experience of fear as a conceptual act. *Psychological Science, 19*, 898–903.

Lindquist, K. A., Barrett, L. F., Bliss-Moreau, E., & Russell, J. A. (2006). Language and the perception of emotion. *Emotion, 6*(1), 125–38. http://dx.doi.org/10.1037/1528-3542.6.1.125

Link, B. G., & Phelan, J. C. (1999). The labeling theory of mental disorder (II): The consequences of labeling. In T. L. Scheid & T. N. Brown (Eds.), *A handbook for the study of mental health: Social contexts, theories, and systems* (pp. 361–76). Cambridge, England: Cambridge University Press.

Luborsky, L., McLellan, A. T., Diguer, L., Woody, G., & Seligman, D. A. (1997). The psychotherapist matters: Comparison of outcomes across twenty-two therapists and seven patient samples. *Clinical Psychology: Science and Practice, 4*(1), 53–65. http://dx.doi.org/10.1111/j.1468-2850.1997.tb00099.x

Malouff, J. M., Thorsteinsson, E. B., & Schutte, N. S. (2005). The relationship between the five-factor model of personality and symptoms of clinical disorders: A meta-analysis. *Journal of Psychopathology and Behavioral Assessment, 27*(2), 101–14. http://dx.doi.org/10.1007/s10862-005-5384-y

Markus, H. R., & Kitayama, S. (1991). Culture and the self: Implications for cognition, emotion, and motivation. *Psychological Review, 98*(2), 224–53. http://dx.doi.org/10.1037/0033-295X.98.2.224

McQueen, D., Cohen, S., St. John-Smith, P., & Rampes, H. (2013). Rethinking placebo in psychiatry: How and why placebo effects occur. *Advances in Psychiatric Treatment, 19*(3), 171–80. http://dx.doi.org/10.1192/apt.bp.112.010405

Mendels, J., & Cochrane, C. (1968). The nosology of depression: The endogenous-reactive concept. *American Journal of Psychiatry, 124*(suppl), 1–11.

Meyer, B., Pilkonis, P. A., Krupnick, J. L., Egan, M. K., Simmens, S. J., & Sotsky, S. M. (2002). Treatment expectancies, patient alliance and outcome: Further analyses from the National Institute of Mental Health Treatment of Depression Collaborative Research Program. *Journal of Consulting and Clinical Psychology, 70*(4), 1051–5. http://dx.doi.org/10.1037/0022-006X.70.4.1051

Michalak, J., Hölz, A., & Teismann, T. (2011). Rumination as a predictor of relapse in mindfulness-based cognitive therapy for depression. *Psychology and Psychotherapy: Theory, Research and Practice, 84*(2), 230–6. http://dx.doi.org/10.1348/147608310X520166

Min, S. K. (2008). Clinical correlates of Hwa Byung and a proposal for a new anger disorder. *Psychiatry Investigation, 5*(3), 125–41. http://dx.doi.org/10.4306/pi.2008.5.3.125

Min, S. K., Suh, S.-Y., & Song, K.-J. (2009). Symptoms to use for diagnostic criteria of Hwa Byung, an anger syndrome. *Psychiatry Investigation, 6*(1), 7–12. http://dx.doi.org/10.4306/pi.2009.6.1.7

Moerman, D. E., & Jonas, W. B. (2002). Deconstructing the placebo effect and finding the meaning response. *Annals of Internal Medicine, 136*(6), 471–6. http://dx.doi.org/10.7326/0003-4819-136-6-200203190-00011

Nathan P. E., Gorman J. M. (Eds.). (2007). *A guide to treatments that work* (3rd ed.). New York, NY: Oxford University Press.

Nolen-Hoeksema, S., Wisco, B. E., & Lyubomirsky, S. (2008). Rethinking rumination. *Perspectives on Psychological Science, 3*(5), 400–24. http://dx.doi.org/10.1111/j.1745-6924.2008.00088.x

Norasakkunkit, V., Kitayama, S., & Uchida, Y. (2012). Social anxiety and holistic cognition: Self-focused social anxiety in the United States and other-focused social anxiety in Japan. *Journal of Cross-Cultural Psychology, 43*(5), 742–57. http://dx.doi.org/10.1177/0022022111405658

Norasakkunkit, V., Uchida, Y., & Toivonen, T. (2012). Caught between culture, society, and globalization: Youth marginalization in post-industrial Japan. *Social and Personality Psychology Compass, 6*(5), 361–78. http://dx.doi.org/10.1111/j.1751-9004.2012.00436.x

Norenzayan, A., Choi, I., & Peng, K. (2007). Perception and cognition. In S. Kitayama & D. Cohen (Eds.), *Handbook of cultural psychology* (pp. 569–94). New York, NY: Guilford Press.

Oyserman, D., Coon, H. M., & Kemmelmeier, M. (2002). Rethinking individualism and collectivism: Evaluation of theoretical assumptions and meta-analyses. *Psychological Bulletin, 128*(1), 3–72. http://dx.doi.org/10.1037/0033-2909.128.1.3

Pasick, R. J., Stewart, S. L., Bird, J. A., & D'Onofrio, C. N. (2001). Quality of data in multiethnic health surveys. *Public Health Reports, 116*(Suppl 1), 223–43. http://dx.doi.org/10.1093/phr/116.S1.223

Pescosolido, B. A., Martin, J. K., Long, J. S., Medina, T. R., Phelan, J. C., & Link, B. G. (2010). "A disease like any other"? A decade of change in public reactions to schizophrenia, depression, and alcohol dependence. *American Journal of Psychiatry, 16*, 1321–30. http://dx.doi.org/10.1176/appi.ajp.2010.09121743

Posey, T. B., & Losch, M. E. (1983). Auditory hallucinations of hearing voices in 375 normal subjects. *Imagination, Cognition and Personality, 3*(2), 99–113. http://dx.doi.org/10.1016/S0022-3999(97)00004-4

Price, D. D., Finniss, D. G., & Benedetti, F. (2008). A comprehensive review of the placebo effect: Recent advances and current thought. *Annual Review of Psychology, 59*, 565–90. http://dx.doi.org/10.1146/annurev.psych.59.113006.095941

Pritzker, S. (2007). Thinking hearts, feeling brains: Metaphor, culture, and the self in Chinese narratives of depression. *Metaphor and Symbol, 22*(3), 251–74. http://dx.doi.org/10.1080/10926480701357679

Pulvermüller, F. (2005). Brain mechanisms linking language and action. *Nature Reviews Neuroscience, 6*(7), 576–82. http://dx.doi.org/10.1038/nrn1706

Purdon, C., & Clark, D. A. (1993). Obsessive intrusive thoughts in nonclinical subjects: Part I. Content and relation with depressive, anxious and obsessional symptoms. *Behaviour Research and Therapy, 31*(8), 713–20. http://dx.doi.org/10.1016/0005-7967(93)90001-B

Rapee, R. M., Kim, J., Wang, J., Liu, X., Hofmann, S. G., Chen, J., ... Alden, L. E. (2011). Perceived impact of socially anxious behaviors on individuals' lives in Western and East Asian countries. *Behavior Therapy, 42*(3), 485–92. http://dx.doi.org/10.1016/j.beth.2010.11.004

Rector, N. A., Kocovski, N. L., & Ryder, A. G. (2006a). Social anxiety and the fear of causing discomfort to others: Conceptualization and treatment. *Journal of Social and Clinical Psychology, 25*(8), 906–18. http://dx.doi.org/10.1007/s10608-006-9050-9

Rector, N. A., Kocovski, N. L., & Ryder, A. G. (2006b). Social anxiety and the fear of causing discomfort to others: Response to Roth Medley and Magee et al. *Journal of Social and Clinical Psychology, 25*, 937–44.

Richardson, M. J., Marsh, K. L., & Schmidt, R. C. (2010). Challenging the egocentric view of coordinated perceiving, acting, and knowing. In B. Mesquita, L. Barrett, E. R. Smith (Eds.), *The mind in context* (pp. 307–33). New York, NY: Guilford Press.

Rimé, B. (2007). Interpersonal Emotion Regulation. In J. J. Gross (Ed.), *Handbook of emotion regulation* (pp. 466–85). New York, NY: Guilford Press.

Robbins, J. M., & Kirmayer, L. J. (1986). Illness cognition, symptom reporting and somatization in primary care. In S. McHugh & T. M. Vallis (Eds.), *Illness behavior: A multidisciplinary model* (pp. 283–302). New York, NY: Plenum Press.

Rumelhart, D. E. (1984). Schemata and the cognitive system. In R. S. Wyer Jr., & T. K. Srull (Eds.), *Handbook of social cognition* (Vol. 1; pp. 161–88). Mahwah, NJ: Lawrence Erlbaum.

Rumelhart, D. E., & Ortony, A. (1977). The representation of knowledge in memory. In R. C. Anderson, R. J. Spiro, & W. E. Montague (Eds.), *Schooling and the acquisition of knowledge* (pp. 99–135). Hillsdale, NJ: Erlbaum.

Ryder, A. G., & Dere, J. (2010). Canadian diversity and clinical psychology: Defining and transcending 'cultural competence'. *CAP Monitor, 35*, 1 and 6–13. Retrieved from www.cap.ab.ca/pdfs/capmonitor35.pdf

Ryder, A. G., Ban, L. M., & Chentsova-Dutton, Y. E. (2011). Towards a cultural–clinical psychology. *Social and Personality Psychology Compass, 5*(12), 960–75. http://dx.doi.org/10.1111/j.1751-9004.2011.00404.x

Ryder, A. G., & Chentsova-Dutton, Y. E. (2012). Depression in cultural context: "Chinese somatization," revisited. *Psychiatric Clinics of North America, 35*(1), 15–36. http://dx.doi.org/10.1016/j.psc.2011.11.006

Ryder, A. G., Dere, J., Sun, J., & Chentsova-Dutton, Y. E. (2014). The cultural shaping of personality disorder. In F. L. Leong, L. Comas-Díaz, G. C. Nagayama Hall, V. C. McLoyd, J. E. Trimble (Eds.), *APA handbook of multicultural psychology, Vol. 2: Applications and training* (pp. 307–28). Washington, DC: American Psychological Association.

Ryder, A. G., Sun, J., Zhu, X., Yao, S., & Chentsova-Dutton, Y. E. (2012). Depression in China: Integrating developmental psychopathology and cultural-clinical psychology. *Journal of Clinical Child & Adolescent Psychology*, *41*(5), 682–94. http://dx.doi.org/10.1080/15374416.2012.710163

Ryder, A. G., Yang, J., Zhu, X., Yao, S., Yi, J., Heine, S. J., & Bagby, R. M. (2008). The cultural shaping of depression: Somatic symptoms in China, psychological symptoms in North America? *Journal of Abnormal Psychology*, *117*(2), 300–13. http://dx.doi.org/10.1037/0021-843X.117.2.300

Saint Arnault, D., & Kim, O. (2008). Is there an Asian idiom of distress? Somatic symptoms in female Japanese and Korean students. *Archives of Psychiatric Nursing*, *22*(1), 27–38. http://dx.doi.org/10.1016/j.apnu.2007.10.003

Schank, R. C., & Abelson, R. P. (1977). *Scripts, plans, goals, and understanding: An inquiry into human knowledge structures*. Hillsdale, NJ: Lawrence Erlbaum.

Schinka, J., Busch, R., & Robichaux-Keene, N. (2004). A meta-analysis of the association between the serotonin transporter gene polymorphism (5-HTTLPR) and trait anxiety. *Molecular Psychiatry*, *9*(2), 197–202. http://dx.doi.org/10.1038/sj.mp.4001405

Segal, Z. V., & Ingram, R. E. (1994). Mood priming and construct activation in tests of cognitive vulnerability to unipolar depression. *Clinical Psychology Review*, *14*(7), 663–95. http://dx.doi.org/10.1016/0272-7358(94)90003-5

Sen, S., Burmeister, M., & Ghosh, D. (2004). Meta-analysis of the association between a serotonin transporter promoter polymorphism (5-HTTLPR) and anxiety-related personality traits. *American Journal of Medical Genetics Part B: Neuropsychiatric Genetics*, *127*(1), 85–89. http://dx.doi.org/10.1002/ajmg.b.20158

Shweder, R. A. (1990). Cultural psychology: What is it? In J. W. Stigler, R. A. Shweder, & G. Herdt (Eds.), *Cultural psychology: Essays on comparative human development* (pp. 1–43). New York, NY: Cambridge University Press.

Skelton, J., & Pennebaker, J. W. (1982). The psychology of physical symptoms and sensations. In G. S. Sanders & J. Suls (Eds.), *Social psychology of health and illness* (pp. 99–128). Hillsdale, NJ: Lawrence Erlbaum.

Sperber, D., & Hirschfeld, L. A. (2004). The cognitive foundations of cultural stability and diversity. *Trends in Cognitive Sciences*, *8*(1), 40–6. http://dx.doi.org/10.1016/j.tics.2003.11.002

Starrs, C. J., Abela, J. R. Z., Shih, J. H., Cohen, J. R., Yao, S., Zhu, X., Hammen, C. L. (2010). Stress generation and vulnerability in adolescents in Mainland China. *International Journal of Cognitive Therapy*, *3*(4), 345–57. http://dx.doi.org/10.1521/ijct.2010.3.4.345

Storms, M. D., & McCaul, K. D. (1976). Attribution processes and emotional exacerbations of dysfunctional behavior. In J. H. Harvey, W. J. Ickes & R. F. Kidd (Eds.), *New directions in attribution research* (Vol. 1, pp. 143–64). Hillsdale, NJ: Erlbaum.

Teasdale, J. D. (1988). Cognitive vulnerability to persistent depression. *Cognition & Emotion*, *2*(3), 247–74. http://dx.doi.org/10.1080/02699938808410927

Tucker, M., & Ellis, R. (2004). Action priming by briefly presented objects. *Acta Psychologica*, *116*(2), 185–203. http://dx.doi.org/10.1016/j.actpsy.2004.01.004

Tyrer, P., Seiveright, H., & Johnson, T. (2003). The core elements of neurosis: Mixed anxiety depression (cothymia) and personality disorder. *Journal of Personality Disorders, 17*(2), 129–38. http://dx.doi.org/10.1521/pedi.17.2.129.23989

Valsiner, J., & Van der Veer, R. (2000). *The social mind: Construction of the idea.* New York, NY: Cambridge University Press.

Vygotsky, L. (1978). *Mind in society: The development of higher mental process.* Cambridge, MA: Harvard University Press.

Wampold, B. E. (2001). *The great psychotherapy debate: Models, methods and findings.* Mahwah, NJ: Lawrence Erlbaum.

Warren, W. H. (2006). The dynamics of perception and action. *Psychological Review, 113*(2), 358–89. http://dx.doi.org/10.1037/0033-295X.113.2.358

Westra, H. A., Dozois, D. J., & Marcus, M. (2007). Expectancy, homework compliance, and initial change in cognitive-behavioral therapy for anxiety. *Journal of Consulting and Clinical Psychology, 75*(3), 363–73. http://dx.doi.org/10.1037/0022-006X.75.3.363

Whitehead, W. E., Crowell, M. D., Heller, B. R., Robinson, J. C., Schuster, M. M., & Horn, S. (1994). Modeling and reinforcement of the sick role during childhood predicts adult illness behavior. *Psychosomatic Medicine, 56*(6), 541–50. http://dx.doi.org/10.1097/00006842-199411000-00010

Whitley, R. (2007). Cultural competence, evidence-based medicine, and evidence-based practices. *Psychiatric Services, 58*(12), 1588–90. http://dx.doi.org/10.1176/appi.ps.58.12.1588

Wiens, S. (2005). Interoception in emotional experience. *Current Opinion in Neurology, 18*(4), 442–7. http://dx.doi.org/10.1097/01.wco.0000168079.92106.99

Wierzbicka, A. (1994). Emotion, language, and cultural scripts. In S. Kitayama, H. Markus (Eds.), *Emotion and culture: Empirical studies of mutual influence* (pp. 133–96). Washington, DC: American Psychological Association.

Willis, G. B. (2005). *Cognitive interviewing: A tool for improving questionnaire design.* Thousand Oaks, CA: Sage.

Willis, G. B., & Zahnd, E. (2007). Questionnaire design from a cross-cultural perspective: An empirical investigation of Koreans and non-Koreans. *Journal of Health Care for the Poor and Underserved, 18*(4 Suppl.), 197–217. http://dx.doi.org/10.1353/hpu.2007.0118

Wilson, A. D., & Golonka, S. (2013). Embodied cognition is not what you think it is. *Frontiers in Psychology, 4*(58), 1–13. http://dx.doi.org/10.3389/fpsyg.2013.00058

Witthöft, M., & Rubin, G. J. (2012). Are media warnings about the adverse health effects of modern life self-fulfilling? An experimental study on idiopathic environmental intolerance attributed to electromagnetic fields (IEI-EMF). *Journal of Psychosomatic Research, 74*(3), 206–12. http://dx.doi.org/10.1016/j.jpsychores.2012.12.002

Wittink, M. N., Dahlberg, B., Biruk, C., & Barg, F. K. (2008). How older adults combine medical and experiential notions of depression. *Qualitative Health Research, 18*(9), 1174–83. http://dx.doi.org/10.1177/1049732308321737

Wong, D. F. K. (2008). Cognitive behavioral treatment groups for people with chronic depression in Hong Kong: A randomized wait-list control design. *Depression and Anxiety, 25*(2), 142–8. http://dx.doi.org/10.1002/da.20286

Zhou, X., Dere, J., Zhu, X., Yao, S., Chentsova-Dutton, Y. E., & Ryder, A. G. (2011). Anxiety symptom presentations in Han Chinese and Euro-Canadian outpatients: Is distress always somatized in China? *Journal of Affective Disorders, 135*(1–3), 111–14. http://dx.doi.org/10.1016/j.jad.2011.06.049

Zhu, X., Yao, S., Dere, J., Zhou, B., Yang, J., & Ryder, A. G. (2014). The cultural shaping of social anxiety: Distress about causing distress to others in Han Chinese and Euro-Canadian outpatients. *Journal of Social and Clinical Psychology, 33*(10), 906–17. http://dx.doi.org/10.1521/jscp.2014.33.10.906

17 Psychiatric Classification Beyond the *DSM*
An Interdisciplinary Approach

Roberto Lewis-Fernández and Neil Krishan Aggarwal

The descriptions of psychiatric disorders in *DSM-5* (APA, 2013) represent only some of the diverse forms of clinical presentations worldwide and throughout history. Cultural variation may help explain why current *DSM* diagnoses only partially map onto their putative biological substrates at the genetic or neurocircuitry level. It is more likely that these biological domains constitute dimensional vulnerability factors that pattern disorder expression more generally (e.g., mood dysregulation), and that specific syndromes arise from the interaction of this general vulnerability with other contextual factors, including culturally patterned illness expressions. This hypothesis raises several questions: How can research on cultural variation help elucidate the full range of underlying mechanisms that culminate in a given illness prototype? What cultural-contextual information can help clarify the relationship between related but diverse presentations of psychopathology? How can cultural variation be included in a universalistic nosology, such as *DSM-5*? This chapter presents a model of interdisciplinary triangulation that suggests how combining findings from sociocultural contextual analysis, neurobiological substrates of mental illness, and psychological dimensions can identify the substrates of illness phenomenology. The model will first be illustrated through an example of research on language, and then applied to a cultural syndrome included in the *DSM-5* Appendix: *ataque de nervios* (attack of nerves). The chapter concludes by discussing how this model helped the *DSM-5* revision process and by suggesting areas for future research.

Psychopathology is experienced, expressed, and interpreted around the world with considerable cultural variation. To date, no blueprint exists that can untangle the contributions to this variation from neurobiological, psychological, and cultural levels of analysis (Kendler, 2008). As a result, classification systems of psychopathology rely almost exclusively on phenomenological description – in its simplest sense of that which is apparent to an external observer (Andreasen, 2007; Hyman,

2010) and with only the barest attention to other aspects of illness phenomenology, such as the sufferer's own subjective description of lived experience and an accounting of the sociocultural environment that helps pattern illness expression (Csordas, Chapter 5, *this volume*; Heidegger, 1962/1927; Merleau-Ponty, 1996/1945; Parnas & Gallagher, Chapter 3, *this volume*). Every nosology based on phenomenology is incomplete, however, because it is a snapshot of what is perceived in a particular time and place as the local ways-of-being-ill, which respond to historically contingent ways of expressing and perceiving illness and are shaped by specific heuristic, social, and therapeutic goals (Kirmayer, 2005; Kleinman 1988). In effect, every nosology to date, including the APA's fourth and fifth editions of the *DSM* (*DSM-IV*; APA, 1994; *DSM-5*; APA, 2013), has been a catalogue elaborating popular illness prototypes.

This local contingency complicates the development of a grand theory of psychopathology that would account for all manifestations of cognitive and emotional illness (Kirmayer, 2005). At the same time, local contingency highlights an irreducible function of all nosologies, which is to organize information from highly localized phenomenological descriptions on how the different domains that produce illness (e.g., sociocultural, neurobiological, psychological) combine to form illness patterns. From this perspective, a valid nosology can be defined as *a classification system that organizes phenomenological data into a comprehensive yet parsimonious set of categories or dimensions that clarify the interrelationships among the domains of illness production*. In this respect, no domain is more fundamental than any other. Psychopathology emerges from the interactions of all the domains, no more from the bedrock of genetics and brain circuitry than from the bedrocks of cognitive processing, emotion regulation, social structure, or culturally mediated concepts of distress.

Cultural variation in the phenomenology of psychopathology thus challenges neuroscientific research that reductively attempts to match the forms of illness expression to underlying biological processes, regardless of their contextual embedding, because the relationship between form and biology (e.g., between depressive disorder and its associated genetics) is influenced by the local sociocultural *context* in which the person's biology has developed (Berrios & Marková, Chapter 2, *this volume*; Choudhury & Kirmayer, 2009; Insel & Wang, 2010). By *context*, we mean the specific environmental and social characteristics in which individuals and groups develop. These include *interpretive* aspects of culture (e.g., traditions for how to ascribe meaning to experience and human interactions); *social structures* such as institutions of collective organization (e.g., home, school, places of occupation, government);

forms of *political economy* that delimit activity and access to resources (e.g., the health consequences of structural discrimination, such as racism); and sociocultural reactions to the *ecological environment*, which sets parameters for engaging natural resources and technology.

The same studies that show the genetic bases of psychiatric disorders also reveal the strong influence of environmental factors in their onset, course, and outcome (Kendler, 2008). Research on *DSM-5 cultural concepts of distress*, such as *cultural syndromes, idioms of distress,* and *explanations* (APA, 2013) documents how much culture patterns the specific somatic, cognitive, and emotional experiences that define psychiatric disorders. The same type of research is being extended to specific *DSM* diagnoses. Culture patterns the modes of interpretation and coping that constitute the underlying mechanisms of *DSM* disorders; the extent to which stimuli are interpreted as catastrophic and lead to panic attacks through cognitive feedback loops (Hinton & Simon, Chapter 14, *this volume*); and the interpretation of what constitutes a traumatic stressor and/or a successful coping response, predisposing to PTSD (Hinton, Hofmann, Pitman, Pollack, & Barlow, 2008; Hinton & Lewis-Fernández, 2011). Thus, to identify the range of biological substrates of psychopathology requires clarifying how the form of the illness relates to the sociocultural context that helps shape it. This is a main goal of the anthropological study of psychopathology, which traces the connections between discrete contextual elements and fine-grained phenomenological descriptions of cognitive/emotional suffering.

Psychiatry is now at a crossroads with respect to illness classification. Contemporary nosologies based on a descriptive, symptom-based paradigm – hegemonic since the publication of *DSM-III* in 1980 – are increasingly being criticized, particularly by neuroscientists and anthropologists, for blocking the development of classificatory approaches that truly illuminate the role of biological and social processes in illness formation (Hansen et al., 2013; Hyman, 2010; Insel et al., 2010). At this watershed moment, the argument presented in this chapter is that promoting the systematic triangulation of neurobiological, psychological, and anthropological perspectives (Choudhury & Kirmayer, 2009) is a crucial step in clarifying the interactions among the multiple domains that culminate in the phenomenology of cognitive/emotional illness (Berrios & Marková, Chapter 2, *this volume*). By *triangulation,* we mean the iterative comparison of evidence from all three levels of analysis in order to achieve the goal of a valid nosology described earlier: elucidating the origin of the emerging phenomenology in the interaction of the domains of illness formation (Figure 17.1). The concept of triangulation provides a heuristic model that illustrates how the analytical

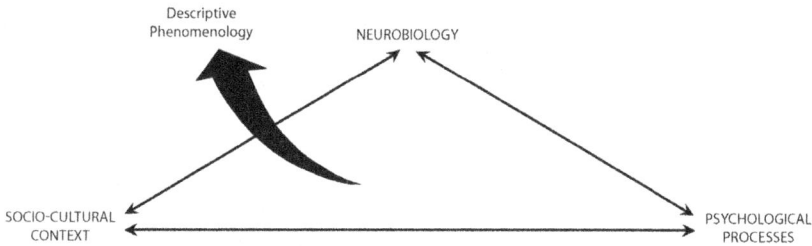

Figure 17.1. General triangulation model. Phenomenology emerges from the interaction of neurobiology, psychological processes, and sociocultural context.

frame is incomplete if it fails to include all key elements that pattern illness. Omitting elements of the triangle overburdens other elements with providing explanations from incomplete information.

This chapter illustrates the triangulation of levels of analysis with two examples, one drawn from published research on language (Han & Northoff, 2008), the other based on a cultural concept of distress, *ataque de nervios* (attack of nerves), which was assessed during the revision of *DSM-IV* leading to *DSM-5* (Guarnaccia, Rivera, Franco, & Neighbors, 1996; Lewis-Fernández, 1998; Lewis-Fernández et al., 2010). The emergence of related but distinct *illness prototypes* across cultures – that is, descriptively similar variants of forms of illness, such as cross-cultural variants of depression-like illness – constitutes an opportunity to further the integrationist agenda (Kendler, 2008), by considering local forms of illness as natural experiments that can elucidate the range of possible psychopathological mechanisms.

Rethinking Psychiatric Nosology

Both neuroscience and anthropology raise challenges that *DSM* diagnoses are over-specified, incomplete, and possibly misleading, emphasizing a reified diagnostic "map" over the more complex "terrain" of local and individual variation (Alarcón et al., 2002; Good, 1996, Hyman, 2007; Kleinman, 1988). The role of dimensions and spectra requires exploration and a different perspective must be applied to clarify the relationships among phenomenological description and underlying processes, conceptualized as biological in one discipline and as cultural-contextual in the other (Bilder, Chapter 8, *this volume*; Hyman, 2010, 2011; Insel et al., 2010). In the language of contemporary epigenetics, the alternative hypothesis is that biological substrates of psychopathology are almost never due to rare genetic variants or simple regulatory abnormalities of the genome, associated one-to-one with particular phenotypes (Labonté, Farah, & Turecki, Chapter 9, *this volume*; McKenzie & Shah, Chapter 13, *this volume*; Happe, Ronald, & Plomin, 2006). More often, they are dimensional vulnerability factors (e.g., brain abnormalities in emotion regulation) that become specific illness forms when this general vulnerability interacts with other contextual factors, ranging from molecular environments affecting the development and functioning of brain circuits to sociocultural elements such as historically patterned modes of illness expression (Insel & Wang, 2010; Kirmayer & Young, 1999; Kleinman, 1986). We suggest that a systematic analytical process of interdisciplinary triangulation may clarify these interactions and transcend the current tendency of analyzing problems with different disciplinary models in separate silos.

The Example of Language

Research on language illustrates the utility of this triangulation process, showing how cultural factors clarify discrepant neurobiological and psychological findings relevant to our disorder classifications. The advantage of language as an example is that there are many starting points of agreement between these disciplines. Language is widely accepted as a universal neurobiological-cognitive capacity of humans whose expression varies on many dimensions, depending on cultural context (Li, 2003). The components of phonemic inventories vary widely across cultures, ranging from clicks and flaps to trills. Some languages are read alphabetically as sounds corresponding to fine-grained phonemic units are shorter than syllables (e.g., English), whereas others are logographic, represented by a pictorial unit that is read at the monosyllabic level (e.g., Mandarin Chinese).

Considering these cultural differences helps to explain the neurobiological and cognitive processes involved in reading (Han & Northoff, 2008; Siok, Perfetti, Jin, & Tan, 2004). Reading an alphabetic language relies on a cognitive process that maps graphemes (visual forms) onto phonemes (minimal phonological units of speech); in this system, the components of words (letters) correspond to the sounds of the read text. Logographic languages, by contrast, require other means of reading, involving cognitive strategies that link orthographical shapes, phonology, and meaning; in other words, the visual representation of the word (e.g., Chinese character) has a complex relationship to the phonology of its associated meaning. Meanings are associated instead with the visual configuration of the logograph (Siok et al., 2004).

These cognitive tasks recruit brain regions that neuroimaging techniques can visualize (Han & Northoff, 2008). If all types of written languages were read using the same brain substrates, neuroimaging should yield consistent findings. Yet research shows considerable variation across alphabetic and logographic languages. Comparing reading patterns between English monolinguals and Mandarin monolinguals, for example, shows that both groups activate the left superior posterior temporal gyrus and the inferior frontal gyrus (Bolger, Perfetti, & Schneider, 2005). When English monolinguals read English, they involve the superior temporal gyrus but when Mandarin monolinguals read Mandarin, activation extends to the middle frontal gyrus, the dorsal extent of the inferior parietal lobe, and the fusiform gyrus (Bolger et al., 2005; Siok et al., 2004; Tan, Laird, Li, & Fox, 2005). These discrepant findings suggest cultural differences in the neurobiological recruitment of reading between these two languages (Tan et al., 2005). Reading alphabetic languages, which relies heavily on moment-to-moment cognitive conversion of graphemes to phonemes, tends to utilize posterior temporoparietal systems that mediate these cognitive tasks. Reading logographic languages, based on meaning retrieval through direct integration of visual-orthographic and semantic processes, tends to activate regions serving these cognitive functions, including the middle frontal gyrus. In other words, the brain substrates of reading appear to vary based on cultural differences in how people read (Han & Northoff, 2008). Limiting research to only one kind of language (e.g., alphabetic) would have resulted in incomplete information on the cognitive and neurobiological mechanisms of reading behavior.

This information helpfully clarifies the substrates of some *DSM-5* diagnoses (Han & Northoff, 2008). Specific learning disorder with impairment in reading (dyslexia) is a *DSM-5* disorder of reading achievement (e.g., accuracy, fluency, or comprehension) that affects children of normal intelligence and schooling (APA, 2013; called Reading Disorder in *DSM-IV*; APA, 1994). As with normal reading, the cognitive and neurobiological substrates of dyslexia vary according to the cultural characteristics of the languages being read. Whereas English-language *DSM-IV* reading disorder is related to difficulties linking orthography and phonology, reading impairments in Chinese appear to be related to a substandard connection between orthography and semantics (Perfetti, Liu, & Tan, 2005; Siok et al., 2004). Neuroimaging studies of individuals with reading disorder can identify these differences. English monolinguals show abnormalities of the left temporoparietal cortex and the left inferior frontal gyrus (Shaywitz et al., 1998; Temple et al., 2003); Mandarin monolinguals show left middle frontal gyrus dysfunction

(Siok et al., 2004). These findings have important therapeutic implications. Whereas behavioral remediation focused on phonological processing appears to normalize temporoparietal brain functioning in English-speaking children with dyslexia (Temple et al., 2003), therapies for Chinese-language readers may require greater attention to visual-orthographic and semantic processing (Siok et al., 2004).

The logical conclusion is that the range of biological and cognitive substrates associated with normal reading extends to pathological reading behavior, similarly driven by cultural characteristics. Without knowing that English and Mandarin Chinese differ in linguistic characteristics, researchers exploring the substrates of dyslexia would be puzzled as to why U.S. and Chinese subgroups of dyslexic individuals differed in behavioral and neuroimaging findings. In other words, the triangulation model shows that research on cultural variation helps clarify the relationship among the other elements in the model. In fact, it would be hard to interpret neurobiological and cognitive findings without cultural information: Understanding the existence of diverse language forms (e.g., alphabetic and logographic) is necessary to explain the variation in brain activation and behavioral patterns in dyslexia.

In effect, the cultural patterning of reading pathology into distinct but related forms of dyslexia constitutes a kind of natural experiment that allows investigators to map interactions across the domains of illness production more fully, by comparing diverse constellations of interactions from the real world as historically constituted clusters of cultural, cognitive, and brain activation processes. Here, a *cluster* is the pattern of associations across domains of illness formation that characterize a local version of a psychopathological illness prototype, such as English and Chinese variants of dyslexia (e.g., the ways a historically evolved form of writing is associated with a particular cognitive way of reading and with a specific brain activation pattern). Interpolation of information on how the domains interact within each local cluster can produce a comprehensive picture of possible interactions associated with the full range of variants characterizing a potentially universal illness prototype. For example, knowledge about *all* the ways in which dyslexia phenomenology can emerge, not just one local variant of the prototype, can be built into a more generally useful psychiatric nosology based on understanding the interplay of neurobiology, culture, and context.

The Example of *Ataque de Nervios*

A second example of the usefulness of the interdisciplinary triangulation model involves *ataque de nervios* ("attack of nerves"), a cultural syndrome common in Latin America and among U.S. Latinos, which was assessed during the *DSM-5* revision process. *Ataque* exemplifies the nosological challenges presented by local forms of psychopathology that do not fit existing diagnostic categories. Triangulating evidence on the sociocultural contexts and psychological processes associated with *ataque* helps clarify how interactions among these domains result in the particular phenomenology of the syndrome. Unfortunately, the lack of neurobiological data on *ataque* precludes our incorporating this domain in the illustration of the triangulation model, but the example will show how far we can get in refining our thinking with a careful cultural-contextual analysis.

Descriptive Phenomenology and Epidemiology

An *ataque de nervios* is a sudden fit of acute emotionality during which the person feels out of control; *ataques* can involve various intense emotions such as fear, rage, or grief (Guarnaccia et al., 1996). Afterward, the person usually disavows the episode as something unintended, frequently something performed "not by me" (*ese no era yo*), as if executed without the person's agency (Lewis-Fernández, 1998; Lewis-Fernández, Guarnaccia, Patel, Lizardi, & Díaz, 2005). Attacks frequently occur as a direct result of a stressful event relating to the family, such as news of the death of a close relative, conflicts with a spouse or children, or witnessing an accident involving a family member (Guarnaccia, 1992). For some individuals, no particular social event triggers *ataques*; instead, the person's vulnerability to losing control comes from the accumulated experience of suffering (APA, 2013; Guarnaccia et al., 1996). Ethnographic research with Puerto Rican *ataque* sufferers in the United States indicates that a key element of the *ataque* experience is the sense of being overwhelmed by an adverse situation. People about to have an attack usually say something like, "I can't take it anymore!" or literally, "I can't/won't hold back anymore!" (*¡No me aguanto más!*). This latter expression indicates the internal struggle with resisting overwhelming emotionality, prior to releasing the accumulated tension in the emotional paroxysm (Lewis-Fernández, 1998). *Ataque* sufferers also typically describe being unsuccessful at containing their emotions in situations that do not give rise to *ataques*, such as their anxiety, worry or irritability over mild conflicts or other stressful situations (Lewis-Fernández et al., 2005).

Qualitative research in Puerto Rico by Guarnaccia and colleagues (1996) revealed that an *ataque* has four basic experiential dimensions: (1) an emotional domain including experiences such as screaming, crying, or being very anxious or angry; (2) a bodily domain experiencing trembling, palpitations, and chest pain; (3) an action domain concerning aggressiveness or suicidal ideation or behavior; and (4) alterations in consciousness such as amnesia, fainting, or hallucinations. Spontaneous accounts of first *ataques* by community-based sufferers in Puerto Rico include symptoms of panic-like anxiety, loss of control, dissociation, anger and aggression, suicidal ideation and behavior, crying, and fainting (Table 17.1). Dissociative symptoms – notably depersonalization, derealization, loss of consciousness, and amnesia – arise in at least 53 percent of first *ataques*. Some *ataque* episodes are dangerous: About 1 in 7 first *ataques* results in a suicide attempt, and 1 in 4 is associated with destruction of property (Guarnaccia et al., 1996). At the symptom level, therefore, *ataques* do not easily conform to a single *DSM-5* category: In some respects they resemble panic attacks, yet they also have elements of acute dissociative reaction, impulse control disorder, or even conversion disorder when the main presentation is "fainting" accompanied by an inability to move.

Moreover, unlike *DSM* disorders, not all *ataques* indicate psychopathology (Guarnaccia, Canino, Rubio-Stipec, & Bravo, 1993). Some *ataques* may be normal expressions of distress occurring after sufficient provocation and in contexts such as funerals, where they represent highly emotional coping reactions (Guarnaccia, Lewis-Fernández, & Rivera Marano, 2003). Although they are associated with transient distress, such *ataques* may have no lasting sequelae. Other *ataques* are recurrent and associated with functional impairment. This dimensional range of severity complicates the psychiatric classification of *ataques* using existing categorical approaches.

Epidemiological studies with representative national samples in Puerto Rico and the United States have found that *ataques* are fairly common among community-based Latinos: The lifetime prevalence in adults ranges between 5 and 15 percent, depending on the Latino group and the measure used (Guarnaccia et al., 1993, 2010). Puerto Ricans consistently show the highest rates, whether assessed in Puerto Rico (15 percent) or the United States (11 percent). *Ataque* prevalence tends to be higher in older adolescent girls and women over forty-five years of age (Guarnaccia et al., 1993; Guarnaccia, Martínez, Ramírez, & Canino, 2005). Being formerly married, being out of the labor force or unemployed, and having less than a high school education are additional risk factors. Research has found no one-to-one relationship between *ataque* and any given psychiatric disorder, although certain disorders, such as *DSM-IV* panic disorder and dissociative disorder not otherwise specified, overlap with *ataque* symptomatology (Guarnaccia et al., 1993; Lewis-Fernández et al., 2002). Yet, 67 percent of Puerto Ricans with

Table 17.1 *Symptom Frequency of First* Ataque de Nervios *in Puerto Rico (N=77)*

Symptom	n	%
Panic-like symptoms		
Became nervous	69	90
Trembled a lot	59	77
Heart beat hard	58	75
Chest tightness	58	75
Frightened	50	65
Felt like was suffocating	47	61
Felt heat in chest	43	56
Afraid of going crazy	41	53
Afraid of dying	30	39
Dizzy	27	35
Loss of control		
Became hysterical	53	69
Lost/Afraid of losing control	49	64
Screamed a lot/Out of control	43	56
Dissociative symptoms		
Surroundings seemed unreal	41	53
Body felt unreal	32	42
Lost consciousness	27	35
Period of amnesia	22	29
Anger and aggression		
Felt anger	40	52
Broke things	20	26
Became aggressive	24	31
Suicide symptoms		
Suicidal thoughts	20	26
Suicide attempt	11	14
Other symptoms		
Cried/Attacks of crying	68	88
Fainted	33	43
Fell to floor	16	21

Note. Adapted from "The Experiences of *Ataques de Nervios*: Towards an Anthropology of Emotions in Puerto Rico," by P. J. Guarnaccia, M. Rivera, F. Franco, & C. Neighbors, 1996, *Culture, Medicine, and Psychiatry, 20*(3), p. 354. Copyright 1996 by Springer. With kind permission from Springer Science and Business Media.

ataque do not meet *DSM-IV* panic disorder criteria. Hence, *ataque* is not simply a culturally patterned or variant form of panic disorder (Lewis-Fernández, Guarnaccia, et al., 2002). *Ataques* are associated instead with diverse anxiety, depressive, dissociative, and somatoform disorders (Guarnaccia et al., 1993, 2005, 2010). In community samples, lifetime endorsement of *ataque* correlates with greater suicidal ideation, disability due to mental health problems, and outpatient psychiatric service utilization, even after adjusting for the contribution of psychiatric diagnoses, traumatic exposure, and other clinical and demographic covariates (Lewis-Fernández et al., 2009). This reinforces the importance of *ataque* as an independent outcome marker in Latino communities.

In sum, *ataque* constitutes a culturally patterned behavioral repertoire common among persons of Latin American descent that indicates a sense of being overwhelmed by stress and adversity. It presents with a range from transient distress to marked psychopathology, yet at the community level it can constitute an independent marker of morbidity. *Ataques* are more prevalent among socially disadvantaged groups, women more than men, and Puerto Ricans more than other Latin Americans. The phenomenology of *ataque* seems to combine types of psychopathology in ways not recognized in the organization of *DSM-5* disorders.

Sociocultural Context

Returning to the interdisciplinary triangulation model: How can information on the sociocultural context help us understand *ataque* phenomenology? What is the rationale for these frequent paroxysmic reactions that do not conform to current psychiatric nosology and that combine diverse emotions, aggressive behaviors, and dissociative symptoms? We will focus particularly on Puerto Rican communities, where nearly all ethnographic research on *ataque* has taken place and where attacks are nearly twice as common as among other Latin American groups. The applicability of these cultural-contextual findings to other Latino groups remains to be examined.

Qualitative interviews with *ataque* sufferers and the first author's participant observation and psychiatric practice over several years in Puerto Rican communities indicate the centrality in these settings of being *controlado/a* (in control) and *tranquilo/a* (tranquil, in equanimity) (Lewis-Fernández, 1998). People in these communities value retaining emotional control as a sign of maturity. A "controlled" person is expected to react with *tranquilidad* even when faced with remarkable adversity. For example, a sixty-six-year-old anxious man seen in a Puerto Rican primary care clinic stated with deliberate exaggeration that he wanted to remain *tranquilo* "even if the sky were to fall" (Lewis-Fernández, 1998:274; all translations from Spanish by RLF). However, maintaining control should not be confused with expressing emotion. Someone may aspire to remain controlled and tranquil even in the midst of strong emotion, as long as the person remains within the appropriate cultural bounds of emotional expression and preserves social harmony. Maintaining this balance or homeostasis requires constant awareness of the impact of verbal or emotional expression on other people and their subsequent reactions (Lewis-Fernández, 1998). That is, individuals constantly monitor the social desirability of reactions, ranging from the intensity of emotions in situational context to the types of emotions deemed socially appropriate. This ideal balance of emotion and restraint is reflected in the popular Puerto Rican saying, "*Salsa y control,*" which has its initial referent in dance music, that is, *salsa*. A band in Puerto Rico, for example, might interrupt its performance to say in unison, "*Salsa y control,*" and then resume playing. This saying conveys the desired balance of passion, *salsa*, and also *control* (here synonymous with coolness and musicianship), illustrated in the band's expert performance and, presumably, that of the dancing audience. The saying has become generalized in Puerto Rican society to indicate a cultural ideal (Quintero Rivera, 1998; see Figure 17.2).

As part of this *control-tranquilidad* complex, many Puerto Ricans believe that intense emotionality that is inappropriately channeled can be dangerous or harmful. This is especially true for certain emotions – including anger, jealousy, or envy – that are considered negative for the individual and community (Lewis-Fernández, 1998). Intense emotionality can lead to the obverse of the *control-tranquilidad* complex, which is a state of *nervios* (nerves). *Nervios* refers to an "alteration" (*alteración*) of the nervous system, and is a pan-Latino idiom of distress characterized by a general state of vulnerability to stressful life experiences and to difficult life circumstances that, if unchecked, can result in diverse psychiatric symptoms and chronic impairment (APA, 2013; Guarnaccia et al., 2003; Koss-Chioino, 1992). In Puerto Rican communities, uncontrolled emotionality can trigger *nervios*. In a clinical ethnography of *ataque de nervios* in New England, one forty-three-year-old male Puerto Rican participant reported that the cause of *estar enfermo de los nervios* (being ill with nerves) was:

Emotions. A good emotion or a bad emotion – both are emotions and alter the nervous system [...] Sometimes people die when ... 'Tell me softly, little-by-little (*suavecito*), if I won the million. I could have an *ataque* and I could die.' (Lewis-Fernández, 1998, p. 274)

Thus, even a "good" emotion can destabilize the nervous system. A forty-nine-year-old participant in the New England study put it succinctly: "Because one gets nervous from happiness and sadness too" (Lewis-Fernández, 1998, p. 274). Another fifty-four-year-old female participant gave an example of a "bad" emotion:

62 EL NUEVO DIA · LUNES 24 DE ABRIL DE 1995

ENTRENOTAS

Salsa y control

Por JAIME TORRES TORRES
REDACTOR DE POR DENTRO

¡Ultima hora! La nueva Puerto Rico All Stars del productor Frankie Gregory está grabando un disco en el estudio de Vinny Urrutia en Carolina.

Se espera que los compactos y casetes sean distribuidos por RMM Records durante el verano, posiblemente en julio.

El director musical del proyecto es Luis García y los arreglistas, Mario Ortiz, Ray Santos, Julito Alvarado y Lenny Prieto.

El concepto de la producción consiste en salsa tradicional.

Los soneros reclutados son Andy Montañez, su hija Lisa, Héctor Tricoche, Tito Nieves, Victor Manuel, Dárvel García y Wichy Camacho.

Tite Curet y Johnny Ortiz aportaron varias composiciones.

Los músicos son Piro Rodríguez, Luis Aquino, Ito Torres, Vicente Castillo, Elías Lopés, Mario Ortiz, Juancito Torres, José Reymundi, Gamalier González, Elliot Cintrón, Furito Ríos, Angel Torres, Cheguito Encarnación, Ernesto Sánchez, Héctor Veneros y Roberto Jiménez, entre otros.

Mario, Elías y Juancito trabajaron con la organización original que grabó los discos "P.R. All Stars", "Los profesionales" y "Tributo al Mesías", los tres disponibles en CD gracias a Combo Records.

Juancito Torres es uno de los músicos que participa en la grabación del nuevo disco de la Puerto Rico All Stars.

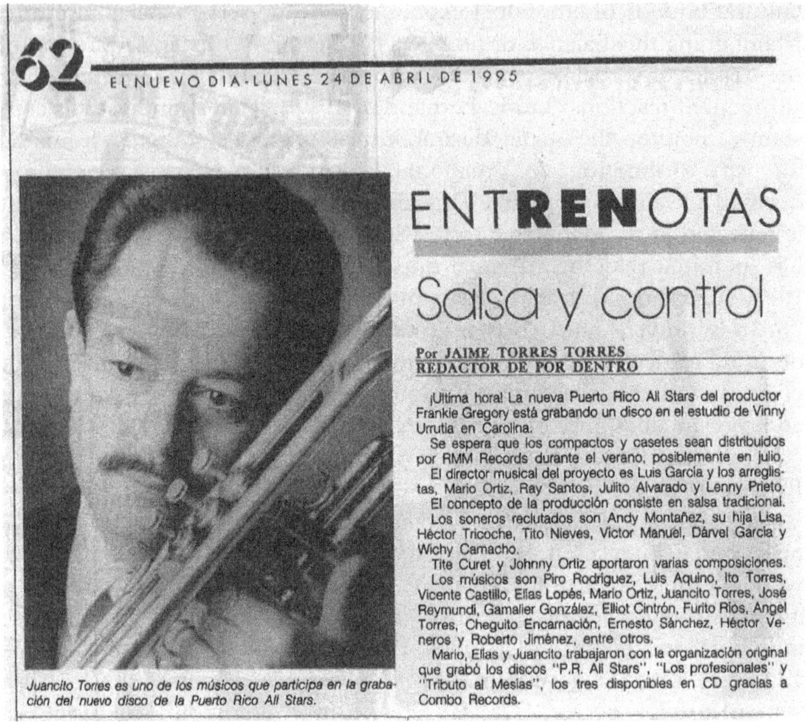

Figure 17.2. Reprinted from "Salsa y control," April 24, 1995, *El Nuevo Día.*

Yes, when one gets a rage (*le da coraje*) one's nerves go out of control (*se le descontrolan los nervios*). I think that is why there are so many deaths . . . because one person starts to argue with another and his nerves are altered (*se le alteran los nervios*) and under that nervousness he can do a terrible thing. How is it? His nerves are altered, so he doesn't know. He says: 'No, I didn't do it, I didn't do it.' Because when I was recently in Puerto Rico, the neighbor killed his wife. (Lewis-Fernández, 1998, p. 275)

Reinforcing the potentially catastrophic nature of strong emotions is the widespread popular view that persistently uncontrolled emotionality can worsen *nervios* and *ataques* to the point of insanity (*locura*) and violence (Harwood, 1987). In other words, the potential downside of the loss of control is terror. In the words of two other research participants:

(Replying to a question on the worst that could happen without treatment for *nervios*) Well, the worst, that I would lose control completely and kill somebody.

Lose my mind completely. (Forty-two-year-old woman; Lewis-Fernández, 1998, p. 281)

And when she (a relative) gets her *ataques de nervios*, she starts to tear her clothes ... tear, too much. As if one is not in one's right mind. As if one is crazy (*Está como si loco*). (Thirty-seven-year-old woman; Lewis-Fernández, 1998, p. 281)

Another element of the *control-tranquilidad* complex is the need to "control" disclosures of certain secrets or personal information, as they might be used against the individual. In the words of a twenty-eight-year-old female patient in Puerto Rico: "the less people know about me, the less they can harm me" (Lewis-Fernández, 1998, p. 276). Accentuating the need for discretion is the interconnection and lack of anonymity that characterizes life on a small island like Puerto Rico. There is a sense that letting people know too much about what you are feeling, some details of your life, leaves you vulnerable to *their* lack of control in misusing this information (Lewis-Fernández & Kleinman, 1993). In fact, disclosure can make you vulnerable not only to others' voluntary lack of control, but also to inchoate spiritual agencies that amplify their lack of control. Seizing the opportunity of a person's uncontrolled thoughts or behaviors, as if a metaphysical doorway had thereby been opened, these agencies can enter the social world to exert their harmful effects. For example, envy, *envidia*, is akin to a disembodied force between people that can harm others, even innocent bystanders, if it is summoned by envious thoughts (Lewis-Fernández, 1998). Praising a newborn, for example, without immediately inserting the verbal formula, "May God bless her" (*Que Dios la bendiga*), might result in the child's death through *mal de ojo* (evil eye), understood as an unwilled (and usually unconscious) transmission of envy to the vulnerable infant (Harwood, 1987). It was not uncommon in Puerto Rico in the 1990s to encounter bumper stickers that read, "Envy Kills," frequently meant very literally (Lewis-Fernández, 1998). The idea is that uncontrolled envy will actually cause dangerous social disruption. People may kill each other over greed, anger, and other "negative" emotions, so the role of a mature person is to rein in and control that envy.

The social desirability of emotions and the expectations around level of control tend to be gendered in Puerto Rican communities. Women are held to higher standards for these behaviors and dangers than are men (Lewis-Fernández, 1998). Women are supposed to go without, pacify the men, educate the children in the social ideal of control, defuse conflict, and restrain themselves sexually to a greater extent than men; men's honor, in turn, is connected to women's sexual restraint. These gendered expectations are changing, as a result of gains in female equality worldwide, but currently Puerto Rican women are still supposed to have more control than men. The 2:1 female-to-male gender ratio in *ataque* prevalence reflects these gendered aspects of the *control-tranquilidad* complex.

Cultural concepts like *control* and *tranquilidad* are not just cognitive experiences, but rather embodied dispositions (Bentley, 1987; Bourdieu, 1977). The embodied aspect of these concepts is evident in the physical symptoms of anxiety, depression, and somatization that characterize the idiom of *nervios* as the antithesis of *control*. It also manifests in other ways-of-being-Puerto-Rican, such as certain ways of moving and pacing oneself (important components of what Bourdieu [1990] calls *habitus*, embodied predispositions that are out of conscious awareness and that represent and communicate cultural priorities); ways of raising children; and the ideal characteristics of the self. For example, *control* and *tranquilidad* may underlie the preference of many Puerto Ricans for walking and talking in a measured fashion; the visceral dislike for *la prisa loca* (the mad rush) and *el ajoro* (being harried); and the ritualized politeness that *evita el roce* connotes (literally: avoid the physical friction of human contact; figuratively: prevent conflict). *Control* and *tranquilidad* may lie behind child-rearing practices in Puerto Rican communities that focus on raising *un/a niño/a tranquilo/a* (a tranquil child) and avoiding *un/a niño/a desinquieto/a*. The grammatically incorrect double negative (*des-in*), as opposed to the usual Spanish term *inquieto* (restless, anxious), emphasizes the intensity of the child's undesired behavior (Harwood, Miller, & Lucca Irizarry, 1995). The *control-tranquilidad* complex may also explain the general acceptance in Puerto Rico of the language of *imperactividad* as a popular gloss of "hyperactivity." The phrase, *"un/a niño/a imperactivo/a"* (an imperative child), combines in one word the restlessness and constant motion of "hyperactivity" (*hiperactividad*) with the demanding nature of an "imperative" child (*imperativo/a*), one who orders others about. The polyvalence of the vernacular term "imperactive" enriches the purely technical term "hyperactive," providing a better gloss for "uncontrolled"; that is, not only lack of equanimity, but also demanding more than one's share are undesirable elements that should be bred out of a child.

The *control-tranquilidad* complex affects many spheres of Puerto Rican community life, indicating its importance. A flyer for a San Juan daycare center for three to five year olds advertised exercises for children's self-control (*autocontrol*; observed January 10, 1997). A radio ad from the Department of Social Services equated lack of parental control with child abuse: "Don't let them watch TV without control, or miss school without a reason. Help us avoid abuse (*maltrato*) due to negligence" (1994).

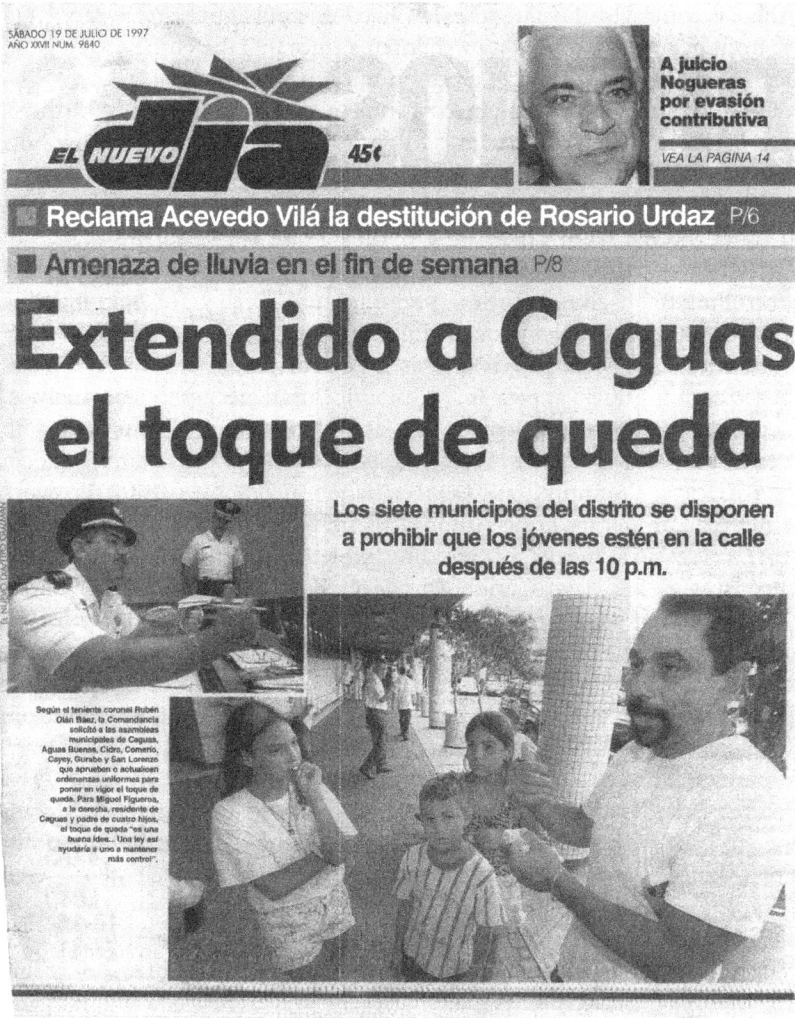

Figure 17.3. Reprinted from "Extendido a Caguas el Toque de Queda," July 19, 1997, *El Nuevo Día*.

The daily newspaper *El Nuevo Día* printed a series of articles about a proposed curfew for adolescents in various small towns in Puerto Rico, as a government strategy to decrease drug violence, often committed by adolescents (see Figure 17.3, "Extendido a Caguas el Toque de Queda," 1997). In the body of the article, the mother of three adolescents was quoted as saying: "Control over children is imposed when they are small, if there is control by the parents, a law like this would not be necessary." On the front page, the father of four children argues that the curfew, "is a good idea. ... A law like that helps a person to keep more control."

Finally, a neighbor explained during a one-year-old girl's birthday party: "When kids are beginning to walk like that, but don't know how to follow instructions, there is no control. They are the ones that control us" (June 15, 1997; all examples from Lewis-Fernández, 1998, p. 278). In other words, from birth, Puerto Ricans are supposed to engage in practices to control their children and teach them internalized ways of controlling themselves in order to raise mature social actors and thereby, in the worst case, prevent social violence.

Additional examples of *control* as a central preoccupation in Puerto Rican communities appear in economic strategies, political analysis, social analysis, ecological planning, and social determinants of health (Lewis-Fernández, 1998). Why is *control* such an important value in Puerto Rican communities? One explanation emerges from the work of the Cuban literary critic Antonio Benítez-Rojo (1992) on the role of *performance* as a means of avoiding violence in Caribbean societies. According to his view, Caribbean people have tended to adopt a non-confrontational stance in order to cope with the tremendous structural violence created by genocide, slavery, colonial despotism, and the Plantation as a social system. Rather than adopting a "do-or-die attitude" that would likely generate civil war and social disintegration, Caribbean societies have privileged instead a "sinuous," "fluid," "rhythmic" response that opposes an image of dance to that of war. In effect, says Benítez-Rojo, Caribbean people turn all confrontations into a perform-ance in order to avoid despairing because of relentless social limitations. This "dance" enables them to integrate disparate cultural elements, such as multiple ethnic groups, into a cohesive quasi-national identity out of the ever-shifting reconciliation of opposite movements into a single collective rhythm. Formally, this grand "rhumba" is composed of recur-ring thematic counterpoints that are never resolved into a permanent and static synthesis (Benítez-Rojo, 1992). One way to understand the con-cept of *control*, then, is as one of these contrapuntal themes in Puerto Rican communities, acting as the thematic opposite of unrestrained emotionality, including anger and aggression, which are considered the first movements in a sequence that frequently ends in anxiety, madness, and violence. The two opposing tendencies (*control* and emotionality) interact without neutralizing each other; out of their "dance" comes a-way-of-being that is typically Puerto Rican.

It is unclear whether Puerto Rican communities rely on the *control-tranquilidad* complex more than other Caribbean societies, reflecting their higher rate of *ataques*. However, Puerto Rico has sustained a longer period of colonialism and direct economic dependency than other Caribbean nations, extending to the present. Since at least the 1930s, Puerto Rican intellectuals have decried the "docility," "passivity," and "obliquity" they see emerging from this history of structural violence (Marqués, 1963; Meléndez Muñoz, 1963; Pedreira, 1934). These labels may reflect their disagreement with the *control-tranquilidad* complex as a folk solution to the colonial situation. Rather than seeing it as a legitimate desire to avoid direct confrontation because of its perceived futility, these canonical authors (Gelpí, 1993) seem to be judging it as a weak, vacillating, nonvirile basis for a national project (Duany, 1991).

To summarize, *ataque* is a gendered expression of distress best understood as a reaction to a cultural ideology of social and personal control that exists in order to prevent direct confrontation and ultimately forestall social violence. In the best circumstances, emotionality that is understood as "negative" (e.g., rage) and personal disclosures considered dangerous are bottled up and processed into equanimity. Faced with overwhelming adversity, however, individuals have access to the *ataque* as a release for the expression of intense feelings that does not rely on verbal disclosure of the circumstances of the event. The gendered aspect of *ataques* and its association with overwhelming distress helps explain why it is more prevalent among women and people with psychiatric disorder, as well as its association not with one particular disorder but with a wide range of disorders.

Psychological Processes

Following our interdisciplinary triangulation model, what can research on psychological processes associated with *ataque* contribute to clarifying the phenomenology of the syndrome? Why, for example, are attacks associated with dissociative symptoms such as depersonalization and amnesia? Why are they performed "not by me"? Why do they occur as acute paroxysms rather than more gradual reactions?

One explanation hinges on the role that dissociation plays in the genesis and phenomenology of *ataque*. *Dissociation* is a psychological process characterized by disruption and/or discontinuity in the normal integration of consciousness, memory, identity, emotion, perception, body representation, motor control, and behavior (*DSM-5*; APA, 2013). Dissociation is a normal psychological response, often triggered by adversity, which becomes a disorder when it is associated with distress and impairment (*DSM-5*; APA, 2013). Repeated studies have associated the presence and severity of *ataque* with higher dissociative symptoms and disorder among Latinos in outpatient mental health care (Hinton, Chong, Pollack, Barlow, & McNally, 2008; Lewis-Fernández, Garrido-Castillo, et al., 2002; Lewis-Fernández, et al., 2010). A study with first-generation Puerto Rican immigrant women in psychiatric care in New England found a direct correlation between the number of lifetime *ataques* the person reported and the presence of dissociation. Whether assessed by self-reported dissociative symptoms or by clinician-administered, semistructured interviews for dissociative disorders, increasing lifetime frequency of *ataques* was associated with higher dissociative symptoms (Lewis-Fernández, Garrido-Castillo, et al., 2002). In examining participants' dissociative diagnoses on the SCID, only the group with many *ataques* met criteria for a *DSM-IV* dissociative disorder – in this case dissociative disorder not otherwise specified: 38 percent of patients in this group had DDNOS (Lewis-Fernández, Garrido-Castillo, et al., 2002).

Confirming these findings, another study conducted with Latino men and women from diverse subethnicities, all of whom had suffered traumatic exposure, found a strong direct correlation between self-reported dissociative symptoms and the presence of *ataque*. Dissociative symptoms were likewise associated with two other Latino cultural concepts of distress: currently ill with *nervios* (*estar enfermo/a de los nervios ahora*) and experiencing altered perceptions (pseudo-hallucinations such as seeing *celajes*, or shadows), both of which are part of the larger *nervios* complex described earlier. In addition, all three *nervios*-related concepts (*ataque, enfermedad de los nervios,* and altered perceptions) were significantly intercorrelated (Lewis-Fernández et al., 2010), confirming ethnographic reports on the folk association among these concepts. Dissociation, therefore, seems to constitute a psychological process basic to the development of *ataque,* in combination with other psychological processes, such as anxiety sensitivity and impulsivity (Hinton et al., 2008). Not all *ataques,* however, correlate with measures of dissociation; some appear to be characterized more by elevated anxiety sensitivity (Hinton et al., 2008), indicating the psychological heterogeneity of the cultural syndrome.

The following descriptions of *ataques de nervios* from our clinical ethnography among Puerto Ricans in New England illustrate the dissociative features of *ataque* accounts (noted by the authors in italics). The first example is a fifty-four-year-old woman, who explained that a major argument between her husband and her father had led to an *ataque*:

That [the argument] made me very nervous. I went to the bedroom and began to cry. Later I went to the bathroom and kept crying. [My husband] went out and, I don't know, *only in my mind* I went and took the medicine and I took many kinds of medicine. To me, in that moment, *I was not (yo no era)*, that is what I call *not being there/not being me (no estar uno)*. Because *if I had been myself (yo misma)* I would have thought that I was going to leave my children, that when I was small, I was only 12 when my mother died and my little siblings were very small, I would have thought of all that and I would not have done that. . . . I imagine it was kind of a crazy behavior (*loquera*), of some kind of crazy (*algo de loca*) that one gets. Because no one who is *conscious of her things (consciente en sus cosas)* does things like that. To me, *it was as if it was not me who did that (no era yo la que hice eso)*. To me, it was like an *ataque de nervios*, or it might be. I couldn't even explain it to myself. (Lewis-Fernández, 1998, p. 282)

A second example involves a rage-like *ataque* in a thirty-eight-year-old, physically active, strong woman recounting the story of a romantic betrayal by her boyfriend (the interviewer's [I] questions to the respondent [R] are interspersed throughout):

R: Then I was arranging some clothes and I grabbed a razor that I have and I put it against his throat. But when the woman [her landlady who lived upstairs] came down . . . the woman of the house came down and found me with him . . . with it against his throat, she yelled at me and then I, you know, dropped the razor, *came back to myself (como que volví en sí)* but I almost cut his throat.

I: What did you feel during that *ataque*?

R: A tremendous rage, but with a desire to kill. If it had not been for that woman, to whom I am grateful today, really, I don't know what I would have done.

I: You said that you came back to yourself at that moment. How were you feeling before you came back to yourself?

R: I don't know, like another person. *As if I was another person*, I don't know. *As if I was not in the world there.* In that instant, *I was not me* until she yelled at me *(No sé, como otra persona. Como si yo fuera otra persona, no sé. Como si yo no estuviera en el mundo ahí. En ese instante yo no era yo, hasta que ella me gritó)*. (Lewis-Fernández, 1998, p. 282)

These examples describe depersonalization, defined as dissociative experiences of unreality or detachment from one's mind, self, or body (APA, 2013). The last example, recounted by a forty-four-year-old woman, describes an *ataque* characterized by abrupt amnesia. Homeless, she and her children were living in the apartment of her relatives who had just asked them to find another place to live. At the beginning of her retelling, the *ataque* had already started and her brother was attempting to "control" her by putting his arms around her:

Well, I remember when he had me like that, I, he was behind me. I remember when that heat flash rose up in me. *He says* that I turned on him – my brother is 6'4" and I'm just 5'4". He says that "I don't know how you were able to turn around on me," because it was a kind of wrestling hold that he was using on me, he cannot explain to himself how I turned around on him. Then he says that what I wanted to get at was his face with my nails. *I don't remember that, doctor,* but he says that when he would not let me get to his face, he says that I tore up his shirt in pieces. I tore it to pieces. ... Then she [her mother] got a Valium and gave it to me. I took it, and I still struggled a little bit but then I started calming down. And that my brother – *that I do remember* – that my brother had me like this, they laid me down, and he had taken hold of my hands, he had me by the hands, to my side... When I was calm, *I do remember* that my brother told me, "I'm going to let you go." And I said to him, *"But why are you holding me like this?"* (Lewis-Fernández, 1998, p. 288)

These examples illustrate the importance of dissociative process in the development of *ataque* phenomenology.

Synthesis

The centrality of dissociation in *ataques* helps to clarify how the cultural-contextual findings described earlier get translated into phenomeno-logical particulars. Dissociative mechanisms allow sufferers to purge negative feelings while still trying to retain their sense of themselves as mature, controlled social actors. It is as if, in order to conform to the cultural *control-tranquilidad* complex, the person's self-experience and public representation of self as a controlled person becomes equated to the totality of the self: because *I* don't lose control, because I am a mature, social actor, the *I* (in the sense of agency and self-consciousness) when I lose control is not me. The *ataque* may be experienced as some-thing that just "happened" to the person while overwhelmed by adversity, an experience that was not part of "him" or "her" but, rather, a totally uncontrolled expression of emotionality from which the person can essentially "return" and ask: "What happened?" Dissociation thus solves the culturally constructed dilemma of how to handle intolerable emo-tionality without losing control. In contexts of severe stress, through the medium of the *ataque* and other *nervios*-related experiences, the person can express intense feeling and in effect protest the situation that pro-voked the reaction, yet protect the self from these confrontational and dangerous demands. The individual avoids both horns of the dilemma by conveying a dissociated message that at once endorses the need to remain in control, yet expresses unrestrained emotionality. In order to make this work, however, the episode of loss of control must be brief, paroxysmic, abrupt; it may be most effective when it places the person at risk (such as through suicidal behavior), because this forcefully demon-strates the person's lack of agency in the episode (Littlewood & Lipsedge, 1987). This temporary break in the person's effortful self-control indicates that the person was struggling all along to retain control and finally can recover it once the affective storm has passed. Acting otherwise would belie one's commitment to control and social responsibility. In the words of a former Secretary of Mental Health of Puerto Rico: "Without dissociation, it would not be an *ataque*, it would be a kind of tantrum" (Dr. Efrén Ramírez, personal communication). Volition and agency are preserved, but the emotionality has been discharged.

This recurrent pattern of explosive expression and effortful emotional containment comprises the full trajectory of the *ataque* experience (clinicians tend to see the "peaks," the attacks, but may not be aware of the "valleys," the episodes of ongoing restraint that are equally basic to understanding the phenomenon). In the words of a fifty-four-year-old New England study participant:

> I call it [*ataque*] that someone feels rage (*que le da coraje a la persona*), that he gets angry about something. And there are people who know how to control themselves about something that happens to them, and there are others that ... that is, there are things that one holds in and holds in (*que aguanta y aguanta*), but then everything that one has held in comes out, and that's how one's *nervios* come out (*se le salen los nervios a uno*). (Lewis-Fernández, 1998, p. 275)

The cultural logic of *ataque* relies on the hope that difficult emotions can be purged all at once rather than slowly and over time, probably because of the social and gendered barriers to expressing "negative" feelings. However, as adverse contexts recur, it becomes difficult to contain hurt and anger, and this partly explains why a person can develop more frequent *ataques* if the situation does not improve. The *ataque* also signifies a call for help. Sufferers usually seek protected settings – within the family or the social network, but many seek therapy for this purpose as well – where they can *desahogarse* (unchoke or unburden themselves) by telling their story of suffering that led up to the *ataque*. This is commonly how many Puerto Ricans understand the work of psychotherapy (Lewis-Fernández et al., 2005).

The interdisciplinary triangulation model helps clarify the descriptive phenomenology of this form of emotional distress. Distress is experienced in the form of *ataque* largely because dissociative processes permit the sufferer to solve a dilemma arising from a cultural construction of the self, an ideal understanding of emotionality, and a set of historically evolved conventions on the social dangers of uncontrolled individual behavior. As in the example of language and dyslexia, without data on the sociocultural context, it would be hard to understand why distress takes this form. Triangulation helps us see how a person's expression can be patterned by the sociocultural context via the medium of an underlying psychological process like dissociation. If we had neurobiological data for experiences such as *ataque*, we could examine how the context – in this case, ideas about control, gendered social roles, and expectations about reacting to adversity – patterns psychopathology at the neurobiological level. Conversely, the absence of a contextual approach in most neuroscientific research may help explain its difficulty in identifying discrete neurobiological underpinnings for many illness prototypes in our current nosology; as in the case of language and reading, the relevant brain substrates may differ as the local variants of the prototype (and even the phenomenological boundaries of the prototype itself) vary in response to contextual elements.

Implications for Diagnostic Nosology: Cultural Concepts of Distress

The interdisciplinary triangulation model informed the recommendations the *DSM-5* Gender and Culture Study Group made on whether and how to include *ataque de nervios* in the revised nosology. Data this model organized were most helpful in clarifying why *ataque* does not fit one *DSM-5* disorder exclusively. *Ataque* instead represents one entry in a different type of classification system that cannot be combined easily with the *DSM* approach, a folk Latino nosology that includes *ataque*, as well as other subcategories of *nervios*, such as altered perceptions (Guarnaccia et al., 2003; Lewis-Fernández et al., 2009, 2010). What holds *ataque de nervios* together as a conceptual category in this folk nosology is its polar opposition to an idealized expression of self and behavior, an outburst of raw, uncontrolled emotionality signaling an experience of being overwhelmed that is deemed inherently dangerous to the person and the social order. This helps explain why *ataque* occurs in the context of diverse *DSM* disorders, all of which increase the person's risk of feeling overwhelmed. But it also explains why attacks can be triggered by experiences of acute adversity, even in the absence of underlying psychopathology, if the stressor is severe enough or if it culminates a series of subthreshold experiences of suffering.

To clarify the relationship between psychiatric diagnoses and local expressions of suffering such as *ataque de nervios*, *DSM-5* introduced the notion of *cultural concepts of distress* (APA, 2013). Whereas diagnoses are intended as heuristic descriptions of proto-universal illness prototypes (e.g., anxiety-dissociative paroxysms), *cultural concepts* present a classificatory framework that, first, problematizes the apparent universality of current diagnosis prototypes by presenting alternate classification systems of cognitive and emotional distress patterned by different contextual and historical factors. Second, cultural concepts show how, even as evidence accumulates for the potential universality of a prototype, local contexts yield variants that respond to cultural-contextual priorities. Ignoring these contexts can lead to misdiagnosis of the underlying prototype.

The data on *ataque* and other local expressions helped clarify for *DSM-5* three ways in which these concepts of distress usually present. The first is as coherent and fairly stereotyped behavioral and cognitive repertoires that correspond to the medical notion of syndromes as co-occurring symptoms and signs understood as representing stable entities with a characteristic course and outcome (Kirmayer & Young, 1999); *ataque* usually conforms to this definition. The second is more akin to languages of suffering, general modes of expressing distress associated with a wide range of possible symptoms. These have been called *idioms of distress* to emphasize their function of communicating distress to others (Nichter, 1981). Examples include ways of expressing distress in terms of particular bodily symptoms or psychological experiences, like the general expressions of *nervios* or the altered perceptions described earlier (Hinton & Lewis-Fernández, 2010). The third way cultural concepts present is as explanations or causes (e.g., "stress," witchcraft, *susto* or "fright illness") that help make etiological sense of various forms of suffering and guide the search for treatment (APA, 2013).

Concepts of distress also provide a framework for understanding how individuals manifest suffering in ways that are phenomenologically similar to an illness prototype, but without rising to the threshold of psychopathology. The illness pattern emerges from the culture as a behavioral repertoire that is experienced not only by individuals with different psychiatric disorders, but also by those without psychopathology (Carr & Vitaliano, 1985). Just as single *ataques* often represent normal adaptations to adversity, individuals who present with protracted dysphoria in the context of ongoing demoralization may be expressing an idiom of distress rather than a diagnosable condition such as *DSM-5*'s "persistent depressive disorder." The framework of cultural concepts of distress provides a heuristic model that locates in cultural-contextual factors a mechanism for the shared phenomenological features between normal and pathological reactions to adversity.

In addition to helping clarify the relationship between cultural concepts and illness prototypes, the triangulation data reveals the centrality of dissociative mechanisms in the development of *ataque de nervios*. Many *ataques* are also strongly patterned by anxiety, the risk of which is associated with traits such as anxiety sensitivity (Cintrón, Carter, Suchday, Sbrocco, & Gray, 2005; Hinton et al., 2008). These psychological processes help explain why epidemiological assessments of *ataque* emphasize its relationship with panic attacks, panic disorder, and acute dissociative reactions (Guarnaccia et al., 1993, 2005, 2010; Lewis-Fernández, Garrido-Castillo, et al., 2002; Lewis-Fernández, Guarnaccia, et al., 2002). One way to look at *ataque* is as a local variant of a potentially universal prototype, of which panic attack is another cultural variant. This prototype may emerge at the intersection of anxiety and dissociation – possibly as a locally constructed dissociative reaction to overwhelming anxiety – that is often precipitated by adversity, though in specific cases it may evolve into a recurrent reaction triggered by milder internal or external stimuli. This category might also include forms of distress such as *indisposition* in Haiti, "falling-out" among southern African Americans, and "blacking-out" among Bahamians, which are local expressions of distress similar to *ataque,* in which afflicted individuals experience a fit of acute emotionality characterized by locally patterned anxiety and dissociative symptoms (Weidman, 1979). As a result of sustained research attention, *DSM* and *ICD* have elevated panic attack from a specific variant of this larger prototype to the status of a universal syndrome. This has resulted in privileging the anxiety component of this type of paroxysm, but cross-cultural research shows that cognate expressions exist across the world with varying phenomenological emphases. For example, some acute variants of this paroxysmic prototype with more prominent dissociative than anxiety features might be labeled instead as instances of "acute dissociative reactions," of the type described in *ICD-10* (e.g., dissociative convulsions; World Health Organization, 1992) and incorporated in *DSM-5* under the revised category of "other specified dissociative disorder." Clearly, a dimensional approach based on anxiety and dissociative dimensions would provide a useful alternative (or complementary) basis to the classification of various local expressions around the world that instantiate this potentially universal prototype in specific cultural contexts (e.g., Hinton & Simon, Chapter 14, *this volume*).

The relationship between this paroxysmic anxiety-dissociative prototype and other psychological dimensions also deserves greater research attention. For example, *ataque* may relate to episodes of loss of impulse control, such as those included under "intermittent explosive disorder." However, lack of research on the relationship between *ataque* and impulsivity precludes the association of the cultural syndrome with this diagnostic grouping. Other associations needing study include the role of anger regulation and conversion processes in the psychological substrates of some *ataques*. Future research should continue to disentangle the relationships among levels of analysis to characterize the constituent components of *ataque* experience.

Ultimately, serious consideration of triangulation data leads to the conclusion that *ataque* should not be subsumed with any single *DSM-5* disorder. Instead, a universalistic nosology such as *DSM-5* could guide clinicians to consider cultural concepts such as *ataque*: (a) under the criteria for the disorder prototype(s) the concept is related to (e.g., panic attacks, acute dissociative reactions) in order to increase the cultural validity of these criteria; (b) in the descriptive text of these disorder prototypes to help clinicians diagnose specific presentations of the cultural concept that meet disorder criteria; and (c) in a separate section on cultural concepts of distress to help clinicians remember that the existing nosology does not capture these cultural concepts and that research using the triangulation model remains necessary to establish valid boundaries for all forms of psychopathology, including cultural concepts of distress.

DSM-5 also includes a novel methodology for assessing cultural-contextual factors that can guide the clinician in obtaining the information necessary to classify expressions of distress with greater contextual validity. This approach, in effect, operationalizes an evaluation of the role that the sociocultural context plays in the interdisciplinary triangulation model. *DSM-5* pushed forward work started in *DSM-IV* on the Outline for Cultural Formulation, a systematic description of how to conduct a cultural assessment, by developing a series of questionnaires for carrying it out, collectively called the Cultural Formulation Interview (CFI). Components include a core sixteen-item interview for use in initial assessments, an informant version to obtain collateral information from caregivers and members of the individual's social network, and twelve supplementary modules for assessing core CFI domains in greater depth and tailoring the assessment for specific groups, such as children and adolescents, immigrants, and refugees (http://www.psych.org/practice/dsm/dsm5/online-assessment-measures#Cultural; Lewis-Fernández et al., 2014). The cultural-contextual information obtained via the CFI is intended to help clinicians calibrate the person's presentation against the appropriate sociocultural background, thereby reducing the risk of overpathologization and of missing cultural variants of illness expression (APA, 2013).

Explicitly, the CFI can help clinicians assessing a person with an episode of *ataque de nervios* to (Lewis-Fernández et al., 2005):

- Elicit phenomenological information on the characteristics of this particular *ataque*, out of the possible range of *ataque* experiences.
- Prepare a safe setting for the patient by promoting trustworthiness (*confianza*), to enable him or her to overcome the cultural barrier to disclosure of potentially dangerous information, so as to recount the events surrounding the *ataque*.
- Obtain the story that led to the *ataque* in order to understand the person's specific sociocultural context, including what the patient has previously done to cope with the situation on his or her own and to seek help for it, as well as the patient's preferences for help at present. The CFI is designed to help the clinician obtain this information. Individuals often experience the process of disclosure itself as therapeutic,

temporarily lifting the cultural prohibition on expressing "negative" emotionality and relieving the person of the internal tension of "holding in" the emotional reaction (*desahogarse*) (Lewis-Fernández et al., 2005).

- Identify one or more *DSM* disorders that best correspond to the *ataque*, as well as the psychological dimensions (e.g., dissociation, anxiety sensitivity, impulsivity, emotion dysregulation) associated with this particular instance of the cultural syndrome.
- Use the sum total of information gathered to formulate a diagnosis and a treatment plan, and negotiate these with the patient and possibly other members of the social network in order to maximize engagement and outcome by tailoring them to the patient's expectations and preferences. Keep in mind that research with community-based populations links the presence of *ataque de nervios* with higher risk of suicidal ideation, disability due to mental health problems, and outpatient psychiatric service utilization. Attention to these potential outcomes can inform treatment planning and patient and family psychoeducation efforts.

Implications for Research and the Development of Psychiatric Nosology

The interdisciplinary triangulation model proposes that a psychiatric classification system at least partially based on categories – as opposed to pure dimensions – remains useful, despite neurobiological and anthropological critiques. Categories correspond to snapshots of psychological and neurobiological dimensions patterned by the sociocultural context in which the person lives. The categories are long-lasting and relatively stable, and provide frames for examining how the dimensions interact: how, for example, particular social pressures pattern an anxiety-dissociation prototype into specific local pathological expressions. A category-based approach acknowledges the "hybrid" nature of psychiatric categories at the intersection of the natural and the human sciences, and attempts to trace the contribution of each formative element – "the essential historicity, regionality, language boundedness, and subjectivity of psychiatry and its objects" (Berrios & Marková, Chapter 2, p. 45, *this volume*) – by focusing on a particular illness form. Categories are, thus, like a series of natural experiments that help identify interactions between relevant domains at different levels of analysis. The concept of triangulation is useful in explaining why the analytical frame is incomplete if it does not include all of the key elements that pattern the pathological condition. If we omitted context, for example, we would find a fair amount of diversity in the neurobiological and psychological correlates of a disorder, but we might not understand the origins of this diversity. Including all levels of analysis clarifies the pattern.

The triangulation model points to future areas for research. One potentially valuable research agenda could examine the range of inter-relationships among dimensions contained in a series of related categories that are cultural variants of each other. As an example, let us take different types of anxiety-dissociative paroxysms such as *DSM-5* panic attack and *ataque de nervios*.

Research on Category 1 (e.g., panic attacks) would show a certain interrelationship between, for example, genes, neural circuits, sociocultural context, emotion regulation, and cognitive processes. Category 2 (e.g., *ataque de nervios*) would reveal a different, related set of interrelationships, and likewise for Category 3 (e.g., *indisposition*). By examining these natural experiments organized as cultural categories – the different local variants of a paroxysmic anxiety-dissociative prototype – we would better understand how the dimensions interact in shaping all expressions of this general prototype. If a person lives in a context imbued with particular notions about self and social control and certain norms for emotional expression, as in Puerto Rican communities, this will prime the person to experience a particular type of anxiety-dissociation paroxysm that emphasizes feelings of loss of control, nonverbal disclosure of conflicts, highly expressive anxiety symptoms (e.g., screaming and crying), and certain dissociative symptoms (e.g., depersonalization and amnesia). Analogously, the interdisciplinary triangulation model could guide research on mood, psychotic, addiction, and other psychiatric disorders as a tool for understanding the mutually reciprocal interactions between culture, psychology, and neurobiology.

Going forward, the clinical and research tasks of global mental health and cultural psychiatry are intimately linked, as we try to understand and assist in the lives of individuals and populations expressing locally developed patterns of suffering. We must clarify the links between local expressions of suffering and existing (or novel) illness prototypes, as well as identify the contexts that pattern this local variation. Frequently, these links reveal fundamental collective concerns that are being expressed in the language of cognitive and emotional suffering. Ignoring these concerns may end up compromising our therapeutic effectiveness and depriving mental health research of a deeper understanding of the relationship between all domains of illness formation.

Acknowledgments

The authors appreciate the assistance of Constance Cummings, Marit Boiler, and John C. Markowitz; the research partnership with Peter J. Guarnaccia on *ataque*; and the editorial recommendations of Laurence J. Kirmayer.

REFERENCES

Akil, H., Brenner, S., Kandel, E., Kendler, K. S., King, M. C., Scolnick, E., Watson, J. D., & Zoghbi, H. Y. (2010). The future of psychiatric research: Genomes and neural circuits. *Science, 327*, 1580–1. http://dx.doi.org/ 10.1126/science.1188654

Alarcón, R. D., Bell, C. C., Kirmayer, L. J., Lin, K. M., Ustun, T. B., & Wisner, K. L. (2002). Beyond the funhouse mirrors: Research agenda on culture and psychiatric diagnosis. In D. J. Kupfer, M. B. First, & D. A. Regier (Eds.), *A research agenda for "DSM-V"* (pp. 219–89). Washington, DC: American Psychiatric Association.

American Psychiatric Association. (1994). *Diagnostic and statistical manual of mental disorders* (4th ed.). Washington, DC: Author.

American Psychiatric Association. (2013). *Diagnostic and statistical manual of mental disorders* (5th ed.). Washington, DC: Author.

Andreasen, N. C. (2007). *DSM* and the death of phenomenology in America: An example of unintended consequences. *Schizophrenia Bulletin, 33*, 108–12. http://dx.doi.org/10.1093/schbul/sbl054

Benítez-Rojo, A. (1992). *The repeating island: The Caribbean and the postmodern perspective*. Durham, NC: Duke University Press.

Bentley, G. C. (1987), Ethnicity and practice. *Comparative Studies in Society and History, 29*, 24–55. http://dx.doi.org/10.1017/S001041750001433X

Berger, P. L., & Luckmann, T. (1967). *The social construction of reality*. New York, NY: Anchor.

Berrios, G. E., & Marková, I. S. (2015). Toward a new epistemology of psychiatry. In L. J. Kirmayer, R. Lemelson, & C. A. Cummings (Eds.), *Re-visioning psychiatry: Cultural phenomenology, critical neuroscience, and global mental health* (pp. 41–64). New York, NY: Cambridge University Press.

Bilder, R. M. (2015). Dimensional and categorical approaches to mental illness: Let biology decide. In L. J. Kirmayer, R. Lemelson, & C. A. Cummings (Eds.), *Re-visioning psychiatry: Cultural phenomenology, critical neuroscience, and global mental health* (pp. 179–205). New York, NY: Cambridge University Press.

Bolger, D. J., Perfetti, C. A., & Schneider, W. (2005). Cross-cultural effect on the brain revisited: Universal structures plus writing system variation. *Human Brain Mapping, 25*, 92–104. http://dx.doi.org/10.1002/hbm.20124

Bourdieu, P. (1977). *Outline of a theory of practice*. Cambridge, England: Cambridge University Press. http://dx.doi.org/10.1017/CBO9780511812507

Bourdieu, P. (1990). *The logic of practice*. Stanford, CA: Stanford University Press.

Brown, T. A., & Barlow, D. H. (2009). A proposal for a dimensional classification system based on the shared features of the *DSM-IV* anxiety and mood disorders: Implications for assessment and treatment. *Psychological Assessment, 21*, 256–71. http://dx.doi.org/10.1037/a0016608

Carr, J. E., & Vitaliano, P. P. (1985). The theoretical implications of converging research on depression and the culture-bound syndromes. In A. Kleinman & B. Good (Eds.), *Culture and depression: Studies in the anthropology and cross-cultural psychiatry of affect and disorder* (pp. 244–66). Berkeley: University of California Press.

Choudhury, S., & Kirmayer, L. J. (2009). Cultural neuroscience and psychopathology: Prospects for cultural psychiatry. *Progress in Brain Research, 178*, 263–83. http://dx.doi.org/10.1016/S0079-6123(09)17820-2

Cintrón, J. A., Carter, M. C., Suchday, S., Sbrocco, T., & Gray, J. (2005). Factor structure and construct validity of the Anxiety Sensitivity Index among island Puerto Ricans. *Journal of Anxiety Disorders, 19*, 51–68. http://dx.doi.org/10.1016/j.janxdis.2003.10.007

Craddock, N., O'Donovan, M. C., & Owen, M. J. (2005). The genetics of schizophrenia and bipolar disorder: Dissecting psychosis. *Journal of Medical Genetics, 42*, 193–204. http://dx.doi.org/10.1136/jmg.2005.030718

Craske, M. G., Kircanski, K., Epstein, A., Wittchen, H. U., Pine, D. S., Lewis-Fernández, R., & Hinton, D. E. (2010). Panic disorder: A review of *DSM-IV* panic disorder and proposals for *DSM-V*. *Depression and Anxiety, 27*, 93–112. http://dx.doi.org/10.1002/da.20654

Csordas, T. J. (2015). Cultural phenomenology and psychiatric illness. In L. J. Kirmayer, R. Lemelson, & C. A. Cummings (Eds.), *Re-visioning psychiatry: Cultural phenomenology, critical neuroscience, and global mental health* (pp. 117–40). New York, NY: Cambridge University Press.

de Bruin, E. I., Ferdinand, R. F., Meester, S., de Nijs, P. F., & Verheij, F. (2007). High rates of psychiatric co-morbidity in PDD-NOS. *Journal of Autism & Developmental Disorders, 37*, 877–86. http://dx.doi.org/10.1007/s10803-006-0215-x

Dell, P. F. (2009). The long struggle to diagnose multiple personality disorder (MPD): Partial MPD. In P. F. Dell & J. A. O'Neil (Eds.), *Dissociation and the dissociative disorders: "DSM-V" and beyond* (pp. 403–28). New York, NY: Routledge.

Duany, J. (1991). *Más allá de la docilidad: La antropología psicológica en Puerto Rico. Avance de Investigación #9, Centro de Investigaciones Académicas*. Santurce, Puerto Rico: Universidad del Sagrado Corazón.

Extendido a Caguas el toque de queda. (1997, July 19). *El Nuevo Día*, p. 1.

Frank, E., Rucci, P., & Cassano, G. B. (2011). One way forward for psychiatric nomenclature: The example of the spectrum project approach. In D. A. Regier, W. E. Narrow, E. A. Kuhl, & D. J. Kupfer (Eds.), *The conceptual evolution of "DSM-5"* (pp. 37–58). Arlington, VA: American Psychiatric Association.

Gelpí, J. (1993). *Literatura y paternalismo en Puerto Rico*. San Juan, PR: La Editorial Universidad de Puerto Rico.

Goldberg, D., Simms, L. J., Gater, R., & Krueger, R. F. (2011). Integration of dimensional spectra for depression and anxiety into categorical diagnoses for general medical practice. In D. A. Regier, W. E. Narrow, E. A. Kuhl, & D. J. Kupfer (Eds.), *The conceptual evolution of "DSM-5"* (pp. 19–36). Arlington, VA: American Psychiatric Publishing.

Good, B. J. (1996). Culture and *DSM-IV*: Diagnosis, knowledge and power. *Culture, Medicine, and Psychiatry, 20*, 127–32. http://dx.doi.org/10.1007/BF00115857

Guarnaccia, P. J. (1992). *Ataques de nervios* in Puerto Rico: Culture-bound syndrome or popular illness? *Medical Anthropology, 15*, 1–14.

Guarnaccia, P. J., Canino, G., Rubio-Stipec, M., & Bravo, M. (1993). The prevalence of *ataque de nervios* in the Puerto Rico disaster study:

The role of culture in psychiatric epidemiology. *Journal of Nervous and Mental Disease, 181*, 157–65. http://dx.doi.org/10.1097/00005053-199303000-00003

Guarnaccia, P. J., Rivera, M., Franco, F., & Neighbors, C. (1996). The experiences of *ataques de nervios:* Towards an anthropology of emotions in Puerto Rico. *Culture, Medicine, and Psychiatry, 20*, 343–67. http://dx.doi.org/10.1007/BF00113824

Guarnaccia, P. J., Lewis-Fernández, R., & Rivera Marano, M. (2003). Toward a Puerto Rican popular nosology: *Nervios* and *ataque de nervios*. *Culture, Medicine, and Psychiatry, 27*, 339–66. http://dx.doi.org/10.1023/A:1025303315932

Guarnaccia, P. J., Martínez, I., Ramírez, R., & Canino, G. (2005). Are *ataques de nervios* in Puerto Rican children associated with psychiatric disorder? *Journal of the American Academy of Child and Adolescent Psychiatry, 44*, 1184–92. http://dx.doi.org/10.1097/01.chi.0000177059.34031.5d

Guarnaccia, P. J., Lewis-Fernández, R., Martinez Pincay, I., Shrout, P., Guo, J., Torres, M., . . . Alegria, M. (2010). *Ataque de nervios* as a marker of social and psychiatric vulnerability: Results from the NLAAS. *International Journal of Social Psychiatry, 56*, 298–309. http://dx.doi.org/10.1177/0020764008101636

Han, S., & Northoff, G. (2008). Cultural-sensitive neural substrates of human cognition: A transcultural neuroimaging approach. *Nature Reviews Neuroscience, 9*, 646–54. http://dx.doi.org/10.1038/nrn2456

Hansen, H. B., Donaldson, Z., Link, B. G., Bearman, P. S., Hopper, K., Bates, L. M., . . . Teitler, J.O. (2013). Independent review of social and population variation in mental health could improve diagnosis in *DSM* revisions. *Health Affairs, 32*, 1–10. http://dx.doi.org/10.1377/hlthaff.2011.0596

Happe, F., Ronald, A., & Plomin, R. (2006). Time to give up on a single explanation for autism. *Nature Neuroscience, 912*, 18–20.

Harris, W. V. (2013). Thinking about mental disorders in classical antiquity. In W. V. Harris (Ed.), *Mental disorders in the classical world* (pp. 1–23). Leiden, Netherlands: Brill. http://dx.doi.org/10.1163/9789004249875_002

Harwood, A. (1987). *RX: Spiritist as needed*. Ithaca, NY: Cornell University Press.

Harwood, R., Miller, J., & Lucca Irizarry, N. (1995). *Culture and attachment: Perceptions of the child in context*. New York, NY: Guilford.

Heidegger, M. (1962). *Being and time* (J. Macquarrie & E. Robinson, Trans.). New York, NY: Harper & Row. (Original work published 1927)

Helzer, J. E. (2011). A proposal for incorporating clinically relevant dimensions into *DSM-5*. In D. A. Regier, W. E. Narrow, E. A. Kuhl, & D. J. Kupfer (Eds.), *The conceptual evolution of "DSM-5"* (pp. 81–96). Arlington, VA: American Psychiatric Publishing.

Henningsen, P., & Kirmayer, L. J. (2000). Mind beyond the net: Implications of cognitive neuroscience for cultural psychiatry. *Transcultural Psychiatry, 37*, 467–90. http://dx.doi.org/10.1177/136346150003700401

Hinton, D. E., Chong, R., Pollack, M. H., Barlow, D. H., & McNally, R. J. (2008). *Ataque de nervios*: Relationship to anxiety sensitivity and dissociation predisposition. *Depression and Anxiety, 25*, 489–95. http://dx.doi.org/10.1002/da.20309

Hinton, D. E., Hofmann, S. G., Pitman, R. K., Pollack, M. H., & Barlow, D. H. (2008). The panic attack-posttraumatic stress disorder model: Applicability to orthostatic panic among Cambodian refugees. *Cognitive Behaviour Therapy, 37*, 101–16. http://dx.doi.org/10.1080/16506070801969062

Hinton, D. E., & Lewis-Fernández, R. (2010). Idioms of distress among trauma survivors: Subtypes and clinical utility. *Culture, Medicine, and Psychiatry, 34*, 209–18. http://dx.doi.org/10.1007/s11013-010-9175-x

Hinton, D. E., & Lewis-Fernández, R. (2011). The cross-cultural validity of posttraumatic stress disorder: Implications for *DSM-5*. *Depression and Anxiety, 28*, 783–801. http://dx.doi.org/10.1002/da.20753

Hinton, D. E., & Simon, N. M. (2015). Toward a cultural neuroscience of anxiety disorders: The multiplex model. In L. J. Kirmayer, R. Lemelson, & C. A. Cummings (Eds.), *Re-visioning psychiatry: Cultural phenomenology, critical neuroscience, and global mental health* (pp. 343–74). New York, NY: Cambridge University Press.

Hyman, S. E. (2007). Can neuroscience be integrated into the *DSM-V*? *Nature Reviews Neuroscience, 8*, 725–32. http://dx.doi.org/10.1038/nrn2218

Hyman, S. E. (2010). The diagnosis of mental disorders: The problem of reification. *Annual Review of Clinical Psychology, 6*, 155–79. http://dx.doi.org/10.1146/annurev.clinpsy.3.022806.091532

Hyman, S. E. (2011). Diagnosis of mental disorders in light of modern genetics. In D. A. Regier, W. E. Narrow, E. A. Kuhl, & D. J. Kupfer (Eds.), *The conceptual evolution of "DSM-5"* (pp. 3–18). Arlington, VA: American Psychiatric Publishing.

Insel, T. R. (2010, April). Faulty circuits: Neuroscience is revealing the malfunctioning connections underlying psychological disorders and forcing psychiatrists to rethink the causes of mental illness. *Scientific American*, 44–51. http://dx.doi.org/10.1038/scientificamerican0410-44

Insel, T. R., & Cuthbert, B. N. (2009). Endophenotypes: Bridging genomic complexity and disorder heterogeneity. *Biological Psychiatry, 66*, 988–9. http://dx.doi.org/10.1016/j.biopsych.2009.10.008

Insel, T. R., Cuthbert, B., Garvey, M., Heinssen, R., Pine, D. S., Quinn, K., . . . Wang, P. (2010). Research domain criteria (RDoC): Toward a new classification framework for research on mental disorders. *American Journal of Psychiatry, 167*, 748–51. http://dx.doi.org/10.1176/appi.ajp.2010.09091379

Insel, T. R., & Wang, P. S. (2010). Rethinking mental illness. *Journal of the American Medical Association, 303*, 1970–1. http://dx.doi.org/10.1001/jama.2010.555

International Schizophrenia Consortium. (2009). Common polygenic variation contributes to risk of schizophrenia and bipolar disorder. *Nature, 460*(7256), 748–52. http://dx.doi.org/ 10.1038/nature08185

Kendler, K. S. (2008). Explanatory models for psychiatric illness. *American Journal of Psychiatry, 165*, 695–702. http://dx.doi.org/10.1176/appi.ajp.2008.07071061

Kendler, K. S., Neale, M. C., Kessler, R. C., Heath, A. C., & Eaves, L. J. (1992). Major depression and generalized anxiety disorder: Same genes, (partly) different environments? *Depression and Anxiety, 49*, 716–22.

Kirmayer, L. J. (2005). Culture, context and experience in psychiatric diagnosis. *Psychopathology, 38*, 192–6. http://dx.doi.org/10.1159/000086090

Kirmayer, L. J., & Young, A. (1999). Culture and context in the evolutionary concept of mental disorder. *Journal of Abnormal Psychology, 108*, 446–52. http://dx.doi.org/10.1037/0021-843X.108.3.446

Kleinman, A. (1986). *Social origins of distress and disease: Depression, neurasthenia, and pain in modern China.* New Haven, CT: Yale.

Kleinman, A. (1988). *Rethinking psychiatry: From cultural category to personal experience.* New York, NY: Free Press.

Koss-Chioino, J. (1992). *Women as healers, Women as patients: Mental health care and traditional healing in Puerto Rico.* Boulder, CO: Westview.

Krueger, R. F., Eaton, N. R., South, S. C., Clark, L., & Simms, L.J. (2011). Empirically derived personality disorder prototypes: Bridging dimensions and categories in *DSM-5*. In D. A. Regier, W. E. Narrow, E. A. Kuhl, & D. J. Kupfer (Eds.), *The conceptual evolution of "DSM-5"* (pp. 97–118). Arlington, VA: American Psychiatric Publishing.

Labonté, B., Farah, A., & Turecki, G. (2015). Early-life adversity and epigenetic changes: Implications for understanding suicide. In L. J. Kirmayer, R. Lemelson, & C. A. Cummings (Eds.), *Re-visioning psychiatry: Cultural phenomenology, critical neuroscience, and global mental health* (pp. 206–35). New York, NY: Cambridge University Press.

Lewis-Fernández, R. (1998). Eso no estaba en mí ... no pude controlarme: El control, la identidad, y las emociones en comunidades puertorriqueñas. *Revista de Ciencias Sociales, 4*, 268–99.

Lewis-Fernández, R., Aggarwal, N. K., Bäärnhielm, B., Rohlof, H., Kirmayer, L. J., Weiss, M. G., ... Lu, F. (2014). Culture and psychiatric evaluation: Operationalizing cultural formulation for *DSM-5*. *Psychiatry: Interpersonal and Biological Processes, 77*, 130–54. http://dx.doi.org/10.1521/psyc.2014.77.2.130

Lewis-Fernández, R., Garrido-Castillo, P., Bennasar, C., Parrilla, E. M., Laria, A. J., Ma, G., & Petkova, E. (2002). Dissociation, childhood trauma, and *ataque de nervios* among Puerto Rican psychiatric outpatients. *American Journal of Psychiatry, 159*, 1603–5. http://dx.doi.org/10.1176/appi.ajp.159.9.1603

Lewis-Fernández, R., Gorritz, M., Raggio, G. A., Peláez, C., Chen, H., & Guarnaccia, P. J. (2010). Association of trauma-related disorders and dissociation with four idioms of distress among Latino psychiatric outpatients. *Culture, Medicine, and Psychiatry, 34*, 219–43. http://dx.doi.org/10.1007/s11013-010-9177-8

Lewis-Fernández, R., Guarnaccia, P. J., Martínez, I. E., Salmán, E., Schmidt, A., & Liebowitz, M. (2002). Comparative phenomenology of ataques de nervios, panic attacks, and panic disorder. *Culture, Medicine, and Psychiatry, 26*, 199–223. http://dx.doi.org/10.1023/A:1016349624867

Lewis-Fernández, R., Guarnaccia, P. J., Patel, S., Lizardi, D., & Díaz, N. (2005). *Ataque de nervios*: Anthropological, epidemiological, and clinical dimensions of a cultural syndrome. In A. M. Georgiopoulos & J. F. Rosenbaum (Eds.), *Perspectives in cross-cultural psychiatry* (pp. 63–85). Philadelphia, PA: Lippincott Williams & Wilkins.

Lewis-Fernández, R., Horvitz-Lennon, M., Blanco, C., Guarnaccia, P. J., Cao, Z., & Alegría, M. (2009). Significance of endorsement of psychotic symptoms by US Latinos. *Journal of Nervous and Mental Disease, 197*, 337–47. http://dx.doi.org/10.1097/NMD.0b013e3181a2087e

Lewis-Fernández, R., & Kleinman A. (1993). Culture, personality, and psychopathology. *Journal of Abnormal Psychology, 103*, 67–71. http://dx.doi.org/10.1037/0021-843X.103.1.67

Li, S. C. (2003). Biocultural orchestration of developmental plasticity across levels: The interplay of biology and culture in shaping the mind and behavior across the life span. *Psychological Bulletin, 129*, 171–94. http://dx.doi.org/10.1037/0033-2909.129.2.171

Link, B. G., & Phelan, J. (1995). Social conditions as fundamental causes of disease. *Journal of Health and Social Behavior, 35*(Extra issue), 80–94. http://dx.doi.org/10.2307/2626958

Littlewood, R. (1991). Against pathology: The new psychiatry and its critics. *British Journal of Psychiatry, 159*, 696–702. http://dx.doi.org/10.1192/bjp.159.5.696

Littlewood, R., & Lipsedge, M. (1987). The butterfly and the serpent: Culture, psychopathology and biomedicine. *Culture, Medicine, and Psychiatry, 11*, 289–335. http://dx.doi.org/10.1007/BF00048517

Marqués, R. (1963). El puertorriqueño dócil. *Revista de Ciencias Sociales, 7*, 35–78.

Martínez-Taboas, A., Lewis-Fernández, R., Sar, V., & Aggarwal, A. L. (2010). Cultural aspects of psychogenic non-epileptiform seizures. In S. C. Schachter & W. C. LaFrance, Jr. (Eds.), *Gates and Rowan's nonepileptic seizures* (pp. 121–30). New York, NY: Cambridge University Press.

Meléndez Muñoz, M. (1963). El jíbaro en el siglo XIX. In *Obras Completas de Miguel Meléndez Muñoz, Vol III*, Barcelona, Spain: Ediciones Rumbos, pp. 453–611.

Merleau-Ponty, M. (1996). *Phenomenology of perception* (Colin Smith, Trans.). London, England: Routledge. (Original work published 1945)

Mezzich, J. E., Kirmayer, L. J., Kleinman, A., Fabrega, H., Parron, D. L., Good, B. J., ... Manson, S. M. (1999). The place of culture in *DSM-IV*. *Journal of Nervous and Mental Disease, 187*, 457–64. http://dx.doi.org/10.1097/00005053-199908000-00001

Nichter, M. (1981). Idioms of distress: Alternatives in the expression of psychosocial distress: A case from South India. *Culture, Medicine, and Psychiatry, 5*, 379–408. http://dx.doi.org/10.1007/BF00054782

Parnas, J., & Gallagher, S. (2015). Phenomenology and the interpretation of psychopathological experience. In L. J. Kirmayer, R. Lemelson, & C. A. Cummings (Eds.), *Re-visioning psychiatry: Cultural phenomenology, critical neuroscience, and global mental health* (pp. 65–80). New York, NY: Cambridge University Press.

Patel, V., & Thornicroft, G. (2009). Packages of care for mental, neurological, and substance use disorders in low- and middle-income countries: PLoS Medicine Series. *PLoS Medicine, 6*(10), e1000160. http://dx.doi.org/10.1371/journal/pmed.1000160.

Pedreira, A. S. (1934). *Insularismo*. San Juan, Puerto Rico: Biblioteca de Autores Puertorriqueños.

Perfetti, C. A., Liu, Y., & Tan, H. T. (2005). The lexical constituency model: Some implications of research on Chinese for general theories of reading. *Psychological Review, 112*, 43–59. http://dx.doi.org/10.1037/0033-295X.112.1.43

Quintero Rivera, A. G. (1998). *Salsa, sabor y control: Sociología de la música tropical.* Coyoacán, México: Siglo Veintiuno Editores.

Radden, J. (2003). Is this dame melancholy? Equating today's depression and past melancholia. *Philosophy, Psychiatry, & Psychology, 10,* 37–52. http://dx.doi.org/10.1353/ppp.2003.0081

Ross, C. A, Heber, S., Norton, G. R., Anderson, D., & Barchet, P. (1989). The dissociative disorders interview schedule: A structured interview. *Dissociation, 2,* 169–89.

Shaywitz, S. E., Shaywitz, B. A., Pugh, K. R., Fulbright, R. K., Constable, R. T., Mencl, W. E., . . . Gore, J.C. (1998). Functional disruption in the organization of the brain for reading in dyslexia. *Proceedings of the National Academy of Sciences of the United States of America, 95,* 2636–41. http://dx.doi.org/10.1073/pnas.95.5.2636

Siok, W. T., Perfetti, C. A., Jin, Z., & Tan, L. H. (2004). Biological abnormalities of impaired reading is constrained by culture. *Nature, 431,* 71–6. http://dx.doi.org/10.1038/nature02865

Spiegel, D., Loewenstein, R., Lewis-Fernández, R., Sar, V., Simeon, D., Vermetten, E., . . . Dell, P. (2011). Dissociative disorders in *DSM-5. Depression and Anxiety, 28,* 824–52. http://dx.doi.org/10.1002/da.20874

Tan, L. H., Laird, A. R., Li, K., & Fox, P. T. (2005). Neuroanatomical correlates of phonological processing of Chinese characters and alphabetic words: A meta-analysis. *Human Brain Mapping, 25,* 83–91. http://dx.doi.org/10.1002/hbm.20134

Temple, E., Deutsch, G. K., Poldrack, R. A., Miller, S. L., Tallal, P., Merzenich, M., & Gabrielli, J. D. E. (2003). Neural deficits in children with dyslexia ameliorated by behavioral remediation: Evidence from functional MRI. *Proceedings of the National Academy of Sciences of the United States of America, 100,* 2860–65. http://dx.doi.org/10.1073/pnas.0030098100

Thumiger, C. (2013). The early Greek medical vocabulary of insanity. In W. V. Harris (Ed.), *Mental disorders in the classical world* (pp. 61–95). Leiden, Netherlands: Brill. http://dx.doi.org/10.1163/9789004249875_005

Verheul, R., Bartak, A., & Widiger, T. (2007). Prevalence and construct validity of personality disorder not otherwise specified (PDNOS). *Journal of Personality Disorders, 21,* 359–70. http://dx.doi.org/10.1521/pedi.2007.21.4.359

Weidman, H. H. (1979). Falling-out: A diagnostic and treatment problem viewed from a transcultural perspective. *Social Science and Medicine, 13B,* 95–112.

Wittchen, H. U., Höfler, M., Gloster, A. T., Craske, M. G., & Beesda, K. (2011). Options and dilemmas of dimensional measures for *DSM-5:* Which types of measures fare best in predicting course and outcome? In D. A. Regier, W. E. Narrow, E. A. Kuhl, & D. J. Kupfer (Eds.), *The conceptual evolution of "DSM-5"* (pp. 119–44). Arlington, VA: American Psychiatric Publishing.

World Health Organization. (1992). *The "ICD-10" classification of mental and behavioural disorders: Clinical descriptions and diagnostic guidelines.* Geneva, Switzerland: Author. Retrieved from http://www.who.int/classifications/icd/en/

18 *Reflections*
The Virtues of Cultural Sameness
The Case of Delusion

Ian Gold

In 1918, Victor Tausk – a lawyer who, under the influence of Freud, had turned to psychoanalysis – read a paper to the Vienna Psychoanalytic Society entitled "On the Origin of the 'Influencing Machine' in Schizophrenia" (published as Tausk 1919 and, in English translation, as Tausk 1933). Tausk reports on a thirty-one-year-old patient Natalija A. who had formed the belief that she, her mother, and her friends were being manipulated by a machine located in Berlin. Although she is uncertain about the nature of the machine, she suspects that it functions by means of telepathy.

In a strange coincidence, a version of the influencing machine delusion also appears in the very first extended description in English of what psychiatry would come to call "schizophrenia." James Tilly Matthews, an inmate in Bethlem at the turn of the nineteenth century, was the subject of a detailed case history by his doctor John Haslam (Haslam, 1988; see also Jay, 2012, and Porter, 1985). In the years before being committed to Bethlem, Haslam had been living in Paris when Franz Mesmer was making the rounds of Parisian salons and demonstrating the new force he believed he had discovered and which he called "animal magnetism." Once in Bedlam, Matthews came to believe that a gang of villains was operating outside the walls of the hospital and using a machine – the "Air Loom" – to torment him with magnetic waves.

Tausk notes that as new technologies enter popular culture, they creep into patients' delusions. In the twentieth century (Linn, 1958) the influencing machine is conceived of as a robot; in the twenty-first, it is replete with contemporary tropes: manipulation by Marilyn Manson; persecutors projecting pornography into a patient's eyes by "laser radiation"; Muslims and Russians monitoring a patient's sexual activities; and airport security tracking someone by means of a computer chip inserted into his neck (Hirjak & Fuchs, 2010).

The chapters in this section provide a variety of arguments for the claim that trying to understand psychiatric disorders or symptoms outside of the appropriate cultural context is deeply problematic.

The influencing machine delusion provides a particularly clear illustration of one more way in which the study of culture can serve a revisioned psychiatry. Despite the historical evolution of the influencing machine, the core idea of manipulation is unmistakable, and its status as a delusion of control is thus relatively uncontroversial. In general, despite the range of delusional ideas patients exhibit, the motifs of delusion are remarkably stable and few in number. Indeed, the fundamental themes of delusion recur so frequently across time and culture that they seem more like chest pain or shortness of breath than cultural scripts or parochial idioms of distress. If any symptom of psychiatric disorder is likely to track a biological category, it is delusion. And yet, culture is ineliminable even here. Lewis-Fernández and Aggarwal argue that cultural differences in the manifestation of psychiatric symptoms provide a way to try to triangulate neurocognitive universals. Cultural *sameness* can be no less useful in the attempt to carve the symptoms of psychiatric illness at the joints. The theory of delusion thus provides an apt companion piece to the case of *ataque de nervios,* or so I will argue.

DSM-IV-TR (American Psychiatric Association [APA], 2000, p. 821) defined a delusion as a "false belief based on incorrect inference about external reality that is firmly sustained despite what almost everyone else believes and despite what constitutes incontrovertible and obvious proof or evidence to the contrary." *DSM-5* (APA, 2013, p. 87) has backed away from most of that in describing delusions merely as "fixed beliefs that are not amenable to change in light of conflicting evidence." Whatever the virtues of these characterizations, their generality should lead one to think that there are delusional beliefs concerning just about any topic one can imagine. In fact however, psychiatric practice makes much finer distinctions among strange beliefs than the *DSM* suggests. A patient who tells her psychiatrist that the National Security Agency (NSA) has put a microphone in her tooth is likely to be diagnosed as delusional, but a patient who tells her psychiatrist that the NSA is putting microphones in the teeth of Americans will be identified as a (nondelusional) conspiracy theorist. An indefinitely large number of superstitions, ideologies, probabilistic biases, spiritual commitments, scientific falsehoods, and outright nonsense that satisfy the *DSM* definitions simply don't look like delusions to clinicians. Indeed, the cross-cultural literature on delusion shows that only a tiny handful of beliefs are recognized by psychiatrists as delusional, and although the taxonomies differ across studies, there is a great deal of agreement among them as Table 18.1 reveals.

Table 18.1 *The Motifs of Delusions Across Cultures (%)*

Form	English	African	Jamaican	Continental Europeans	English speaking Non-Europeans*	Asian	Midddle Eastern	Far Eastern	Caribbean
Persecutory	26	45	37	14	11	22	9	7	31
Reference	16	11	9	8	3	12	6	13	11
Grandiose and religious	11	19	21	8	8	8	6	7	8
Sexual and fantastic	14	6	15	7	3	4	0	27	10

*North Americans, White South Africans, Australians, and New Zealanders.

471

Table 18.1 (*cont.*)

Form	Sydney	Form	Tokyo	Vienna	Tübingen	Form	Seoul	Shanghai	Taipei
Persecutory	80.0	Persecution/Injury	75.9	70.3	72.7	Persecutory	72.3	78.9	79.1
Religious	26.7	Poisoning	8.0	14.9	18.0	Reference	6.0	54.2	59.0
Grandiose	23.3	Jealousy	1.9	1.0	6.0	Grandiose	48.2	27.5	38.8
Reference	15.6	Being stolen from	4.9	2.0	2.7	Control	35.5	23.9	30.9
Somatic	14.4	Parasitosis	0.9	3.0	2.0	Somatic	23.4	14.1	24.5
Mind control	4.4	Mission/grandeur/ special ability	19.4	19.8	18.7	Guilt	31.2	4.9	5.8
Guilt	4.4	Erotomania	6.5	5.9	6.7	Jealousy	17.0	8.5	3.6
Mind reading	4.4	Descent	4.4	1.0	0.7	Poverty	2.1	4.2	5.0
Thought broadcasting	3.3	Pregnancy	0.9	3.0	0.7	Nihilism	0.7	2.1	3.6
Transmitting devices	3.3	Resurrection	0	1.0	0				
Thought withdrawal	3.3	Invention	0.3	0	0.7				
Believing that a stranger is a close relative	2.2	Hypochondria/ dying	8.6	19.8	9.3				
Believing that they are someone else	2.2	Guilt/sin	4.9	20.8	15.3				
Believing someone is in love with them	2.2	Being dead	0.3	5.9	0.7				
Extraterrestrial	2.2	Poverty	0	1.0	2.0				
Other delusions	6.7	Death of relations	3.4	1.0	2.7				
		World catastrophe	2.5	2.0	4.7				
		Separation of being	1.5	3.0	1.3				
		Homosexual	0	0	0				
		Others	5.9	10.9	8.0				
		Religious	6.8	19.8	21.3				

Table 18.1 (cont.)

Form	White	British Pakistani	Pakistani	Form	Western Turkey	Central Turkey
Persecution	48	60	62	Persecutory	74.6	83.7
Control	50	26	13	Reference	57.7	70.9
Reference	48	43	11	Poisoning	9.5	26.2
Grandiose Ability	26	19	28	Religious	10.9	20.9
Grandiose identity	14	23	42	Grandiosity	10.0	19.8
Religious	14	21	11	Being controlled	6.0	19.8
Sexual	14	13	16	Mind reading	4.5	17.4
Depersonalization	18	11	2	Jealousy	3.5	14.0
Hypochondriacal	8	17	5	Guilt/sin	0.5	13.4
Misinterpretation	8	6	8	Hypochondria	1.0	12.2
				Erotomania	2.5	9.3
				Thought broadcasting	0.5	11.1
				Thought insertion	1.0	9.3
				Nihilistic	4.0	5.2
				Thought withdrawal	0.5	5.2
				Nobility	0	3.5
				Inferiority	0	3.5
				Homosexual	0	3.5
				Parasitosis	0	1.2
				World catastrophe	0	1.2
				Resurrection	0	1.2
				Others	4.5	0.6

Note. Reprinted with permission from *Suspicious Minds: How Culture Shapes Madness*, by J. Gold & I. Gold, 2014, p. 64. Copyright 2014 by Simon & Schuster. Original data taken from Brakoulias & Starcevic, 2008, p. 90; Gecici et al., 2010, p. 207; Kim et al., 2001, p. 90; Ndetei & Vadher, 1984, p. 74; Suhail & Cochrane, 2002, pp. 130–1; and Tateyama et al., 1998, p. 62.

There are a number of different ways that one could classify the delusional themes identified cross-culturally, and the choice is, at the moment, largely arbitrary. Here is one taxonomy:

> *Persecution*: that others are conspiring to harm you;
>
> *Jealousy*: that your partner is cheating;
>
> *Grandiosity*: that you are particularly powerful or special;
>
> *Erotomania*: that someone of high social status is in love with you;
>
> *Religion*: that divine forces are persecuting you or have anointed you for some purpose;
>
> *Control*: that your actions are being manipulated by an external agency;
>
> *Thought*: that thoughts can be inserted or extracted from your mind, read, or heard by others;
>
> *The Body*: that you are ill or your body is abnormal or incomplete;
>
> *Nihilism*: that the body, the self or others do not exist;
>
> *Guilt or sin*: that you are responsible for a terrible event or state of affairs;
>
> *Reference*: that events in the world have a special significance for you;
>
> *Misidentification*: that the identities of others are not what they appear to be.

Two observations about the motifs of delusion are in order. First, they are all restricted to one corner of the irrational, namely to thoughts about oneself (including one's body) or other people. Second, within this broad domain of social thoughts, some secondary themes are apparent. The most obvious is social threat. Persecutory delusions are ubiquitous across time and culture and the most common form of delusion everywhere by a significant margin (Bentall & Udachina 2013). Jealousy is persecution writ small – harm caused by a loved one and the lover – and some religious delusions are persecution writ large, with God, for example, cast as persecutor. Delusions of control and of thought also have a persecutory flavor insofar as the body and mind of the patient are being manipulated against his will.

Another secondary theme is social power, represented most broadly by grandiose delusions which are often expressions of the kind of power granted by social status: "I could find the key to the cure to cancer"; "I am a special athlete, and I run a national charity"; "I am also a famous DJ. I have Superman-type powers" (Knowles et al., 2011, p. 685). One way in which high social status can be conferred is by means of relations to others of high status. When grandiosity is characterized this way, erotomania turns out to be one of its variants, rather than an independent motif. Similarly, religious delusions in which one may be represented as an important religious figure or on a mission from God are variants of grandiosity, as divine persecution is a variant of ordinary paranoia. Finally, if grandiosity is the assertion of social status and power, then delusions of illness or bodily distortions, delusions of guilt, and some nihilistic delusions can be hypothesized to be expressions of social subordination.

Mapping the themes of delusion in this way supports a general hypothesis. While illness accounts for the vast majority of human death (Heron, 2013), the quotidian dangers of life – loss of relationships, property, and other resources – are those that are posed by other people. Although living in social groups supports the cooperative engagements characteristic of the human form of life, we pay a price for cooperation in an increased risk of exploitation by others. "Free-riding" is the most obvious of these. From the drinking buddy who never gets around to picking up the tab to the tax cheat sustained by the state, cooperation makes it possible for some of us to reap the benefits of group living without contributing anything in return.

Because cooperation is profoundly beneficial, it would be irrational to avoid it in order to protect oneself from exploitation. Instead, human beings have developed cognitive strategies designed to avoid dangerous people. Gossip may be one such strategy (Dunbar, 2004). An interest in malicious stories about others serves to bring to our attention those people who might be best avoided. A second strategy is suspicion (Enquist & Leimar, 1993). A rapid, automatic disposition to a differential mistrust of strangers would serve the purpose of distinguishing those who are likely to be good cooperative partners from those who are not. And, indeed, despite the fact that only extensive experience of someone's behavior can support a confident assessment of their trustworthiness, human beings appear to have an impressive, largely unconscious, cognitive capacity to make nonrandom judgments (though not necessarily *true* ones) about the kindness of strangers. One line of evidence for this ability comes from the study of faces. In a series of elegant experiments, Alexander Todorov and his colleagues (see Oosterhof & Todorov, 2008 and Todorov et al., 2009) have demonstrated that people are able to make extremely rapid trustworthiness judgments. When asked to select the most trustworthy face from a group (see Figure 18.1), Todorov and his colleagues found that at a thirty-three-millisecond exposure, participants made nonrandom choices. At one hundred milliseconds, they were indistinguishable in their judgments from those made without any time restriction.

A second line of evidence regarding the human capacity for suspicion comes from studies of amygdala function. In 1990, Daniel Tranel and Bradley Hyman (Tranel & Hyman, 1990) reported on a patient with bilateral amygdala lesions known as SM. Investigation of SM and other amygdala patients suggested at first that the primary deficit associated

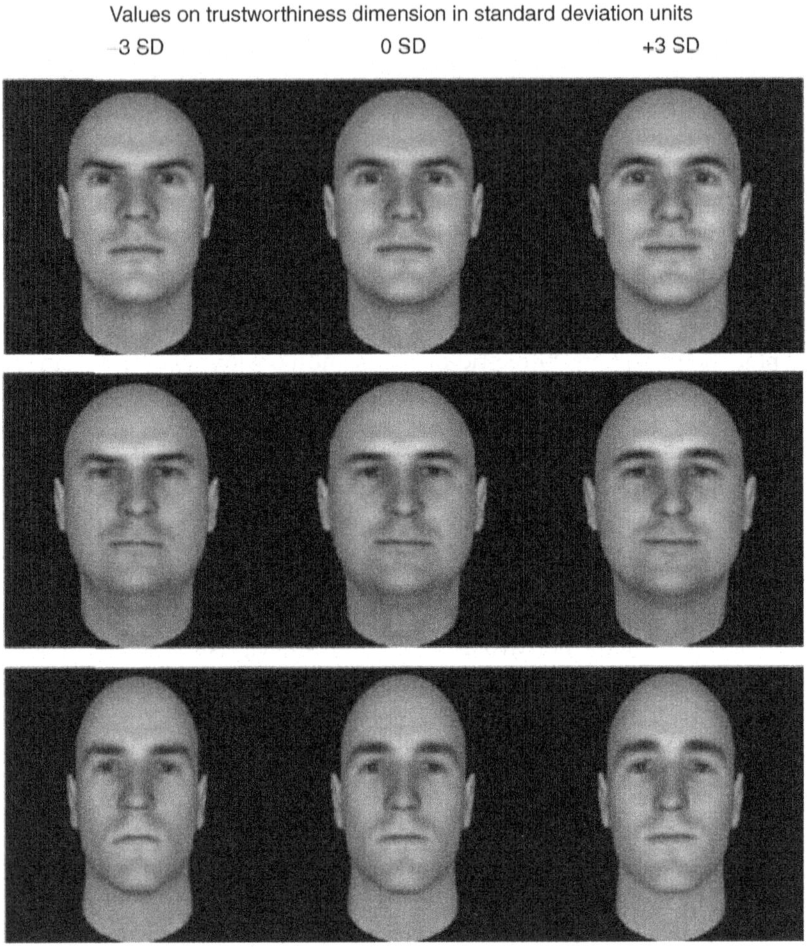

Values on trustworthiness dimension in standard deviation units

-3 SD   0 SD   +3 SD

Figure 18.1. More and less trustworthy faces. Reprinted with permission of Guilford Press and Alexander Todorov, from "Evaluating Faces on Trustworthiness After Minimal Time Exposure," by A. Todorov, M. Pakrashi, & N. Oosterhof, 2009, *Social Cognition, 27*(6), p. 823.

with the lesions was an inability to recognize facial expressions of fear. In recent years, however, it has begun to seem that the deficit is better described as social. In a 1998 study, Ralph Adolphs and his colleagues showed SM and other patients a set of faces and asked them to rank the faces according to their "trustworthiness" or "approachability." SM's judgments largely agreed with the healthy controls regarding the trustworthy faces, but diverged on the untrustworthy ones; she perceived all the faces as trustworthy or approachable. And in a subsequent study, SM was evaluated by a psychotherapist (ignorant of her condition) who observed that SM "did not seem to have a normal sense of distrust and 'danger'" (Buchanan et al., 2009, p. 310). The parents of another amygdala lesion patient AP observe that "she tends to 'trust' people too easily" and have encouraged her to be "more wary of strangers" (Buchanan et al., 2009, p. 301). Amygdala lesions thus appear to abolish the capacity for adaptive suspicion.

Given the themes of delusion sketched above, a hypothesis worth considering is that neurocognitive disorders could cause healthy suspicion to become paranoia. Further, grandiosity and its variants– erotomania and religion – can be conceptualized as a pathological attempt to *respond to* a social threat. When faced with aggressors, animals engage in a variety of behaviors designed to make themselves look bigger in an effort to highlight their capacity for defense and retaliation (Eibl-Eibesfeldt, 1970). In social interactions, status and evidence of social power play the role of physical size. Grandiosity may be a distorted attempt to warn a putative aggressor of the price of social exploitation. Delusions of social subordination may play a parallel role as the pathological expression of the kind of submissiveness that defuses a threat by the assertion that one is not a worthy target. The belief that you are morally bad or physically damaged is a way of telling an aggressor that you are not worth his effort, and the conviction that you are sick conveys a subtle threat of infection into the bargain.

Whatever the virtues of this sketch of a hypothesis about delusions, the exercise shows that while cultural difference can be revealing, so can the *sameness* that is visible beneath the surface of cultural difference. Two secondary conclusions are also in order. Culture is at the heart of the hypothesis I have sketched to the extent that delusions are hypothesized to be the manifestation of a neurocognitive mechanism directed at *other people*. If the view is correct, there cannot be a theory of delusion that ignores culture anymore than there could be a theory of vision that omits the physics of light. Even if this social theory of delusion is completely wrong, there is good reason to think that social relations are central to other forms of psychiatric disorder (Mendez & Manes, 2011). Psychiatric theory uninformed by anthropology is thus likely to be blind to some of the most important phenomena it seeks to explain. I agree with Luhrmann (Chapter 12, *this volume*), therefore, that there is an optimistic reading of the RDoC approach that could see psychiatric research focus on what is essentially social in mental disorder.

Finally, a word about "meaning" in a revisioned psychiatry. The medical model of psychiatric diagnosis represented by the *DSM* has led

to what Nancy Andreasen (2007) has lamented as the "death of phenomenology" in psychiatry. The checklist approach to diagnosis has
rendered the meanings of the patient's symptoms otiose. It makes a great
difference to an emergency room psychiatrist whether her patient has a
delusional thought, but the particular content of the thought is taken
to be irrelevant. In contrast, the hypothesis sketched earlier supports the
presupposition implicit in the papers in this section that one cannot
ignore the meanings of psychiatric symptoms. If culture is to play its
proper role in the future of psychiatry, then we cannot dispense with the
thought contents of symptoms – whether in delusion, auditory voice
hallucination, depressive cognitions, obsessive rumination, or whatever.
Getting to neurocognitive bedrock may require going through the messy
but informative sediment of patients' thinking.

REFERENCES

Adolphs, R., Tranel, D., & Damasio, A. (1998). The human amygdala in social
    judgment. *Nature, 393,* 470–4. http://dx.doi.org/10.1038/30982
American Psychiatric Association. (2000). *Diagnostic and statistical manual of
    mental disorders* (4th ed., text rev.). Washington, DC: Author.
American Psychiatric Association. (2013). *Diagnostic and statistical manual of
    mental disorders* (5th ed.). Washington, DC: Author.
Andreasen N. 2007. *DSM* and the death of phenomenology in America:
    An example of unintended consequences. *Schizophrenia Bulletin, 33,*
    108–12. http://dx.doi.org/10.1093/schbul/sbl054
Bentall, R., & Udachina, A. (2013). Social cognition and the dynamics
    of paranoid ideation. In D. Roberts & D. Penn (Eds.), *Social cognition
    in schizophrenia* (pp. 215–44). Oxford, England: Oxford University
    Press.
Brakoulias V, Starcevic V. 2008. A cross-sectional survey of the frequency and
    characteristics of delusions in acute psychiatric wards. *Australasian
    Psychiatry, 16*: 87–91. http://dx.doi.org/10.1080/10398560701633176
Buchanan, T., Tranel, D., & Adolphs, R. (2009). The human amygdala in
    social function. In P. Whalen & E. Phelps (Eds.), *The human amygdala*
    (pp. 289–318). New York, NY: Guilford Press.
Dunbar, R. (2004). Gossip in evolutionary perspective. *Review of General
    Psychology, 8,* 100–10. http://dx.doi.org/10.1037/1089-2680.8.2.100
Eibl-Eibesfeldt, I. (1970). *Ethology: The biology of behavior* (E Kinghammer,
    Trans.). New York, NY: Holt, Rinehart, & Winston.
Enoch, M., & Ball, H. (2001). *Uncommon psychiatric syndromes.* London,
    England: Arnold.
Enquist, M., & Leimar, O. (1993). The evolution of cooperation in mobile
    organisms. *Animal Behaviour, 45,* 747–57. http://dx.doi.org/10.1006/
    anbe.1993.1089
Gecici O, Kuloglu M, Guler O, Ozbulut O, Kurt E, Onen S, Ekinci O,
    Yesilbas D, Caykoylu A, Emül M, Alatas G, Albayrak Y. 2010.

Phenomenology of delusions and hallucinations in patients
with schizophrenia. *Bulletin of Clinical Psychopharmacology, 20*, 204–12.

Gold, J., & Gold, I. (2014). *Suspicious minds: How culture shapes madness.*
New York, NY: Free Press.

Haslam, J. (1988). *Illustrations of madness*, (R. Porter, Ed.). London, England:
Routledge.

Heron, M. (2013). Deaths: Leading causes 2010. *National Vital Statistics Reports,
62*, 1–96.

Hirjak, D., & Fuchs, T. (2010). Delusions of technical alien control:
A phenomenological description of three cases. *Psychopathology, 43*, 96–103.
http://dx.doi.org/10.1159/000274178

Jay, M. (2012). *The influencing machine: James Tilly Matthews and the air loom.*
London, England: Strange Attractor Press.

Kim, K., Hwu, H., Zhang, L., Lu, M., Park, K., Hwang, T., . . . Park, Y. (2001).
Schizophrenic delusions in Seoul, Shanghai and Taipei: A transcultural
study. *Journal of Korean Medical Science, 16*, 88–94. http://dx.doi.org/
10.3346/jkms.2001.16.1.88

Knowles, R., McCarthy-Jones, S., & Rowse, G. (2011). Grandiose delusions:
A review and theoretical integration of cognitive and affective perspectives.
Clinical Psychology Review, 31, 684–96. http://dx.doi.org/10.1016/j.
cpr.2011.02.009

Lewis-Fernández, R., & Aggarwal, N. K. (2015). Psychiatric classification
beyond the *DSM*: An interdisciplinary approach. In L. J. Kirmayer,
R. Lemelson, & C. A. Cummings (Eds.), *Re-visioning psychiatry: Cultural
phenomenology, critical neuroscience, and global mental health* (pp. 434–68).
New York, NY: Cambridge University Press.

Linn, L. (1958). Some comments on the origin of the influencing machine.
Journal of the American Psychoanalytic Association, 6, 305–8. http://dx.doi.org/
10.1177/000306515800600209

Luhrmann, T. M. (2015). Reflections: Hearing voices – How social context
shapes psychiatric symptoms. In L. J. Kirmayer, R. Lemelson, &
C. A. Cummings (Eds.), *Re-visioning psychiatry: Cultural phenomenology,
critical neuroscience, and global mental health* (pp. 305–13). New York, NY:
Cambridge University Press.

Mendez, M., & Manes, F. (2011). The emerging impact of social neuroscience
on neuropsychiatry and clinical neuroscience. *Social Neuroscience, 6*, 415–19.
http://dx.doi.org/10.1080/17470919.2011.624806

Ndetei, D., Vadher, A. (1984). Frequency and clinical significance of delusions
across cultures. *Acta Psychiatrica Scandinavica, 70*, 73–6. http://dx.doi.org/
10.1111/j.1600-0447.1984.tb01184.x

Oosterhof, N. N., & Todorov, A. (2008). The functional basis of face evaluation.
*Proceedings of the National Academy of Sciences of the United States of
America, 105*, 11087–92. http://dx.doi.org/10.1073/pnas.0805664105

Porter, R. (1985). Under the influence: Mesmerism in England. *History Today,
35*, 22–9.

Suhail, K., Cochrane, R. (2002). Effect of culture and environment on the
phenomenology of delusions and hallucinations. *International Journal of*

Social Psychiatry, 48, 126–38. http://dx.doi.org/10.1177/
002076402128783181

Tateyama, M., Asai, M., Hashimoto, M., Bartels, M., & Kasper, S. (1998).
Transcultural study of schizophrenic delusions. *Psychopathology, 31*, 59–68.
http://dx.doi.org/10.1159/000029025

Tausk, V. (1919). Über die Entstehung des Beeinflussungsapparates" in der
Schizophrenie. *Internationale Zeitschrift für Ärztliche Psychoanalyse V*, 1–33.

Tausk, V. (1933). On the origin of the "influencing machine" in schizophrenia.
Psychoanalytic Quarterly, 2, 519–56.

Todorov, A., Pakrashi, M., Oosterhof, N. (2009). Evaluating faces on
trustworthiness after minimal time exposure. *Social Cognition, 27*(6),
813–33. http://dx.doi.org/10.1521/soco.2009.27.6.813

Tranel, D., Hyman, B. (1990). Neuropsychological correlates of bilateral
amygdala damage. *Archives of Neurology, 47*, 349–55. http://dx.doi.org/
10.1001/archneur.1990.00530030131029

Yip, K.-S. (2003). Traditional Chinese religious beliefs and superstitions in
delusions and hallucinations of Chinese schizophrenic patients. *International
Journal of Social Psychiatry, 49*, 97–111. http://dx.doi.org/10.1177/
0020764003049002003

Section Four

Psychiatric Practice in Global Context

19 Afflictions
Psychopathology and Recovery in Cultural Context

Robert Lemelson and Annie Tucker

> I would usually hear sounds like the wind, like the rain. Then I would feel I was going to get sick again. I would try to remember [my] face from when [I was] young. Because when I was young, I was happy.
> —Ni Ketut Kasih, an elderly Balinese woman diagnosed with paranoid schizophrenia

> The most important thing for Javanese is their true identity. "It's true man, you may have a brilliant brain like Americans." I remember the message of Mister Suharto our smiling general. Let's take the doctor's advice. The doctors said that I suffered from ... not schizophrenia, but schizoaffective. I'll just change "a" with "e" and it'll become effective, right?
> —Bambang, A young Javanese man diagnosed with schizoaffective disorder

A central question of this volume concerns how to integrate social and biological models to better understand the nature and meaning of mental illness. Although identifying the interactions of social and biological factors is key to a comprehensive theory of mental illness, the implications of an integrative view are not merely theoretical. As work elsewhere in this volume has shown, integrative theories that can guide how we respond to and treat the mentally ill are extraordinarily important. For the seriously mentally ill, their families, communities, and those who care for and treat them, one of the most pressing questions is: "What factors are the most salient contributors to a better overall outcome and recovery?" To answer this question, we must address a series of fundamental research problems, including the role of biology, family, and community in the causes, courses, and outcomes of illness. Multiple theories postulate that many of these illnesses are influenced, mediated, and in some cases caused by complex neurobiological processes – and complementary or competing theories about the roles multiple social and cultural factors play in differential outcomes and recovery abound. This chapter will explore issues of outcome and recovery for the severely mentally ill in developing Southeast Asia, as seen through the lens of two in-depth case studies of people with mental illness in Indonesia.

Advancing an Integrative View of Mental illness Through Ethnography

Specific methodologies are required to address the complexity of the lives of people diagnosed with mental illness. Much work in medical and psychological anthropology has been devoted to examining the influence of culture on all aspects of human experience and society, including development, deviance, and illness. Psychological anthropology has developed methodologies to explore the complex dynamics of subjectivity, intersubjectivity, phenomenology, and interpretation that shape mental illness in social situations based on local models and understandings of illness and social behavior (Csordas, 2002; Chapter 5, *this volume;* Desjarlais & Throop, 2011; Kirmayer, Lemelson, & Cummings, Chapter 1, *this volume;* White & Marsella, 1982). Engaging the lifeworlds of patients may lead to better understanding of the course and outcome of illness than is afforded by the measures typically employed in psychiatric research and practice (Kleinman, 1988, p. 66).

Ethnographic research shows how culture pervades the subjective experience of psychiatric illness, including psychosis, mediating aspects that might be considered "hard-wired," not only by influencing the content of hallucinations, obsessions, and anxieties, but also by shaping the basic processes of cognition and affect, providing local idioms for personal expressions of distress, and offering frameworks for interpreting the meaning of illness. Culture structures the events that may act as causes or triggers of mental illness and shapes the personal narratives and embodied experiences that organize and express suffering. In addition to influencing the pathophysiological processes that underlie major mental illness, family and the immediate psychosocial environment play key roles in the degree of disability, morbidity, and mortality associated with major mental illness; and family and the environment are major factors influencing outcome and recovery. The influence of culture on these and other facets of mental health and illness presents an important challenge to those who argue for a global psychiatry that relies on biological treatments as its mainstay.

The *Afflictions* Film Series: Integrating Visual and Medical Anthropology to Understand the Course of Psychiatric Illness in the Developing World

The potential of ethnographic methods to clarify cultural contexts essential to understanding mental illness is illustrated by the film series

Afflictions: Culture and Mental Illness in Indonesia (www.afflictionsfilm
series.com). The first documentary film series on mental illness in the
developing world, *Afflictions* integrates visual ethnography with a longitudinal person-centered approach to studying severe mental illness in
cultural context. The films examine the lives of six people with thought
and neuropsychiatric disorders on the islands of Bali and Java and
consider the impact of personal experience, family, culture, and community on the course of their illness. In this series, an ethnographic
frame offers a holistic perspective to otherwise clinically oriented
research, encompassing broader dimensions of the lived experience of
select individuals. In doing so, it captures some of those areas of experience and aspects of culture that are often elided or inadequately
attended to in psychiatric research and practice, yet that ultimately
prove to be the central issues at stake in the lives of those with major
mental illness.[1]

Two individuals, each the subject of their own film in the *Afflictions*
series, are representative of contemporary Indonesia's striking diversity
and the complexity of this research. The main character in the
film *Ritual Burdens* is Ni Ketut Kasih (Ketut), a rural agrarian
Balinese Hindu grandmother who never finished elementary school
and has been diagnosed with paranoid schizophrenia. The main character in the film *Memory of My Face* is Bambang Rujito (Bambang), a
highly educated urban Javanese Muslim and young father, with
a diagnosis of schizoaffective disorder. Their case studies are connected by similar diagnoses and histories of colonialism, political
violence, and globalized mental health discourses that inform and
influence the intersubjective interpretation of their illnesses. Yet,
Ketut and Bambang were born on different islands a generation apart –
with Ketut growing up as Indonesia achieved independence in the
1940s and Bambang coming of age during the economic boom
of the 1980s and later collapse of President Suharto's "New
Order" authoritarian regime in the late 1990s. Furthermore, Ketut
lives in an agricultural village that is predominantly grounded in
local traditional beliefs and practices, whereas Bambang lives in a
rapidly changing urban environment that has been significantly
impacted by globalization. Consequently, they live in different
local worlds, and they and their families make sense of their

[1] Additional ethnographic films by the first author addressing related areas of interest to
psychological anthropologists and transcultural psychiatrists can be found at www.
elementalproductions.org.

predicaments in different ways, calling on the imagery, resources, and ethos of those worlds.

This chapter includes links to short videos, excerpted from the longer documentary films about Ketut and Bambang, in order to provide access to the visual methods crucial to this project.[2]

Ni Ketut Kasih: The Power of "Traditional" Culture in Shaping Outcome

Ketut was born in the early 1940s, the eighth child of twelve in a small village in Central Bali. She has lived her life surrounded by the rhythms and requirements of the dense Balinese ritual calendar, with temple observances, holy days, and village and regional festivals occurring on a weekly or sometimes daily basis.

Ketut remembers a happy early childhood (http://vimeo.com/album/3014164/video/104655295). Her father was a weapons specialist who fought against both Japanese and Dutch occupiers during World War II and Indonesia's struggle for independence. In 1947, when Ketut was still a child, her father was captured and held in a prison camp for months. Ketut's mother was sick, and the family was financially hard-pressed, so Ketut was forced to postpone her education and to help support her family by working as a seamstress and a peddler. After her father returned home, Ketut was able to attend elementary school; but ongoing financial difficulties once again forced her to abandon her education – this time for good – after completing the sixth grade.

As Ketut grew into a young woman, she became a successful fish merchant, but a market crisis in 1965 left her with significant debts. Meanwhile, her family was reeling from the national violence that followed a purported communist coup and subsequent counter-coup and governmental takeover by Suharto-directed military and paramilitary, in which Ketut's uncle and cousin were killed. After this difficult time, Ketut's family arranged for her to marry a distant relative. Ketut wished she could pick her own husband, but she didn't dare resist. Her feelings of resentment soon diminished as she settled into a loving relationship with her husband.

---

[2] These videos are all on the website http://vimeo.com/album/3014164, freely available to readers of this volume with the password "book." Full-length films and supplemental study guides are available at www.der.org/films/afflictions.html and www. afflictionsfilmseries.org.

Ketut gave birth to the couple's first child in 1969, three days after a family ritual ceremony. Ketut exhibited postpartum distress, which was the first of many episodes of what she described as an "inner sickness" (B.I. [Bahasa Indonesia], *sakit dalam*); she rejected her son, refused to breastfeed, and exhibited symptoms of dissociation and disorientation (http://vimeo.com/album/3014164/video/104656427). She was ill for about three and a half months, during which her family sought a variety of traditional treatments. One healer conducted a religious ceremony and gave Ketut oil to drink, causing mucous to pour out of her mouth and nose, a commonly recognized sign of recovery in Bali. Ketut returned to her "normal self" within a month of this treatment and lived her life fairly free of incident for over fifteen years. She gave birth to three more children and took care of the household, while selling staples at the nearby market.

Then in 1986, Ketut attended a large-scale family ritual marking both a tooth-filing ceremony, a Balinese rite of passage, and her brother-in-law's wedding. Soon after arriving she suddenly felt weak, couldn't speak, began to weep, and ultimately collapsed. She was taken to a psychiatrist, diagnosed with schizophrenia, prescribed chlorpromazine, and returned to her village with her symptoms substantially in remission within eleven days. However, she soon relapsed, at which point her family brought her to the psychiatric ward at a nearby hospital. Over the following decades, Ketut was hospitalized more than thirty-five times, either at a local hospital in the capital, Denspasar, or at a large state psychiatric hospital in rural central Bali, sometimes briefly and sometimes for a month or more. During a relapse, Ketut might wander; behave in a social deviant and disruptive manner, such as disrobing in public; act aggressively toward family members or strangers; or remain prostrate and mute for days at a time.

Ketut and her family both believe that the triggers for her episodes are the emotional burdens posed by ritual events and family obligations, as Ketut worries that her family will be unable to meet expectations and demands. A large portion of ritual responsibilities fall heavily on Balinese women, who often contribute financially and must spend countless hours crafting offerings by hand. It is a common belief that if these complex and costly rituals are not followed exactly, the spirits being propitiated will become upset, leading to a variety of misfortunes, such as illness or financial hardship. Ketut's speed and mastery in preparing offerings had earned her high public status. Yet privately, these preparations and ceremonies filled her with dread and acted as triggers for illness episodes (http://vimeo.com/album/3014164/video/104657208).

When her husband died in 2006, Ketut took over his duties as a village ritual specialist (B.B. [Bahasa Bali], *pemangku*). Although this role commanded an even higher degree of respect in the village, it added to her burden, and the frequency of her relapses seemed to increase. After years of struggle, Ketut's family relieved her of the task of preparing offerings, and her role as a *pemangku* went to her eldest son. Her children and grandchildren now assume the responsibility for the family's ritual requirements, sometimes even receiving help from other villagers, in an attempt to protect Ketut's peace of mind. Ketut still experiences an occasional relapse, but taking the empathetic view that anyone can become overly stressed, the family actively rejects any stigmatization of her symptoms, instead calmly facing each episode as it comes (http://vimeo.com/album/3014164/video/104658235).

Bambang: The Pervasive Effects of Globalization in Shaping Mental Illness Experience

Bambang was born in 1969, a generation after Ni Ketut Kasih across the Bali Strait on the island of Java. He grew up surrounded by siblings and a warm extended family near Borobudur, a rural area in Central Java that is home to the world-famous temple of the same name. His father was a sailor who traveled the trade route from Jakarta to Japan, and his mother sold traditional health tonics.

When Bambang was only four, his father was killed in a violent fight in a distant port. Bambang's mother moved to Jakarta, Indonesia's largest metropolis, to make her living at a food stall. At first, Bambang stayed behind with relatives so as not to disrupt his education, but later he joined his mother for middle school, where he rose to the top of his class. In recognition of his promise, he was accepted into a prestigious local high school.

When he was a sophomore, Bambang became troubled and exhausted. His religious studies began to disturb him; characters from Islamic cosmology seemed almost uncomfortably vivid in his imagination, and he was frustrated that the moral ideals he encountered in religious doctrine were rarely realized in everyday life. When his first girlfriend broke up with him, he was devastated (http://vimeo.com/album/3014164/video/104658584). One night he decided to pray for guidance, but instead lost consciousness and awoke into a frightening world where his sins had come alive to pursue him. At first, he was diagnosed with a fever and a thyroid condition, but after the more delusional elements of his illness became apparent, he was hospitalized for a month.

Bambang recovered, resumed his academic life, and enrolled at the University of Indonesia in Jakarta. He did well academically, but relapsed frequently, rarely sleeping, believing himself to be a great Imam, and declaring his own political parties. These feelings of power were sometimes countered by splitting headaches, bouts of weeping, and tremendous anxiety. He was hospitalized once more in Bogor, but was lonely and returned home, where he slowly returned to a stable condition.

Bambang then met his wife, Yatmi, who was impressed by his education and English skills. They married and were soon expecting a child. He found employment in the stock market, where he often worked overnight monitoring the *Reuters* news feed; he developed the habit of taking energy supplements and drinking many cups of coffee to stay awake. In 1999, the mounting stress of his work caused him to resign. He went home, and believing that it was Independence Day, took his young toddler on a very long walk to join in the "celebration." The two wandered the streets of South Jakarta for a full twenty-four hours. Bambang's mother decided that his condition was unsafe for the family, so she brought Bambang back to Central Java with her. In 2000, the family ultimately committed him to the psychiatric ward of a large state hospital in Central Java, where he stayed for the greater part of three years. It was here that he introduced himself to the first author and film team during a hospital folk dance performance (http://vimeo.com/album/3014164/video/104662116).

Bambang returned to his wife and child in 2003. From that time, he has intermittently experienced major relapses that have required hospitalization. Between episodes, he maintains his religious and civic duties but has withdrawn from more casual friendships. The family has moved five or six times after neighbors witnessed his out-of-control behavior. Yatmi supports the family as a manager in a multinational garment factory.

Beyond Diagnosis: Culture and the Subjective Experience of Psychotic Disorders

During their periods of hospitalization, Ketut was diagnosed with paranoid schizophrenia and Bambang with schizoaffective disorder. The recent reconfiguration of diagnoses in the *DSM-5* – which has eliminated the subtypes of schizophrenia (APA, 2013, p. 810) and kept schizoaffective disorder with the proviso that there is growing evidence it is not a distinct nosological category (APA, 2013, p. 90) – underscores the fact that these are complex disorders with probable genetic, biological, and symptomatic overlap (Bilder, Chapter 8, *this volume*;

Berrettini, 2003; Blackwood et al., 2001; Kelsoe, 2003; Smoller et al., 2013). The dominant current models of such psychotic disorders emphasize their biological underpinnings by focusing on neurobiological processes, psychopharmocological treatments, and genetic research; however, biological approaches do not obviate the need for understanding the environmental, psychosocial, and/or cultural factors that influence the course, content, and outcome of these disorders.

Content of Hallucinations: Symptomatology and Idioms of Distress

The idioms used to describe the symptomatology of mental illness utilize the ideas, sensations, and images most meaningful to those experiencing them, and thus reflect the rhythms, activities, and ecologies of daily life. Ketut lives in rural Bali and is steeped in traditional agrarian Balinese culture. The idioms of distress she uses to describe her prodromal symptoms include a heightened sensitivity toward the culturally significant features of her natural environment. She describes becoming acutely sensitive to "the voice of the wind" or the sound of rain falling on leaves, and feels like her head is filled with rice or that she has been pummeled with a bamboo spear. Preceding her manic episodes, she may have visions of light that she interprets as being that of the full moon, a powerful image in Balinese culture associated with ritual and festivity. Alternately, her relationship to the sun and her own shadow might serve to presage an episode of depression. As Ketut described it, "If I couldn't see my own shadow I was going to have a relapse" (http://vimeo.com/album/3014164/video/104662835).

In Indonesia, the penetration of Western biomedical and psychiatric models is not evenly spread or understood in daily cultural life. To explain and frame an illness, people in rural Indonesia like Ketut continue to rely on local explanatory models for guidance. Certainly, this is variably the case in other places as well, including in the West, where biomedical understanding of mental illness may be fragmented or reinterpreted and folk models and local metaphors for mental illness remain active – at times complementary, at times conflicting, but not coterminous with biomedical models (Estroff, Lachicotte, Illingworth, & Johnston, 1991; Martin, 2007). However, compared with both urban Indonesians and many in the West (Jenkins, 2010), on the whole biomedical models in rural Indonesia have not substantially displaced local metaphors (Good, 2010).

Unlike Ketut, Bambang lives in the megalopolis of Jakarta with constant exposure to globalized media. His manic psychosis and paranoid delusions incorporate elements of these, mixed with local, regional, and national tropes and imagery. He explains,

I opened newspapers and magazines all night long. I can conclude that my hallucinations were about what I read, what I heard, things I deeply felt. I was totally obsessed by the war between Palestine versus Israel. [...] Or if I saw a funeral procession, I would see that as a Soviet battalion. In my imagination, it was like a war [...] In my mind, there was chaos. I was scared all the time. (http://vimeo.com/album/3014164/video/104663220)

These distinct internal and projected worlds indicate that hallucinations are not meaningless sequelae of psychopathology, but learned and shaped both by "cultural invitation and by biological constraint" (Luhrmann, 2011, p. 71). Furthermore, Ketut and Bambang's vastly different imagery and idioms of symptomatology illustrate a dialectic and agentic model of mental disorders, wherein a person actively attends to and interprets experienced changes in perception or sensation in accordance with engagement in a culturally shared world, while at the same time infusing culturally available symbols with a personal or psychological dimension in addition to their public, culturally sanctioned roles (Obeyesekere, 1981). Variations in the content of hallucinations, then, may be more the effect of different elaborations or interpretations than of different underlying transformations of bodily experience (Sass, 2007; Stanghellini, Bolton, & Fulford, 2013). Whether these hallucinations are pleasurable, neutral, or persecutory may be determined in part by available cultural imagery and attitudes toward such changes in perception or sensation (Luhrmann, Padmavati, Tharoor, & Osei, 2014). This kind of cultural phenomenological account implies a basic neurophenomenology with a secondary cultural elaboration, a concept central to descriptions of a cultural phenomenology grounded in embodiment (Csordas, 1997, 1999); cultural neurophenomenology (Kirmayer, 2009; Laughlin & Throop, 2006); and an epistemology of psychiatry and mental symptoms (Marková & Berrios, 2012, 2009).

Cultural Regulation and Interpretation of Cognition and Affect

A preponderance of the psychocultural ethnographic literature emphasizes that in Indonesian cultures generally, and in Balinese and Javanese cultures specifically, the experience and expression of conflict, anger, and grief are negatively valenced in many (but not all) contexts. This literature also emphasizes how individuals strive to maintain a smooth and nonreactive composure, even when experiencing internal strife; and highlights various key idioms that encapsulate these values and ideals of comportment, which are manifested in childrearing practices, personal demeanor, and interpersonal relationships (Bateson & Mead, 1942; Belo, 1970; Browne, 2001; H. Geertz, 1961, 1974; Hollan, 1988, 1992; Hollan & Wellenkamp, 1994; Keeler, 1983, 1987; Subandi, 2006; Wikan, 1990).

This down-regulation of anger or conflict is active for all members of Balinese culture in most contexts, but is gendered as it applies most strongly to women, who are expected to be decorous and deferent. In describing her episodes of mental illness, Ketut says problems arise "when my heart wants me to go to the mountain and my family wants me to go to the sea" (http://vimeo.com/album/3014164/video/104663438), a muted metaphor for conflict that calls upon Balinese topographical features.[3]

Anger may be equally inappropriate for a Javanese man. In the Javanese *habitus*, expressions of anger indicate a loss, not an exercise, of power as the Javanese view power as an "attractive rather than coercive force" (Keeler, 1987), more typically exhibited through self-mastery, restraint, and the modeling of refined behavior (Anderson, 1972; Stange, 1984). Counter-hegemonic readings of Javanese masculinity suggest that while lauded for their leadership in public, in private, Javanese husbands should defer to their wives (Brenner, 1995). In times of frustration or mood instability, Bambang does not fit either of these models of Javanese masculinity; instead, his temper flares. Yatmi sees these outbursts as indicative of Bambang's difficulty in comporting himself as a proper man (http://vimeo.com/album/3014164/video/104663549).

The complex interplay of personal subjectivity and cultural context constructs a phenomenology of mental illness in relationship to anger and conflict. A certain level of conflict is an unavoidable part of life; yet, because of its psychocultural construction, the expression of anger that in other cultures might seem healthy (e.g., "blowing off some steam") in Java and Bali can be read as disordered or sick. Classic and contemporary arguments in social anthropology have attempted to link the repression of anger and conflict in Indonesia with functional or nonfunctional dissociation, mental illness, and psychotic symptoms (Bateson & Mead, 1942; Browne, 2001; Connor, 1979; Good, 2012; Good & Good, 2008; Good, Good, & Subandi, 2007; Hollan, 2000; Suryani, 1984). Of course, in the case of major mental illness, symptoms of aggression, poor

---

[3] The directions of *kaja*, toward the holy mountain of *Gunung Agung* located inland, and *kelod*, outward toward the water, are potent organizers of physical, social, and spiritual space in Bali (Eiseman & Eiseman, 1989).

impulse control, and the like are significantly biologically driven, mean-ing that culture is not "causing" psychosis. Yet, neither is it irrelevant; anger *is* likely to be viewed as pathological in both the community at large and by Javanese and Balinese clinical staff. The loss of control and detachment from social norms signaled by explicit expressions of conflict may indicate that a person's emotional states are unmanageable or that he or she has lost touch with a cultural reality, and thus may be a sign of mental illness (Browne, 2001; Hollan, 1988).

In addition to anger, Ketut explicitly experiences shame (B.I., *malu*) as a trigger, saying, "If I have too much shame I go crazy"(http://vimeo.com/album/3014164/video/104664358). *Malu* may in some contexts be similar to the Western understanding of shame, a negative reactive emotional state associated with embarrassment and guilt when a person cannot uphold social norms or requirements. But *malu* may also connote active and vigilant processes of preventing shame, a kind of "stage fright" or anxiety over the possibility of social awkwardness, insult, or poor role performance in the ongoing negotiation of status, signaling the complex emotional and mental labor associated with shame in Balinese (C. Geertz, 1973) and Javanese (Keeler, 1983) cultures.

Religious systems and related ideologies, practices, and *habitus* may provide shared and positively valenced frameworks to interpret and manage conflict, shame, and/or mental distress in Indonesia (Browne, 2001), and both Ketut and Bambang report drawing strength from their faith (http://vimeo.com/album/3014164/video/104664708). But religion may also be a source of distress; Bambang's religious obsessions provided context for hallucinations that were suffused with anxiety, while for Ketut, gendered expectations embedded into religious practice overlapped with her own personal histories of burden. Therefore, religious beliefs, practices, and institutions influence patients' emotions, states of consciousness, and sense of self in myriad complex ways; and they intersect with different components of mental illness subjectivity and symptomatology.

Gendered Responsibilities and Gender Identities as Stressors

Bali is known as one of the most ritually dense cultures in the world, with a calendar marked by annual, monthly, and bimonthly rituals, as well as holy days, honor days, and large-scale rituals to mark important life cycle events (Lansing 1994). An integral element of Balinese ritual is the making of *sesajen*, or devotional offerings, from flowers, food, coins, and incense. These offerings are rich with symbolic references to the life cycle and Hindu philosophy and are believed to confer wellbeing and prevent suffering (Bateson, 1972).

As previously mentioned, a wide variety of personal and family ills are interpreted as having their etiology in improperly performed rituals (Lemelson, 2004) and therefore many families go into debt ensuring that a ritual ceremony, complete with many offerings, is performed in a timely and appropriate manner. This places a significant responsibility on Balinese women, who are tasked with making the offerings and, by extension, preserving the health of their families and communities. Given the required physical labor; time; and spiritual, emotional, and financial investment required to make offerings and fulfill family obligations – combined with the over-determined significance of ritual in Balinese family and community life – ceremonies may become not just culturally elaborated festivities, but also culturally marked stressors (Connor, 1995; Wikan, 1990). Ketut identifies rituals as her biggest triggers of psychotic episodes, as she worries about whether her family can make the necessary preparations and contributions, anticipates shame if they cannot, and experiences flashbacks to her childhood where she felt overwhelmed with burdens. When she is having a "fit" or manic episode, Ketut often channels her extra energy into industriously making offerings for the gods (http://vimeo.com/album/3014164/video/104665935).

Bambang's illness experience is similarly colored by gendered expectations and responsibilities, although his challenges arise in the context of Jakarta's rapidly globalizing economy and the corollary new middle-class ideal of the masculine provider. Historically, in many Javanese households, women have been valued entrepreneurs and primary breadwinners (Brenner, 1995). However, the Indonesian urban middle class has grown exponentially over the last decade, along with the globalized ideal of the nuclear family, now heavily promoted in the media and popular culture, with father as sole provider of modern consumer goods (Nilan, 2001, 2009). Bambang frequently voices the tensions and discomforts that emerge around his perceived economic failures as a husband. He says,

Bill Gates himself started in his garage, but he's been able to take over the world. ... What makes me feel a bit negative is that I just stay at home, my income is just a fraction of what my wife makes. [...] Why, as a husband, can I not meet the needs of my family?

Unfortunately, the tasks required to fulfill the role obligations of a middle-class Indonesian man, such as working long hours in a high-pressure office environment, have triggered Bambang's illness. Bambang wants to reenter the workforce, but has low self-confidence and worries about future relapses. The family has successfully adjusted by allowing Bambang to care for his son at home while his wife supports them by working in a factory. The domestic tasks that Bambang performs are integral to the functioning of the family, but they make him feel "useless" because doing "women's work" feels demeaning, and he is no longer treated as a decision-making "head of the household." Therefore, beyond a sense of economic failure, Bambang laments the loss of gendered role status, which compounds his depressive episodes. Bambang's return in 2006 to teaching English part-time seems to have been therapeutic in easing some of these tensions. Although this job is neither full-time nor particularly lucrative, its prestige allows Bambang to feel like his wife "has a husband" again (http://vimeo.com/album/3014164/video/104665064).

Cultural Influences on Recovery: Tradition and Globalization

In both Ketut's and Bambang's lives, we can see the complex, contextualized, and at times unexpected interplay of gender, cultural life, and mental illness. Understanding the local and global dynamics of shifting gender roles within the family and cultural niches as sources of personal competence and self-esteem may be essential for promoting the recovery of individuals with severe mental disorders.

Family Interpretations and Accommodations

Families may act as stressors, especially in sociocultural contexts like those described above, in which negative emotions must be internally managed and carefully suppressed. However, families often act as protective buffers as well. Three types of family-related factors appear over and over to explain better course and outcome: destigmatizing illness beliefs, supportive kin networks, and flexible and accommodating work routines (Beels, 1989; Cohen, Hammen, Henry & Daley, 2004; Corin, 1998; Corin & Lauzon, 1992; Corrigan & Watson, 2002; Evans & Repper, 2000; Hopper, 1991; Jenkins, 1991; Link et al., 2001; Waxler, 1979). These three traits have consistently been found in Indonesian and Malay families of the mentally ill (Kraeplin, 1921; Jilek, 1995; Pfeiffer 1967), and all three are clearly operative in the cases of Ketut and Bambang.

Western psychiatric nosology is variably changing the ways that people think about their own health and penetrating into local social concepts of mental illness and recovery. To a certain extent, both Ketut and Bambang have accepted psychiatric labels for themselves;

Ketut describes herself as periodically mentally ill (B.I., *sakit jiwa*), and Bambang identifies both as being "schizoaffective" (using the English term) and as someone with a "mental disability" (B.I., *cacat mental*), having deeply internalized globalized frameworks for selfhood and mental illness. However, labels are not only the result of self-identification; they are also negotiated in strategic decision-making by family members (Jenkins & Karno, 1992). Significantly, despite mobilizing a diagnosis to procure medication and periodic institutional care when needed, both families actively avoided stigmatizing labels for Ketut and Bambang, instead normalizing their experiences and behaviors. Ketut's son explained,

> In Indonesia it's "crazy." But we don't make assumptions like that. We see our mother as having too many burdens on her thoughts, and anyone can experience such a thing. My mother's family still says, 'This woman is sick like this because she indeed has many burdens.' There isn't a problem.

Bambang's aunt similarly normalizes his experience by saying,

> He was taken back to the family community in Central Java because he was ill, suffering from stress. How could he live in Jakarta, if he suffered from stress it would be hard to live there. [...] But in Java, in this region, most people still have pity on a person who suffers from stress, that's the point.

In avoiding conflating symptoms with selves, both families emphasize the transient quality of mental illness, leaving room for periods of stability and lucidity and underscoring a sense of continuity to Bambang and Ketut's daily lives. This keeps a variety of social roles open to them during periods of recovery, in contrast to the progressive role restriction that often comes to define those with major mental illness elsewhere (Corrigan, 2005; Goffman, 1959; Goldberg, 2012; Estroff, 1989; Perry, 2011; Sarbin & Mancuso, 1970, p. 168; Schomerus et al., 2012).

Furthermore, in the collectivist and interdependent societies of Java and Bali, the kin network is considered profoundly significant in determining the behavior or outcome of any individual, and therefore the responsibility for cure is shared. While both Bambang's and Ketut's families did obtain institutional care, they *themselves* also played a key therapeutic role, exhibiting a collective approach to recovery and offering flexible adaptations to allow for ongoing contribution to family life and fulfillment of meaningful duties. Ketut's son says, "*We* make efforts for her to recover," emphasizing the investment and effort of the family unit evident in actions like monitoring Ketut, keeping her away from potential triggers, and striving to foster her balanced state. Bambang's family responded to his illness collectively as well. His aunt explained, "I guess when he gets sick, as Indonesians, we can't let him suffer by

himself." Indeed, traditional healing throughout Indonesia often incorporates the entire family unit (Ferzacca, 2001; Salan & Maretzki, 1983;
Jensen & Suryani, 1992). In such instances of collective approaches
to health and well-being, family members will mobilize to help cure
the sick person, rather than blaming, punishing, or isolating them
(Estroff, 1981, p. 246); this is significant since critical attitudes or hostile
interactions seem to increase the rate of relapse or negative outcome
(Barrowclough & Hooley, 2003; Bebbington & Kuipers, 1994; Kuipers &
Moore, 1995).

These forgiving explanations and accommodations are bolstered by
local understandings of the etiologies of mental disturbance. As evident
above, both families interpret mental illness as the result of "stress" and/
or "too many burdens," conditions to which practically everyone is seen
as being vulnerable. Accordingly, both families respond by trying to
preserve the peace of mind of their disturbed member. Kin and villagers
adapt to Ketut's shifting needs and capabilities, affording her duties when
she can handle them and easing such expectations when she cannot. The
ritual, childcare, and other responsibilities that Ketut and her family
undertake as part of their daily labor provide opportunities for a gradual
and successful reintegration after episodes of mental illness. Indeed, in
traditional village settings and agrarian subsistence economies, work is less
segmented from other areas of social life, less competitive and often
collectively organized, and undertaken alongside kin networks, making it
more accommodating than industrial or office labor. Despite the fact that
Bambang was working in a wage economy and unable to keep his office
job due to his episodes, his family allowed him to take responsibility at
home until he found more flexible employment. Both families seem to
understand that the ability to continue doing meaningful work with a
schedule that accommodates periods of disability is essential to supporting
mental health; indeed WHO and others have demonstrated that a flexible
work routine is a main predictive factor of better outcome (Hopper et al.,
2007).

The integral role of family and community support points to urban
migration as a potential stressor for those with mental illness because it
removes individuals from stable, accommodating, and supportive networks (Lin & Kleinman, 1988), as well as the chance for an ongoing
sense of relevant and successful contribution. Urban migration also
requires migrants to contend with new economic and social models of
self-reliance and competition and potential sensory overstimulation
(McKenzie & Shah, Chapter 13, *this volume*). Indeed, in other narratives
of mental illness in Indonesia, a disappointing or otherwise upsetting
relocation to urban centers is similarly associated with psychotic episodes

(cf. Good, Good & Subandi, 2007). This has implications not just for onset of mental illness, but also for treatment and recovery. Institutionalized care in Indonesia is often only available in urban centers (Pols, 2006). Although the better institutions are able to provide integrated treatment (including medication and psychotherapy), they may still be experienced as deeply isolating. Bambang abandoned institutional care numerous times – failing to complete a full course of treatment – because he was lonely. Meanwhile, being treated at home or nearby, if home is in a small town where people have known a patient their whole lives, allows for the restoration of social support and therefore may be instrumental in a return to stability (Hopper et al., 2007, p. 279).

Bambang's and Ketut's experiences attest to the benefits of family care; however, this, too, comes with challenges as people with major mental illness may upset others, especially if their symptoms do not fit with vernacular models of disturbance (e.g., spirit possession). During previous illness episodes, Bambang has switched off his neighbors' electricity in an attempt to "save" them from rising energy costs, urinated inside a mosque, and made obscene gestures at schoolgirls, for which he was beaten to the point of having his front teeth knocked out. Even family members with the best intentions may not know how to respond to such behavior, occasionally resorting to shackling or confinement (B.I., *pasung*) (Minas & Diatri, 2008) to keep their family member safe and out of trouble.

Post-Colonial Subjectivities and Mental Health

Ketut and Bambang's lives, including their episodes of illness and recovery, have unfolded not only within their family context but also within the broader sweeping socioeconomic and political changes that Indonesia has experienced over the past half-century, illustrating the personal repercussions of political and economic instability. Major events, such as the war for independence, the mass killings of 1965, the economic crisis and political chaos of 1998–9 – and the culturally inflected reactions to these – have deep personal effects on the lives of individual Indonesians suffering from mental illness (Dwyer & Santikarma, 2007; Lemelson, 2008; Lemelson, Kirmayer, & Barad, 2007). Although it is quite possible that Ketut or Bambang had genetic and other biological vulnerabilities – Bambang in particular postulated that his father's death in a brawl may have been the result of manic behavior – these traumatic historical events have influenced each individual's developmental trajectory, alongside their personal, familial, and communal resources and responses to illness and recovery.

The Dutch colonized Indonesia for centuries, although their domination and influence was regionally variable. Where they did have solid control, they instituted labor exploitation, segregation, and discrimination that kept many Indonesians impoverished. As a revolutionary Indonesian nationalist movement was growing, the country was swept into World War II; independence was declared in 1945, but the country remained occupied and the indigenous population fought against Japanese, Dutch, and British forces until 1949. The entire nation was strained by wartime conditions of extreme food shortages, ongoing violence, and instability.

Ketut's father was captured and imprisoned while fighting for Indonesian independence. Rituals are triggering for Ketut, particularly because they evoke this formative episode in her childhood when these historical and personal circumstances forced her into a role of premature responsibility. The neurobiology of stress has provided insight into the seemingly atypical chronology of trauma, where past and present distresses are folded into one another through flashbacks, reexperiencing events, or "kindling" (Hinton, Howes, & Kirmayer, 2008). Culturally, personally, and historically determined frameworks of attribution and interpretation intertwine and interact with emerging sensations, thoughts, or emotions in complex loops that can amplify, mute, link, or generate new sensations and create meaning for the person experiencing them (Hinton & Kirmayer, 2013; Kirmayer & Sartorius, 2007; Kirmayer & Young, 1998). The loop of anxiety and attention is most significant; certain feelings or sensations are unpleasant and cause high alert, yet constantly scanning for, thinking about, or attending to such feelings may cause them to intensify. Factors that affect which feelings or sensations deserve such close attention include ethnopsychology, traumatic memory, interpersonal relationships, and self-image.

In Ketut's case, current family obligation stressors are amplified by her personal history of trauma and responsibility, confounding present with past anxieties, and reminding Ketut of her grief at being forced to abandon her schooling, causing her to say she feels "empty and mournful" at the lost opportunity. Furthermore, the ritual and economic burdens Ketut was forced to undertake were folded into the emotional and physical stressors of war: both the sociohistorical milieu of anxiety and violence and physiological responses to hunger and starvation may have amplified her stress at that time. Meanwhile, as described above, feelings of shame are particularly weighted in Balinese culture; therefore, the threat of shame is likely to lead to heightened attention and arousal.

In an interesting counterpoint to Ketut's direct embodied experience, some of Bambang's recurring anxieties speak to histories of colonization that he did not personally undergo. In one extended episode, he calls Indonesia "the Dutch territory," and ironically muses, "The Dutch occupied us in order to teach us." Yet he simultaneously references a history of resistance, claiming, "I am the 13th grandson of Prince Diponegoro," assuming the identity of a Mataram Prince who fought against Dutch colonization from 1825 to 1830 and was exiled. When Bambang meets Lemelson, the film's director – a Euro-American – he at first teases, "You want to invade my country!" Later, he enacts a fascinating metonymic transfer of mental illness, saying "Bye-bye, schizophrenia," symbolically relocating pathology onto the surrogate colonizing body in order to banish it. Yet at the same time, Bambang gleefully welcomes the opportunity to practice his English and perform his broad cosmopolitan knowledge that just might have the power to change him from being "schizoaffective" to being "effective."

His continuous verbal productions weave together such diverse threads as lyrics from 1980s pop songs, Qur'anic verse, Sukarno's development maxims, global trade, and local news, creating a strikingly insightful lexical fabric of historical and political commentary. Although from a strictly diagnostic perspective these seeming nonsequiturs might be read as the epiphenomena of more fundamental cognitive changes associated with manic and psychotic processes, the cultural context for these verbal productions allows for a more meaningful interpretation of them than merely as symptoms of loose associations or a flight of ideas (http://vimeo.com/album/3014164/video/104665174).

There is a long literature exploring the connections between mental illness and the oppression of colonial subjugation, which may lead to hypervigilance, an inferiority complex, and the sense of an unstable split identity or "dual consciousness" (Fanon, 1952; Jameson, 1991; Nandy, 1983, 1995). Ironically, colonial discourses often framed the indigenous subject as "disordered" or "mad" and occupying powers as there to impose "order"; but of course, this pretext of "order" was used to carry out all kinds of violence (Good, Hyde, Pinto, & Good, 2008). In Indonesia, those who protested the Dutch order – such as domestic servants who rebelled against their masters or plantation workers who organized – were labeled as madly "running amok" (Browne, 2001; Good & Good, 2008; Simons, 2001). In this milieu of oppression, some registered their discontent through passive resistance and verbal rebellion. In listening to Bambang, historians might be reminded of the Samins, nineteenth-century Indonesian plantation workers, who wore down the resolve of their Dutch overseers through evasive double entendres and cryptic puns. For example, a Samin who was ordered to work might not outright refuse, but rather reply, "Sorry, I am already in service, my work is sex with my wife" (Vickers, 2005, p. 43).

The references to colonial domination and resistance folded into Bambang's manic monologues indicate that painful histories continue to "haunt" (Good, 2012) the subjective worlds of citizens who did not directly experience colonial rule.[4] In twenty-first-century urban Indonesia, these persistent hauntings collide with the excesses of global-ized culture, its alternate narratives of development and possibility, and its own structural inequalities. As Homi Bhabha puts it, the "colonial shadow falls across the successes of globalization" as economic policies create and perpetuate divided worlds (Bhabha, 2004, p. xii). Especially since Suharto's fall in the late 1990s, when censorship loosened and a sense of liberating self-expression bloomed, Indonesian citizens have enthusiastically participated in global discourses of identity politics and capitalistic self-fashioning (Boellstorff, 2005; Heryanto, 1999, 2008; Vickers, 2005). Yet access to far-reaching global media networks also implicates ordinary citizens in global struggles, stoking everyday worry with unrelenting representations of enduring violence and inequality, which then take root in personal experiences of distress. For Bambang, ambivalence about colonialism, globalization, and his own subject position seems to trigger interpenetrating affects that cycle quickly. It is worth noting that his most severe episode of mental illness in 1999 corresponded with a pan-Asian economic crisis and a national political transition, when markets were starting to "collapse" and everything was "going crazy" all over the country, as frustrated Indonesians rioted en masse. During his "flight of ideas," Bambang negotiates the euphoria and grief of a globalized subjectivity saying, "The most disturbed patient, his name is 'The World.'" His poignant diagnosis points to contemporary society's "com-plex, conflicting, and potentially disorienting cognitive requirements" and the harrowing assignment of individual responsibility in negotiating these (Sass, 1992) as precipitating either a vertiginous psychosis or an unsettling insight into the workings of the contemporary world (Sass, 2007), or both.

---

[4] The postcolonial political violence that erupted in Indonesia's early national history, which led to Suharto's New Order regime, is equally traumatic. Many families experienced violence and stigma during the mass killings of 1965 and afterwards (Cribb, 1990, 2002; Lemelson, 2008; Lemelson, Kirmayer, & Barad, 2007; Lemelson, Supartini, & Ng, 2010), traumas that are woven into both Ketut and Bambang's stories; for example, Yatmi says that she felt well-equipped to deal with Bambang's mental illness because her own father had a condition – making him uncomfortable around strangers, reluctant to leave the house, and persistently afraid – that she believes stemmed from the 1965 purge of communists, during which many of his friends were imprisoned or killed.

Global Mental Health Economies

Throughout the course of their illnesses, Bambang and Ketut have received various therapeutic interventions: family care in the home, institutional treatment, ongoing outpatient pharmacological therapy, traditional healing (http://vimeo.com/album/3014164/video/104665326), and occasional counseling. In this diverse landscape of mental illness response, they and their families have mobilized both globalized and locally coherent concepts of health and disturbance and participated in local and global economies of care and recovery, which variably influence ideas and behaviors relating to preferred treatment, self-concept, and course of mental illness.

Both Ketut and Bambang avail themselves of pharmaceutical treatment to manage their symptoms, but the use of medication is not unproblematic for them. Ketut is being treated with the long-term antipsychotic, Thorazine, which is most useful in treating schizophrenia. Ketut does have some symptoms that overlap with schizophrenia; when she is having an episode, Ketut starts to feel that "this world is a world of treachery," and fears that people aim to harm her (http://vimeo.com/album/3014164/video/104665465). However, in this case, disentangling paranoid ideations from the local context is a complex endeavor. Psychological anthropologist Theodore Schwartz coined the notion of the "paranoid ethos" (Schwartz, 1973) to indicate a generalized response to uncertainty prevalent amongst Melanesian and Pacific societies, and, to a certain extent, operative in Indonesia: Misfortune is attributed to the ill intent of other community members and supernatural beings. In Bali, there is pervasive belief in black magic, and black magic may be one of the most commonly understood causes of illness in traditional healing, with the illness onset or abnormal behavior often interpreted as the result of jealous extended family members using magic to cause harm or exact revenge (Connor, 1982; Watson & Ellen, 1993; Lemelson, 2003, 2004; Wikan, 1990). This vernacular understanding of black magic as a causal factor for symptoms of mental illness explains why Ketut would feel suspicious when she starts to feel ill, and why rituals involving contact with relatives and in-laws who might harbor secret bad intentions against her would cause fear, without requiring recourse to biological explanations.

It is possible that bipolar disorder, which causes unusual shifts in mood, energy, sleep patterns, and the ability to carry out day-to-day tasks, is the more accurate diagnosis for Ketut's condition. Bipolar disorder is usually treated with a mood-stabilizer such as lithium. However, lithium treatment is more difficult to implement than an antipsychotic regimen because its narrow range of efficacy and potential toxicity require regularly monitoring blood levels. Currently, the few laboratories capable of measuring blood lithium levels in Indonesia are in urban areas, making such monitoring expensive and inconvenient. The first generation of antipsychotic medications, the phenothiazines, have been used for decades instead of lithium, but they do not have the same efficacy in bipolar disorder, and they cause other side effects, including tardive dyskinesia (TD), which in Ketut's case involves uncontrollable movements of the mouth and eyebrows. These side effects are stigmatizing in her community, and have led to long-term stiffness and pain in Ketut's jaw. It has been said that the "injudicious chronic use" of antipsychotics produces much higher rates of TD in the developing world (Burns, 2009); in fact, Ketut perceives this iatrogenic harm as her most troubling symptom (http://vimeo.com/album/3014164/video/104665715).

Although not leading to noticeable physical side effects, Bambang's use of medication has also deeply affected his sense of self. Along with internalizing an identity of someone who is "mentally handicapped," Bambang has also accepted an ongoing dependency on medication, saying that he must take medication as ordered by the doctors and admit to himself that he is ill and will never fully recover. This echoes the psychopharmacological discourse stressed and repeated in multiple contexts such as medication advertisements, sales pitches by drug company representatives, research and training conferences paid for by the pharmaceutical industry, and the orientation of hospitals and clinics where medical staff have been trained in Western biomedical treatment modalities (Applbaum, Chapter 21, *this volume*).

Clearly, globalized models of mental health care provision and the global psychopharmacological trade penetrate deeply into subjects' lives, causing physical and/or psychological side effects (Jenkins, 2010). The WHO's Determinants of Outcomes of Severe Mental Disorders (DOSMD) study ended in 1992, before the rush of globalization and its onslaught of new media, technology, and economic systems, which have deeply influenced peoples' personal imagery, goals, and sense of efficacy and worth in reorganized labor markets, family systems, and responses to mental distress. Globalized health care has brought with it a host of hegemonic symbols and messages that inform individuals' ideas about the chronicity of mental illness and its formative relationship to the self. Indeed, a failure of patients to incorporate these ideas or to agree with the "medical-model, disease-entity perspective of oneself" as having a psychiatric illness is often interpreted as an additional symptom, quite commonly found in schizophrenic patients, as "lack of insight" (Sass,

2007); this despite evidence that insight, defined as the attitude toward changes in the self due to mental illness, is culturally construed and frequently contested by patients and their families (Kirmayer, Corin, & Jarvis, 2004; Tranulis, Corin, & Kirmayer, 2008).

The comparison between Ketut and Bambang becomes particularly compelling in relationship to globalization. Although there is a strong influence of Western ideas, culture, and "modernization" on Bali, particularly in the south, much of the island has maintained the integrity of traditional cultural beliefs. In many ways, Ketut's experience of mental illness is deeply "Balinese": her illness is triggered by temple ritual obligations; her symptoms are expressed in agrarian and geographical imagery of place and orientation; and she wrestles with negatively valenced emotions of anger, suspicion, and shame. Perhaps most significantly, while accepting a biomedical label and biomedical treatment for her troubles, Ketut and her family have not accepted mental illness as an inherent part of her identity. Meanwhile, the many globalized features of Bambang's experience are quite central to his illness and recovery narrative, including institutionalized care, economic expectations in a rapidly changing urban environment, and the pervasive presence of global popular culture in his imagination. Along with these other influences, Bambang clearly has internalized his "mental disability" and identifies with his Western psychiatric diagnosis, leading him to think of himself as "mentally handicapped." Despite this, certain elements of Bambang's illness experience could be considered "Javanese," perhaps most significantly the active role and recuperative power that family support has played in his recovery.

Even amidst rapid globalization and socioeconomic change, therefore, certain cultural models of response may persist because they are effective for coping with illness or achieving other personal and socially important goals and values. Indeed, in many ways Ketut and Bambang's situations very closely resemble the WHO IPSS and DOSMD's description of ideal "communities of recovery" as "stigma-free havens, blessed by forgiving beliefs [about] psychiatric disorder, and ready stores of supportive kin and accommodating work" (Hopper et al., 2007, pp. 278–9). In trying to close the treatment gap for people living with mental and neurological disorders, service providers need to build on these local models in order to ensure that cultural benefits, as we have been able to outline them in this chapter, are not threatened or eroded by efforts to provide "better" care. Scholars and service providers need to look beyond the clinical confines of psychiatry in order to incorporate the benefits of these local models of support; if we do not, the disruption of social networks that often accompanies economic growth and increasing globalization, and the instantiation of the biomedical psychiatric illness model, may result in increased disability and diminished quality of life for those with major mental illnesses, despite increasing access to institutional and pharmacological treatment (Hopper et al., 2007). Bambang's case suggests that the narrowed vision of globalized psychiatric care, which emphasizes neurophysiological monitoring of symptoms and biological models of mental illness, may bring with it restrictive labels and a narrowing sense of self and possibility (Haslam, 2000, 2005; Harré & Read, 2001; Walker & Read, 2002).

Conclusion

A number of factors play differing roles in the life course and illness outcome of Ketut and Bambang: family support; labeling of illness; access to different forms of treatment; community understandings and interpretations of illness symptoms and course; individual expression of illness phenomenology; the effects of a changing political economy; and, finally, the increasingly ever-present effects of globalization. These two cases show that cultural milieu colors the content of symptomatology and shapes idioms of expression, while cultural values determine the regulation and interpretation of affect and influence labels and social roles that are available to the ill person. The two families we have discussed support and accommodate their mentally ill members through empathetic responses to distress, collective and collaborative approaches to illness and recovery, and occupational accommodations to preserve self-worth and community integration. These accommodations are crucial, although certainly not seamless. Meanwhile, broader processes of change interact with embodied systems of knowledge and culture, as well as with personal vulnerabilities, to trigger mental illness as individual psyches (already challenged with complex tasks such as nation building or negotiating the disruptions of urbanization) deal with the residues of colonialism and historical trauma. Amidst these complex conditions, globalized mental health treatment – pharmaceuticals, institutionalization, and the mobilization of "psychiatric illness" in self-concept – is taken up and put to use in various ways that may support or threaten recovery and long-term well-being.

Ethnographic methods in general, and the *Affliction* film series in particular, go against reductive trends in the provision of psychiatric care to consider a wide range of factors salient to the experience, study, and treatment of mental illness. The case studies discussed here illustrate key issues that join individual biological and biographical vulnerabilities, society, and culture in the phenomenology, study, and treatment of mental illness in a global context. They also model longitudinal visual ethnographic methods that are particularly useful in illustrating such connections. Indeed, this analysis reinforces the notion that culture is critical in nearly every aspect of major mental illness experience (Jenkins & Barrett, 2004), providing compelling evidence for why ethnographic methodologies remain crucial for understanding psychiatric illness in the twenty-first century (Roepstorff, 2013). Meanwhile, the integration of visual material with the written text serves as a model for innovation within this methodology and invites other ethnographers to "revision" the work of psychological anthropology and transcultural psychiatry. Visual methods of data collection and presentation are able to capture the "particularities of the 'local,'" (Hopper et al., 2007, p. 280) individual, and subjective experiences of mental illness, evoking internal and cultural worlds and presenting subjects within complex lives that are affected, but not delimited, by their mental illness diagnoses.

Ethnography remains crucial for creating integrative social and neuroscientific methodologies that can encompass the complexity of the social worlds and phenomenology of mental illness. Ethnography is needed to identify crucial issues and tell how they are related to each other in particular social contexts. If, as we have suggested, the categories, issues, factors, and domains that are identified in the course of detailed, experience-near, person-centered ethnography are directly related to better health outcomes, then attending to these dimensions will provide an essential component of policies that aim to positively affect the treatment and care of the mentally ill.

REFERENCES

American Psychiatric Association. (2013). *Diagnostic and statistical manual of mental disorders* (5th ed.). Washington, DC: Author.
Anderson, B. R. O'G. (1972). The idea of power in Javanese culture. In C. Holt (Ed.), *Culture and politics in Indonesia* (pp. 1–70). Ithaca, NY: Cornell University Press.
Applbaum, K. (2015). Solving global mental health as a delivery problem: Toward a critical epistemology of the solution. In L. J. Kirmayer, R. Lemelson, & C. A. Cummings (Eds.), *Re-visioning psychiatry: Cultural phenomenology, critical neuroscience, and global mental health* (pp. 544–74). New York, NY: Cambridge University Press.
Barrowclough, C., & Hooley, J. M. (2003). Attributions and expressed emotion: A review. *Clinical Psychology Review, 23*(6), 849–80. http://dx.doi.org/10.1016/S0272-7358(03)00075-8
Bateson, G. (1972). *Steps to an ecology of mind.* New York, NY: Ballantine.
Bateson, G., & Mead, M. (1942). *Balinese character: A photographic analysis.* New York, NY: New York Academy of Sciences.

Bebbington, P., & Kuipers, L. (1994). The predictive utility of expressed emotion in schizophrenia: An aggregate analysis. *Psychological Medicine, 24*(3), 707–18. http://dx.doi.org/10.1017/S0033291700027860

Beels, C. C. (1989). The invisible village. *New Directions for Mental Health Services, 1989*(42), 27–40. http://dx.doi.org/10.1002/yd.23319894205

Belo, J. (1970). *Traditional Balinese culture.* New York, NY: Columbia University Press.

Berrettini, W. (2003). Evidence for shared susceptibility in bipolar disorder and schizophrenia [Special issue: The genetics of bipolar disorder]. *American Journal of Medical Genetics Part C: Seminars in Medical Genetics, 123C*(1), 59–64. http://dx.doi.org/10.1002/ajmg.c.20014

Bhabha, H. (2004). *The location of culture* (2nd ed.). Oxford, England: Routledge Classics.

Bilder, R. M. (2015). Dimensional and categorical approaches to mental illness: Let biology decide. In L. J. Kirmayer, R. Lemelson, & C. A. Cummings (Eds.), *Re-visioning psychiatry: Cultural phenomenology, critical neuroscience, and global mental health* (pp. 179–205). New York, NY: Cambridge University Press.

Blackwood, D., Fordyce, A., Walker, M. T., St. Clair, D. M., Porteous, D. J., & Muir, W. J. (2001). Schizophrenia and affective disorders: Cosegregation with a translocation at chromosome 1q42 that directly disrupts brain-expressed genes: clinical and P300 findings in a family. *American Journal of Human Genetics, 69*(2), 428–33. http://dx.doi.org/10.1086/321969

Boellstorff, T. (2005). *The gay archipelago: Sexuality and nation in Indonesia.* Princeton, NJ: Princeton University Press.

Brenner, S. (1995). Why women rule the roost: Rethinking Javanese ideologies of gender and self-control. In A. Ong (Ed.), *Bewitching women, pious men: Gender and body politics in Southeast Asia* (pp. 19–50). Berkeley, CA: University of California Press.

Browne, K. (2001). (Ng) amuk revisited: Emotional expression and mental illness in Central Java, Indonesia. *Transcultural Psychiatry, 38*(2), 147–65. http://dx.doi.org/10.1177/136346150103800201

Burns, J. (2009). Dispelling a myth: Developing world poverty, inequality, violence and social fragmentation are not good for outcome in schizophrenia. *African Journal of Psychiatry, 12*(3), 200–5. http://dx.doi.org/10.4314/ajpsy.v12i3.48494

Cohen, A. N., Hammen, C., Henry, R.M., & Daley, S.E. (2004). Effects of stress and social support on recurrence in bipolar disorder. *Journal of Affective Disorders, 82*(1), 143–7. http://dx.doi.org/10.1016/j.jad.2003.10.008

Connor, L. (1979). Corpse abuse and trance in Bali: The cultural mediation of aggression. *Mankind, 12*(2), 104–18.

Connor, L. (1982). The unbounded self: Balinese therapy in theory and practice. In A. J. Marsella & G. M. White (Eds.), *Cultural conceptions of mental health and therapy* (pp. 251–67). Boston, MA: Kluwer.

Connor, L. (1995). The action of the body on society: Washing a corpse in Bali. *Journal of the Royal Anthropological Institute, 1,* 537–59. http://dx.doi.org/10.2307/3034574

Corin, E. (1998). The thickness of being: Intentional worlds, strategies of identity, and experience among schizophrenics. *Psychiatry, 61*(2), 133–46.

Corin, E., & Lauzon, G. (1992). Positive withdrawal and the quest for meaning: The reconstruction of experience among schizophrenics. *Psychiatry: Interpersonal and Biological Processes, 55*(3), 266–78.

Corrigan, P. W. (2005). *On the stigma of mental illness: Practical strategies for research and social change.* Washington, DC: American Psychological Assocation.

Corrigan, P. W., & Watson, A. C. (2002). Understanding the impact of stigma on people with mental illness. *World Psychiatry, 1*(1), 16–20.

Cribb, R. B. (Ed.). (1990). *The Indonesian killings of 1965–1966: Studies from Java and Bali.* Clayton, Australia: Monash University Centre of Southeast Asian Studies.

Cribb, R. (2002). Unresolved problems in the Indonesian killings of 1965–1966. *Asian Survey, 42*(4), 550–63. http://dx.doi.org/10.1525/as.2002.42.4.550

Csordas, T. J. (1997). *The sacred self: A cultural phenomenology of charismatic healing.* Berkeley: University of California Press.

Csordas, T. J. (1999). Embodiment and cultural phenomenology. In G. Weiss & H. F. Haber (Eds.), *Perspectives on embodiment: The intersections of nature and culture* (pp. 143–62). New York, NY: Routledge.

Csordas, T. J. (2002). *Body/meaning/healing.* New York, NY: Palgrave Macmillan.

Csordas, T. J. (2015). Cultural phenomenology and psychiatric illness. In L. J. Kirmayer, R. Lemelson, & C. A. Cummings (Eds.), *Re-visioning psychiatry: Cultural phenomenology, critical neuroscience, and global mental health* (pp. 117–40). New York, NY: Cambridge University Press.

Desjarlais, R., & Throop, C. J. (2011). Phenomenological approaches in anthropology. *Annual Review of Anthropology, 40*, 87–102.

Dwyer, L., & Santikarma, D. (2007). Post-traumatic politics: Violence, memory, and biomedical discourse in Bali. In L. J. Kirmayer, R. Lemelson, & M. Barad (Eds.), *Understanding trauma: Integrating biological, clinical, and cultural perspectives* (pp. 403–32). New York, NY: Cambridge University Press. http://dx.doi.org/10.1017/CBO9780511500008.025

Edgerton, R. B. (1980). Traditional treatment for mental illness in Africa: A review. *Culture, Medicine, and Psychiatry, 4*(2), 167–89. http://dx.doi.org/10.1007/BF00051433

Edgerton, R. B. (1999). Perspectives from a varied career. *Ethos, 27*(1), 49–53. http://dx.doi.org/10.1525/eth.1999.27.1.49

Eiseman, F. B., & Eiseman, M. H. (1989). *Bali: sekala and niskala,* Hong Kong: Periplus Editions.

Estroff, S. (1981). *Making it crazy: An ethnography of psychiatric clients in an American community.* Berkeley: University of California Press.

Estroff, S. E. (1989). Self, identity, and subjective experiences of schizophrenia. *Schizophrenia Bulletin, 15*(2), 189–96. http://dx.doi.org/10.1093/schbul/15.2.189

Estroff, S. E., Lachicotte, W. S., Illingworth, L. C., & Johnston, A. (1991). Everybody's got a little mental illness: accounts of illness and self among people with severe, persistent mental illnesses. *Medical Anthropology Quarterly, 5*(4), 331–69. http://dx.doi.org/10.1525/maq.1991.5.4.02a00030

Evans, J., & Repper, J. (2000). Employment, social inclusion and mental health. *Journal of Psychiatric and Mental Health Nursing, 7*(1), 15–24. http://dx.doi.org/10.1046/j.1365-2850.2000.00260.x

Fanon, F. (1952/1994). *Black skin, white masks* (C. Farrington, Trans). New York, NY: Grove Press.

Ferzacca, S. (2001). *Healing the modern in a central Javanese city.* Durham, NC: Carolina Academic Press.

Geertz, C. (1973). Person, time, and conduct in Bali. In Geertz, *The interpretation of cultures* (pp. 360–411). New York, NY: Basic Books.

Geertz, H. (1961). *The Javanese family: A study of kinship and socialization.* New York, NY: Free Press of Glencoe.

Geertz, H. (1974). The vocabulary of emotion: A study of Javanese socialization process. In R. A. LeVine (Ed.), *Culture and personality: Contemporary readings* (pp. 249–64). Chicago, IL: Aldine.

Goffman, E. (1959). The moral career of the mental patient. *Psychiatry, 22*(2), 123–42.

Goldberg, S. G. (2012). Becoming the denigrated other: Group relations perspectives on initial reactions to a bipolar disorder diagnosis. *Frontiers in Psychology: Psychoanalysis and Neuropsychoanalysis, 3*(347). http://dx.doi.org/10.3389/fpsyg.2012.00347

Good, B. J. (2010). Medical anthropology and the problem of belief. In P. Shipton (Series Ed.), *Blackwell Anthologies in Social and Cultural Anthropology: Vol. 14. A reader in medical anthropology: Theoretical trajectories, emergent realities* (pp. 64–76). West Sussex, England: Wiley-Blackwell.

Good, B. J. (2012). Phenomenology, psychoanalysis, and subjectivity in Java. *Ethos, 40*(1), 24–36.

Good, M.-J. D., & Good, B. J. (2008). Indonesia sakit: Indonesian disorders and the subjective experience and interpretive politics of contemporary Indonesian artists. In M.-J. D. Good, S. T. Hyde, S. Pinto, & B. J. Good (Eds.), *Postcolonial disorders* (pp. 62–108). Berkeley: University of California Press.

Good, B. J., Good, M.-J. D., & Subandi. (2007). The subject of mental illness: Psychosis, mad violence, and subjectivity in Indonesia. In J. Biehl, B. Good, & A. Kleinman (Eds.), *Subjectivity: Ethnographic investigations* (pp. 243–72). Berkeley, CA: University of California Press.

Good, M.-J. D., Hyde, S. T., Pinto, S., & Good, B. J. (Eds.). (2008). *Postcolonial disorders.* Berkeley: University of California Press. http://dx.doi.org/10.1525/california/9780520252233.001.0001

Harré, N., & Read, J. (2001). The role of biological and genetic causal beliefs in the stigmatisation of 'mental patients'. *Journal of Mental Health, 10*(2), 223–35. http://dx.doi.org/10.1080/09638230123129

Haslam, N. (2000). Psychiatric categories as natural kinds: Essentialist thinking about mental disorder. *Social Research, 67*, 1031–58. www.jstor.org/stable/40971424

Haslam, N. (2005). Dimensions of folk psychiatry. *Review of General Psychology, 9*(1), 35–47. http://dx.doi.org/10.1037/1089-2680.9.1.35

Heryanto, A. (1999). The years of living luxuriously: Identity politics of Indonesia's new rich. In M. Pinches (Ed.), *Culture and privilege in capitalist Asia* (pp. 159–87). London, England: Routledge.

Heryanto, A. (Ed.). (2008). *Popular culture in Indonesia: Fluid identities in post-authoritarian politics.* London, England: Routledge.

Hinton, D. E., Howes, D., & Kirmayer, L. J. (2008). Toward a medical anthropology of sensations: Definitions and research agenda. *Transcultural Psychiatry, 45*(2), 142–62. http://dx.doi.org/10.1177/1363461508089763

Hinton, D. E., & Kirmayer, L. J. (2013). Local responses to trauma: Symptom, affect, and healing. *Transcultural Psychiatry, 50*(5), 607–21. http://dx.doi.org/10.1177/1363461513506529

Hollan, D. (1988). Staying "cool" in Toraja: Informal strategies for the management of anger and hostility in a nonviolent society. *Ethos, 16*(1), 52–72. http://dx.doi.org/10.1525/eth.1988.16.1.02a00030

Hollan, D. (1992). Emotion work and the value of emotional equanimity among the Toraja. *Ethnology, 31*(1), 45–56. http://dx.doi.org/10.2307/3773441

Hollan, D. (2000). Culture and dissociation in Toraja. *Transcultural Psychiatry, 37*(4), 545–59. http://dx.doi.org/10.1177/136346150003700404

Hollan, D. W., & Wellenkamp, J. (1994). *Contentment and suffering: Culture and experience in Toraja.* New York, NY: Columbia University Press.

Hopper, K. (1991). Some old questions for the new cross-cultural psychiatry. *Medical Anthropology Quarterly, 5*(4), 299–330. http://dx.doi.org/10.1525/maq.1991.5.4.02a00020

Hopper, K., Harrison, G., Janca, A., & Sartorius, N. (Eds.). (2007). *Recovery from schizophrenia: An international perspective.* A report from the WHO Collaborative Project, The International Study of Schizophrenia. Oxford, England: Oxford University Press.

Jablensky, A. (1990). Public health aspects of social psychiatry. In D. Goldberg & D. Tantam (Eds.), *The public health impact of mental disorder* (pp. 5–13). Toronto, ON: Hogrefe & Huber.

Jameson, F. (1991). *Postmodernism, or, the cultural logic of late capitalism.* Durham, NC: Duke University Press.

Jenkins, J. H. (1991). Anthropology, expressed emotion, and schizophrenia. *Ethos, 19*(4), 387–431. http://dx.doi.org/10.1525/eth.1991.19.4.02a00010

Jenkins, J. H. (Ed.). (2010). *Pharmaceutical self: The global shaping of experience in an age of psychopharmacology.* Sante Fe, NM: School for Advanced Research Press.

Jenkins, J. H., & Barrett, R. J. (2004). *Schizophrenia, culture, and subjectivity: The edge of experience.* Cambridge, England: Cambridge University Press.

Jenkins, J. H., & Karno, M. (1992). The meaning of expressed emotion: Theoretical issues raised by cross-cultural research. *American Journal of Psychiatry, 149*, 9–21.

Jensen, G. D., & Suryani, L.K. (1992). *The Balinese people: A reinvestigation of character.* Singapore: Oxford University Press.

Jilek, W. G. (1995). Emil Kraepelin and comparative sociocultural psychiatry. *European Archives of Psychiatry and Clinical Neuroscience, 245*(4–5), 231–8. http://dx.doi.org/10.1007/BF02191802

Keeler, W. (1983). Shame and stage fright in Java. *Ethos, 11*(3), 152–65. http://dx.doi.org/10.1525/eth.1983.11.3.02a00040

Keeler, W. (1987). *Javenese shadow plays, Javanese selves*. Princeton, NJ: Princeton University Press.

Kelsoe, J. R. (2003). Arguments for the genetic basis of the bipolar spectrum. *Journal of Affective Disorders, 73*(1), 183–97. http://dx.doi.org/10.1016/S0165-0327(02)00323-3

Kirmayer, L. J., (2009). Nightmares, neurophenomenology and the cultural logic of trauma. *Culture, Medicine, and Psychiatry, 33*(2), 323–31. http://dx.doi.org/10.1007/s11013-009-9136-4

Kirmayer, L. J., Corin, E., & Jarvis, G. E. (2004). Inside knowledge: Cultural constructions of insight in psychosis. In X. F. Amador & A. S. David (Eds.), *Insight and psychosis: Awareness of illness in schizophrenia and related disorders* (2nd ed., pp. 197–229). New York, NY: Oxford University Press.

Kirmayer, L. J., & Sartorius, N. (2007). Cultural models and somatic syndromes. *Psychosomatic Medicine, 69*(9), 832–40. http://dx.doi.org/10.1097/PSY.0b013e31815b002c

Kirmayer, L. J., Thombs, B. D., Jurcik, T., Jarvis, G. E., & Guzder, J. (2008). Use of an expanded version of the *DSM-IV* outline for cultural formulation on a cultural consultation service. *Psychiatric Services, 59*(6), 683–6. http://dx.doi.org/10.1176/appi.ps.59.6.683

Kirmayer, L. J., & Young, A. (1998). Culture and somatization: Clinical, epidemiological, and ethnographic perspectives. *Psychosomatic Medicine, 60*(4), 420–30. http://dx.doi.org/10.1097/00006842-199807000-00006

Kleinman, A. (1988). *The illness narratives: Suffering, healing and the human condition.* New York, NY: Basic Books.

Kleinman, A., & Kleinman, J. (1996). The appeal of experience; the dismay of images: Cultural appropriations of suffering in our times. *Daedalus 125*(1), 1–23.

Kraepelin, E. (1921). Manic-depressive insanity and paranoia [Book review]. *The Journal of Nervous and Mental Disease, 53*(4), 350. http://dx.doi.org/10.1097/00005053-192104000-00057

Kuipers, E., & Moore, E. (1995). Expressed emotion and staff–client relationships: Implications for community care of the severely mentally ill. *International Journal of Mental Health, 24*(3), 13–26.

Lansing, J. S. (1994). *The Balinese*. Stamford, CT: Cengage Learning.

Laughlin, C. D., & Throop, C. J. (2006). Cultural neurophenomenology: Integrating experience, culture and reality through fisher information. *Culture & Psychology, 12*(3), 305–37. http://dx.doi.org/10.1177/1354067X06067143

Lemelson, R. (2003). Obsessive-compulsive disorder in Bali: The cultural shaping of a neuropsychiatric disorder. *Transcultural Psychiatry, 40*(3), 377–408. http://dx.doi.org/10.1177/13634615030403004

Lemelson, R. (2004). Traditional healing and its discontents: Efficacy and traditional therapies of neuropsychiatric disorders in Bali. *Medical Anthropology Quarterly, 18*(1), 48–76. http://dx.doi.org/10.1525/maq.2004.18.1.48

Lemelson, R. (Producer & Director). (2008). *40 years of silence: An Indonesian tragedy* [Motion picture]. Watertown, MA: Documentary Educational Resources.

Lemelson, R. (2009). Dissatisfied seekers: Efficacy in traditional healing of neuropsychiatric disorders in Bali. In M. Incayawar, R. Wintrob, & L. Bouchard (Eds.), *Psychiatrists and traditional healers: Unwitting partners in global mental health* (pp. 179–96). West Sussex, England: Wiley.

Lemelson, R. (Producer & Director). (2011). *Memory of my face* [Motion picture]. Watertown, MA: Documentary Educational Resources.

Lemelson, R. (Producer & Director). (2011). *Ritual burdens* [Motion picture]. Watertown, MA: Documentary Educational Resources.

Lemelson, R., Kirmayer, L. J., & Barad, M. (2007). Trauma in context: Integrating biological, clinical, and cultural perspectives. In L. J. Kirmayer, R. Lemelson, & M. Barad (Eds.), *Understanding trauma: Integrating biological, clinical, and cultural perspectives* (pp. 451–74). New York, NY: Cambridge University Press.

Lemelson, R., Supartini, N., & Ng, E. (2010). Ethnographic case study. In C. M. Worthman, P. M. Plotsky, D. S. Schechter, & C. A. Cummings (Eds.), *Formative experiences: The Interaction of caregiving, culture, and developmental psychobiology* (pp. 378–89). New York, NY: Cambridge University Press. http://dx.doi.org/10.1017/CBO9780511711879.034

Lin, K.-M., & Kleinman, A. M. (1988). Psychopathology and clinical course of schizophrenia: A cross-cultural perspective. *Schizophrenia Bulletin, 14*(4), 555–67. http://dx.doi.org/10.1093/schbul/14.4.555

Link, B. G., Struening, E. L., Neese-Todd, S., Asmussen, S., & Phelan, J. C. (2001). Stigma as a barrier to recovery: The consequences of stigma for the self-esteem of people with mental illnesses. *Psychiatric Services, 52*(12), 1621–6. http://dx.doi.org/10.1176/appi.ps.52.12.1621

Luhrmann, T. M. (2011).Hallucinations and sensory overrides. *Annual Review of Anthropology, 40*, 71–85. http://dx.doi.org/10.1146/annurev-anthro-081309-145819

Luhrmann, T. M., Padmavati, R., Tharoor, H., & Osei, A. (2014). Differences in voice-hearing experiences of people with psychosis in the USA, India and Ghana: An interview-based study. *British Journal of Psychiatry, 205*(2). http://dx.doi.org/10.1192/bjp.bp.113.139048

Marková, I. S., & Berrios, G. E. (2009). Epistemology of mental symptoms. *Psychopathology, 42*(6), 343–9. http://dx.doi.org/10.1159/000236905

Marková, I. S., & Berrios, G. E. (2012). Epistemology of psychiatry. *Psychopathology, 45*(4), 220–7. http://dx.doi.org/10.1159/000331599

Martin, E. (2007). *Bipolar expeditions: Mania and depression in American culture.* Princeton, NJ: Princeton University Press.

McKenzie, J., & Shah, J., (2015). Understanding the social etiology of psychosis. In L. J. Kirmayer, R. Lemelson, & C. A. Cummings (Eds.), *Re-visioning psychiatry: Cultural phenomenology, critical neuroscience, and global mental health* (pp. 317–42). New York, NY: Cambridge University Press.

Mezzich, J. E., Caracci, G., Fabrega, H., Jr., & Kirmayer, L. J. (2009). Cultural formulation guidelines. *Transcultural Psychiatry, 46*(3), 383–405. http://dx.doi.org/10.1177/1363461509342942

Minas, H., & Diatri, H. (2008). Pasung: Physical restraint and confinement of the mentally ill in the community. *International Journal of Mental Health Systems, 2*(1), 1–5. http://dx.doi.org/10.1186/1752-4458-2-8

Nandy, A. (1983). Towards an alternative politics of psychology. *International Social Science Journal, 35*(2), 332–8.

Nandy, A. (1995). *The savage Freud and other essays on possible and retrievable selves.* Princeton, NJ: Princeton University Press.

Nilan, P. (2001). Gendered dreams: Women watching sinetron (soap operas) on Indonesian TV. *Indonesia and the Malay World, 29*(84), 85–98. http://dx. doi.org/10.1080/713672783

Nilan, P. (2009). Contemporary masculinities and young men in Indonesia. *Indonesia and the Malay World, 37*(109), 327–44. http://dx.doi.org/10.1080/13639810903269318

Obeyesekere, G. (1981). *Medusa's hair: An essay on personal symbols and religious experience.* Chicago, IL: University of Chicago Press.

Perry, B. L. (2011). The labeling paradox stigma, the sick role, and social networks in mental illness. *Journal of Health and Social Behavior, 52*(4), 460–77. http://dx.doi.org/10.1177/0022146511408913

Pfeiffer, W. (1967). Psychiatric peculiarities in Indonesia. *Bibliotheca Psychiatrica et Neurologica, 132,* 102–42.

Pols, H. (2006). The development of psychiatry in Indonesia: From colonial to modern times. *International Review of Psychiatry, 18*(4), 363–70. http://dx. doi.org/10.1080/09540260600775421

Roepstorff, A. (2013). Why am I not just lovin' cultural neuroscience? Toward a slow science of cultural difference. *Psychological Inquiry, 24*(1), 61–3. http://dx.doi.org/10.1080/1047840X.2013.768058

Salan, R. & Maretzki, T. (1983). Mental health services and traditional healing in Indonesia: Are the roles compatible? *Culture, Medicine, and Psychiatry, 7*(4), 377–412.

Sarbin, T. R., & Mancuso, J. C. (1970). Failure of a moral enterprise: Attitude of the public toward mental illness. *Journal of Consulting and Clinical Psychology, 35*(2), 159–73.

Sass, L. A. (1992). *Madness and modernism: Insanity in the light of modern art, literature, and thought.* New York, NY: Basic Books.

Sass, L. A. (2007). "Schizophrenic person" or "person with schizophrenia"? An essay on illness and the self. *Theory & Psychology, 17*(3), 395–420. http://dx.doi.org/10.1177/0959354307073152

Schomerus, G., Schwahn, C., Holzinger, A., Corrigan, P. W., Grabe, H. J., Carta, M. G., & Angermeyer, M. C. (2012). Evolution of public attitudes about mental illness: a systematic review and meta-analysis. *Acta Psychiatrica Scandinavica, 125*(6), 440–52. http://dx.doi.org/10.1111/j.1600-0447.2012.01826.x

Schwartz, T. (1973). Cult and context: the paranoid ethos in Melanesia. *Ethos 1*(2), 153–74.

Simons, R. C. (2001). Introduction to culture-bound syndromes. *Psychiatric Times, 18*(11), 283–92.

Smoller, J. W., Craddock, N., Kendler, J., Lee, P. H., Neale, B. M., Nurnberger, J. I., ... Sullivan, P. F. (2013). Identification of risk loci with shared effects on five major psychiatric disorders: A genome-wide analysis. *Lancet, 381,* 1371–9. http://dx.doi.org/10.1016/S0140-6736(12)62129-1

Stange, P. (1984). The logic of rasa in Java. *Indonesia, 38,* 113–34. http://dx.doi. org/10.2307/3350848

Stanghellini, G., Bolton, D., & Fulford, W. K. (2013). Person-centered psychopathology of schizophrenia: Building on Karl Jaspers' understanding of patient's attitude toward his illness. *Schizophrenia Bulletin, 39*(2), 287–94. http://dx.doi.org/10.1093/schbul/sbs154

Subandi (2006). *Psychocultural dimensions of recovery from first episode psychosis in Java* (Doctoral dissertation). University of Adelaide, Adelaide, Australia.

Suryani, L. K. (1984). Culture and mental disorder: The case of Bebainan in Bali. *Culture, Medicine, and Psychiatry, 8*(1), 95–113. http://dx.doi.org/ 10.1007/BF00053103

Tranulis, C., Corin, E., & Kirmayer, L. J. (2008). Insight and psychosis: Comparing the perspectives of patient, entourage and clinician. *International Journal of Social Psychiatry, 54*(3), 225–41. http://dx.doi.org/ 10.1177/0020764008088860

Vickers, A. (2005). *A history of modern Indonesia* (1st ed.). New York, NY: Cambridge University Press.

Walker, I., & Read, J. (2002). The differential effectiveness of psychosocial and biogenetic causal explanations in reducing negative attitudes toward "mental illness." *Psychiatry: Interpersonal and Biological Processes, 65*(4), 313–25. http://dx.doi.org/10.1521/psyc.65.4.313.20238

Watson, C., & Ellen, R. F. (1993). *Understanding witchcraft and sorcery in Southeast Asia.* Honolulu: University of Hawaii Press.

Waxler, N. (1979). Is outcome for schizophrenia better in nonindustrialised societies? The case of Sri Lanka. *Journal of Nervous and Mental Disease, 167,* 144–158.

White, G. M., & Marsella, A. J. (1982). Introduction: Cultural conceptions in mental health research and practice. In A. J. Marsella & G. M. White (Eds.), *Cultural conceptions of mental health and therapy* (pp. 1–38). Boston, MA: Reidel.

Wikan, U. (1990). *Managing turbulent hearts: A Balinese formula for living.* Chicago, IL: University of Chicago Press.

World Health Organization. (1974). *Report of the international pilot study of schizophrenia, volume I: Results of the initial evaluation phase.* Geneva, Switzerland: Author.

20 Eating Pathology in Fiji
Phenomenologic Diversity, Visibility,
and Vulnerability

Anne E. Becker and Jennifer J. Thomas

> *Mental disorders are invisible in most societies and we need to make our cause*
> *visible to everyone by our numbers and by public action.*
> —Vikram Patel and colleagues (2011)

Introduction

In 2004, members of our research team sat cross-legged in a community
hall of a rural village in Western Fiji after offering our ceremonial kava root
to introduce ourselves and our request. We were there to report study
findings about eating disorder symptoms among *iTaukei* Fijian schoolgirls
after the recent introduction of broadcast television to Fiji.[1] We sought to
inform the community about worrisome study findings and engage them
in a focus group discussion in response. Among the participants were men
and women, as well as parents and community leaders, including many
with strong opinions about television's impact on their community.

We had also come with an offer to follow up on our initial pilot study
with another study to better understand the health and social impacts of
televised media on youth. The participants had many thoughtful comments and insights, and we found their reception of the findings about
disordered eating to be polite, but lukewarm, in contrast with their
enthusiasm for discussing other concerns about perceived impacts of
the media and social change. Perhaps this could be ascribed to their
unfamiliarity with the problem of eating disorders. What appeared to
occupy their thoughts instead, was the apparent increase in youth risk
behaviors and associated consequences, including theft and teenage
pregnancy. Paramount among these concerns was the diminishing
respect for tradition perceived among *iTaukei* Fijian youth.

---

[1] The preferred term for the population original to Fiji is "iTaukei." This term replaces
previous nomenclature including, "Fijian," "indigenous Fijian," and "ethnic Fijian." In
this chapter, we use "iTaukei Fijian" or "iTaukei" to clarify the ethnicity of the population
discussed (see http://www.fijianaffairs.gov.fj/iTaukei.html).

Although most of the adults professed to have observed few signs of disordered eating among young women, a traditional *iTaukei* Fijian healer reported that some young women were using *dranu* (traditional *iTaukei* Fijian herbal medicines) as purgatives to manage their weight. He made it clear that he did not consider the unsupervised use of *dranu* for this purpose to be appropriate. Our previous work on disordered eating in Fiji had failed to identify herbal purgative use, possibly because the behavior was relatively new and we had not known to pose this question.

Apart from this rather oblique reference to eating pathology, the disordered eating symptoms described in Western clinical settings seemed utterly unfamiliar to our respondents. However, the initial consensus among adults that eating pathology was not prevalent among adolescent *iTaukei* Fijian girls was belied by study findings in 1998, and subsequently in 2007, indicating that, in fact, young women in Fiji were quietly engaging in behaviors that threatened their health and emotional well-being.

On the one hand, this lack of awareness was surprising since *iTaukei* Fijian indigenous medical nosology clearly recognizes appetite and weight loss afflictions. *Macake* is characterized by poor appetite that can be complicated further by weight loss. "Going thin" indexes bereavement or social loss in visible weight change. Despite these recognized conditions, the eating pathology had not registered as a problem among the parents' generation. On the other hand, this lack of awareness in Fiji is not such an outlier from the responses to eating pathology in many other countries, where it can commonly be marginalized, trivialized, or even glamorized. Even in the United States, 48 percent of newspaper stories about eating disorders appear in the arts and entertainment sections, while only 13 percent are found in the health section (O'Hara & Smith, 2007). The tenor of this popular response is evident in the lack of funding directed to eating disorders research, as well as in the low prestige of working with eating disorder patients, who are seen as difficult or recalcitrant, and stigmatized by professionals (Thompson-Brenner, Satir, Franko, & Herzog, 2012). Paradoxically, eating disorders continue to have relative invisibility – in patients, populations, and policy – despite their serious medical comorbidity and potential lethality.

This chapter interrogates the low profile of eating disorders in both Fiji and in global mental health *writ large*. Features intrinsic to the disorders, as well as the social position of the most vulnerable group – typically young females – diminish their visibility. The heterogeneity of eating disorders, in particular, may limit their recognition across diverse cultures. Despite numerous studies documenting how the etiology and phenomenology of body image and eating disturbances are embedded in local social contexts, few studies have addressed the clinical utility of diagnostic criteria for eating disorders outside of the high-income countries in which they were developed. This chapter will critique the application of standard diagnostic criteria for eating disorders across culturally diverse populations by considering epidemiologic, clinical narrative, and ethnographic data from Fiji. This evidence suggests that cultural variations in symptom expression and vulnerabilities that undermine access to care for eating disorders – not just in Fiji, but around the globe – may result in underestimates of prevalence, which, in turn, result in a lack of attention in public health and clinical settings.

Visibility and the Global Mental Health Agenda

Despite their associated serious morbidity and high mortality (Klump, Bulik, Kaye, Treasure, & Tyson, 2009), eating disorders are virtually absent from the global mental health agenda. Eating disorders are a latecomer to reports on the world burden of disease, having only recently made their debut on the ledger of years lived with disability (YLDs; Vos et al., 2012). Indeed, the prevalence of eating disorders has not routinely been assessed in low- and middle-income countries (LMICs), even though they had been flagged by the World Health Organization (WHO) as a priority area for adolescent mental health (WHO, 2003). This absence can be partially attributed to intrinsic features of their psychopathology that result in a low profile in clinical settings. When the World Health Report 2001 drew unprecedented attention to global mental health, the WHO called upon member states to commit resources to surveillance and documentation of mental health problems (WHO, 2001). Estimating prevalence, however, was premised on valid diagnostic criteria that were considered comparable across regions with vastly different social contexts and cultural traditions. The epidemiologic, anthropologic, and psychiatric literatures provide ample documentation of how case ascertainment of mental disorders is problematic. Eating disorders present a special challenge in this regard for several reasons.

Notwithstanding the disorders' potentially devastating health and social impacts, individuals with an eating disorder commonly avoid treatment, either because they do not recognize their behaviors as threatening their social, psychological, and physical health, or because they choose not to seek help for – or perhaps even not to reveal – their symptoms and suffering (Becker, Thomas, Franko, & Herzog, 2005; Becker, Perloe, & Eddy, 2009). Numerous social barriers to care also exist (Becker, Arrindell, Perloe, Fay, & Striegel-Moore, 2010), as indicated by documented disparities in service utilization across the major U.S. ethnic groups (Marques et al., 2011). Opportunities for clinicians to intervene are limited by the frequently inconspicuous clinical presentation of eating disorder symptoms. Bulimia nervosa (BN) and binge-eating disorder can present without any physical findings at all, and symptomatic behaviors characterizing anorexia nervosa (AN), BN, and binge-eating disorder can easily elude observation. Even when physical findings do occur, they frequently are relatively nonspecific, such as weight changes or laboratory abnormalities. In other words, the diagnostician must rely on observational data, which may be difficult to come by, or self-disclosure, which may not be forthcoming (Hunt, Becker, Guimaraes, Stemmer-Rachamimov, & Misdraji, 2012). Indeed, patients are frequently disinclined to volunteer information to their doctors (Becker et al., 2005; Becker, Perloe, et al., 2009), and evidence supports that eating disorders frequently are not recognized in clinical settings.

The visibility of eating disorders may also be obscured by their diverse modes of expression. When symptoms present in unfamiliar ways, and when diagnostic criteria do not fully encompass these diverse phenotypic outliers, eating disorders may be more likely to evade clinical detection.

Discarding the Unfamiliar

Beginning in the second half of the twentieth century, several major cross-national studies settled some important questions about whether major mental disorders were culture-bound to the West, but universalizing criteria for mental disorders did not emerge until the 1960s (Sartorius, 1978). Several studies, for example, supported the cross-national occurrence of schizophrenia and depressive disorders (Jablensky et al., 1992; Thornicroft & Sartorius, 1993). These studies have had important pragmatic impact, redirecting the focus from debating the presence of mental disorders at all to the delivery of effective mental health care (Becker & Kleinman, 2014).

However, these landmark studies also identified important heterogeneity with respect to the risk and course of mental disorders. Although these findings generated interest in the impact of social environment on risk and prognosis, relatively less attention was paid to diversity in the presentation of major mental disorders across these populations. In fact, selection bias embedded in the study design made it more likely that cases corresponding to common presentations in Western settings were included, whereas cases with unfamiliar presentations were excluded. In other words, these studies were not designed to limn the full scope of phenotypes, but rather to ascertain the presence of cases resembling those familiar to Western investigators. Although the findings had relevance and importance in the populations that were studied, the

Western diagnostic criteria were reified in a potentially misleading way by excluding cases that looked different. If these cases, which would have looked like outliers in Western populations, had been the norm in the populations assessed, the studies would presumably not have unearthed that fact (see Becker & Kleinman, 2014, for a review).

The limited representativeness of a nosology of mental disorders developed from clinical and epidemiologic data drawn primarily from Western populations has been widely critiqued (e.g., Patel & Sumathipala, 2001; Patel & Kim, 2007). The selective publication of clinical trials and other research from high-income countries constructs and reifies "ideal types" and perpetuates assumptions about their uniformity, thereby preempting a full understanding of cultural diversity in the phenomenology, risk, and course of mental disorders. That the vast majority of first authors hail from affluent Western countries, and draw their study samples from their demographic backyard, systematically excludes nearly 90 percent of the world's population from top psychology journals (Henrich, Heine, & Norenzayan, 2010).

Psychiatric epidemiological work during the second half of the twentieth century ferreted out phenotypic commonalities that could establish that the footprint of mental disorders was global. Although making an invaluable contribution, this discernment of core psychopathology represented only a partial truth, in contrast to the protean nature of mental illness encountered in lived experience and clinical practice. Variations in clinical presentations across cultures have received little serious attention in constructing nosologies of mental disorders. Presentations unfamiliar in the West were sometimes understood as "culture-bound syndromes" and quite literally marginalized. Even in 1994, when the *DSM-IV* was published, the painstaking efforts of cultural psychiatrists and medical anthropologists were relegated to two pages of text in a remote appendix (Mezzich et al., 1999). The glossary of culture-bound syndromes was disconnected from the well-thumbed sections in the body of the book, giving the impression that they were regarded as exotica (Alarcon et al., 2009).

Although half a century has passed since universal psychiatric criteria were forged, diagnostic screening questionnaires are still widely regarded as having uncertain validity across diverse social contexts (Kessler, Wang, & Wittchen, 2010). This leaves ambiguity about the prevalence and associated burden of less clinically and socially visible mental disorders. In particular, when the form that symptoms take is shaped by social context, we should expect great cultural diversity and, in turn, many clinical presentations that fall outside the perimeters of existing diagnostic criteria. There may be no better example of this than the "fat phobia" criterion intrinsic to the *DSM-IV* diagnosis of AN.

Anorexia Nervosa: Culturally Bounded or Culturally Moderated?

The early narrative about AN located it at a culturally and historically particular crossroads, positing that it might be culturally bound to the West (Prince, 1985), or to "culture[s] of modernity" (Lee, 1996). By definition, AN has been characterized by an "intense fear" of fatness (APA, 1994). Setting aside the subjectivity of an emotional response like fear, it is self-evident that the construction of fat as *fearsome* must be anchored in social norms. The historical record, for example, is clear that self-starvation resembling AN made an early appearance (for instance, in the fourteenth century; Bell, 1987), but that the cultural valuation of thinness did not emerge until the twentieth century (Brumberg, 1988). Likewise, cultural variation in the expressed fear of fatness has been well documented (Becker, Thomas, & Pike, 2009). The crux of the debate is whether AN can exist in the absence of fat phobia.

Lee and colleagues first described non-fat-phobic AN (NFP-AN) and proposed that it was a variant of AN. Their findings demonstrated that NFP-AN is similar to AN, except for the absence of an intense fear of fatness. NFP-AN was subsequently identified in other geographically diverse settings, including South Asia, Africa, and the United States (see Becker, Thomas, et al., 2009, for a review). The absence of fat phobia in these cases was attributed to the relatively low salience of weight and shape concerns in the immediate cultural context, in contrast with the expressed rationales for restricting dietary intake. Since then, other explanations for food restriction have been identified in low-weight eating disorder patients who minimize or deny fat phobia. These include desire for control (Fairburn, Cooper, & O'Connor, 2008), religious asceticism (Banks, 1992), and post-prandial discomfort (Lee, Lee, Ngai, Lee, & Wing, 2001).

NFP-AN raises an interesting challenge to the centrality of body shape and weight concerns to the core psychopathology of AN. Two meta-analyses comparing NFP-AN to AN have supported its association with milder eating pathology (Thomas, Vartanian, & Brownell, 2009), even when excluding the specific weight concerns that already distinguish the two (Becker, Thomas, et al., 2009). This milder psychopathology is consistent with Fairburn and colleagues' (1999) prediction that NFP-AN should have a better prognosis than typical AN, because a critical maintaining mechanism of the disorder (i.e., extreme vigilance for even minor changes in shape and weight) is absent. A proportional increase in conventional AN presentations in Hong Kong across the past two decades has also been demonstrated and lends support to a close link between AN cognitive symptoms and cultural resonance (Lee, Ng, Kwok, & Fung, 2010).

In addition to this observed historical trend within a Hong Kong Chinese population, evidence suggests that an individual's own stated rationale for food restriction in NFP-AN may be flexible over time, further illustrating its biosocial basis. On the one hand, the emergence of fat phobia during the course of AN may be explained by a lack of either insight or willingness to recognize or disclose fear of weight gain, a common observation in patients with AN presenting in culturally Western settings (Becker, Perloe, et al., 2009; Bravender et al., 2007; Thomas, Weigel, Lawton, Levendusky, & Becker, 2012). The disinclination to disclose symptoms should also be understood as culturally patterned. For example, such disclosure requires a level of autonomy and self-agency relative to clinical or parental authority that is not universal. On the other hand, Lee has also argued that illness narratives regarding AN can be socially constructed through the clinical encounter (Lee, 1995). In this scenario, intensive fear of weight gain could plausibly follow, rather than drive, the initial weight loss (or failure to gain weight with linear growth) associated with an episode of AN. According to Hacking's (1995) looping hypothesis, "to create new ways of classifying people is also to change how we can think of ourselves, to change our self-worth, even how we remember our own past. This in turn generates a looping effect, because people of the kind behave differently and so are different" (p. 369). In the case of AN, popular descriptions of the class (i.e., as having a pathological desire for thinness) may alter the way individuals within the class (i.e., those with AN) perceive themselves (i.e., as too fat). Thus, dissemination of AN as a legitimate – and even prestigious – idiom of distress could conceivably cultivate and propagate the fat-phobic variant of AN in social contexts even where the desirability of thinness is novel.

If "fat phobia" is culturally and socially plastic, then AN might be more aptly regarded as a *culturally moderated* disorder rather than a *culture-bound* syndrome. In this reframing, NFP-AN could be understood as falling within a spectrum of phenotypic variations of AN – rather than being categorically distinct from AN – with the social environment patterning its manifestation, and quite possibly, its prognosis. That is, the same proto-disorder is present, but it looks different and unfolds differently in contextually specific ways. Likewise, the social environment provides the contextual basis for a communication strategy for engaging or avoiding caregivers and therapeutic intervention.

With the globalizing exposure to consumer culture, entertainment media, and Western values, the salience of body and weight management to self-presentation has diffused and unprecedented worldwide distribution. Uptake of the attitudes that would be expected to result in high levels of concern, how these valorize or motivate behaviors, and how this relation is formulated and articulated, will doubtless involve complex biosocial interactions. Two examples of emerging eating pathology in Fiji will serve to illustrate recognizably disordered eating with distinctive cultural features.

The Emergence of Eating Pathology in Fiji

An archipelago located in the Western Pacific, Fiji has an indigenous population (previously termed "ethnic Fijians" and now termed "iTaukei") that draws its cultural legacy from Polynesia, where a traditional preference for large body size is documented (Becker, 1995), and which has been of interest as a foil to modern ideals common to populations of Anglo-European descent residing in industrialized countries. In the traditional *iTaukei* Fijian setting, aesthetic body ideals were not the impetus for personal cultivation of body size and shape, as they are easily seen to be in populations residing in societies characterized by Western cultural traditions (Becker, 1995). Body size in Fiji was traditionally understood as the proper domain of the family, not the individual, a fact with relevance to constraints on expression and pursuit of a personal health agenda. This historical context is also germane since encroaching images and narratives embedded in media exported from the United States, United Kingdom, Australia, and New Zealand provided access to ideas that began to circulate among adolescent girls soon after television (TV) was introduced and there was an initial broad exposure to it in the late 1990s. Prior to that time, eating disorders – as operationalized in *DSM-IV* (APA, 1994) – were not described in *iTaukei* Fijian nosology and were also absent from Western clinical settings in Fiji. Many features of *iTaukei* Fijian cultural traditions could be seen as contributing to this apparent resilience, not least the social valuation of abundant feasting, robust body size, frequent food exchange, and communal eating, as well as attunement to weight changes that reflected the wealth of kin and social communities (Becker, 1995).

After TV was introduced, however, a shift in ideal body size could be discerned among *iTaukei* Fijian girls. Concomitantly, disordered eating appeared to emerge. The latter was perhaps best illustrated in a two-wave cohort study finding approximately three years after the community had gained access to TV that 11 percent of participants had used purging to control weight, compared with none when TV broadcasts first began in the region (Becker, Burwell, Gilman, Herzog, & Hamburg, 2002). The impact of TV on body ideals may have been profound, but it was anything but temporally stable. Initial evidence supported a keen interest in TV actresses as role models, as they were perceived to embody success across several social domains. The *iTaukei* Fijian girls surveyed found the consistently thin bodies portrayed in TV shows most remarkable. Some expressed a desire to emulate these characters, in part by managing their weight (Becker et al., 2002; Becker, 2004).

Intentional weight management in rural Fiji is difficult to keep private. Conventionally, there is close surveillance of weight changes among children and adults, and comments about poor appetite are frequent. Intervention with small children is swift, often with traditional herbal treatments for *macake*, an indigenous *iTaukei* syndrome heralded by loss of appetite (Becker, 1994). Interventions are common for adults, too. Herbal prophylaxis to forestall appetite loss is routine, and concern is liberally expressed when adults do not appear to eat well. Criticism is not spared when expectations are unmet. Eating secretly is equally subject to criticism, as evidenced in the locally searing insult that someone is *kanakana lo* (a secret eater). Young women can hardly count on privacy for either exercise or purging within the rhythm of routine village life. In this regard, behaviors aimed at weight loss require effortful circumvention of convention.

In this respect, young *iTaukei* women lack opportunity for charting a course toward weight management. In fact, their self-agency around restrictive eating and other weight management behaviors is highly constrained, much as it is around other pursuits. This kind of restrictive milieu may in fact reduce eating pathology among *iTaukei* women, although there is no simple way to test this hypothesis. There are noteworthy similarities to some of the therapeutic surveillance and behavioral restrictions enforced in residential treatment settings for eating disorders. Eating disorders in Western settings are commonly characterized by surreptitious behaviors. But the high level of attunement to appetite and weight in Fiji, and lack of privacy, make such behaviors extremely difficult. The level of community scrutiny of weight and appetite in Fiji, coupled with the traditional preference for robust size, may have contributed to the resilience to eating pathology that characterized the *iTaukei* Fijian population prior to the ensuing rapid economic development (Becker, 1995). Perceived lack of legitimation of self-agency, moreover, presumably delimits articulation and disclosure of personal weight management goals, just as it constrains expression of distress (Becker, 1998). As a result, the deeply subjective experience of "fat phobia" or body dissatisfaction may not be expressed by *iTaukei* Fijian women as readily as in other social settings.

Robust bodies in Fiji have traditionally been regarded as a community asset. Body size ideals are closely tied to perceived capacity to contribute to household and community labor, which, in turn, influences social approbation and respect. Oftentimes, this capacity is tied to physical labor essential to farming and performing other domestic chores without the benefit of motorized transport or labor-saving appliances. In this respect, there is little social advantage to being either too thin or too large, since either end of the spectrum may be read as potentially disabling. This fluctuation in ideal body size, from large to thin, and then back to something in the middle, renders the social meaning of "fatness" highly variable. On the one hand, routine greetings enshrine the enduring social valuation of robust size (*urouro*, *levulevu*) and cue the disdain for thinness (*li la*); on the other hand, there is new social currency for body size, one that is slimmed down from traditional ideals over the last two decades. Following *iTaukei* Fijian tradition, it would not be within a young woman's purview to formulate weight management as a personal goal, because it is her family and community who are charged with governing her size. And finally, fatness is a highly subjective and culturally relative construct. In affluent social contexts, fatness or obesity may be tied to a specific weight, clothing size, or a specific value of the body mass index (BMI). In Western settings, normative data about BMI, may be used by pediatricians, parents, schools, and health policy-makers as a metric to gauge overweight. Fatness in the *iTaukei* context (and doubtless many others) has a more fluid and less quantitative nature.

Following the focus group discussions during which community stakeholders were apprised, we sought to document whether eating pathology – and additional youth risk behaviors important to parents – were present in a large, representative group of *iTaukei* Fijian girls. The study design, methods, and validation of pertinent assessments, as well as the relevant ethnographic context, are described in detail elsewhere (Becker, 1995; Becker, Bainivualiku, et al, 2009; Becker et al., 2010a; Becker et al., 2010b; Becker, Roberts, et al., 2010); here we focus on findings salient to the culturally distinctive presentation of eating pathology. Self-report assessments included the Eating Disorder Examination-Questionnaire (EDE-Q; Fairburn & Beglin, 2008), and interview assessments included content based on the Eating Disorder Examination (EDE; Fairburn, Cooper, & O'Connor, 2008). Our clinical assessment of eating disorders was informed by the criteria outlined in *DSM-IV* (APA, 1994), the diagnostic system in use at the time of data collection.

Fear of Fatness: A Categorical or Dimensional Feature of AN?

Previous literature addressing cultural influences on eating disorders has posited fear of fatness as a *categorical* difference between NFP-AN and conventional AN. In contrast, we suggest here that it might also be regarded as differentiator along a *dimensional* spectrum, moderated by the nature and intensity of environmental pressures. Excerpts from clinically oriented interviews with four low-weight *iTaukei* adolescents illustrate this possibility. These four young women were among the 523 schoolgoing *iTaukei* Fijian study participants (ages fifteen to twenty) in the previously mentioned study of eating pathology in Fiji. Following the study protocol, participants with a BMI of 17.5 kg/m^2 or below were sought for an interview to evaluate possible AN. Four of the five respondents meeting this criterion were available for in-person interviews with the first author, an eating disorders specialist. The fifth respondent met this screening criterion but was unavailable for an interview, which was designed to explore the respondents' symptoms, including whether consistent with AN.

We report here on the problematic – but very interesting – effort to assess "fear of fatness" in this cultural context. Far from confirming or disconfirming the symptom of "fat phobia," the interviews raised questions about whether a committed and unqualified phobia is a valid construct in this context. Because of this, the presence or absence of this diagnostic criterion for AN could not consistently be established with confidence.

Case 1. Asenaca* (all names are pseudonyms) was a fifteen-year-old girl who attended school in a rural area. Her BMI was very low: below the fifth percentile based on international age- and gender-matched norms (WHO, 2007). Asenaca's interview responses were remarkable for multiple inconsistencies relating to her concerns about weight gain and the intentionality of her dietary restriction. Whereas she affirmed her wish to be thinner in her first interview in response to EDE-based questions (Fairburn, Cooper, & O'Connor, 2008) posed by an *iTaukei* Fijian non-clinician, she recanted her expressed desire to restrict her diet and avoid weight gain in a subsequent interview with the first author. However, even during the second, more clinically oriented interview, she continued to contradict herself regarding her feelings about her weight, resulting in ambiguity about whether or why she was intending to undermine weight gain.

For example in the first interview, when asked if she was trying to reduce what she was eating, she replied she was "cutting down on it presently." She also indicated this was to lose weight and that her present low weight was fine with her. When asked how much weight she would like to lose, she indicated she wanted to weigh "thirty kilograms" (an implausibly low and unhealthful weight for her from a clinical perspective), and she also reported that she wanted her belly to be smaller. During her second interview, however, she denied a wish to lose any weight and affirmed that she thought that her weight should increase a little bit. On the other hand, when asked if she was afraid of becoming "too large" ("*levulevu hivisia*") she replied in the affirmative. When probed about this further, she said she was afraid that people would make fun of her if she gained weight. Although denying a fear of weight gain per se (at least at one point in the interview), she stated that her current weight was "adequate" *(rauta)*. Whereas she first recanted her report in the previous interview that she had restricted her diet to lose weight, she later admitted that she sometimes did reduce her diet in order to prevent weight gain. She also allowed that she could gain just a little bit ("*Levulevu tale va hewa*"). Over the course of her interviews, she rationalized her poor dietary intake as a means of avoiding weight gain and also attributed it to sometimes being too tired or busy to eat dinner because of studying and afterschool activities. By the end of the interviews, Asenaca had contradicted herself several times, and there was great ambiguity about her investment in either losing or gaining weight. Whereas she seemed to endorse restriction in the first interview, she mitigated this position during the ensuing clinically focused interview. In retrospect, this may have been in response to concern expressed by the interviewers about her low weight.

Considering the contradictory interview responses, the presence of *DSM-IV-TR* AN criterion B (an "intense fear of weight gain"; APA, 2000) could neither be established nor excluded in this case. Asenaca's illness narrative can best be described as equivocal with respect to concern about gaining weight. Although she confirmed her worry about becoming *levulevu hivisia* ("too fat"), she also indicated her willingness to gain some weight, did not endorse an intense fear of weight gain in the EDE interview, and reported taking *dranu* (an indigenous *iTaukei* folk medicinal preparation) to prevent *macake*. From a clinical perspective, given her extremely low weight, Asenaca's initial responses reflecting her interest in maintaining a low weight and her affirmation of dietary restriction and weight concerns – even if partially recanted and in the end leaving a somewhat muddled understanding of her intent to reduce her weight – warranted concern.

The inconsistencies in Asenaca's expressed commitment to fat phobia are not unusual in themselves. Ambivalence about working toward a more healthful body weight is a common presentation in Western clinical settings. What appeared culturally novel in this setting, however, was the way Asenaca's potential eating pathology was organized around maintaining a weight within social norms, while apparently misjudging how her own weight matched those. In other words, Asenaca was neither fully committed to thinness nor fully opposed to weight gain. Instead, she sought to achieve a weight in the middle: one that would not be ridiculed. What is not fully transparent in this brief interview encounter is whether the ambiguities in Asenaca's responses reflect an intended communication strategy, ambivalence about weight and fatness, feelings that remain contradictory and unformulated, and/or constraints on self-agency.

Case 2. Kesaia was a nearly sixteen-year-old girl who attended a school in a rural setting. Her BMI was well below the fifteenth percentile for her age. Whereas she initially reported that she had not tried to lose weight, she admitted that she was pleased with her current low weight and affirmed that she was "afraid" of gaining weight. Her interview responses revealed her history of intentional dietary restriction that contributed to weight loss and confirmed her fat phobia:

INTERVIEWER:	You are perhaps afraid of being large? [*O iko bara matakucia na levulevu?*]
KESAIA:	Yes [*Io*]
INTERVIEWER:	Very afraid? [*Matakucia d'jina?*]
KESAIA:	Yes [*Io*]
INTERVIEWER:	Strongly? [*Vakaikai?*]
KESAIA:	Yes [*Io*]

Although she initially denied wanting to lose weight, she acknowledged that, "I always cut down on my eating," ostensibly so that "my size should not become too big."

In addition to endorsing this aversion to weight gain, Kesaia provided multiple alternate rationales for her dietary restriction: (1) as a means of exerting control (in response to specific EDE items probing control); (2) avoiding becoming too large to work efficiently; and (3) avoiding becoming fat because it would adversely affect her appearance. She referenced her concerns about weight gain against local social norms that equate very large size with inadequate capacity to perform household responsibilities. For example, she explained that, "I should not become too large, so that I am able to do my work." She referenced diverse *iTaukei* Fijian norms and guidance relating to socially ideal weight in her responses, noting that her parents wished for her to eat more: "[My parents] always say that I should eat a lot so that I can gain weight. I always say that I do not want to get big." She also perceived that her dietary restriction was congruent with her grandmother's advice not to become too big. For example, she referenced a conversation with her grandmother discussing the pros and cons of weight gain: "I always say shall I get large or not? She [my grandmother] always says, don't because being large causes laziness and not doing a lot of housework." However, when asked whether she was concerned about weight gain because of her appearance or because she might not be a good worker, she replied, "I only don't want to gain weight at all because my appearance is bad that way." Finally, and seemingly paradoxically, Kesaia also stated that she took folk medicine twice monthly to prevent *macake*, explaining that she was afraid of *macake* since it caused extreme weight loss. Notwithstanding her low weight, she reported that her weight was: "currently right" (*donu koto*). In response to feedback during her interview that her weight was actually very low, she agreed to work to address her eating saying, "I will have to change." While still admitting that she was afraid of getting fat, she said that she would not be afraid of gaining a "little" weight and was amenable to gaining weight as part of the study team's recommendation.

Case 3. Tamarisi was a fifteen-year-old girl attending a school located in a rural setting. Her BMI was below the fifteenth percentile for her age. Tamarisi was clear and consistent about her desire to avoid weight gain. Although she acknowledged that she was presently "too thin" (*hewahewa hivisia*), she admitted to restricting her food intake lest she become too large, stating, "I cut down on my eating so that I would not become too fat."

She affirmed fear of gaining *too much* weight, but also denied wanting to lose more weight. Tamarisi was aware that her wish to stay thin contradicted her parents' wish that she gain weight. She acknowledged skipping meals and also admitted that she had been resisting her parents' interventions to make her eat more. Tamarisi said she felt she looked good at her present weight, reporting that she had disagreed with her parents about it ("My mother always tells me to eat a lot, so that my body will get larger. I always say no").

She provided several rationales for her current dietary restriction. Although these included non-fat-phobic rationales such as (1) lack of hunger and (2) skipping breakfast to catch the school bus, she also endorsed fat phobia. Similar to Kesaia (Case 2), Tamarisi explained her fat phobia by relating overweight to interference with responsibilities for domestic and other chores, explaining, "[as a result of overweight] we can't always do our work well." Despite this, she also reported having taken *dranu* to prevent *macake*. In response to the recommendation that she should gain weight for her health, she thought that would be "difficult" (*dredre*), but said she would be willing to work on it and accepted a referral for help with this.

Case 4. Anaseini was a fifteen-year-old girl who attended a school in a rural location. Her BMI was below the fifth percentile for her age. During the interview, she neither "refused" to gain weight (e.g., as framed in *DSM-IV-TR* criterion B for AN; APA, 2000) nor was worried about being too thin, but rather stated she simply wanted her weight to be "just enough." While expressing a desire for a "just right" weight might be regarded as a sign of health, she admitted that it would bother her to gain weight, despite her very low weight, suggesting that she held a distorted view of a healthful body weight. Although she claimed not to worry about her weight much, she admitted to avoiding eating too much and framed her concern in terms of eating "just enough." For example, she stated that, "I always want to stop being too small, so I should gain only a little bit of weight, so that it will be just enough." She acknowledged that people had advised her to gain weight. "I always eat slowly, so that the amount of food I eat is small; they always say I should eat a lot; they say: Look at your shape, you are small." She explained her position this way: "Yes it's true, I should eat so that I can be large, but my size should not become too large [...] I always say, I should gain weight, but I should not gain too much weight; I should be just big enough."

In summary, interview evaluation of these respondents yielded uncertainty about whether "fear of fatness" (1) was endorsed as a primary or stable rationale for inadequate dietary intake, (2) was experienced in the same way as conventionally described in Euro-American populations, and (3) deviated substantially from local social norms linking overweight to inadequate capacity to work. The clinical presentations of the four young women interviewed were also atypical for conventional representations of AN, given their expressed willingness to gain some weight and their routine use of folk medicine to avoid appetite loss.

Overall, each of these narratives did not give clear evidence of fat phobia as a committed rationale for inadequate dietary intake. With the exception of Tamarisi, each of the respondents reported considering the input of family or friends in rationalizing her weight goals, highlighting a common element of social desirability in responses and intentions unifying these cases. Respondents differed from Euro-American individuals with AN by denying singular concern with extreme thinness, instead insisting that they would accept a modest amount of weight gain.

Setting aside whether or not these four respondents would meet full diagnostic criteria for AN, they expressed a novel cultural variant of fear of weight gain. Three of these underweight participants reported taking herbal medication to prevent *macake*, the condition associated with appetite and weight loss, notwithstanding concerns about weight gain. In this respect, they were engaging in behavior that countered appetite loss, even while they endorsed a concern about gaining too much weight. Narrative data also illustrated how respondents acknowledged their low weight, but simultaneously expressed a culturally syntonic concern about becoming *levulevu hivisia* ("too fat"). In general, we observed an investment in being a normative size rather than concern with being thin.

These concerns were consistent with the strong cultural valuation of robust appetite and the perceived importance of embodying capacity and willingness to work hard. In recent years, the ideal body shape in Fiji appears to have toggled from robust and large to thin and back to "about right." Notably, the new cultural ideal reflects how "fitting in" is valued in Fiji, rather than "standing out." This desire to conform to local social norms for body size contrasts with Western AN presentations, in which thinness is more often viewed as a pathway to exceptionalism (i.e., becoming "special" or "different" from others; Serpell, Teasdale, Troop, & Treasure, 2004). This dimension of the clinical presentation of disordered eating in Fiji resonates with study findings from Belize described by Anderson-Fye in which, "family expectations of thinness" appeared to drive behaviors rather than a cognitive or affective stance toward weight or fatness (Anderson-Fye, 2004).

It is not uncommon for Euro-American patients with AN to present with superficial compliance about their need to gain weight; in such cases, a more overt fear of weight gain frequently emerges as patients engage in nutritional rehabilitation and experience weight gain in the concrete sense (e.g., Thomas et al., 2012). Without the benefit of longitudinal follow-up and collateral data, we cannot be certain what the course of weight gain would be for these underweight young women or whether a greater willingness or capacity to articulate weight concerns would have emerged. By contrast, these clinical narratives suggest a departure from typical AN presentations in Euro-American clinical settings. In particular, respondents endorsed prophylactic folk medicine use to prevent appetite loss, consistent with local social norms, but seemingly contradictory to a concern with maintaining a low weight. This herbal medicine use was congruent with their expressed desire not to lose too much weight. Finally, the noncommittal nature of these clinical narratives is consistent with social taboos on excessive expression of personal needs or autonomy. This finding is congruous with ethnographic research in Fiji finding that women are discouraged from overt expression of distress, in favor of using somatic idioms instead (see Becker, 1995; Becker 1998).

These narrative data illustrate the complexity of ascertaining AN in a non-Euro-American population. This is unlikely to be solely attributable to a language barrier but, rather, also to cultural styles in expressing distress and social norms encouraging consensus and conformity. The ethnographic context is also critical to rendering seemingly paradoxical behaviors clinically meaningful. The willingness of these respondents to protect their appetite and weight through use of traditional medicines to prevent *macake* suggests a useful therapeutic hook in this cultural environment that warrants research. This is an empirical question, and future research on the course of AN in diverse social environments can inform diagnostic assessment and therapeutic strategies. Until those data are available, clinicians will benefit from evaluating how particular cultural orientations inform patient clinical narratives.

Finally, prevalence estimates of AN that are premised on universal core symptoms risk missing cases that present with phenomenologic variation. The classification of eating disorders in *DSM* – and especially in its previous iterations – invites consideration of potential limitations in its global relevance. In particular, opportunities for identifying cultural diversity in phenotypes and prevalence are pre-empted by case detection that applies diagnostic criteria largely developed with reference to Euro-American populations.

Combining Herbal Purgatives and Appetite Stimulants: Another Paradoxical Narrative?

In summary, the rationales for dietary restriction of these low-weight respondents are strikingly unfamiliar – at least from the perspective of an American eating disorder clinician. The narratives are notable for the absence of an expressed commitment to a very low weight and their tacit endorsement of compromise to accommodate the multiple opinions within their social universe. Far from presenting the rationale for dietary restriction as a *rigid*, self-referential concern about weight, the views expressed are comparatively more flexible and relational. This cognitive flexibility is somewhat unexpected, given that the presentation of AN in the United States, Europe, and Australia/New Zealand is typically characterized by cognitive rigidity (i.e., making significantly more perseverative errors than healthy controls on behavioral tasks that require switching back and forth between strategies; Tchanturia et al., 2012). It may be that, consistent with Hacking's (1995) looping hypothesis, the *iTaukei* Fijian participants presenting with low weight and possible AN had had insufficient impetus to formulate a unifying rationale for their food restriction in response to intervention or commentary by individuals who viewed their low weight as a sign of a mental illness prior to the study interviews.

The expressed concerns about avoiding both thinness and fatness were not the only paradoxical weight management behaviors illuminated by this study. Indeed, we made a similar observation among the *iTaukei* Fijian respondents who self-reported purging. A latent profile analysis conducted among the 222 respondents who self-reported vomiting, taking herbal purgatives, or both behaviors in the past month also revealed a picture of eating pathology with kinship to, but incomplete overlap with, BN (Thomas, Crosby, Wonderlich, Striegel-Moore, & Becker, 2011). Four notable findings emerged in this second analysis. First, the self-reported prevalence of purging by one or both of these two methods within the past month was unexpectedly high, affecting 42 percent of this representative sample of school-going adolescent girls. Second, although one of the latent profiles associated with vomiting looked very similar to subthreshold BN (which would be classified as - eating disorder, not otherwise specified [EDNOS] under *DSM-IV* criteria; APA, 2000), the other was distinguished by the use of traditional *iTaukei* Fijian purgatives to induce vomiting or diarrhea. Third, among the respondents who self-reported purging, more than half (53 percent) also had taken traditional herbal medicine to treat or prevent *macake* within the same timeframe. Finally, some of the respondents had been supplied with herbal purgatives by an adult relative (i.e., a mother or a grandmother), who encouraged their use.

Because traditional herbal purgatives are also used medicinally in Fiji, we considered whether the herbal purgative use could have been misclassified as pathological when it was, in fact, a culturally sanctioned behavior. However, the phrasing of the question specified that the behavior was used "as a means of controlling your weight." Moreover, we found convincing evidence in follow-up interviews that at least some respondents acknowledged their use of herbal purgatives as a weight control tool (Thomas et al., 2011). In addition, the latent profile characterized by traditional purgative use was associated with significantly greater eating pathology, as measured by the EDE-Q (Fairburn & Beglin, 2008) – as was the profile resembling BN – than nonpurging respondents. The "herbal purgative use" respondents also showed greater clinical impairment (as measured by the Clinical Impairment Assessment; Bohn et al., 2008) than either non-purging respondents or the BN-like group. In other words, our findings suggested that this distinctive *iTaukei* Fijian variant of eating pathology was associated with greater impairment than a more conventional presentation, even though it would not have been consistently identified by the unmodified version (Fairburn & Beglin, 2008) of the EDE-Q (Thomas et al., 2011).

As noted above, the contemporaneous use of herbal therapies for both purging and *macake* is, on the surface, paradoxical. Each of these would be expected to have an opposite effect on weight since the purgatives would result in weight loss and the *macake* therapy in weight gain or stabilization. So how can we understand the use of both? Since we did not pose this question to the respondents who used both, we propose five plausible explanations. First, we have no reason to believe that the girls themselves regarded these two behaviors as inconsistent. It is possible that they were practicing both behaviors without formulating them as goal-directed, and thus did not perceive them as contradictory. The self-report questionnaire and interview may have been their first opportunity to sequence the behaviors and attribute motivation to them. This possibility has important implications for the interpretation of the coherence or consistency of expressed behavioral symptoms. Second, both the purgatives and *macake* remedy may have overlapping utility in the *iTaukei* Fijian pharmacopeia, with impact on a dimension other than weight, referencing the indigenous (*iTaukei*) explanatory model for the pathogenesis of *macake*, such as cleansing the gastrointestinal tract. In this respect, the practices may have variable motivation across and even within respondents; in some cases, the behaviors may be wholly or partially driven by interests outside of the realm of weight concerns. Third, the respondents may have been aiming at a culturally "safe" middle ground for their weight. Similar to the narratives of the low-weight respondents detailed above, they may have been using two herbal therapies to prevent both weight gain and weight loss: aiming for the *levulevu varausia* (just-right) size rather than for either the traditional *iTaukei* Fijian ideal of robust or the Western ideal of thin: an uncontroversial middle ground. That is, their behavior may have reflected that they both understood and wished to avoid the social costs of being either too thin or too large. Fourth, these young women may have been accommodating conflicting expectations imposed by their social network. Young women have very little license to decline parental instructions, at least overtly. Autonomy is discouraged and self-agency is concomitantly low. Both behaviors leading to weight control and appetite restoration may have been reactive: they represented acquiescence and even a strategy for calibration in titrating between too much food and too little. Finally, the respondents may have felt little agency to decline the *macake* treatment or prophylaxis, and may have used purgatives to subvert the associated weight gain. In this way, they could both accommodate the wishes of their parents and convention for protecting appetite, while neutralizing unwanted weight gain with purgatives.

There is another possibility, which is culturally grounded but unrelated to weight management, and which is also consistent with the confusing (to the investigators) narratives of the low-weight respondents. The research study protocol imposed a requirement to declare intentionality (in the self-report questionnaire) and formulate a causal narrative in response to interview questions. Formulating a narrative of intent – and concomitantly motivation to achieve personal goals – is second nature to Americans, who value self-direction and achievement.

A narrative of agency, however, may not be a practiced route for *iTaukei* girls, who are expected to respect authority and who value conformity and social harmony. It is plausible that the *iTaukei* Fijian respondents had no preexisting narrative to explain their behavior, but accommodated the research protocol by providing one.

In their seminal cognitive-behavioral account, Fairburn and colleagues (1999) propose three maintaining mechanisms for AN: (1) dietary restriction increases one's sense of being in control; (2) sequelae of starvation (e.g., increased satiety) encourage further dietary restriction; and (3) extreme concerns about shape and weight fuel further dietary restriction. They argue that the first two mechanisms are almost always present, whereas the third mechanism is culturally optional: "It is argued that an extreme need to control eating is the central feature of the disorder, and that in Western societies a tendency to judge self-worth in terms of shape and weight is superimposed on this need for self-control" (p. 1). However, "need for control" as a putative maintaining mechanism for AN may also be culturally moderated, since both the valuation and experience of being "in control" (as described clinically for AN) and the motivation and capacity to "be in control" of one's appetite and eating are structured by opportunities to exercise agency and autonomy over diet (relatively constrained in Fiji, compared with the United States), as well as by social norms that set expectations for decision-making rights about a young woman's body and comportment. By tradition, for example, a young *iTaukei* woman in Fiji would defer to her family to decide how she should wear her hair or clothing. However, new opportunities to pursue education and employment in the commercial sector expand the scope of decision-making for *iTaukei* Fijian women; presumably, concomitant shifts in social norms governing agency and autonomy are in play vis-à-vis weight management and self-presentation, as well.

Outliers: Diagnostic Criteria and the Inner Circle

Available evidence supports the claim that fat phobia characterizing AN is anchored in particular historical and cultural contexts. It is also an historical fact that BN – or at least its visibility – was a relative latecomer to Western psychiatric nosology. It was first described as "an ominous variant" of AN in a 1979 paper (Russell, 1979). More phenotypes of eating pathology have subsequently come to light: binge-eating disorder, now formalized as an eating disorder in *DSM-5* (APA, 2013, p. 350) was previously described in the back matter of *DSM-IV* in 1994 (APA, 1994). Purging disorder, moreover, which was initially described as an "ominous variant of bulimia nervosa" (Keel, Haedt, & Edler, 2005), now appears as an example of an "other specified feeding or eating disorder" (OSFED) in *DSM-5* (APA, 2013), in light of accumulating empirical data. In fact, the pronounced heterogeneity of eating pathology might best be captured in the data that indicated that the residual category of EDNOS in *DSM-IV* was the most frequently presenting clinical diagnosis (Zimmerman, Francione-Witt, Chelminski, Young, & Tortolani, 2008). Although revised criteria presented in *DSM-5* redefine the diagnostic boundaries of AN, BN, and EDNOS so that fewer cases are relegated to the new residual category (OSFED), the heterogeneity of eating pathology is remarkable and also defies attempts to encompass it neatly into discrete diagnostic categories. Indeed, available data suggest that, even under *DSM-5*, a substantial proportion of eating disorder cases will still fall in the residual category (Thomas et al., 2014).

The literature documenting the variability of expressed fat phobia has focused on the cultural salience of prevailing cultural norms governing style and aesthetics. Evidence supporting the observation that men with eating pathology tend to be motivated by contemporary masculine ideals of visible and bulky musculature (Pope, Phillips, & Olivardia, 2000) has also emphasized the pathogenic influence of aesthetic ideals. These examples are convincing but have largely left out another salient dimension of cultural variability that may govern local variation: self-agency. It is unsurprising that self-agency to appropriate a personal narrative of intent – or expression of distress – would be absent among *iTaukei* Fijian adolescent girls. Undocumented illness, in this respect, can be seen as a dimension of structural violence that undermines the well-being of these young women.

Compounding Vulnerabilities

The discourse on global health is dominated by questions about efficiency and fairness in the distribution of scarce resources. Attempts to set priorities and corresponding resource allocation are rationalized by the proportional burden of disease, cost-effectiveness, and collateral impacts of intervention, as well as by the pursuit of social justice for the economically and socially marginalized. There are strong arguments for protecting the socially vulnerable, including the mentally ill, who are frequently among the most socially disenfranchised because of economic poverty, social stigma, and discrimination (WHO, 2010).

Because most of the evidence base pertaining to mental disorders and their treatment has been generated in high-income countries (Patel & Thornicroft, 2009), engaging local knowledge about priorities and healthcare delivery strategies is essential to ensuring local relevance and effectiveness. It is widely recognized that achieving health equity requires that health consumers be empowered not just to access services (WHO, 2008) but also to influence policy (WHO, 2010). Indeed, the success of the Movement for Global Mental Health is premised on strong partnerships of mental health consumers with clinicians, researchers, and policy-makers (Patel et al., 2011). Notwithstanding the power of a strategy that mobilizes and organizes diverse groups with a vested interest in health policy and reform, it is not clear whether or how the diverse constituencies comprising health consumers will all find a voice among these stakeholders.

Furthermore, there may be unrecognized problems among marginalized demographic groups, including ethnic minorities, adolescents, and women, whose legitimacy to speak is either consistently challenged or undermined. When they do not have a voice, it is uncertain whether their interlocutors – if they have any – will have adequate information and motivation to advocate effectively on their behalf. Education itself is a precondition for understanding that one is in poor health (Sen, 1994).

Considering the vast unmet needs in global mental health that have a high profile, it is easy to understand how some could regard ferreting out undeclared eating disorders as a frivolous exercise. For example, a person might ask, "Why should mental health service providers uncover disorders they are not equipped to treat?" Sadly, this logic enters into a vicious cycle of perpetual deficits as knowledge of illness burden may be the impetus for developing a full complement of appropriate mental health services. Even the ethical basis of assessing prevalence for a disorder absent resources to respond by offering services may be challenged. Why commit resources to look for a problem without a workable plan to deploy a remedy? This ethical conundrum surely has another side, however, as it hardly seems defensible or wise to avoid probing the contours of a problem that could be substantial, even if out of view. Expanded access to interventions and training resources for eating disorders through delivery of clinical training and supervision and guided self-help via a web-based platform, to name two examples, is on the horizon (Fairburn & Wilson, 2013; Bauer & Moessner, 2013). Indeed, solving the health-delivery challenges in low-income regions may ultimately offer solutions toward resolving inequities in health care access in the rich world as well.

More importantly, when few community-based resources are available, social structural barriers such as affordability of services or poor access to transportation especially impact adolescents, who may not routinely access care in LMICs and among whom signs of mental disorders may have low visibility. Many symptoms of mental disorders are dimensional (see Bilder, Chapter 7, *this volume)*. At one end of the spectrum, they may overlap with mood and physical states that are continuous with normative experience. In this respect, measurement of distress, disability, and impairment may resist absolute or universal standards when a mental disorder is incipient or presents in unfamiliar ways. Mental health needs should not be overlooked for low visibility of disorders or communities. For disorders that often begin in adolescent populations like these, there may be strong arguments for active case detection and treatment of mental disorders and for preventative interventions. For example, mental disorders that strike in adolescence may start the individual on a path to economic and social vulnerability.

Finally, as our data from Fiji illustrate, we must be prepared to recognize that for social structural, economic, and cultural reasons, afflicted individuals may not always have the agency or platform to articulate their own needs so as to inform health policy makers. When research agendas are set and resources are committed, we must ensure that the voices and needs of even the most marginalized are encompassed if we are to safeguard the human right to health among the vulnerable.

Acknowledgments

This study was supported in part by K23 MH068575 (AEB) and a Harvard University Research Enabling Grant (AEB). We gratefully acknowledge the assistance at the time of data collection of Dr. Lepani Waqatakirewa, CEO, Fiji Ministry of Health, and his team; the Fiji Ministry of Education; the late Joana Rokomatu, *Tui Sigatoka*; Dr. Jan Pryor, Chair of the FN-RERC; Dr. Tevita Qorimasi; Nisha Khan; Asenaca Bainiliku; the late Kesaia Navara; and members of the Senior Advisory Group for the HEALTHY Fiji Study (Health-Risk and Eating Attitudes and Behaviors in Adolescents Living through Transition for Healthy Youth in Fiji Study), including Bill Aalbersberg, Alumita Taganesia, Livinai Masei, Pushpa Wati Khan, and Fulori Sarai. Finally, we thank all the Fiji-based principals and teachers who facilitated this study. The content is solely the responsibility of the authors and does not necessarily represent the official views of the National Institutes of Health or other consultants.

REFERENCES

Alarcon, R. D., Becker, A. E., Lewis-Fernández, R., Like, R. C. Desai, P., Foulks, E., ... Cultural Psychiatry Committee of the Group for the Advancement of Psychiatry. (2009). Issues for the *DSM-V*: The role of culture in psychiatric diagnosis. *Journal of Nervous and Mental Disease*, *197*(8), 559–660. http://dx.doi.org/10.1097/NMD.0b013e3181b0cbff

American Psychiatric Association. (1994). *Diagnostic and statistical manual of mental disorders* (4th ed.). Washington, DC: Author.

American Psychiatric Association. (2000). *Diagnostic and statistical manual of mental disorders* (4th ed., text rev.). Washington, DC: Author.

American Psychiatric Association. (2013). *Diagnostic and statistical manual of mental disorders* (5th ed.). Washington, DC: Author.

Anderson-Fye, E. P. (2004). A "Coca-Cola" shape: Cultural change, body image, and eating disorders in San Andres, Belize. *Culture, Medicine, and Psychiatry, 28*(4), 561–95. http://dx.doi.org/10.1007/s11013-004-1068-4

Banks, C. G. (1992). "Culture" in culture-bound syndromes: The case of anorexia nervosa. *Social Science & Medicine, 34*(8), 867–84. http://dx.doi.org/10.1016/0277-9536(92)90256-P

Bauer, S., & Moessner, M. (2013). Harnessing the power of technology for the treatment and prevention of eating disorders. *International Journal of Eating Disorders, 46*(5), 508–15. http://dx.doi.org/10.1002/eat.22109

Becker, A. E. (1994). Nurturing and negligence: Working on others' bodies in Fiji. In T. Csordas (Ed.), *Embodiment and experience* (pp. 100–15). Cambridge, England: Cambridge University Press.

Becker, A. E. (1995). *Body, self, and society: The view from Fiji.* Philadelphia: University of Pennsylvania Press.

Becker, A. E. (1998). Postpartum illness in Fiji: A sociosomatic perspective. *Psychosomatic Medicine, 60*, 431–8.

Becker, A. E. (2004). Television, disordered eating, and young women in Fiji: Negotiating body image and identity during rapid social change. *Culture, Medicine, and Psychiatry, 28*(4), 533–59. http://dx.doi.org/10.1007/s11013-004-1067-5

Becker, A. E., Arrindell, A. H., Perloe, A., Fay, K., & Striegel-Moore, R. H. (2010). A qualitative study of perceived social barriers to care for eating disorders: Perspectives from ethnically diverse health care consumers. *International Journal of Eating Disorders, 43*(7), 633–47. http://dx.doi.org/10.1002/eat.20755

Becker, A. E., Bainivualiku, A., Khan, A. N., Aalbersberg, W., Geraghty, P., Gilman, S. E., ... Striegel-Moore, R. H. (2009). Feasibility of a school-based study of health risk behaviors in ethnic Fijian female adolescents in Fiji: The HEALTHY Fiji Study. *Fiji Medical Journal, 28*, 18–34.

Becker, A. E., Burwell, R. A., Gilman, S. E., Herzog, D. B., & Hamburg, P. (2002). Eating behaviours and attitudes following prolonged television exposure among ethnic Fijian adolescent girls. *The British Journal of Psychiatry, 180*, 509–14. http://dx.doi.org/10.1192/bjp.180.6.509

Becker, A. E., & Kleinman, A. (2014). The history of cultural psychiatry in the last half-century. In S. Bloch, S. Green, & J. Holmes (Eds.), *Psychiatry: past, present, and prospect* (pp. 74–95). Oxford, England: Oxford University Press.

Becker, A. E., Perloe, A., & Eddy, K. (2009). Clarifying criteria for cognitive signs and symptoms for eating disorders in *DSM-V*. *International Journal of Eating Disorders, 42*(7), 611–19. http://dx.doi.org/10.1002/eat.20723

Becker, A. E., Roberts, A. L., Perloe, A., Bainivualiku, A., Richards, L. K., Gilman, S. E., & Striegel-Moore, R. H. (2010). Youth health risk behavior assessment in Fiji: The reliability of Global School-based Student Health Survey content adapted for ethnic Fijian girls. *Ethnicity & Health, 15*, 181–97. http://dx.doi.org/10.1080/13557851003615552

Becker, A. E., Thomas, J. J., Bainivualiku, A., Richards, L., Navara, K., Roberts, A. L., … Striegel-Moore, R. H. for the HEALTHY Fiji Study Group. (2010a). Validity and reliability of a Fijian translation and adaptation of the Eating Disorder Examination Questionnaire. *International Journal of Eating Disorders, 43*, 171–8. http://dx.doi.org/10.1002/eat.20675

Becker, A. E., Thomas, J. J., Bainivualiku, B. A., Richards, A., Navara, K., Roberts, A. L., … Striegel-Moore, R. H. for the HEALTHY Fiji Study Group. (2010b). Adaptation and evaluation of the Clinical Impairment Assessment to assess disordered eating related distress in an adolescent female ethnic Fijian population. *International Journal of Eating Disorders, 43*, 179–86. http://dx.doi.org/10.1002/eat.20665

Becker, A. E., Thomas, J. J., Franko, D. L., & Herzog, D. B. (2005). Disclosure patterns of eating and weight concerns to clinicians, educational professionals, family, and peers. *International Journal of Eating Disorders, 38*(1), 18–23. http://dx.doi.org/10.1002/eat.20141

Becker, A. E., Thomas, J. J., & Pike, K. (2009). Should non-fat-phobic anorexia nervosa be included in *DSM-V*? *International Journal of Eating Disorders, 42*(7), 620–35. http://dx.doi.org/10.1002/eat.20727

Bell, R. M. (1987). *Holy anorexia*. Chicago, IL: University of Chicago Press.

Bilder, R. M. (2015). Dimensional and categorical approaches to mental illness: Let biology decide. In L. J. Kirmayer, R. Lemelson, & C. A. Cummings (Eds.), *Re-visioning psychiatry: Cultural phenomenology, critical neuroscience, and global mental health* (pp. 179–205). New York, NY: Cambridge University Press.

Bohn, K., Doll, H. A., Cooper, Z., O'Connor, M., Palmer, R. L., & Fairburn, C. G. (2008). The measurement of impairment due to eating disorder psychopathology. *Behaviour Research and Therapy, 46*(10), 1105–10. http://dx.doi.org/10.1016/j.brat.2008.06.012

Brumberg, J. J. (1988). *Fasting girls: The history of anorexia nervosa*. Cambridge, MA: Harvard University Press.

Bravender, T., Bryant-Waugh, R., Herzog, D., Katzman, D., Kreipe, R. D., Lask, B., Workgroup for Classification of Eating Disorders in Children and Adolescents. (2007). Classification of child and adolescent eating disturbances. *International Journal of Eating Disorders, 40*(Suppl), S117–22. http://dx.doi.org/10.1002/eat.20458

Fairburn, C. G., & Beglin, S. J. (2008). Eating Disorder Examination Questionnaire (6.0). In C. G. Fairburn (Ed.) *Cognitive Behavior Therapy and Eating Disorders* (pp. 309–13). New York, NY: Guilford Press.

Fairburn, C. G., Cooper, Z., & O'Connor, M. E. (2008). Eating disorder examination (Edition 16.0D). In C. G. Fairburn (Ed.), *Cognitive behavior therapy and eating disorders* (pp. 265–308). New York, NY: Guilford.

Fairburn, C. G., Shafran, R., & Cooper, Z. (1999). A cognitive behavioural theory of anorexia nervosa. *Behaviour Research and Therapy, 37*(1), 1–13. http://dx.doi.org/10.1016/S0005-7967(98)00102-8

Fairburn, C.G., & Wilson, C.T. (2013). The dissemination and implementation of psychological treatments: Problems and solutions. *International Journal of Eating Disorders, 46*(5), 516–21. http://dx.doi.org/10.1002/eat.22110

Hacking, I. (1995). The looping effects of human kinds. In D. Sperber, D. Premack, & A. J. Premack, *Causal cognition: A multidisciplinary approach* (pp. 351–83). New York, NY: Oxford University Press.

Harris, E. C., & Barraclough, B. (1998). Excess mortality of mental disorder. *British Journal of Psychiatry, 173*, 11–53. http://dx.doi.org/10.1192/bjp.173.1.11

Henrich, J., Heine, S. J., & Norenzayan, A. (2010). The weirdest people in the world? *Behavioral and Brain Sciences, 33*, 61–83. http://dx.doi.org/10.1017/S0140525X0999152X

Hunt, D. P., Becker, A. E., Guimaraes, A. R., Stemmer-Rachamimov, A., Misdraji, J. (2012). Case 21–2012: A 27-year-old man with fatigue, weakness, weight loss, and decreased libido. [Case records of the Massachusetts General Hospital]. *New England Journal of Medicine, 367*(2), 157–69. http://dx.doi.org/10.1056/NEJMcpc1110053

Jablensky, A., Sartorius, N., Ernberg, G., Anker, M., Korten, A., Cooper, J. E., ... Bertelsen, A. (1992). Schizophrenia: Manifestations, incidence and course in different cultures. A World Health Organization ten-country study [Monograph supplement]. *Psychological Medicine, 20*, 1–97. http://dx.doi.org/10.1017/S0264180100000904

Keel, P. K., Haedt, A., & Edler, C. (2005). Purging disorder: An ominous variant of bulimia nervosa? *International Journal of Eating Disorders, 38*(3), 191–9. http://dx.doi.org/10.1002/eat.20179

Kessler, R. C., Wang, P. S., & Wittchen, H.-U. (2010). The social epidemiology of mental disorder. In C. Morgan & D. Bhugra (Eds.), *Principles of social psychiatry* (2nd ed.; pp. 91–101). West Sussex, England: John Wiley & Sons, Ltd. http://dx.doi.org/10.1002/9780470684214.ch8

Klump, K. L., Bulik, C. M., Kaye, W. H., Treasure, J., & Tyson, E. (2009). Academy for eating disorders position paper: Eating disorders are serious mental illnesses. *International Journal of Eating Disorders, 42*(2), 97–103. http://dx.doi.org/10.1002/eat.20589.

Lee, S. (1995). Self-starvation in context: Towards a culturally sensitive understanding of anorexia nervosa. *Social Science & Medicine, 41*(1), 25–36. http://dx.doi.org/10.1016/0277-9536(94)00305-D

Lee, S. (1996). Reconsidering the status of anorexia nervosa as a western culture-bound syndrome. *Social Science and Medicine, 42*(1), 21–34. http://dx.doi.org/10.1016/0277-9536(95)00074-7

Lee, S., Lee, A. M., Ngai, E., Lee, D. T. S., & Wing, Y. K. (2001). Rationales for food refusal in Chinese patients with anorexia nervosa. *International Journal of Eating Disorders, 29*(2), 224–9.

Lee, S., Ng, L. K., Kwok, K., & Fung, C. (2010). The changing profile of eating disorders at a tertiary psychiatric clinic in Hong Kong (1987–2007). *International Journal of Eating Disorders, 43*(4), 307–14. http://dx.doi.org/10.1002/eat.20686

Marques, L., Alegria, M., Becker, A. E., Chen, C.-N., Fang, A., Chosak, A., & Diniz, J. B. (2011). Comparative prevalence, correlates of impairment, and service utilization for eating disorders across US ethnic groups: Implications for reducing ethnic disparities in health care access for eating disorders. *International Journal of Eating Disorders, 44*(5), 412–20. http://dx.doi.org/10.1002/eat.20787

Mezzich, J., Kirmayer, L. J., Kleinman, A., Fabrega, H., Jr., Parron, D. L., Good, B. J., . . . Manson, S. M. (1999). The place of culture in *DSM-IV. Journal of Nervous and Mental Disease, 187*(8), 457–64. http://dx.doi.org/10.1097/00005053-199908000-00001

O'Hara, S. K., & Smith, K. G. (2007). Presentation of eating disorders in the news media: What are the implications for patient diagnosis and treatment? *Patient Education and Counseling, 68*(1), 43–51. http://dx.doi.org/10.1016/j.pec.2007.04.006

Patel, V., Collins, P. Y., Copeland, J., Kakuma, R., Katontoka, S., Lamichhane, J., . . . Skeen, S. (2011). The movement for global mental health. *British Journal of Psychiatry, 198*(2), 88–90. http://dx.doi.org/10.1192/bjp.bp.109.074518

Patel V., & Kim Y.-R. (2007). Contribution of low- and middle-income countries to research published in leading psychiatry journals, 2002–2004. *British Journal of Psychiatry, 190*, 77–8. http://dx.doi.org/10.1192/bjp.bp.106.025692

Patel, V., & Sumathipala, A. (2001). International representation in psychiatric literature: Survey of six leading journals. *British Journal of Psychiatry, 178*, 406–9. http://dx.doi.org/10.1192/bjp.178.5.406

Patel V., & Thornicroft G. (2009). Packages of care for mental, neurological, and substance use disorders in low- and middle-income countries: PLoS Medicine Series. *PLoS Medicine, 6*(10), e1000160. http://dx.doi.org/10.1371/journal/pmed.1000160

Pope, H. G., Phillips, K. A., Olivardia, R. (2000). *The adonis complex: The secret crisis of male body obsession.* New York, NY: Free Press.

Prince, R. (1985). The concept of culture-bound syndromes: Anorexia nervosa and brain fag. *Social Science and Medicine, 21*(2), 197–203. http://dx.doi.org/10.1016/0277-9536(85)90089-9

Russell, G. (1979). Bulimia nervosa: An ominous variant of anorexia nervosa. *Psychological Medicine, 9*(3), 429–48. http://dx.doi.org/10.1017/S0033291700031974

Sartorius, N. (1978). Diagnosis and classification: Cross cultural and international perspectives. *Mental Health and Society, 5*(1–2), 79–85.

Sen, A. (1994). Objectivity and position: Assessment of health and well-being. In L. Chen, A. Kleinman, & N. Ware (Eds.), *Health and social change in international perspective.* Boston, MA: Harvard School of Public Health.

Serpell, L., Teasdale, J. D., Troop, N. A., & Treasure, J. (2004). The development of the P-CAN, a measure to operationalize the pros and cons of anorexia nervosa. *International Journal of Eating Disorders, 36*(4), 416–33. http://dx.doi.org/10.1002/eat.20040

Tchanturia, K., Davies, H., Roberts, M., Harrison, A., Nakazato, M., Schmidt, ... Morris, R. (2012). Poor cognitive flexibility in eating disorders: Examining the evidence using the Wisconsin Card Sorting Task. *PLoS One, 7*(1), e28331. http://dx.doi.org/10.1371/journal.pone.0028331

Thomas, J. J., Crosby, R. D., Wonderlich, S. A., Striegel-Moore, R. H., & Becker, A. E. (2011). A latent profile analysis of the typology of bulimic symptoms in an indigenous Pacific population: Evidence of cross-cultural variation in phenomenology. *Psychological Medicine, 41*(1), 195–206. http://dx.doi.org/10.1017/S0033291710000255

Thomas, J. J., Koh, K. A., Eddy, K. T., Hartmann, A. S., Murray, H. B., Gorman, ... Becker, A. E. (2014). Do *DSM-5* feeding and eating disorder criteria overpathologize normative eating patterns among individuals with obesity? *Journal of Obesity, 320803*, 1–8.

Thomas, J. J., Vartanian, L. R., & Brownell, K. D. (2009). The relationship between eating disorder not otherwise specified (EDNOS) and officially recognized eating disorders: Meta-analysis and implications for *DSM. Psychological Bulletin, 135*(3), 407–33. http://dx.doi.org/10.1037/a0015326

Thomas J. J., Weigel, T. J., Lawton, B., Levendusky, P. G., & Becker, A. E. (2012). The cognitive-behavioral treatment of body image disturbance in a congenitally blind patient with anorexia nervosa. *American Journal of Psychiatry, 169*(1), 16–20. http://dx.doi.org/10.1176/appi.ajp.2010.10040555

Thompson-Brenner, H., Satir, D. A., Franko, D. L., & Herzog, D. B. (2012). Clinician reactions to patients with eating disorders: A review of the literature. *Psychiatric Services, 63*(1), 73–8. http://dx.doi.org/10.1176/appi.ps.201100050

Thornicroft, G., & Sartorius, N. (1993). The course and outcome of depression in different cultures: 10-year follow-up of the WHO Collaborative Study on the Assessment of Depressive Disorders. *Psychological Medicine, 23*(4), 1023–32. http://dx.doi.org/10.1017/S0033291700026489

Vos, T., Flaxman, A. D., Naghavi, M., Lozano, R., Michaud, C., Ezzati, M., ... Murray, C. J. (2012). Years lived with disability (YLDs) for 1160 sequelae of 289 diseases and injuries 1990–2010: A systematic analysis for the Global Burden of Disease Study 2010. *The Lancet, 380*(9859), 2163–96. http://dx.doi.org/10.1016/S0140-6736(12)61728-2

World Health Organization. (2001). *The world health report 2001: Mental health – New understanding, new hope.* Geneva, Switzerland: World Health Organization.

World Health Organization. (2003). *Caring for children and adolescents with mental disorders: Setting WHO directions.* Geneva, Switzerland: Author.

World Health Organization. (2007). BMI-for-age: Girls 5 to 19 years (percentiles). Retrieved from WHO website: http://www.who.int/growthref/bmifa_girls_5_19years_per.pdf

World Health Organization. (2008). *Closing the gap in a generation: Health equity through action on the social determinants of health.* Geneva, Switzerland: Author.

World Health Organization. (2010). *Mental health and development: Targeting people with mental health conditions as a vulnerable group.* Geneva, Switzerland: Author.

Zimmerman, M., Francione-Witt, C., Chelminski, I., Young, D., & Tortolani, C. (2008). Problems applying the *DSM-IV* eating disorders diagnostic criteria in a general psychiatric outpatient practice. *Journal of Clinical Psychiatry, 69*(3), 381–4. http://dx.doi.org/10.4088/JCP.v69n0306

21   Solving Global Mental Health as a Delivery Problem
Toward a Critical Epistemology of the Solution

Kalman Applbaum

Introduction to the Problem

WHO [World Health Organization] is making a simple statement: mental health – neglected for far too long – is crucial to the well-being of individuals, societies and countries and must be universally regarded in a new light. (WHO, 2001, p. ix)

WHO has received an increasing number of requests from countries for assistance and country-specific action. The need for – and relevance of – an economic perspective in planning, provision, and assessment of services, and for scaling up care for MNS [Mental, Neurological and Substance use] disorders is another reason to revise the focus of the mental health strategy. Moreover, a comprehensive programme for action can inspire stakeholders and accelerate progress by bringing together partners with a common purpose. (WHO Mental Health Gap Action Programme, 2008, p. 9)

How does a term such as "global mental health" become a normative object of medical and epidemiological evaluation and estimation to the degree that remedial strategies can be deployed toward its improvement? When WHO reports that, worldwide, "Depression is the leading cause of disability as measured by YLDs [years lost due to disability]" and that "by the year 2020, depression is projected to reach 2nd place of the ranking of DALYs [disability adjusted life years] calculated for all ages, both sexes,"[1] how does WHO wish us to understand the object so as to act on it?

We move closer to the intended object with the WHO estimate that the treatment gap for mental, neurological, and substance abuse disorders is greater than 75 percent (Barbui et al., 2010), and through comorbidities is linked further, as cause and consequence, to primary health concerns in those locales (Prince et al., 2007, p. 1). The opening quote from WHO

---

[1] http://www.who.int/mental_health/management/depression/en/. See also www.who.int/healthinfo/global_burden_disease/metrics_daly/en/.

frames their engagement with global mental health as a response to pleas for help from low- and middle-income countries (LMICs).

In a podcast interview of three of the founders of the new global mental health movement, including Shekhar Saxena, coordinator for mental health at WHO, Graham Thornicroft estimated that every year a quarter of all adults will have a mental illness, with a lifetime prevalence of 50 percent.[2] These same authors were involved in two more fronts for advocacy of the movement: six "pioneering" articles in a 2007 *Lancet* issue on global mental health (Prince et al., 2007) and the same number in a follow-up issue (Patel, Boyce, Collins, Saxena, & Horton, 2011); as well as six articles in a 2009 *PLOS Medicine* issue on the same subject, entitled "Packages of Care" (Patel & Thornicroft, 2009). "Crisis of epidemic proportions" is the first impression made visible when we encounter "global mental health." These figures of 25, 50, and 75 percent (for annual, lifetime, and untreated incidence, respectively) and first and second place (rankings for depression's contribution to disability today and tomorrow) are not just epidemiological estimates, but large, rounded numbers intended to spur action.

Where there is crisis, the solution must be found nearby. The troubling uncertainties voiced in at least some quarters over the definition/prevalence estimate (combined per the Latin etymology: *definio ire*, meaning "to limit, bound") of mental wellness and its obverse, and the circumstances in which the current battery of therapies are deemed to achieve (or not achieve) successful amelioration of suffering, must shrink before the scale of the untreated anguish and the moral clarity behind the call to *do something*. Qualitative misgivings must yield to quantitative certainties. At least one group of psychiatrist activists propose sacrificing anthropology, presumably as the representative of qualitative prudence, to the locomotive of quantitative urgency. Melanie Abas, a psychiatrist and experienced global mental health researcher, writes in the cross-cultural forum of the *Harvard Review of Psychiatry*: "It would be wrong to delay the implementation of evidenced-based treatments for distressing and disabling CMDs [common mental disorders] while awaiting extensive anthropological work in all countries of the globe" (2003, p. 168).

---

[2] http://www.audiomedica.com/global-health-issues/lshtm-audio-news-special-global-mental-health-september-15th-2007/ This interview took place in the context of the launch of a website for the "new global mental health movement" (www.globalmentalhealth.org/). The new movement can be construed as a rebranding maneuver insofar as it is a renewed attempt to gain attention and status for mental health in the crowded but underserved global health world.

Introduction to the Solution

In recent decades, pharmaceutical modalities have come to occupy an ever larger portion of biomedical interventions. Global health initiatives now fully reflect this emphasis, stressing the poor access that people in LMICs have to "essential drugs" (Greene, 2011). The expanded importance of pharmaceuticals, combined with their transportability, has translated into a new attentiveness to solving problems associated with effective delivery. The tactic of disseminating medicines through more diverse channels (rural clinics, trained community health workers, for example), sometimes referred to as "task shifting," and the implementation of new technologies of compliance through these agencies, have proven successful strategies for enhancing outcomes in the treatment of infectious, diarrheal, and parasitic diseases, as well as improving uptake in immunization programs.[3]

Apparently inspired by these successes, a comparable treatment model with an emphasis on delivery underlies a recently updated WHO mental health initiative for the psychiatrically underserved LMICs. The mental health Gap Action Programme (mhGAP) *Intervention Guide* states:

There is a widely shared but mistaken idea that all mental health interventions are sophisticated and can only be delivered by highly specialized staff. Research in recent years has demonstrated the feasibility of delivery of pharmacological and psychosocial interventions in non-specialized healthcare settings. (2010, p. 1)[4]

Framing the remedy in terms of delivery on the scale implied – to a quarter or half of three-quarters of the world's population – partly prefigures the realized solution, I will argue, as a market-based one with psychopharmaceuticals at its nucleus. "Delivery" implies building distribution networks of intermediaries capable of bringing a standard product, if customized in some superficial way to meet local requirements, to the end user. Of all possible psychiatric solutions to mental

---

[3] See, for example, http://www.pih.org/blog/task-shifting.
[4] The day after the mhGAP program was introduced, several of the authors launched a website for the "new global mental health movement" (www.globalmentalhealth.org/). The new movement can be construed as a rebranding maneuver insofar as it is a renewed attempt to gain attention and status for mental health in the crowded but underserved global health world. These same authors were involved in two more fronts for advocacy of the movement: six articles in a 2007 *Lancet* issue on global mental health, and six articles in a 2009 *PLOS Medicine* issue on the same subject, entitled "Packages of Care."

illness, drugs are by far the most amenable to this logistic goal. Abas and colleagues, who told us that there is no time for anthropological research, are not troubled by the dearth of local knowledge because they conceive of mental health care delivery in a *consumer* idiom: "The WHO South-East Asia Regional Office expressly supports consumer involvement in the delivery of mental health services. Little is known, however, about the way that consumers would like services to be delivered" (2003, p. 168). The language of consumer preference (how they would "like services to be delivered") and "involvement" comes explicitly from consumer marketing. A recent *Journal of Marketing* article explains, "strive to maximize consumer involvement in the customization [because this leads] *to opportunities for expanding the market by assisting the consumer in the process of specialization and value creation*" (Vargo & Lusch, 2004, p. 12, emphasis added).

We can decide later about the hazards of purposely or inadvertently sharing language and delivery models with consumer marketers (see Applbaum 2009a, 2009b, 2009c).[5] We also need not dwell for the moment on the question of whether the current standard of pharmacotherapy is or is not the best solution to this or that mental disorder. What concerns me here is the likelihood that a plan to dispense Western psychiatric solutions continuously (since mental illnesses tend to get managed, not cured) to hundreds of millions or perhaps billions of people is not going to favor nuanced psychosocial interventions, but pill distribution. In high-income countries (HICs), pharmacotherapy has become the de facto gold standard for treatment; resources permitting, is this not the solution Western psychiatry would also ultimately envision for LMICs?

The first concern one might raise is not the insufficiency of knowledge about the context for etiology, diagnosis, and care among the LMIC billions, but an inattention to the ambiguous state of knowledge regarding treatment outcomes at the industrialized core, from which

---

[5] Dominique Behague has been astute to point out to me, "In the broader history of public health ... even in the most 'public' of public health's corners, neoliberal models of development have been creeping in since the 1980s with structural adjustment, the decline of national and regional governments, and the rise of the big donors, all with their own separate visions and aims and accountability structures. Even in health issues where pharma is not as central a player, some actors have been bemoaning the infiltration of technocratic and market-oriented rationales (e.g., DALYs)." One must, she suggests, "tackle some of the core reasons market principles have been able to infiltrate into public health in a first instance, which I think relates not only to the pharmaceutical industry finding its way in through PPV [private public ventures] amongst other routes, but also to the whole cost-effectiveness model upon which most global and national public health action is now based" (personal communication).

Table 21.1 *Psychiatric Drug Sales US (1990–2008)*

	1990	2000	2008
Antidepressants	$950 million	$8.9 billion	$9.6 billion
Antipsychotics	$250 million	$3.5 billion	$14.6 billion
Psychostimulants	$76 million	$600 million	$4.8 billion
Total	$2.5 billion	$15.2 billion	n/a

Note. $1 in 2008 = $0.80 in 2000 = $.60 in 1990 (approx.).
Source: IMS Health.

the endeavor to export solutions originates. A frank look not at individual drug studies, which somehow miraculously always show progress, but at the overall situation for mental health in HIC environments – where resources invested and awareness are high and seekers encounter fewer impediments to accessing state-of-the-art psychiatric services – should give us pause: Rates of disability from mental illness in treatment-rich environments remain discouragingly high.

Using U.S. Department of Health Services data on "patient care episodes" for mental illness, and cross-checking the data with SSDI (Social Security Disability Insurance) and SSI (Supplemental Security Income) rolls that code for mental illness in individuals under age sixty-five, Robert Whitaker estimates that the number of mentally ill in America actually doubled between 1987 and 2005 (Whitaker, 2005). A static view of the same puzzling picture is visible on world DALY maps, which appear to confirm that many of the countries with the highest investment in mental health care nevertheless continue to suffer from high rates of disability.

We can compound the paradoxical figures with another set describing trends in the prescription and sales of psychopharmaceuticals in the United States: The selective serotonin reuptake inhibitors (SSRIs) grew from a $2.5 billion business in 1990 to a $15.2 billion business in 2000 (Table 21.1). In 1997, 88.3 million prescriptions for antidepressants were written. The number nearly tripled to 232.7 million in just ten years. In the 2000s, as SSRI blockbusters like Prozac and Paxil came off patent, profit leadership was assumed by the atypical antipsychotics (Risperdal, Zyprexa, for example) and ADHD medicines, the sales of which grew 3,500 and 3,800 percent, respectively, between 1990 and 2008. In 2008 and 2009 such a rarefied agent as atypical antipsychotics were the best-selling class of drugs in the United States at $14.6 billion (Abraham, 2010), or roughly 1.5 times the total public expenditure for all healthcare in India in 2010; worldwide sales of the drugs in this class are approaching $22 billion in revenues. The number of antipsychotic prescriptions in the United States tripled between 1995 and 2008, and nearly half those were written for unapproved (that is, off-label) uses (Alexander et al., 2011; see also Friedman, 2012). Prescription/sales of select benzodiazapines such as Xanax (alprozolam) and Klonopin (clonazepam) continued to grow during this period (Xanax alone enjoyed 44 million U.S. prescriptions in 2009), despite recurrent warnings about dependency, and insomnia medications rose from relative obscurity to become a $3.6 billion business.[6]

Given the triumphant propagation of the most modern psychiatric treatments in the HICs, why is the DALY map representation of these countries still beet red? Is the upsurge in prescriptions written for these classes of drugs the outcome of advancements in science and public health, or is it the result of an agent-driven enlargement of markets?

Critics hold that the meteoric expansion of psychopharmaceuticals since 1990 has little to do with progress in psychiatry, but is the fruit of marketing campaigns devised to distort psychiatric epidemiology and evidence of drug effectiveness in the furtherance of pharmaceuticalization, defined in the current context as "the process by which social, behavioural or bodily conditions are treated or deemed to be in need of treatment with medical drugs," at a pace that outstrips actual biomedical advances to justify such expansion (Abraham, 2010). The upshot is what Robert Rosenheck (2005), one of psychiatry's most prominent clinical researchers, has decried as the triumph of "irrational exuberance" over evidence-based practice, leading to inappropriate, excessive, and ultimately iatrogenic prescription of psychopharmaceuticals by psychiatrists and even more pronouncedly by primary care physicians (PCPs) through much of the industrialized world.

To our temporary relief, the architects of the new global mental health movement and of the mhGAP guideline appear to express no overt favoritism for pharmacological over psychosocial interventions. The guideline rather seems to be recommending against a quick trigger appeal to pharmaceuticals to address conditions that in the United States or the United Kingdom, for instance, would almost reflexively incur this algorithm of treatment. This already demonstrates an important new thoughtfulness in comparison with earlier recommendations regarding the applicability and/or cost effectiveness of Western

---

[6] See http://dbt.consultantlive.com/display/article/1145628/1404717; www.healthcarefinance news.com/press-release/pipeline-antipsychotic-drugs-drive-next-market-evolution; and http://psychcentral.com/lib/2010/top-25-psychiatric-prescriptions-for-2009/.

treatments in LMIC environments. Others of a more anthropological bent who may have lent a hand in informing the recommendations advocate for the foregrounding of locally sensible solutions (Desjarlais et al., 1995; Cohen et al., 2002, for example).

One might therefore be optimistic and supportive of the plan to scale up mental health in the new global health agenda. Yet there is reason to fear that the forces of global diffusion of the Western psychiatric imaginary, well-established in the systemic habits of the profession in more affluent countries and middle-class areas of LMICs, may overwhelm more delicate, human-centered intentions. The movement's apparently unexamined use of the terms "delivery" and "packages of care" (Patel & Thornicroft, 2009) as merely logistical constructs may betray an unreflexive pragmatism insufficiently troubled by historical, transcultural psychiatric, ethnographic, or political economic dimensions. Confidence in the comparability-of-outcomes evidence derived from HICs (for example, "It is heartening to note that where attempts to replicate evidence on effectiveness have been attempted in low and middle income countries, the findings are consonant with those from high income countries, suggesting that such evidence may be generalizable across cultures" (Patel & Thornicroft, 2009, p. 2) echo earlier inattentions to cultural considerations in the compilation of the *DSM-IV* (Mezzich et al., 1999) and do not initially inspire optimism that the new program will incorporate a necessary "critical epistemology" (Farmer, 1999; Berrios & Marková, Chapter 2, *this volume*) to inform this most complex undertaking.[7] Mental illness is more contextually embedded than other sicknesses. It requires, therefore, a higher degree of familiarity with cultural features and with articulations to what Arthur Kleinman calls "local moral worlds" (1999). The complexities of globalization itself set the facts of mental wellness/illness and psychiatry's reaction to them in new motion, rendering the already tenuous assessment of illness manifestation, course, and treatment outcomes more vulnerable to uncertainty (Kirmayer & Minas, 2000).

The transmission of conditions, practices, and cultures endemic to medicine in wealthy nations may be poised to extend to LMICs by means of the targeted exertions of both multinational companies ("big pharma"), which already report massively expanding sales of their

---

[7] Das and Rao also point out, "Patel and colleagues' (Prince et al., 2007) review of treatment and prevention in LMIC, in aggregate, reveals that more than 80% of trials for depression were for psychopharmaceuticals alone. This suggests a bias in the research agenda, when evidence from high income countries (HIC) indicates that both pharmacological and psychological interventions are equally efficacious" (2012, p. 3).

products in what they graspingly call "pharmerging countries" in Asia and Latin America, and of local entrepreneurs ("little pharma") who trade on the generic leftovers of the branded blockbusters.

One is justified in speaking of the commercial globalization of psychiatry through the medium of the pill, or "psychopharmaceutical globalization." The delivery channels of psychopharmaceutical globalization is facilitated by international trade agreements such as TRIPS (Trade Related Aspects of International Property Rights) and the ICH (International Committee on Harmonization) (Timmermans, 2007). More actively, psychopharmaceutical globalization is encouraged by the pervasive implementation of global public-private partnerships (GPPPs) between states and pharmaceutical companies based on the interested argument that pill solutions are more efficient, cheaper, and scientifically sounder than the alternatives. The adoption of simplified mental health screens and rating scales, often traceable to initiatives sponsored by drug companies to increase drug sales (Healy, 1997), is used to support this claim. GPPPs thrive in the context of market-directed health reforms being undertaken by budget-strapped (and often indebted) governments; together with international trade mechanisms, GPPPs are outgrowths of neoliberal globalization itself (Panitch & Leys, 2010; Buse & Walt, 2000). Finally, the independent trend towards deinstitutionalization of the mentally ill naturally tilts unfolding treatment paradigms toward drug use in a difficult-to-regulate fashion.[8] Studies from the field suggest that in the implementation of recent mental health policy objectives, care is already being task-shifted to pills:

As institutional care becomes increasingly outsourced to entrepreneurs and local communities, and as powerful medications circulate without even a doctor visit, human relationships to medical technology are increasingly constituted outside the clinical encounter. New populations and forms of intimacy are now emerging around technology at community and domestic levels, as in the case of ... the massive and often unregulated dissemination of psychiatric drugs worldwide. (Bichl & Moran-Thomas, 2009, p. 274)

The process is abetted by the commercial motivation of local entrepreneurs, often including physicians, to favor dispensing drugs over other forms of treatment. As we will see, through the dissemination of local branded generics in particular, psychopharmaceuticals may not be as inaccessible as the WHO reports suggest.

---

[8] De Menil and Cohen (2009) have argued that irrational overprescription practices may be common in psychiatric hospitals as well.

Commercial Biopower and Global Psychiatry

Commercial globalization[9] is contingent on the power of firms to standardize product, message, and most importantly – but imperceptibly – to help flatten trade structures and the perceived context for product utility (Applbaum, 2004a). I encountered an impressive example of this "megamarketing" (Kotler, 1986) in the introduction of SSRIs in Japan in the early 2000s. The effort to launch SSRIs in Japan was more than just another case study in export marketing or adaptation to medical cultural particularities. The European/American firms endeavoring to penetrate the Japanese market with SSRIs were not seeking to merely adapt their drugs and marketing programs to local situations, nor did they relate to one another mainly as competitors. Instead, with the help of the industry trade representative, PhRMA, they formed an oligopolistic front to alter the total environment in which these drugs were to be sold and used (Applbaum, 2006; see also Kitanaka, 2006, and Kirmayer, 2002).

Once multiple markets are primed for one's product category, the next step is to adapt specific products into local schemes of meaning and practice – a procedure sometimes called mass customization. In the case of psychopharmaceuticals (mood stabilizers, antidepressants, etc.), bio- and ethical-universalism serve as standardizing conveyances, while adaptation consists of tailoring not the advertising but the *science* to meet local perceptions of product value through positioning, targeting, and other marketing tools (Matheson, 2008). In my research into the progress of atypical antipsychotics in the Japanese market (Applbaum, 2010), I learned how Eli Lilly diverted attention away from the side effects of its drugs by using doctors' misperceptions of the drugs as the basis for fresh scientific publication programs in defense of the brand. In other words, the company treated the medical concerns associated with its drugs as a relative and fungible truth – as a brand truth that the company had ownership rights and resources to control. Eli Lilly assembles perceptual data by country and setting. The science is adjusted in each

---

[9] I use Waitzkin et al.'s (2007, p. 209, fn. 1) definition of globalization as "the process by which interconnected economic transactions increasingly occur throughout the world, facilitated by (*a*) technological changes in communication and transportation that have dramatically changed the speed of financial and commercial transactions; (*b*) international agreements that encourage 'free trade,' with a shift of regulatory authority from governments to international financial institutions and trade organizations; (*c*) expanded investments, sales, and collaborations by multinational corporations; (*d*) increased movement of private finance capital across national boundaries; and (*e*) privatization of enterprises previously administered in the public sector."

market to meet specific challenges of that market; the company does not make the same pronouncement regarding side effects in each locale, as might be expected by medical standards or those of regulatory authorities.

If this is a sample view from the bridge of drug companies solving the strategic problem of "how to go global," conversely, biopsychiatric globalization as a totalizing proposition, and not just one of shreds and patches, depends upon commercial pharmaceutical globalization. Without the drugs, biopsychiatry is little more than an inert theory,[10] and without pharmaceutical companies that are striving to go global, and local companies seeking to compete with products comparable to those marketed by big pharma, the engine for global dissemination is weak. Commodity globalization is a strong force, to borrow the language of physics, while psychiatric globalization is, when unaided, a weak one.

A glimpse into this relationship presented itself to me at the WPA (World Psychiatric Association) meeting in Yokohama in 2002. I attended an open meeting where conference organizers discussed plans for the next conference in Cairo. They consistently demonstrated subservience to the pharmaceutical industry's demands since many of the amenities and the costs of bringing many of the "delegates" were borne by companies. "Let us get better organized in how we approach industry, so we can continue to have credibility as a whole," one of the organizers said. At a minimum, the relationship between the association and big pharma was symbiotic, particularly as both contemplated the prospect of their needs in face of the challenges of globalization.

The WPA is competing with other organizations for success in organizing glorious congresses—in the words of one of the organizers, "Globalization is happening everywhere. There's more competition. People know all about the

---

[10] Thomas Ban argues that from a scientific standpoint the prioritization of drug developers' self-serving methodologies in evaluating the effectiveness of various treatment modalities has rendered inert both psychiatry and psychopharmacology ("the scientific discipline dedicated to the detection of psychopathologic symptoms and syndromes, and the identification of nosologic entities that are affected by psychotropic drugs" [2006, p. 434]):

As decisions regarding the choice of treatment were to become based increasingly on findings in the clinical development of psychotropic drugs, psychiatric nosology was replaced by consensus-based classifications and psychopathology by rating scale variables used in the clinical studies conducted for the demonstration of therapeutic effects. … Since one of the essential prerequisites for the development of neuropsychopharmacology is the identification of a treatment responsive form of illness, consensus-based classifications and sensitized rating scales blocked the development of the combined discipline. (Ban, 2006, pp. 434, 435)

conference all over the world." The WPA, however, is "on the way up." It is targeting developing countries more aggressively than ever in the attempt to increase the association's enrollment and to bring superior mental health care to the developing world. The next congress will be held in Cairo. The organizers already speak of a new method for advertising their meeting: asking drug company sales reps to carry news of the conference to every doctor they visit. The geographic expansion of the WPA is likewise good for the drug companies who sponsor it. The treatment of depression and anxiety with SSRIs is new business in most places outside of the triad of the U.S., Europe, and more recently Japan. The WPA, both with its non-sponsored and sponsored scientific programs, will carry the message to new destination markets. (Applbaum, 2004b, p. 309)

It is true that specialized agents such as chlorpromazine that came on line in the 1950s represented a revolutionary advance over prior technologies for treating schizophrenic psychosis and required no specific marketing program to encourage their export around the world. There was marketing, but use of the drugs was limited to the most severely ill within the restricted environment of the asylum. The projected broad base for adoption of psychopharmaceuticals and other psychiatric treatments is not comparable. To get 25 to 50 percent of the world into some kind of psychiatric treatment, which is what the WHO statistics would suggest is called for, a medicalization project of vast proportions will be necessary. The linked belief in scientific progress and the free market as sources of divine providence may indeed be widespread, and can be a powerful opening for commercial medicalization. Only under the coordination of commercial biopower might 1.7 to 3.5 billion individuals come to self-identify as mentally ill and to consume psychiatric treatments. Pharmaceutical companies will gain nothing from promoting nonpharmacological treatments, much less from reconfiguring their mission to alleviate the poverty that, more fundamentally than disease processes, is the precipitate to so much emotional suffering.

The global commodity nature of psychopharmaceuticals and psychiatry's inseparable linkage to it can be seen in empirical examples of how drugs actually travel. If the classification of disease in the *DSM* at one time preceded the drugs that are now implicitly linked to them, the same is not true in much of the world where the two, the *DSM* (or *ICD*) and the associated drug list, arrive in a single envelope. In that case, the *DSM* functions as a decoder and a user's manual to the "system of objects" (Baudrillard, 1968/1996) that constitute the psychopharmacopeia. We can expect modification to abstractions about the culture of drugs (as commodities, for instance) to emerge from further ethnographic investigation, but the process of their dissemination in diverse environments is already in motion. We must take the above into consideration when evaluating claims made by the new global mental health movement regarding the treatment gap.

Pharmerging Examples: India, Brazil, and the Globalization of Psychiatry Through the Medium of the Pill

Where some have argued that big pharma acts as the dominant partner to psychiatry in creating and demonstrating pharmaceutical value in home markets (Applbaum, 2011; Ban, 2006; Healy, 1997, 2008; Sismondo, 2007), affecting the configuration of psychiatric truths around the world, ethnographic research shows that big pharma's influence in the actual distribution of psychopharmaceuticals in LMICs is highly mediated, and sometimes resisted, by local thinking and social forces (Lakoff, 2006, for example). To make sense of how other places may become "psychophar-macological societies," as Nikolas Rose terms it (2004), we need to temper our respect for global sales figures and big pharma's strategic intent, and instead pay closer attention to "local cultural codes, everyday concerns and diverse epidemiological realities" (Behague, 2008, p. 143). Reformist states or small market players, possibly ignorant of or indiffer-ent to debates over the efficacy of drugs and the scientific status of biological psychiatry, can be lured by the promise of magic-bullet cures. The examples of India and Brazil, which are centers of attention for both multinational drug companies and for the new global mental health movement, offer enlightening case studies.

Little Pharma and Un/Regulated Proliferation of SSRIs in India

Stefan Ecks directly confronts estimates of WHO and the global mental health *Lancet* authors (see Footnote 2) concerning the supposed treat-ment gap in West Bengal, India. Ecks is a member of a collaborative project entitled "Tracing Pharmaceuticals in South Asia," which followed production, distribution, retail sales, prescription, and regula-tion of fluoxetine (the SSRI marketed as Prozac in the United States). He says, "It is widely believed that depression goes largely untreated in India. ... If a methodology is used that starts with the actual availability of antidepressant drugs rather than the availability of medical personnel and institutions, a drastically different picture emerges" (Ecks, 2009). The WHO and *Lancet* authors, he points out, calculate for both burden of disease and treatment gap on the basis of economic measures. "Cal-culations of how much money *should* be spent by national health systems on mental health treatments are contrasted with data on how much money is *actually* spent, and the difference between the two is taken to evince a huge 'treatment gap.'"

Rather than finding a dearth of psychopharmaceuticals in rural areas, as predicted by the WHO reports, Ecks and his colleagues discovered the opposite. There is a "stunning proliferation" of psychopharmaceuticals available, especially SSRIs and above all, fluoxetine, of which they were able to trace sixty-six brands. Twenty-three of these combined fluoxetine with alprazolam (the benzodiazepine marketed as Xanax in the United States), while three combined fluoxetine with olanzapine (the antipsychotic marketed as Zyprexa in the United States). A Kolkata NGO that publishes the *Rational Drug Bulletin* found that "generic fluoxetine is highly available and affordable across all cities and districts of West Bengal" (Ecks, 2009) – more available through some forty thousand medicine shops, in fact, than vital drugs such as the anti-inflammatory ibuprofen or the antibiotic ciprofloxacin.

It is useful to recount the mechanisms by which this situation has come about in Bengal because some of these same conditions may apply to other places where WHO findings presume the unavailability of these drugs. The most important factor giving rise to the hyper-availability of psychopharmaceuticals such as fluoxetine is India's large manufacture and trade in generic pharmaceuticals. Prior to 2005, when India became a full signatory to TRIPS under the WTO, the domestic industry benefitted from a patent law that recognized process patents, but not product patents. This law effectively lowered barriers to entry for domestic competitors to companies such as Eli Lilly, original maker of fluoxetine (Prozac). Second, the dearth of prescription enforcement contributed to the ready availability of psychopharmaceuticals. SSRIs, for instance, are "Schedule H" drugs: they cannot be sold over the counter. In practice, however, they are easily available over the counter, and unlicensed prescribers, ranging from medicine shopkeepers to rural medical practitioners (RMPs), routinely dispense them. Patients are given "floating prescriptions," which permit unrestricted refills (Ecks & Basu, 2009).

Ecks and Basu explain how suggested use of such medicines is communicated. Although there are drug reps who approach licensed and unlicensed prescribers and offer them market-specific narratives and kickbacks, the primary means of information and motivation to adopt new drugs comes "from psychiatrists to licensed generalists, and subsequently to unlicensed practitioners" (Ecks & Basu, 2009, p. 99). This communication is not even from practitioner to practitioner, but instead, doctors and RMPs learn about new treatments from patients who bring prescriptions from other sources. This pattern suggests the importance to marketers of cultivating key opinion leaders in this market, where the "trickle down" of accepted practices is so powerful that potential prescribers will adopt new medicines merely upon learning that some other practitioner is doing so. Of course, prescribers profit from the trade, and this commercial motivation is the last factor behind the trade's liveliness. "The boundaries between production, marketing, distribution, retail, and prescription of drugs can be surprisingly porous. Each of these areas offers its own profit opportunities" (Ecks, 2009, p. 99).

Ecks and his colleagues have been tracing the commercial lines of the availability of psychopharmaceuticals in Bengal. Sumeet Jain and Sushrut Jadhav have studied the political sources of drug availability in Uttar Pradesh. What they find is that "community psychiatry has, in practice, become an administrative psychiatry focused on effective distribution of psychotropic medication" (2009, p. 61). Although many psychiatrists there may have retained an interest in psychosocial approaches to treatment, pills have been the most implementable solution and thus became the most common accommodation to the 2002 "re-strategized" National Mental Health Program. The adoption of a pharmacological solution, Jain and Jadhav suggest, was in any case inevitable.

The implementation of a biologically-oriented psychiatry appeals to health professionals as a way to both achieve desired professional outcomes (e.g., satisfied patients, income, and credibility among peers) and cement linkages with the dominant discourses and institutions of international psychiatry. ... In short, this process of replication and mirroring along a chain that links Geneva, New Delhi and the Kanpur clinic is a cultural dynamic that directly affects the rural patient population. (Ecks, 2009, p. 76)

The end results for rural patients of pills "swallowing policy" are the opposite of what reformers, who the authors say were directly influenced by the earlier mhGAP initiative, might have intended: "Silencing community voices, reinforcing existing barriers to care, and relying on pharmacological solutions to address psychosocial concerns" (2009, p. 61).

Psychopharmaceutical Un/Certainties and the Consequences for Brazilian Ecologies of Care

The rise in medicine's dependency on pharmaceuticals and increasing global/local impetuses to pharmaceuticalization have consequences for more than just general health and health budgets. Consequences also include effects on family and other social bonds, political affiliations, experiences of illness, and even personal identity. Medical anthropologists have responded with a renewed interest in inter-subjectivity (for example, Jenkins & Barrett, 2004; Biehl et al., 2007a). Few drugs may be perceived as treating a person's body completely independently of social associations – the "local ecologies of care" (Das & Das, 2006), in which "meanings of suffering and disease intersect with local providers, labor regimes and families" (Petryna & Kleinman, 2006). Psychiatric drugs, however, are particularly important to investigate in this light; they are somato-, psycho-, and socioactive agents with subjective and intersubjective experiential dimensions that are not secondary to treatment but inherent qualities of the agents themselves. Because someone taking psychopharmaceuticals is often seen as mad, users are put at risk for social exclusion; conversely, a person who is already enduring social exclusion is liable to be prescribed psychopharmaceuticals. The drugs' sometimes visible side effects alone can place their takers at social risk. Combining these hazards with the fact that psychopharmaceuticals are typically used to improve psychological well-being in a tradeoff against physical health (use of antipsychotic agents, for example, is positively correlated with morbidity [Joukamaa et al., 2006]) gives us further reason to delve into the question of how interaction with drugs is a socially-consequential process. Just as institutionalization has never been merely a socially isolated form of therapy, and given that drugs are prone to mis/ overuse, if we focus on the relationship between medication experience and local ecologies of care, we can compare current trends in drug intervention with institutional encasement, and hypothesize the transition of one to the other as another kind of trans-institutionalization.

João Biehl's ethnographic portrayals of the interface between psycho-pharmaceuticals, national health policies, domestic economies, and individual subjectivities in a "zone of social abandonment" in southern Brazil clearly demonstrate the combined risks of the above factors. Biehl recounts that the efforts of mental health workers in the 1990s to bring about the "progressive closure of psychiatric institutions and their replacement by local networks of community- and family-based psycho-social care [were] exemplary" (2007a, p. 403). What happened, however, sounds eerily familiar to those who have studied the progress of deinstitutionalization in the United States:

[T]he demands and strategies of the mental health movement became entangled in and even facilitated local government's neoliberalizing moves in public health: the mad were literally expelled from overcrowded and inefficient institutions, and the government allocated little new funding for the alternative services that had been proposed. (2007a, p. 403)

The caretakers for the mentally ill were now families, who "have learned to act as proxy psychiatrists" (2007a, p. 404; compare Pinto,

2009) and volunteers in the zones of social abandonment. The volunteers will "at [a] whim" give the unfortunate residents antidepressants to take (2007a, p. 404). Consequent upon the coeval neoliberal reforms that swept Brazil in the 1990s (Harvey, 2005), there is "widespread availability of new biochemical treatments. Brazil is now one of the world's ten largest pharmaceutical markets. The pharmaceuticalization of public health has run parallel with ... the overall demise of clinical infrastructures" (2007a, p. 403).

Biehl closely follows the case of one woman through her varied encounters with the mental health system. Again, the words he chooses to relate her situation are sadly familiar – this time, I interject, in concord with my own findings in ongoing clinical ethnographic research in an urban psychiatric hospital in the U.S. Midwest.

> At the Caridade and São Paulo Hospitals, the diagnoses of Catarina's condition varied from "schizophrenia" to "postpartum psychosis," "unspecified psychosis," "mood disorder," and "anorexia and anemia."
>
> In tracing Catarina's passage through these medical institutions, I saw her not as an exception but as a patterned entity. Caught in struggles for deinstitutionalization, lack of public funding, and the proliferation of new classifications and treatments, the local psychiatry didn't account for her particularity or social condition. . . .
>
> [S]he continued to be overmedicated with powerful antipsychotics and all kinds of drugs to treat neurological side effects ... As I read her files, I could not separate the symptoms of the psychiatric illness from the effects of the medication, and I was struck that doctors did not bother to differentiate between the two in Catarina. (2007a, p. 411)[11]

Where Biehl depicts the tragic experiential side of uncertain diagnoses and pharmacological treatments for the patient, Annette Leibing (2009) observes the evolution of Brazilian psychiatrists' certainty in the application of atypical antipsychotics for Alzheimer's disease. These psychiatric drugs were a relatively new entry in the Alzheimer's market, joining the "cognitive enhancers." Some of the physicians Leibing interviews in Rio de Janeiro are already informed about the risks associated with use of atypical antipsychotics in the elderly and about the research regarding

---

[11] As a relevant aside, one can notice in Biehl's account that as psychiatric health policy on the ground shifts to a reliance on pharmacotherapy, the tendency is for the acting caregiver to blame the patient for her own failure to recover due to real or supposed noncompliance with treatment. A subset of studies focusing specifically on compliance reveals a pattern in which noncompliant "others" are labeled by doctors or public health actors as irrational, backwards, traditional, dangerous, or the like (for example, Hunt & Arar, 2001; Whitmarsh, 2009; Jain & Jadhav, 2009; Rouse, 2010; Glick & Applbaum, 2010; see also Greene, 2004).

the drugs' doubtful efficacy for "treating" dementia. Brazilian psychiatrists are not, Leibing says, "passive recipients of internationally circulating knowledge. Particularly since the Brazilian psychiatrist Jorge Alberto Costa e Silva became the director of the WHO mental health division ..." (2009, p. 185). Nevertheless, Leibing's psychiatrist interviewees continue to prescribe the drugs and to switch patients from one brand to another when they feel a given drug is not producing the desired effect. "In their answers, the psychogeriatricians showed little doubt in regard to their treatment of dementia, and reflected none of the tension that surrounds the contradictory information about medications" (2009, p. 187).

Overconfidence may be an occupational hazard in medicine, but Leibing is interested in deeper causes for this paradoxical certitude. She finds it in the debate, internal to geriatric health studies, over the relative significance of two separate impairments associated with dementia: cognitive and noncognitive, the second of which includes behavior, functionality, and quality of life measures. While both have always received treatment attention, Leibing discerned that in contrast with research in the same locale a decade earlier, "the notion of dementia itself had changed, as non-cognitive symptoms had become core symptoms." The doctors "had internalized the new focus on non-cognitive symptoms and notions like quality of life or functionality" (2009a, p. 188).

To understand this shift, Leibing studied the scientific literature on Alzheimer's. She found that the change in focus among her Brazilian informants to behavioral aspects of dementia had occurred a few years earlier in the United States. Janssen Pharmaceuticals, maker of the atypical antipsychotic, Risperdal:

provided an unrestricted grant for a consensus conference organized by the International Psychogeriatric Association (IPA) in Landsdowne, VA in 1996, the event that was central to the development of the new category BPSD. "The development of the Consensus Statement on Behavioral and Psychological Symptoms of Dementia (BPSD) represents a first step towards recognizing that *these are core symptoms of dementia* and that it is as essential to study and treat them as it is to study and treat any other aspects of dementing disorders," wrote one of the organizers. ... A second conference followed in 1999, resulting in more publications (IPA, 1996a, 1996b, 1996c, 2000, 2002). Afterwards updated educational materials were regularly mailed to all IPA members, in an effort which gradually changed the way health professionals understand and define dementia.

How to Serve Brandkind

In her investigation of how Alzheimer's patients came to be treated with atypical antipsychotics in Brazil, Leibing discovered a mechanism familiar to students of pharmaceutical marketing. BPSD became what some marketers call the "white space" surrounding Risperdal, understood as the territory available for brand expansion, which, not incidentally to our interests, may or may not contribute to the medical value of the drug. From a medical standpoint, the bounds or incidence of a given condition can only be determined through investigations that have psychiatric and epidemiological reference points. From a marketing standpoint, the scope or incidence of a condition is *a priori* a subset of those things that can be made relevant to the company's product offering. Like a Kantian category of understanding, for marketers the brand is a whole reality: Whatever fits under the brand umbrella is a fact. All other information is either irrelevant or becomes the object of future incorporation into brand reality – the target of future "branding." Too literal an understanding of brands as a name, symbol, or trademark will cause us to miss the point of how brands are the essence of contemporary commercialization (Klein, 2000). The word *brand* is far more compelling to marketers as a verb than as a noun since, in keeping with the very nature of capitalism, brands must grow in order to survive. Everything that lies in the potential ambit of the product thus must be thought of as potentially branded space that will become useful or real once it is colonized for the brand.

David Healy has shown how drug companies invent new medical terminology as part of creating a market around a psychiatric drug. The expression *SSRI* was coined in the marketing department of SmithKline Beacham (Healy, 2004). The terms *atypical antipsychotics* (applied to products that are not really atypical, since they block dopaminergic receptors just as the "typicals" do [Tyrer & Kendall, 2009]) and *mood stabilizers* are examples of class nomenclature that, if not directly coined in marketing departments, have at least as much marketing as psychiatric provenience (Healy, 2002, 2008).

In a brandchannel.com article entitled "Brand Matters: The Lingua Franca of Pharmaceutical Brand Names," Rebecca Robins describes the field or space around the brand that is not itself seen as "white space." She says, "The battle for brand-stand out [*sic*] is hard won and defining that crucial 'white space' around which to develop the beginnings of that relationship is key." The relationship Robins cites lies between the drug brand and the other definable elements in the non-branded space around it, including diseases (which would be condition-branded) and the terminology that organizes scientific research into cures for that disease. In both cases, the authority – the "share of voice," as marketers say – of medical scientists is regarded as a competitive threat relative to that of marketers and must be diminished. Robins says:

The position of being first in a new class is a privileged one, and thus one to be signaled in clear and distinctive terms. This extends beyond the development of a brand name, to leveraging supportive language, such as class nomenclature. A new class will serve as a positioning tool to separate out the compound from other treatments in the same therapeutic category. In so doing, a company gives itself the opportunity of fighting the marketing battle on new terms, which affords the advantage of a platform for differentiation and a means by which to take ownership of "newness" and of the story behind the science. Pharmaceutical companies that are proactively creating this nomenclature give themselves this edge, *instead of having a classification handed to them.*[12]

While disease expansion has long animated pharmaceutical company dreams of profit-taking (Greene, 2007), and psychiatric drug marketing always enjoyed the possibility of unanticipated runaway best-sellers such as meprobamate/Miltown (Tone, 2009), such expansion developed distinctive possibilities and consequences with the relatively new recognition that the conjoint entity of drug + disease could be a brandable target.

Though the mechanism remains curiously opaque to most psychiatrists, *Money Magazine* could write the following about SSRIs in 2005:

"Ownable syndromes"
Drug marketers have been extraordinarily adept at selling SSRIs – even to people who may not need them. Consider that the drugs, once limited to treating major depression, are now prescribed for everything from shyness about peeing in public restrooms to shopoholism. (Such uses aren't approved by the FDA, but there's no law against doctors prescribing SSRIs and other drugs for "off label" indications.)

The explosive growth of the drugs' market is largely a story of clever branding as makers of "me too" SSRIs sought to replicate Prozac's success. Pfizer, for example, positioned Zoloft, launched in 1992, as a versatile antidepressant that could also treat ills such as post-traumatic stress disorder. Glaxo targeted Paxil, launched in 1993, at anxiety disorders such as SAD (social anxiety disorder, or excessive shyness) and GAD (generalized anxiety disorder, or unremitting angst) – ills that had received little attention before Glaxo began promoting Paxil to treat them. Lilly countered by expanding Prozac's indications to include PMDD (premenstrual dysphoric disorder, or very bad moods some women suffer before their periods) and depression in children.

Indeed, to marketers, SSRIs have been the pharmaceutical equivalent of Play-Doh. In a remarkably forthright 2003 article, Vince Parry, now a branding expert at Ventiv Health, a Somerset, NJ, health-care marketing firm, waxed euphoric about psychiatry's "ownable syndromes." Published in a trade journal, the article laid out strategies "for fostering the creation of a [medical] condition and aligning it with a product" like an SSRI. Wrote Parry: "No therapeutic category is more accepting of condition branding than the field of anxiety and depression, where illness is rarely based on measurable physical symptoms." He cites Lilly's

[12] http://www.expectad.com/white_paper/Brand_Matters_Expect_Advertising_Inc.pdf. Emphasis added.

positioning of Prozac to treat premenstrual woe as an excellent example of condition branding – the company reinvigorated its aging antidepressant by repackaging it in a lavender pill, dubbed Sarafem, for women with PMDD.[13]

In scientific circles, the serotonin hypothesis that escorted these label extensions has been discredited (Lacasse and Leo, 2005). As a clinical/ brand entity materialized in SSRIs, SNRIs, and so on, the theory has proven to be one of the most protean and profitable in the history of capitalism. The model continues to inspire both pharmaceutical product marketing and, for its parsimony and its moral attractions, popular explanations for psychiatric diagnoses – the chemical imbalance thesis.[14] Many physicians still hold to this theory and they tell it to their patients (Lacasse & Leo, 2005). Patient advocacy groups such as NAMI (National Alliance for the Mentally Ill) continue to endorse it. Rose says, "It seems that individuals themselves are beginning to recode their moods and their ills in terms of the functioning of their brain chemicals, and to act upon themselves in the light of this belief" (2004, p. 121; see also Leibing, 2009).

We are living in the age of the annual $22 billion ownable syndrome market for antipsychotic medicines. Several researchers have documented the strategic enlargement of bipolar disorder and the extension

---

[13] http://money.cnn.com/magazines/fortune/fortune_archive/2005/11/28/8361973/index.htm. As I was writing this chapter, the *New York Times* reported the following:

> Two prominent authors of a 1999 book teaching family doctors how to treat psychiatric disorders provided acknowledgment in the preface for an "unrestricted educational grant" from a major pharmaceutical company. But the drug maker, then known as SmithKline Beecham, actually had much more involvement than the book described, newly disclosed documents show. The grant paid for a writing company to develop the outline and text for the two named authors, the documents show, and then the writing company said it planned to show three drafts directly to the pharmaceutical company for comments and proposed a timeline for the writing company to furnish the doctors and SmithKline with draft text and final page proofs for approval. The 269-page book, *Recognition and Treatment of Psychiatric Disorders: A Psychopharmacology Handbook for Primary Care*, is so far the first book among publications, namely medical journal articles, that have been criticized in recent years for hidden drug industry influence, colloquially known as ghostwriting. "To ghostwrite an entire textbook is a new level of chutzpah," said Dr. David A. Kessler, former commissioner of the Food and Drug Administration, after the letter and other documents were described to him. "I've never heard of that before. It takes your breath away" (www.nytimes.com/2010/11/30/business/30drug.html).

[14] From a buyer's standpoint, some reasons for the attraction of this notion include its simplicity as a form of explanation for a complex phenomenon; its shifting the burden of blame to "the brain" rather than to the actions or character of the individual; its transportability and low cost relative to psychological or other therapies; and its simpler conformity to bureaucratic needs for assessing reimbursements and for comparing costs of different treatments.

of antipsychotics to new indications and off-label uses in as many different markets as possible: psychotic depression; personality disorder with psychotic features; non-drug-induced organic mental disorders; drug-induced mental disorders; attention deficit disorder; and dementia with psychosis. There is scant evidence that the drugs perform better than a placebo for these conditions (Applbaum, 2009; Healy, 2006, 2008; Spielmans, 2009). An extension of the Clinical Antipsychotic Trials of Intervention Effectiveness (CATIE) study,[15] demonstrated this failure of efficacy explicitly for Alzheimer's patients (Rosenheck et al., 2007), yet atypical antipsychotics are routinely prescribed in this population. Dr. David Graham of the FDA testified before Congress that the atypical antipsychotics were being promoted illegally for off-label use in nursing homes, resulting in some fifteen thousand deaths annually.[16] Over fifty million prescriptions for atypical antipsychotics are written in the United States every year, a significant and growing number to children, including preschoolers, under the newly marketed category of "mood stabilizers." It is not that drug companies are constructing mental illness, but that much of the considerable propagation of science devoted to discovering new uses for these highly potent and toxic drugs would not have come about were there not vast treasures to be won in doing so.

This, then, is the fuller context of Risperdal and Alzheimer's in Brazil. BPSD was not invented from scratch by the drug companies. The non-cognitive symptoms of dementia are serious, and inattention to them can lead to "immense suffering and early institutionalization" (Leibing, 2009a, p. 194). However, given the unreliable benefits and the potential harms creditable to the use of common atypical drugs for Alzheimer's disease (Gill et al., 2005), to understand their widespread adoption in Rio, one must return to tracing the lines of influence from drug companies to Brazilian psychiatrists. Brazil is a country in which big pharma invests heavily. It is rewarded with prescriptions for branded drugs, despite the government's attempts to keep drug prices down. Leibing writes:

[A]ll of the leading Brazilian psychogeriatricians – who are also the producers of knowledge in their specialty – receive generous funding for congress organization, international travel, research, or other activities. One rarely finds an opinion critical of the pharmaceutical industry in Brazilian journals or scientific

---

[15] This study showed that first-generation antipsychotics introduced in the 1950s equaled the second-generation drugs on every measure: efficacy, side effect profile, and the tendency of patients given the drug to continue taking it (Lieberman et al., 2005).
[16] www.sptimes.com/2007/11/18/Worldandnation/Dementia_relief_with.shtml

meetings. On any given day, one could find several sales representatives from pharmaceutical companies in front of the psychogeriatric unit where part of this research was undertaken. (2009, p. 197)

Conclusion: Four Recommendations

The new global mental health movement, which overlaps the WHO mental health division, undertakes to raise the status of mental health within the global health agenda. Most of what its proponents say, starting with their slogan, "No health without mental health," is laudable and worthy of the highest subscription. But while it is possible that mental illness remains underserved by global health initiatives, the utility of a global mental health movement may be even more threatened by the prospect that an overconfident and under-informed psychiatry may inadvertently transmit commercially rather than medically mediated solutions to needy populations around the world.

I have argued here that "global mental health" is a universalizing construct that is inadvertently liable to expanding the province of psychopharmaceutical globalization. Big and small pharma's construction of the problem embeds a solution that serves their purpose rather than the purposes of public health. To short-circuit the progression of this logic to unwanted outcomes – from the unregulated proliferation of psychopharmaceuticals to the ominous trending toward Rose's "psychopharmacological societies" – and based upon insights gained from general reading in the anthropology of mental health, I wish modestly to propose four immodest, linked paths to remediation.

1) A closer (ethnographic) examination of the liabilities in our own mental health systems.

The new global mental health movement assumes that high per capita investment in psychiatric care, along with the presence of more psychiatrists, will self-evidently result in improvements to mental health. It is by no means clear, however, that those countries with the highest investments in psychiatric care have the lowest rates of disability resulting from mental disorders – even for illnesses such as schizophrenia, where the diagnosis and treatment are the least open to question.

In a recent study of poor recovery from schizophrenia in the United States, Tanya Luhrmann revisits the famed WHO International Pilot Study of Schizophrenia (IPSS) from the 1960s–1980s, which seemed to show, "No matter whether you look at symptoms, disability, clinical profile, or the ability to do productive work, people diagnosed with schizophrenia are far more likely to meet criteria for recovery in the developing world than they do in the developed world" (2007, p. 145). Various interpretations have been discussed, including that studies in developing countries contained subjects who did not really have schizophrenia, or that stronger family ties and other "cultural" factors contributed to better outcomes. Luhrmann, however, proposes a different interpretation: "The normative treatment for schizophrenia in our culture may make things significantly worse, and possibly even turn psychotic reactivity (the possibility for a brief psychotic reaction) into chronic clienthood" (2007, p. 146).

Long-term observation of the mentally ill is difficult, and yields small numbers of cases rather than large quantifiable samples. Yet these are the sorts of studies that may yield the greatest insights into the recovery process.

A second dimension to self-examination starts with observing that our own system focuses on efficacy of drug treatments to the detriment of needed attention to side effects, which in psychiatry are sometimes not on the other side of the coin but on the same side. The problem is compounded by the fact that it is often difficult to distinguish the effects of drugs from those of the sickness; also, studies regarding the effects of dependency and withdrawal associated with long-term application of psychiatric drugs are unpopular.[17]

The lack of systematic clinical research into side effects and withdrawal syndromes, combining into what Healy and Tranter (1999) call "pharmacotherapy-induced stress syndromes," is vexing. Healy connects the lack of information on treatment-induced stress syndromes to normative conduct in clinical trials and the benefits accruing to pharmaceutical companies from current trial practices:

[D]rug withdrawal trials in control subjects ... are needed to distinguish between treatment-induced changes and the supposed effects of treatment on an underlying condition. Without such trials it is not possible to say what the benefits of active agents are, particularly as ... there is a clear bias to seeing any effects emerging on discontinuation as evidence of clinical effectiveness rather than evidence for a treatment-induced problem. Unrecognized, treatment-induced stress syndromes may generate a long-term demand for drugs by converting acute disorders into chronic conditions, or by creating new disease categories with indications for treatment using the provoking agent, or by

---

[17] As Cosgrove and Bursztajn point out, "Only 2 of more than 700 pages of text of the main body of *DSM-IV-TR* deal with diagnosing adverse effects of psychotropic medications" (2010, p. 3). The proposed *DSM-5*, they warn, bodes similar neglect. They relate this conclusion to the fact that 68 percent of the *DSM-5* task force members have ties to the pharmaceutical industry – a 20 percent increase over the *DSM-IV*.

reducing the threshold sensitivity for prescribing the agent as for instance when withdrawal effects of psychotropic drugs are taken as manifestations of an original anxiety or depression. (Healy n.d.)

2) Begin by concentrating on the most severe mental illnesses, such as psychosis and major depression.

Medical anthropology's leading contributor to our understanding of global mental health and its possible solutions is Arthur Kleinman, who has developed his positions in considered detail in many serious venues. I offer the following quote, which appeared in *Harvard Magazine* in 2006, with a note of caution as to its original intended audience:

By medicalizing ordinary unhappiness," says professor of psychiatry and medical anthropology Arthur Kleinman, who is also Rabb professor of anthropology, "we risk doing a disservice to those people who have severe mental illnesses." Kleinman fears that including mild forms of anxiety and depression under an ever-widening umbrella of mental disorders will divert attention and resources from diseases like schizophrenia and major depression, which remain undertreated and stigmatized across much of the world. In his view, "We may turn off the public, who are a huge source of support for mental health research, by telling them that half of them are mad.[18]

Separating severe mental disorders from more common ones makes sense not just in terms of prioritizing resource allocation, but because certain manifestations of illness, such as psychosis, appear also to be the most straightforwardly diagnosable and the most responsive to available therapies. (I do not wish to fall into my own trap by suggesting that psychopharmaceuticals are effective therapies on their own, but the evidence for their utility is more robust in some classes of illness than in others.)

3) Encourage collective (population-based) "public mental health" rather than aggregated individuated mental health models, de-medicalize many common mental disorders, and cultivate a prevention orientation to these.

A study conducted by Parkar, Fernandes, and Weiss (2003) was the specific inspiration for the above suggestion. Their research was conducted in Mumbai, with the aim of sorting out "the impact of common life experience in slums, including poverty, bad living conditions, unemployment, and crowding." The authors hardly reject "effective clinical interventions" for psychiatric disorders, but they conclude that these "cannot directly affect the conditions of urban slums that impair mental health" (2003, p. 291).

---

[18] http://harvardmagazine.com/2006/07/psychiatry-by-prescripti.html

As a mental health study, our approach is somewhat unusual, insofar as it is concerned with non-specific mental health issues (e.g. emotional distress, subjective quality of life of poor people living in deprived conditions) and the role of poor hygiene and sanitation, population density, hutment demolition, homelessness, violence and crime – rather than rates and determinants of psychiatric disorders *per se*. ... New public health initiatives of the 19th century brought about substantial decline in deaths from infectious diseases through sanitary reform, and we now need to consider how analogous population-based measures may be adapted to promote mental health. (2003, p. 306)

The implication of this briefly stated but powerful insight is that by over-medicalizing not only do we risk labeling everyday sadness, for instance, as a treatable disorder (with what iatrogenic effect we do not really know), but we also fail to notice the ways in which it might be better to address the problem on a different level (Kirmayer, 2006). The discernment of social sources of suffering is not new to medical anthropology; however, refinement of the concept to interventionist purposes in psychiatry seems a rarer suggestion. The living circumstances that give rise to cholera and to substance abuse and domestic violence may be the same, but the vectors are quite different, and this is what a public mental health program might address. We associate cholera not so much with its treatment (rehydration, for example) as with the historical success of its prevention through sanitation measures; how might the common mental disorders we have come to treat with antidepressants, for instance, be targeted primarily for prevention?

4) Take into adequate account the mutual embeddedness of psychiatry and commercial biopower.

The expanding corporate intervention in medicine should not be analytically separated from the investigation of clinical practice in any of its aspects, ranging from testing and diagnosis of disease states, to clinician-patient relations, and even to patients' subjective experiences of illness. These are not so much influenced in some abstract, sociological sense by corporate participation in medicine, as co-constituted by it. Commercial and medical cultures are, to borrow the language of economic sociology, "embedded" in one another (Granovetter, 1985).

An earlier generation of medical anthropologists unmasked the partially hidden "moral project of medicine ... obscured by the use of a rhetoric of science that portrays clinical practice as primarily technical, evidence-based, and neutral or value-free" (Kirmayer, 2006, p. 128). Thus was revealed a discord between the universalizing assertions of science and the particularizing, contextualizing work of medical anthropology. Since that time, we have observed an ascendant, interposing, and harmonizing force between universal medical science and the particular objects of its intervention. This is the market sometimes portrayed as a manipulated partnership between doctors, scientists or regulators, and pharmaceutical companies; sometimes as public-private administrative initiatives in healthcare or in biomedical research regimes that are motivated by and result in the marketization of national healthcare systems (Biehl, 2007b; Petryna, 2009); and sometimes as an organizing force in the midst of the disordered contingencies that characterize everyday life in many health care settings around the world. How, specifically, might a deeper familiarity with the market dynamics of healthcare in diverse locales inform our mission to reduce suffering associated with mental illness?

REFERENCES

Abas, M., Baingana, F., Broadhead, J., Iacoponi, E., & Vanderpyl, J. (2003). Common mental disorders and primary health care: Current practice in low-income countries. *Harvard Review of Psychiatry, 11,* 166–73. http://dx.doi.org/10.1080/10673220303954

Abraham, J. (2010). Pharmaceuticalization of society in context: Theoretical, empirical and health dimensions. *Sociology, 44,* 603–22. http://dx.doi.org/10.1177/0038038510369368

Alexander, G. C., Gallagher, S. A., Mascola, A., Moloney, R. M., & Stafford, R. S. (2011). Increasing off-label use of antipsychotic medications in the United States, 1995–2008. *Pharmacoepidemiology and Drug Safety, 20*(2), 177–84. http://dx.doi.org/10.1002/pds.2082

Applbaum, K. (2011). Broadening the marketing concept: Service to humanity, or privatization of the public good? In D. Zwick & J. Cayla (Eds.), *Inside marketing* (pp. 269–98). New York, NY: Oxford University Press. http://dx.doi.org/10.1093/acprof:oso/9780199576746.003.0013

Applbaum, K. (2010). Shadow science: Zyprexa, Eli Lilly and the globalization of pharmaceutical damage control. *BioSocieties, 5,* 236–55. http://dx.doi.org/10.1057/biosoc.2010.5

Applbaum, K. (2009a). Is marketing the enemy of pharmaceutical innovation? *The Hastings Center Report, 39*(4), 13–17. http://dx.doi.org/10.1353/hcr.0.0157

Applbaum, K. (2009b). Getting to yes: Corporate power and the creation of a psychopharmaceutical blockbuster. *Culture, Medicine, and Psychiatry, 33,* 185–215. http://dx.doi.org/10.1007/s11013-009-9129-3

Applbaum, K. (2009c). Consumers are patients! Shared decision making and treatment non-compliance as business opportunity. *Transcultural Psychiatry, 46,* 107–30. http://dx.doi.org/10.1177/1363461509102290

Applbaum, K. (2006). Educating for global mental health: American pharmaceutical companies and the adoption of SSRIs in Japan. In A. Petryna, A. Lakoff, & A. Kleinman (Eds.), *Pharmaceuticals and globalization: Ethics, markets, practices* (pp. 85–110). Durham, NC: Duke University Press.

Applbaum, K. (2004a). *The marketing era: From professional practice to global provisioning* London, England: Routledge.

Applbaum, K. (2004b). How to organize a psychiatric congress. *Anthropological Quarterly, 77*, 303–10. http://dx.doi.org/10.1353/anq.2004.0067

Ban, T.A. (2006). Academic psychiatry and the pharmaceutical industry. *Progress in Neuro-Psychopharmacology and Biological Psychiatry, 30*, 29–41. http://dx. doi.org/10.1016/j.pnpbp.2005.11.014

Barbui, C., Dua, T., van Ommeren, M., Yasamy, T., Fleischmann, A., Clark, N., … Saxena, S. (2010). Challenges in developing evidence-based recommendations using the GRADE approach: The case of mental, neurological, and substance use disorders. *PLOS Medicine, 8*, e1000322. http://dx.doi.org/10.1371/journal.pmed.1000322

Baudrillard, J. (1996). *The system of objects* (J. Benedict, Trans.). London, England: Verso. (Original work published 1968)

Behague, D. P. (2008). The domains of psychiatric practice: From centre to periphery. *Culture, Medicine, and Psychiatry, 32*, 140–51. http://dx.doi.org/10.1007/s11013-008-9096-0

Berrios, G. E., & Marková, I. S. (2015). Toward a new epistemology of psychiatry. In L. J. Kirmayer, R. Lemelson, & C. A. Cummings (Eds.), *Re-visioning psychiatry: Cultural phenomenology, critical neuroscience, and global mental health* (pp. 41–64). New York, NY: Cambridge University Press.

Biehl, J. (2007a). A life: Between psychiatric drugs and social abandonment. In J. Biehl, B. Good, & A. Kleinman (Eds.), *Subjectivity: Ethnographic investigations,* (pp. 397–421). Durham, NC: Duke University Press. http://dx.doi.org/10.1525/california/9780520247925.003.0015

Biehl, J. (2007b). Pharmaceuticalization: AIDS treatment and global health politics. *Anthropological Quarterly, 80*, 1083–1126. http://dx.doi.org/10.1353/anq.2007.0056

Biehl, J., Good, B., & Kleinman, A. (Eds.). (2007). *Subjectivity: Ethnographic investigations.* Durham, NC: Duke University Press. http://dx.doi.org/10.1525/california/9780520247925.001.0001

Biehl, J., & Moran-Thomas, A. (2009). Symptom: Subjectivities, social ills, technologies. *Annual Review of Anthropology, 38*, 267–88. http://dx.doi.org/10.1146/annurev-anthro-091908-164420

Buse, K., & Walt, G. (2000). Global private-public partnerships: A new development in health? *Bulletin of the World Health Organization, 78*(4), 1–19.

Cohen, A., Kleinman, A., & Saraceno, B. (Eds.). (2002). *World mental health casebook: Social and mental health programs in low-income countries.* New York, NY: Kluwer Academic. http://dx.doi.org/10.1007/b112400

Cosgrove, L., & Bursztajn, H. (2010). Undue pharmaceutical influence on psychiatric practice. *Psychiatric Times, 27*, 1–6.

Das, V., & Das, R. (2006). Urban health and pharmaceutical consumption in Delhi, India. *Journal of Biosocial Science, 38*, 69–82. http://dx.doi.org/10.1017/S002193200500091X

Das, A., & Rao, M. (2012). Universal mental health: Re-evaluating the call for global mental health. *Critical Public Health, 22*(4), 383–89. http://dx.doi.org/10.1080/09581596.2012.700393

de Menil V, Cohen A. (2009). Rational use and rationale for use: psychiatric medication at an Argentine institution for intellectual disability. *Transcultural Psychiatry, 46*(4), 651–71. http://dx.doi.org/10.1177/1363461509351377

Desjarlais, R., Eisenberg, L., Good, B., & Kleinman, A. (1995). *World mental health: Problems and priorities in low-income countries.* New York, NY: Oxford University Press.

Ecks, S. (2009). *Unseen drug dissemination: Rethinking the "treatment gap" for antidepressants in India.* Paper presented at the Society for Medical Anthropology Conference, Yale University, New Haven, CT.

Ecks, S., & Basu, S. (2009). The unlicensed lives of antidepressants in India: Generic drugs, unqualified practitioners, and floating prescriptions. *Transcultural Psychiatry, 46*, 86–106. http://dx.doi.org/10.1177/1363461509102289

Farmer, P. (1999). *Infections and inequalities: The modern plagues.* Berkeley: University of California Press.

Friedman, R.A. (2012, September 24). A call for caution on antipsychotic drugs. *New York Times.* Retrieved from http://www.nytimes.com/2012/09/25/health/a-call-for-caution-in-the-use-of-antipsychotic-drugs.html

Gill, S. S., Rochon, P. A., Herrmann, N., Lee, P. E., Sykora, K. Gunraj, N., ... Mamdani, M. (2005). Atypical antipsychotic drugs and risk of ischaemic stroke: Population based retrospective cohort study. *BMJ, 330.* http://dx.doi.org/10.1136/bmj.38330.470486.8F

Glick, D., & Applbaum, K. (2010). Dangerous noncompliance: A narrative analysis of a CNN special investigation into mental illness. *Anthropology & Medicine, 17*, 229–44. http://dx.doi.org/10.1080/13648470.2010.493605

Granovetter, M. (1985). Economic action and social structure: The problem of embeddedness. *American Journal of Sociology, 91*(3), 481–510.

Greene, J. (2011). Making medicines essential: The emergent centrality of pharmaceuticals in global health. *BioSocieties, 6*(1), 10–33. http://dx.doi.org/10.1057/biosoc.2010.39

Greene, J. (2007). *Prescribing by numbers.* Baltimore, MD: Johns Hopkins University Press.

Greene, J. (2004). Therapeutic infidelities: "Noncompliance" enters the medical literature, 1955–1975. *Social History of Medicine, 17*, 327–43. http://dx.doi.org/10.1093/shm/17.3.327

Harvey, D. (2005). *A brief history of neoliberalism.* New York, NY: Oxford University Press.

Healy, D. (n.d.). Enforced compliance: The role of treatment induced stress syndrome. Unpublished manuscript.

Healy, D. (2008). *Mania: A short history of a disorder.* Baltimore, MD: Johns Hopkins University Press.

Healy, D. (2006). The latest mania: Selling bipolar disorder. *PLOS Medicine, 3*(4), e185. http://dx.doi.org/10.1371/journal.pmed.0030185

Healy, D. (2004). *Let them eat Prozac.* New York, NY: New York University Press.

Healy, D. (2002). *The creation of psychopharmacology.* Cambridge, MA: Harvard University Press.

Healy, D. (1997). *The antidepressant era.* Cambridge, MA: Harvard University Press.

Hunt, I., M., & Arar, N.H. (2001). An analytical framework for contrasting patient and provider views of the process of chronic disease management. *Medical Anthropology Quarterly,* New Series, *15,* 347–67.

Jain, S. & Jadhav, S. (2009). Pills that swallow policy: Clinical ethnography of a community mental health program in Northern India. *Transcultural Psychiatry, 46,* 60–85. http://dx.doi.org/10.1177/1363461509102287

Jenkins, J. H., & Barrett, R. (Eds.). (2004). *Schizophrenia, culture, & subjectivity.* New York, NY: Cambridge University Press.

Joukamaa, M., Heliövaara, M., Knekt, P., Aromaa, A., Raitasalo, R., & Lehtinen, V. (2006). Schizophrenia, neuroleptic medication and mortality. *British Journal of Psychiatry, 188,* 122–7. http://dx.doi.org/10.1192/bjp.188.2.122

Kirmayer, L. J. (2002). Psychopathology in a globalizing world: The use of antidepressants in Japan. *Transcultural Psychiatry, 39,* 295–312. http://dx.doi.org/10.1177/136346150203900302

Kirmayer, L. J. (2006). Beyond the "New Cross-Cultural Psychiatry": Cultural biology, discursive psychology and the ironies of globalization. *Transcultural Psychiatry, 43,* 126–44. http://dx.doi.org/10.1177/1363461506061761

Kirmayer, L. J., & Minas, H. (2000). The future of cultural psychiatry: An international perspective. *Canadian Journal of Psychiatry, 45,* 438–46.

Kitanaka, J. (2006). *Society in distress: The psychiatric production of depression in contemporary Japan.* Doctoral dissertation, Department of Anthropology, McGill University, Montréal, Québec.

Klein, M. (2000). *No logo.* New York, NY: Picador.

Kleinman, A. (1999). The new bioethics. *Daedalus, 128,* 69–99.

Koberstein, W. (2002, September 1). When worlds collide: The unleashed power of marketing/R&D collaboration. *Pharmaceutical Executive.* http://www.pharmexec.com/node/242598?rel=canonical

Lacasse, J. R., and Leo, J. (2005). Serotonin and depression: A disconnect between the advertisements and the scientific literature. *PLOS Medicine, 2*(12), e392. http://dx.doi.org/10.1371/journal.pmed.0020392

Lakoff, A. (2006). *Pharmaceutical reason: Knowledge and value in global psychiatry.* Cambridge, England: Cambridge University Press.

Leibing, A. (2009). Tense prescriptions? Alzheimer's medications and the anthropology of uncertainty, *Transcultural Psychiatry, 46,* 180–206. http://dx.doi.org/10.1177/1363461509102297

Lieberman, J. A., Stroup, T. S., McEvoy, J. P., Swartz, M. S., Rosenheck, R. A., Perkins, D. O., … Hsiao, J. K. (2005). Effectiveness of antipsychotic drugs in patients with chronic schizophrenia. *New England Journal of Medicine, 353,* 1209–23. http://dx.doi.org/10.1056/NEJMoa051688

Luhrmann, T. M. (2007). Social defeat and the culture of chronicity: Or, why schizophrenia does so well over there and so badly here. *Culture, Medicine, and Psychiatry, 31,* 135–72. http://dx.doi.org/10.1007/s11013-007-9049-z

Matheson, A. (2008). Corporate science and the husbandry of scientific and medical knowledge by the pharmaceutical industry. *BioSocieties, 3,* 355–82. http://dx.doi.org/10.1017/S1745855208006297

Mezzich, J. E., Kirmayer, L. J., Kleinman, A., Fabrega, H., Jr., Parron, D. L., Good, B. J., ... Manson, S. M. (1999). The place of culture in *DSM-IV*. *The Journal of Nervous and Mental Disease, 187*(8), 457–64. http://dx.doi.org/ 10.1097/00005053-199908000-00001

Panitch, L., & Leys, C. (2010). *Morbid symptoms: Health under capitalism.* New York, NY: Monthly Review Press.

Patel, V., Boyce, N., Collins, P. Y., Saxena, S., & Horton, R. (2011). A renewed agenda for global mental health. *Lancet, 378*(9801), 1441–2. http://dx.doi. org/ 10.1016/S0140-6736(11)61385-8

Parkar, S. R., Fernandes, J., & Weiss, M. G. (2003). Contextualizing mental health: Gendered experiences in a Mumbai slum. *Anthropology & Medicine, 10*, 291–308. http://dx.doi.org/10.1080/1364847032000133825

Patel, V., & Thornicroft, G. (2009). Packages of care for mental, neurological and substance abuse disorders in low- and middle-income countries [PLOS series]. *PLOS Medicine, 6*, 1–2.

Petryna, A. (2009). *When experiments travel: Clinical trials and the global search for human subjects.* Princeton, NJ: Princeton University Press.

Petryna, A., & Kleinman, A. (2006). The pharmaceutical nexus. In A. Petryna, A. Lakoff, & A. Kleinman (Eds.), *Pharmaceuticals and globalization: Ethics, markets, practices* (pp. 1–32). Durham, NC: Duke University Press.

Pinto, S. (2009). Crises of commitment: Ethics of intimacy, kin, and confinement in global psychiatry. *Medical Anthropology, 28*, 1–10. http://dx. doi.org/10.1080/01459740802631718

Prince, M., Patel, V., Saxena, S., Maj, M., Maselko, J., Phillips, M. R., & Rahman, A. (2007). No health without mental health. *The Lancet, 370*, 859–77. http://dx.doi.org/10.1016/S0140-6736(07)61238-0

Rose, N. (2004). Becoming neurochemical selves. In N. Stehr (Ed.), *Biotechnology, commerce and civil society* (pp. 89–128). New York, NY: Transaction Press.

Rosenheck, R. A., Leslie, D. L., Sindelar, J. L., Miller, E. A., Tariot, P. N., Dagerman, K. S., ... Schneider, L. S. (2007). Cost-benefit analysis of second-generation antipsychotics and placebo in a randomized trial of the treatment of psychosis and aggression in Alzheimer disease. *Archives of General Psychiatry, 64*, 1259–68. http://dx.doi.org/10.1001/ archpsyc.64.11.1259

Rosenheck, R. (2005). The growth of psychopharmacology in the 1990s: Evidence-based practice or irrational exuberance? *International Journal of Law and Psychiatry, 28*, 467–83. http://dx.doi.org/10.1016/j.ijlp.2005.08.005

Rouse, C. (2010). Patient and practitioner noncompliance: Rationing, therapeutic uncertainty, and the missing conversation. *Anthropology & Medicine, 17*, 187–200. http://dx.doi.org/10.1080/13648470.2010.493602

Sismondo, S. (2007). Ghost management: How much of the medical literature is shaped behind the scenes by the pharmaceutical industry? *PLOS Medicine, 4*(9), e286. doi:10.1371/journal.pmed.0040286. http://dx.doi.org/10.1371/ journal.pmed.0040286

Spielmans, G. (2009). The promotion of olanzapine in primary care: An examination of internal industry documents. *Social Science and Medicine, 69,* 14–20. http://dx.doi.org/10.1016/j.socscimed.2009.05.001

Timmermans, K. (2007). Monopolizing clinical trial data: Implications and trends. *PLOS Medicine, 4*(2), e2. http://dx.doi.org/10.1371/journal.pmed.0040002

Tone, A. (2009). *The age of anxiety: A history of America's turbulent affair with tranquilizers.* New York, NY: Basic Books.

Vargo, S. L., & Lusch, R. F. (2004). Evolving to a new dominant logic for marketing. *Journal of Marketing, 68,* 1–17.

Waitzkin, H., Jasso-Aguilar, R., & Iriart, C. (2007). Privatization of health services in less developed countries: An empirical response to the proposals of the World Bank and Wharton School. *International Journal of Health Services, 37*(2), 205–27. http://dx.doi.org/10.2190/A1U4-7612-5052-6053

Whitaker, R. (2005). Anatomy of an epidemic: Psychiatric drugs and the astonishing rise of mental illness in America. *Ethical Human Psychology and Psychiatry, 7,* 23–35.

Whitmarsh, I. (2009). Medical schismogenics: Compliance and "culture" in Caribbean biomedicine. *Anthropological Quarterly, 82,* 453–82.

World Health Organization. (2001). *World Health Report 2001. Mental health: New understanding, new hope.* Retrieved from WHO website: http://www.who.int/whr/2001/en/whr01_en.pdf

World Health Organization. (2008). *Mental Health Gap Action Programme: Scaling up care for mental, neurological, and substance use disorders.* Retrieved from WHO website: http://whqlibdoc.who.int/publications/2008/9789241596206_eng.pdf

World Health Organization. (2010). *mhGAP Intervention guide for mental, neurological and substance use disorders in non-specialized health settings.* Retrieved from WHO website: www.who.int/mental_health/mhgap/en/

22 Global Mental Health Praxis
Perspectives from Cultural Psychiatry on Research and Intervention

Brandon A. Kohrt and James L. Griffith

Introduction

As psychiatric discourse continues to spread throughout the world, there is a need to ask how psychiatric knowledge is generated, what forms of psychiatric knowledge hold power in different settings, and what determines how knowledge is transformed into practice. In this chapter, we explore the issues of knowledge and practice at the intersection of cultural psychiatry and global mental health (GMH) to guide the revisioning of psychiatry, with special attention to how psychiatric care is delivered in low- and middle-income countries (LMICs).

The 2001 *World Health Report* entitled *Mental Health: New Understanding, New Hope* outlined the state of the mental health around the world and proposed key steps forward (World Health Organization, 2001). This was followed by the 2007 *Lancet* series, "Global Mental Health," which established goals and approaches for research and intervention to address worldwide disparities in care (Chisholm et al., 2007; Prince et al., 2007). Broadly, this GMH movement has the mission to reduce the gap between the burden of mental illness and the availability of effective mental health services. This mission entails advocating for increased funding for mental health services and personnel, expanding research to develop evidence-based practices for LMICs and low-resource settings, developing government mental health policies, and advancing the rights of persons with mental illness (Collins et al., 2011; Drew et al., 2011; Patel, Collins, et al., 2011; World Health Organization, 2010). The GMH field includes clinicians, government policy makers, public health researchers, mental health consumers, and members of development agencies and the World Health Organization (WHO). The formal Movement for GMH (MGMH) emerged from the 2007 *Lancet* call to action on scaling up GMH.

Along with practitioners and researchers in the general field, MGMH emphasizes improving services in LMICs, where an estimated additional 1.2 million healthcare providers are needed to deliver adequate mental health services (Kakuma et al., 2011). This shortage has led to support of *task-sharing*, also referred to as task-shifting, as a delivery solution. Task-sharing is the process of training primary care and community health workers to assume some care responsibilities that are traditionally the province of mental health specialists (World Health Organization, 2010). In large part, in the areas of implementation, advocacy, policy development, and task-shifting, the field of GMH has followed lessons from the global public health approach to combat infectious disease, most notably HIV/AIDS, malaria, and tuberculosis (Aggarwal & Kohrt, 2013; Raviola, Becker, & Farmer, 2011; World Health Organization, 2008).

Current initiatives in GMH occur against a backdrop of more than a century of cultural psychiatry and medical anthropology research (Littlewood & Dein, 2000). Cultural psychiatry understands human experience as socially situated and demonstrates the ways in which culture shapes illness, healing, and recovery (Kirmayer, 2006; Kirmayer & Jarvis, 1998; Kleinman, 1988; Kleinman, 1987; Littlewood, 1990; Sapir, 1932; Wittkower, 1970; Yap, 1951/2000). Anthropologists, psychologists, psychiatrists, neuroscientists, and researchers from related fields have deployed tools ranging from ethnography to brain imaging to explore relationships between socially patterned experience and mental illness (Choudhury & Kirmayer, 2009; Hollan, 1997; Kleinman & Good, 1985). Cultural psychiatry provides a forum for a range of critiques, such as the generalizability of psychiatric diagnoses, the role of political and economic forces in shaping diagnostic categories and treatments, the use and misuse of the concept of culture in psychiatric research and clinical care, and the boundaries between health and illness (Bracken et al., 2012; Bracken, 2003; Gaines, 1992; Kleinman, 1988; Luhrmann, 2000; Young, 1995).

Cultural psychiatrists, social scientists, human rights advocates, and others have generated critiques of GMH (Swartz, 2012). Patel (2014) identifies four categories of critiques, contending that: (1) psychiatric diagnostic categories are not valid cross-culturally (Fernando, 2011; Summerfield, 2008, 2012); (2) biomedical interventions have a limited role for socially determined health problems (Kleinman, 2012a, 2012b; Summerfield, 1999); (3) pharmaceutical companies drive the agenda and practice for the GMH movement (Applbaum, 2009, 2010; Biehl, 2004; Han, 2013; Petryna, Lakoff, & Kleinman, 2006); and (4) GMH is a form of medical imperialism (Summerfield, 2012). At a conceptual level, these critiques relate to power, knowledge, and practice. For example, who has the authority to generate knowledge and evidence? What forces endow different systems of knowledge with greater power for dissemination and implementation? Who within healthcare systems and beneficiary communities is culturally authorized to provide feedback and critique in reshaping practice? How is such feedback provided and incorporated into practice, and ultimately? What medical, social, and economic ends are served by cross-cultural, international, and global efforts in psychiatry? These debates are not unique to GMH, as global health struggles with similar challenges regarding power relations in diagnostic labeling, practice, policy, and funding (Biehl & Petryna, 2013; Farmer, Kim, Kleinman, & Basilico, 2013).

Our goal in this chapter is to discuss existing and untapped intersections between cultural psychiatry and GMH to develop a framework for understanding and advancing GMH *praxis*, that is, the application of psychiatry, public health, and social science to effective mental health care from the perspective of persons suffering from psychological distress, their families, and their communities. Building on cultural psychiatry's history of reflection and critique about the generation of knowledge, power relations, and disparities in care along cultural, economic, and geographic lines, we discuss GMH praxis drawing attention to four concepts: (1) dialogical practices and the therapeutic alliance; (2) ecological systems; (3) spaces, places, technology, and discourse; and (4) tradeoffs and unintended consequences.

Four Key Concepts for Praxis in GMH

1. *Establish a therapeutic alliance through dialogical practices.* Our starting point for GMH praxis is *dialogical practice*, which forms the core of effective interpersonal healing relationships. Dialogical practice refers to the intentional structuring of interactions so that each participant experiences the empowerment necessary to express his or her perspective, expecting that each perspective will be responded to respectfully during discussion, reflection, and the joint design of goal-directed activities. Dialogical practice can be contrasted with monological practice, in which a single dominant perspective commands or instructs the behaviors of the other participants. Dialogical practice seeks individual expressions of identity, values, and commitments by participants who are active agents; monological practice seeks docility and compliance by participants who are passive agents (Habermas, 1987; Shotter, 1993a, 1993b). In psychotherapy, the building of a robust alliance between clinician and patient is powerfully facilitated by dialogical practices embedded within the treatment relationship (Wampold, 2011, 2012).

The interactions between a healer of any tradition, ranging from biomedical primary care workers to psychotherapists to traditional healers, and a person in suffering ultimately determines whether a healer and healing system accomplish the goal of alleviating suffering. Dialogical practices are not limited to psychotherapy, but are considered to be a universal component of healing across disciplines and cultures (Dow, 1986; Frank & Frank, 1991; Kirmayer, 2004; Kleinman, 1988; Levi-Strauss, 1949/2000). Forming a therapeutic alliance in GMH requires attention to culture, mental health status, healthcare structure, and power differentials across these domains. Cultural psychiatry and medical anthropology can help practitioners recognize and address power differences and cross-cultural expectations in the clinical encounter between healer and sufferer (Kleinman, 1980, 1988; Lewis-Fernandez & Kleinman, 1995); the same concepts can inform alliances between and among health care workers, policy makers, and community stakeholders in LMICs and high-income countries (HICs).

2. *Frame therapeutic alliances within and across ecological levels.* Our second key concept is an *ecological systems approach*. Different system levels and actors within health care systems, social groups, and political economic structures interact within an ecological system that determines both how knowledge is generated and how it is implemented in practice. By synthesizing individual-level work done in psychotherapy with broader, often collective, ritual processes studied in anthropology, a dialogical approach can also address therapeutic alliances at multiple societal ecological levels: families, communities, health infrastructures, policy makers, and international organizations. Public rituals across cultures have direct effects on persons with psychological suffering, as well as indirect effects through changes at family or social levels (Kirmayer, 2004). Given the GMH focus on task-sharing responsibility with lower levels of healthcare workers and paraprofessionals, it is crucial to know about their existing roles and relationships in the community and to address their respective positions within community relations and health systems, that is, where do they fall in terms of providing resources, support, and knowledge, and shaping the care and experience of others?

3. *Use of spaces, places, technologies, and documents to facilitate dialogue within and across ecological levels.* The third core concept relates to factors that shape the settings and tools through which praxis occurs. Dialogue occurs within a specific context and is shaped by the *space (social structures), place (physical locations with specific histories and meaning), technologies,* and the *discourses,* with which they are in transaction. Technologies include diagnostic guidelines such as the *DSM* and the *mental health Gap Action Programme Implementation Guideline (mhGAP-IG)*. Discourses are the broader concepts that both emanate from and lead to modification

and production of technologies. Spaces, places, technologies, and discourse transact to shape praxis. As new relationships and new components of relationships come about through proliferation of public health approaches to GMH, key technologies and structures to foster dialogical practices – ranging from iterative clinical guideline development to physical infrastructure and virtual meeting spaces – need to be identified or created.

4. *Awareness of tradeoffs and unintended consequences within and across ecological levels:* The final concept is *tradeoffs and unintended consequences.* Because all knowledge generation and intervention activity occur within social-ecological systems, it follows naturally that there will be effects throughout the system based on any targeted activities. This leads to tradeoffs such as diversion of energies and attention and transformation in cultural models. GMH activities, as with any health intervention, lead to unintended consequences that may be positive or negative in other parts of the ecological system (Kleinman, 2010). The proliferating public health approach to GMH likewise potentially introduces unintended consequences and tradeoffs, which may result from expanded access to mental health care, ranging from an increased burden among low-level health providers to new spaces for stigmatization.

In this chapter, we discuss these four concepts for GMH praxis (see Table 22.1). We ground our discussion in Critical Medical Anthropology (CMA) models of interacting levels that ultimately shape healer–sufferer interactions (see Figure 22.1). CMA employs systems-based approaches to illuminate how policies, economics, and institutions, across ecological levels, ultimately shape the interaction between healer and sufferer (Baer, Singer, & Susser, 2003; Singer, 1989; Singer, 1995). We provide examples based on our experiences in Kosovo, Liberia, Uganda, and Nepal. Ultimately, this framework can contribute to re-visioning psychiatry in GMH by promoting an ethical stance for action that allows an adaptive flexibility that is only possible through dialogue.

Concept 1: Dialogical Practice and Therapeutic Alliance

Ultimately, any practice or critique related to GMH needs to consider the interaction between healer and sufferer. For a critique to be relevant and constructive, a pathway to influence this interaction needs to be outlined. Similarly, any new intervention, new technology or guideline, or training program must be investigated as it relates to changing some aspect of interaction between healers and sufferers. This interaction is the focus whether one is discussing traditional healers, community health volunteers, or psychiatrists and psychologists.

Table 22.1 *Key Concepts for GMH Praxis*

COMPONENTS	TOPICS	APPLICATIONS
1. Establishment of a therapeutic alliance through dialogical practices	• Current roles and proposed responsibilities • Beneficiaries of services and beneficiaries of training • Potential for "disruption of self" through use of or provision of services	• Use of dialogical practices to develop therapeutic alliance • Outcome of mutual goal setting and implementation plan • Address cultural influences on exchange at patient-provider level and health workforce level that may facilitate or impede dialogical practices
2. Framing therapeutic alliances within and across ecological levels	• Interactions at multiple ecological levels: (a) patients/clients and families; (b) among health care workers; (c) consumer groups and advocates with healthcare workers and policy makers; (d) healthcare workers with policy makers; (e) health care workers from HICs with LMICs • Cultural expectations of interactions of patient/clients and families with health care workers • Cultural expectations of hierarchy, transmission of knowledge, and constructive dialogue	• Ecological mapping of beneficiaries, healthcare workers, policy makers, and other stakeholders • Create opportunities for unmet exchanges across ecological levels • Mapping of HICs and LMICs interactions
3. Use of spaces, places, technologies, and discourse to facilitate dialogue within and across ecological levels	• Current and potential spaces for interaction among persons within and across levels • Documents used to facilitate dialogue • Current and potential use of technologies for dialogical practices • Current and potential supervision processes • Gaps in spaces, technologies, and documents for dialogue across levels	• Identify ecological relationships with limited interaction • Propose new spaces, technologies or documents to facilitate dialogue • Identify avenues for sustainable supervision

Table 22.1 (*cont.*)

COMPONENTS	TOPICS	APPLICATIONS
4. Awareness of tradeoffs and unintended consequences within and across ecological levels	• Tradeoffs across ecological levels related to service provision and demand • Potential unintended consequences of interventions, treatments, and policies, including ripple effects of expectation of services • Potential for stigmatization or discrimination through new programs • Current and potential monitoring systems for unintended or negative sequelae of new programs	• Propose systems for revision and updating of documents, policies, and procedures • Propose systems of monitoring include who would be responsible for types of information to record • Plans for empowerment of most vulnerable groups to increase dialogical opportunities

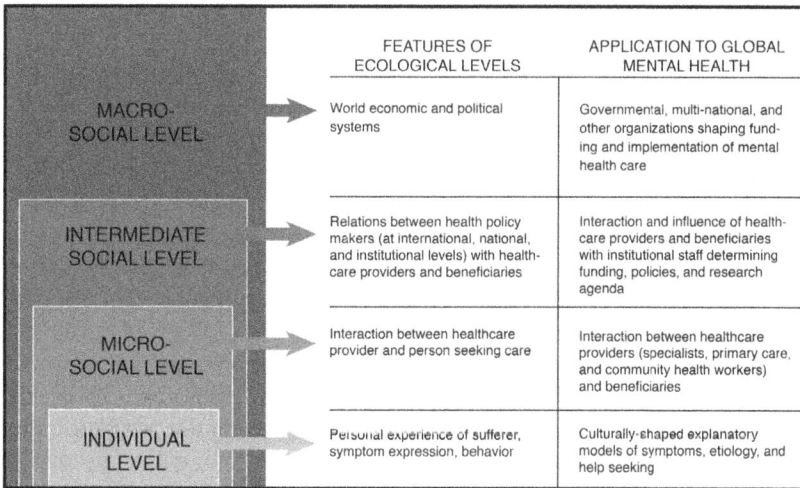

Figure 22.1. Critical medical anthropology levels of health care systems applied to global mental health.

Research on the interaction between therapists and patients is a useful starting point for considering this interaction. Among psychotherapists, there has been long debate about which elements of the therapeutic encounter are most effective in promoting change (Duncan, Miller,

Wampold, & Hubble, 2010). In psychotherapy, *common factors* are those therapeutic elements utilized across psychotherapies that predict positive outcomes, regardless of specific therapy technique (Wampold, 2011). Research on common factors illustrates the importance of a *therapeutic alliance* as the salutogenic aspect of this interaction between healer and sufferer. The therapeutic alliance reflects mutual goal setting between therapist and client or patient, empathy, and the absence of hostility and judgment (Baldwin, Wampold, & Imel, 2007).

A primary tension has been whether specific therapeutic techniques (e.g., cognitive behavior therapy versus mindfulness training) or the quality of the relationship between psychotherapist and patient, that is, the therapeutic alliance, ultimately determines the success of psychotherapy. Psychotherapy outcome studies have repeatedly found that specific methods unique to particular types of psychotherapy matter relatively little. Rather, 85 percent or more of effectiveness resides not in treatment methods unique to a specific school of psychotherapy, but in generic "common factors," including (1) "extracontextual factors" – noticing and building upon a patient's strengths and competencies; (2) "therapeutic alliance" – patient-defined goals, an environment of empathy and support; and (3) "mobilizing hope and expectancy of change" – a shared belief that change in a mutually agreed upon outcome is possible (Frank & Frank, 1991; Lambert & Bergin, 1994; Wampold, 2011).

Ultimately, the *process* of a therapeutic alliance explains more variance in the success of an intervention than does the specific *content* of the intervention, (Barth et al., 2013; Del Re, Fluckiger, Horvath, Symonds, & Wampold, 2012; Duncan et al., 2010; Fluckiger, Del Re, Wampold, Symonds, & Horvath, 2012; Lambert & Bergin, 1994; Wampold, 2011, 2012). In summary, effective psychotherapy can characterized by the following three conditions: (a) engagement of the patient as an active, collaborative agent who helps shape both the agenda and the form of interaction; (b) the patient's acceptance of therapeutic methods drawn from the psychotherapist's expertise; and (c) beginning the psychotherapy with a primary focus on (a), with the expectation that (b) will be produced in time as a by-product of the interaction.

Anthropologists and cultural psychiatrists have considered whether these psychotherapy models can be generalized to ritual and symbolic healing in non-Western cultural settings (Csordas & Kleinman, 1996). Echoing Frank's (1961/1974) assertion that all mental illness represents demoralization, Kleinman argues that healing efficacy depends not on eradicating pathology, but upon the relationship in which healer and sufferer are convinced that the sufferer has changed for the better (1988,

p. 137). Kleinman's work thus elaborates the social realm of healing and psychopathology, and extends the healing process beyond the ritual itself to long-term changes in one's social space.

Ethical Frameworks for Intervention

There are ethical challenges within global health, and health care in general, involving the power differentials between healer and sufferer. Recent critiques of GMH have raised concern that Western psychiatric categories are not applicable to non-Western cultural groups, and thus medicalize and pathologize culturally normal experience (Summerfield, 2008). A second critique, which extends from the first, is that the financial motives of pharmaceutical companies drive healer–sufferer interactions to commodify suffering, by tying it to the purchase of psychotropic medications (Applbaum, 2009, 2010, *this volume;* Biehl, 2004; Han, 2013; Petryna et al.). Another key issue is the impact of the healer–sufferer interaction on a sufferer's social positioning and the risk of stigma through help-seeking behavior and the type of label received.

The philosopher Emmanuel Levinas (1961) provides a way to approach these ethical questions through the concept of "the Other," Levinas (1961) characterizes all human interactions occurring between the self and "the Other," whereby the Other is acknowledged as separate and not fully knowable; it is only through dialogue that one engages the Other, and the "I" only becomes known through the relationship with the Other. Levinas advocates for "the nonmutual, asymmetrical character of self-other relationships without relinquishing a commitment to dialogue" (Griffith, 2010, p. 247). For Levinas, there is an ethical duty to engage with the Other. Ethical responsibility in the form of engagement precedes any "objective searching after truth." For Levinas, the interaction with the Other is not about erasure of difference or denial of power differentials; it demands that we be in conversation with the Other. Levinas emphasizes the presence of the Other as having an emotional impact that causes an "interruption of self," that disrupts habitual or conventional forms of self-awareness. This creates the conditions for a new and deeper level of recognition and dialogue.

The dialogical process intrinsic to Levinas's approach to the Other has direct application to discussions about the evidence-base and ethical frameworks for intervention in GMH. For most practitioners within the GMH movement, the responsibility is felt as the need to provide care where it is currently unavailable. Evidence only comes after ethics; that is, evidence serves to clarify how service to alleviate psychological suffering may be provided, but the pursuit of evidence can only occur after committing to an ethic of responsibility. This ethic calls critics concerned with the lack of evidence in GMH to engage in research to determine how labels and other aspects of power are deployed in the interaction. It also calls for specific training, supervision, and intervention approaches that directly address the dialogical practices that occur in healer–sufferer interactions. In this case, GMH critiques would be better served by considering the process of engagement with the Other rather than the content of specific diagnoses or interventions. This calls for a critique and re-visioning of how groups and individuals engage in the context of the GMH movement rather than solely focusing on the elements (e.g., diagnostic tools and labels) of that engagement. For example, the processes by which technologies such as the mhGAP are implemented are equally important areas of study as the content of the document itself.

Engaging in treatment can be experienced by some as a greater disruption of self than living with untreated psychiatric symptoms. Participating in treatment often involves engaging with a view of the self connected to larger cultural models of mental illness, which implicate aspects of social positioning, worthiness, expectations of self-control and risk of violence, and other social experiences related to stigma and discrimination; all of these factors are influenced by specific cultural values and orientations (Yang, Thornicroft, Alvarado, Vega, & Link, 2014). Thus, taking medication, participating in psychotherapy, or accepting a mental health diagnosis may be resisted or rejected. For others, taking medication or participating in psychotherapy is seen as a pathway to greater realization of the desired self. For example, motivational interviewing promotes the known or desired self, develops discrepancy with the current self, and helps forge a path from the current state to the desired state (Martino, Canning-Ball, Carroll, & Rounsaville, 2011).

The risks of disrupting the self through participation in treatment need to be addressed in terms of how treatment is designed, implemented, and described (Han, 2013). In the majority of task-shifting randomized controlled trials conducted to date, labels related to psychiatric diagnostic categories (e.g., *DSM* or *ICD* [International Classification of Diseases] diagnoses) have not been used for training or psychoeducation (Patel, Chowdhary, Rahman, & Verdeli, 2011). Instead, labels related to "stress" or "tension" have been chosen by interventionists and treatment designers in order to reduce stigma and promote participation in the programs. Service providers in a number of GMH and cross-cultural psychiatry studies have favored labels related to physiological problems – for example, "nerves" – or to psychosocial problems, over psychiatric terms.

These issues are also important for care providers. In LMIC settings, caregivers often have had little professional training; the new roles they are thrust into can make exceptional demands on their competence and challenge their sense of self (Maes, 2012; Maes & Kalofonos, 2013). For health care providers engaged in taking on mental health care responsibilities through task-shifting, training can be experienced as disruption of self if they feel incompetent to address the issues or stigmatized in the engagement (Kane, Gerretsen, Scherpbier, Dal Poz, & Dieleman, 2010). One of the concerns about task-sharing is that it may be simply *"task dumping"* of stigmatized health care activities (e.g., delivering HIV or mental health services) on persons who have less power to refuse these jobs. Ethnographic studies suggest that participation in such programs by nonspecialists is sometimes an act of desperation given the lack of other means for livelihood (Maes, Closser, & Kalofonos, 2014; Maes & Kalofonos, 2013).

Conversely, taking on the task of providing mental health care when one is properly trained and motivated can be experienced as a greater realization of self because the individual feels more empowered to alleviate suffering. However, health workers may draw their sense of self from cultural frames that are quite different from those that underlie mental health care. In systematic review of task-shifting in child health interventions in LMICs, community health volunteers were found to be less likely to adopt new interventions if they felt that the tasks they had mastered did not augment their value in the community, improve their social status, or give them a sense of relatedness to the beneficiaries (Kane et al., 2010). The review found that formalizing ties with the existing health system provided legitimacy that was associated with success of the intervention, whereas interventions that did not confer an identity associated with the existing health system did not show positive outcomes. Systems issues also play a role in health care providers' experience of self. If task-shifting or other health care system restructuring leads to a greater burden on providers, they may feel incompetent, leading to blaming and stigmatizing the most vulnerable members in the system: patients and their families.

Dialogical practices are key to building a therapeutic alliance, whether between clinician and patient, community health volunteer and mental health specialist, or health workers in LMICs and HICs. Such practices structure interactions so that conversations reflect essential features of Jürgen Habermas's "ideal speech situation" (1987). The ensuing communicative acts of listening, reflecting, and responding give form to a social encounter in which: each participant has an opportunity to speak openly and fully; each participant feels assured that he or she will be heard, understood, and seriously considered in ensuing conversations; decision making to determine courses of action reflects democratic processes of dialogue, reflection, and "seeking the best argument"; and work products and program leadership reflect the joint actions of such dialogical processes. We describe a project conducted in Kosovo in which these dialogical practices structured a conversational domain between international professionals and members of local cultures.

Dialogical Practices with Kosovar Mental Health Professionals and Families

At the end of the 1999 war, Kosovo was in a precarious position regarding the mental health of its population, despite its political success in gaining international protection against Serbian violence. During the war, 800,000 of the 1.8 million Kosovar Albanians had fled the country and another 150,000 had been internally displaced. Approximately two-thirds of the Kosovar Albanian population had suffered lack of food or water, combat exposure, and threat of death, and nearly half reported abuse or torture. One-fourth had witnessed murder of a family or friend. Homes and property of Kosovar Albanians were largely destroyed (Lopes Cardozo, Vergara, Agani, & Gotway, 2000). Planning a mental health response was daunting. Kosovo had long been the poorest and least well-educated region of Europe, with a 60 percent postwar rate of unemployment. There was no community mental health system. The twenty psychiatrists in the country had trained only in inpatient psychiatric wards of Serbian and Croatian hospitals. There were two psychologists and no psychiatric nurses or social workers.

Recognizing that the only resources Kosovo had in abundance were the strengths of their large, closely knit families and family clans, leaders of the Kosovar psychiatric community solicited the assistance of the American Family Therapy Academy and its members to develop family-focused mental health services. In 2000, the Kosovar Family Professional Educational Collaborative (KFPEC) formed as a collaboration between sixteen American mental health professionals (with each employed full-time in an academic position or private clinical practice, representing the American Family Therapy Academy) and the faculty and psychiatry residents of the University of Prishtina Department of Psychiatry (Griffith et al., 2005; Pulleyblank-Coffey, Griffith, & Ulaj, 2006; Weine et al., 2005). Relationships between Kosovar and American mental health specialists were founded initially on face-to-face meetings in Kosovo. During the span of the project, Americans made fifteen two-person trips to work onsite in Kosovo, typically five to nine days at a time, with internet supervision of Kosovar clinicians' study and training between visits.

The design of the KFPEC followed the dialogical principles described above. Collaboration between American and Kosovar professionals was structured at each level of project administration, education, and scholarship. Each administrative, clinical, teaching, and writing activity was conducted jointly by paired Kosovar and American colleagues. Workshop topics, teaching priorities, and timing of visits were set by the Kosovars, while American consultants developed didactic curricula and workshop training in evidence-based clinical methods that responded to these priorities. Clinical and research presentations were jointly presented by Americans and Kosovars at international conferences. Publications in professional journals alternated American and Kosovar coauthors, facilitating development of long-term collegial relationships (Griffith et al., 2005; Weine et al., 2005). Control over project funding was jointly divided between American and Kosovar project leadership. Within the scope of a jointly constructed budget, Kosovar partners maintained budgetary control over project expenditures within Kosovo.

The power of dialogic practice was illustrated by a key redirection in the project strategy during its third year. American members of the KFPEC had entered the project under the assumption that their primary mission was to teach family therapy skills for addressing trauma and loss. At this juncture, however, the Kosovar psychiatric society requested that the project refocus on community-based care of persons with chronic mental illness who were being repatriated from psychiatric hospitals in Serbia and Macedonia after the war's end. Poor and uneducated families were unable to afford care for newly arrived relatives whom they had not seen in many years. They did not understand what was needed for such care, and they feared stigmatization. With no community mental health system or hospital for inpatient care of persons with severe mental illness, a public health crisis was looming.

The American team members followed the Kosovar lead and redirected the project toward community mental health services for individuals with severe mental illnesses, focusing on family-centered care and family psychoeducation, including multi-family psychoeducation groups, whose efficacy had been empirically validated (Anderson, Reiss, & Hogarty, 1986; Dixon et al., 2001; McFarlane, 2002; McFarlane, Link, Dushay, Marchal, & Crilly, 1995). The American team reorganized its leadership and structure so that it could effectively train and supervise Kosovar clinicians, according to this new mandate.

Dialogical practices were structured at multiple ecological levels within the KFPEC. Dialogue between Kosovar and American mental health specialists, as well as with families, community members, and other stakeholders, determined the overall goals and methods for the program. Typically, Americans visiting Kosovo initially spent time in villages interviewing families, teachers, and health services providers, as well as Prishtina-based NGOs and government ministries, in order to identify salient issues of concern within the Kosovar communities. Subsequent didactic lectures and workshop trainings for Kosovar psychiatric nurses and other health workers focused on those issues. At the clinical level, the key ecological engagement was between psychiatric nurses and families. This was motivated by several local factors. Family-centered mental health services, rather than a system organized for symptomatic individuals, were prioritized in recognition that families were the fundamental social unit of Kosovar Albanian culture. Resilience-building therapeutic methods, rather than programs for treating psychopathology, were utilized in recognition that resources were far too limited to treat symptomatic individuals one at a time. Nurse teams provided in-home family assessment and emotional support, psychoeducation about mental illnesses and their treatments, crisis intervention, and medication-monitoring. Weekly to monthly multifamily psychoeducation group meetings were held. In addition, day treatment programs were provided for persons with severe mental illness who needed increased stabilization before attempting to optimize the home environment's therapeutic benefits. Protective residential housing was provided for individuals without families.

Ultimately, over a five-year period, the KFPEC helped develop family-centered mental health services at seven new regional mental health centers. A decade later, these family-centered programs have continued to provide care for the chronically mentally ill, and they are now a mandated standard of care that is funded by the Kosovar Ministry of Health.

Concept 2: Ecological Systems Approaches

A therapeutic alliance coexists with other relationships – both current and historical – that impact on the clinical exchange. In common-factors research in psychotherapy, these other relationships are referred to as "extracontextual factors," and they may explain a large part of the variance of effective therapy (Lambert & Bergin, 1994). These relationships form dynamic systems that can be thought of as a social ecology.

The child development literature has been at the forefront of applying ecological models. Bronfenbrenner (1979) pioneered the ecological-transactional model of child development. Critical medical anthropologists similarly have developed a social-determinant-of-health model that views ecological levels as having a range of influences on health outcomes (Baer et al., 2003; see Figure 22.1). Figure 22.2 depicts how a patient or client exists within multiple ecological levels at the intersection of local and international health care systems. The patient is part of a family existing within a community existing within a culturally shaped government and

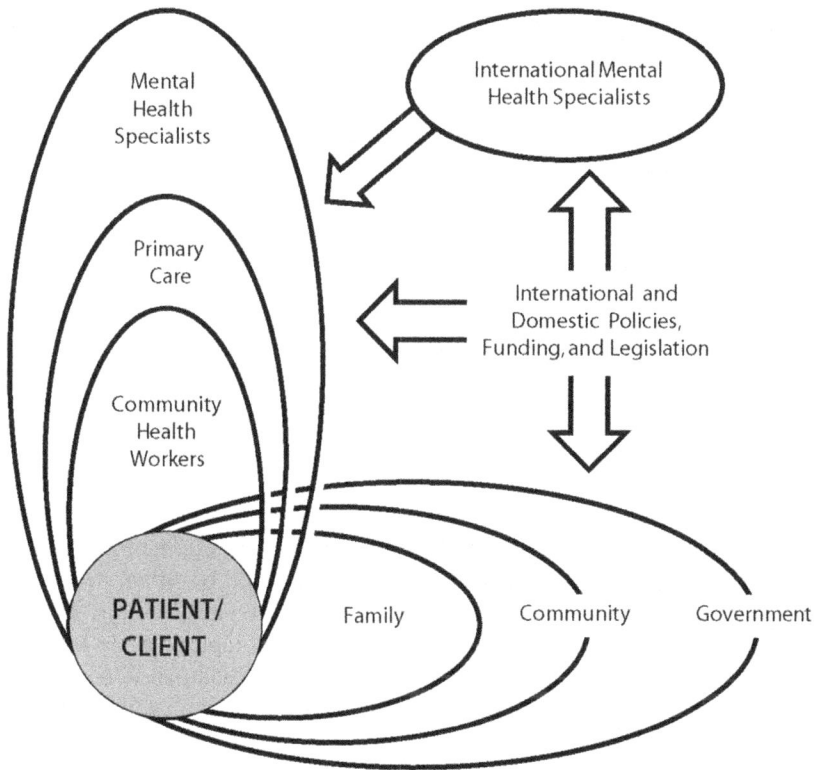

Figure 22.2. Community and health care ecological levels in GMH. The horizontal embedded ecological layers represent the social structures impacting the health and experience of the patient. The vertical layers are different levels of mental health specialization among care providers. Both horizontal and vertical layers are influenced by other sociopolitical-economic processes, such as policies, legislation, and funding.

political economic system. Simultaneously, through participation in treatment, the individual is part of a health care system that has its own multi-
leveled ecology, including community, primary care, and mental health
specialty services. Through GMH endeavors, the health care ecology also
is influenced by international mental health experts. Both international
and domestic policies, funding, and programs shape the structure and
nature of contacts at community and health care levels. Social epidemiology and cultural psychiatry support the importance of social-ecological
models with respect to the course, severity, and functional implications of
mental illness (Betancourt, 2005; Brown et al., 2008; Earls & Carlson,
2001; Kohrt, Jordans, et al., 2010).

Working at the intersection of anthropology and health, Gregory
Bateson (1971) developed an ecological theory of mind and applied
it to thinking about mental health and illness. As general aspects of
Bateson's work and other similar systems-based models, each bit of
information has influences throughout an entire system, and all forms
of information are influenced by immediately preceding forms, as well as
the length of time for information to complete a cycle through the
system. For Bateson, epistemology – how we know what we know –
dominates the ecology of mind. The system is triggered into action by
recognition of *difference*, which sets in motion self-corrective mechanisms. Bateson's ecological model aimed to account for both how psychopathology arises and how treatments can be effective.

These different ecological approaches together are complementary.,-
Bronfenbrenner's work helps conceptualize the different levels that influence individual experience. The critical medical anthropology model of
Singer and Baer applies the ecological perspective to the functioning
of health systems and considers how healer–sufferer interactions always
occur in the context of space and place determined by other structural
factors. Bateson's model calls attention to how information moves
through ecological systems and how different ecological levels operate
with different epistemologies or ways of knowing. A shaman in Mongolia
uses a different epistemology than a neurologist in treating a woman with
severe fatigue because they have different world views and educational
backgrounds with respect to healing practices (Kohrt, Hruschka, Kohrt,
Panebianco, & Tsagaankhuu, 2004). Bateson's model suggests that
introducing new approaches to treatment, such as task-shifting, will have
implications for epistemologies across multiple levels in ecological
systems. The introduction of task-shifting may lead to new ways of
learning and observing, especially for low-level and volunteer health
workers, who have limited prior contact with mental health care. Because
of their roles in the community, the experience of these individuals can

then have ripple effects with regard to how others in the family and community understand mental illness.

Another point that Bateson raises, which is crucial to task-shifting, is the need to consider both the immediate prior position of a cycle of information and its duration. A person's activity prior to participating in mental health training will influence the knowledge gained during the training, and how it is applied. The specific roles that are assigned in task-shifting will influence the conception of mental health and illness and the corresponding epistemologies. With task-shifting to teachers, religious practitioners, and social workers, mental illness might be presented in terms of psychosocial issues. Primary care doctors accustomed to treating malaria, HIV, asthma, and hypertension who become mental health care providers could invite focus on a more biomedical model of pathology.

Biomedical models, especially those in which the primary treatment is medication, center the locus of pathology on the individual. Other healing systems, including some psychotherapies, view mental illness as occurring at the intersections of families and communities (Ensink & Robertson, 1999; Griffith & Griffith, 1987; Gutlove & Thompson, 2004; Parsons, 1984; Rutter, 1999). If evidence-based practices are predominantly drawn from the cultural context of HICs, rather than developed in the cultural context of LMICs, the role of family also may be limited. The clinical culture of healing in an HIC typically is dominated by a focus on the individual. For example, in a randomized control trial that included a family-based intervention for bipolar disorder in the United States, less than 40 percent of patients had family available to participate in the intervention (Miklowitz et al., 2007); therefore, the feasibility and demand for family-based interventions will be considerably lower in the cultural context of some HICs and there will be a bias toward individualized therapies. In contrast, in most hospitals in LMICs, including psychiatric facilities, the family plays a large role. Families purchase medication from outside pharmacies and take laboratory samples to outside facilities for testing; they also assume many of the roles that a nurse would play. In these settings, family-based interventions are more salient (Chatterjee et al., 2011; de Jesus, Razzouk, Thara, Eaton, & Thornicroft, 2009).

A key to developing sustainable interventions with maximum uptake is to embed dialogical practices within and across multiple ecological levels. Dialogical practices embedded within a public health program can ensure that the program meets targeted objective measures to reduce symptoms, respects and empowers the persons who bear the symptoms, and empowers family members and community health workers with the greatest contextual understanding of patients' experiences to act as advocates (Griffith & Griffith, 1994, pp. 65–93). Psychotherapy outcome research further suggests *where* dialogical practices can have the most pivotal impacts. Eliciting ongoing patient feedback during psychotherapy regarding a patient's assessment of the therapeutic alliance, readiness for change, and strength of existing extratherapeutic supports increases the effect size of psychotherapeutic change and the number of patients who achieve a clinically meaningful outcome. In Bateson's terms, the ongoing feedback from each session – rather than waiting for completion of therapy to evaluate progress – accelerates the rate with which information cycles through the system. Dialogical practices also can be embedded within GMH programs so that beneficiaries can reconfigure and redirect program initiatives in a collaborative and ongoing manner, while judiciously adopting Western evidence-based practices.

Dialogical practices would be most beneficial occurring across *multiple ecological levels*. Strategic psychotherapists have observed that a single behavioral change may be countered by homeostatic processes in family systems, so that lasting change in a family often requires interventions that target multiple family members and multiple family relationships (Selvini-Palazzoli, Boscolo, Prata, & Cecchin, 1978). Similarly, a therapeutic alliance that involves individuals, families, community agencies, religious and educational professionals, and government health and social welfare ministries multiplies the relationships that can be activated to initiate change, while also contributing to the maintenance of change. Ultimately, it is possible to incorporate all of these elements into an ecologically based approach to healing as suggested in Kirmayer's (1989, 2004; see also Figure 24.4) model of healing, which includes interactions among the brain, family, community, and the broader social environment.

Designing an Ecological Intervention for Child Soldiers in Nepal

After a decade-long civil war between the Hindu monarchy of Nepal and the Communist Party of Nepal-Maoists, the nongovernmental organization Transcultural Psychosocial Organization (TPO-Nepal) was contracted to identify traditional healing rituals to help former child soldiers reintegrate into families and communities. The work of TPO-Nepal demonstrates beginning with a dialogical approach and then developing an ecologically based intervention. Although the funder had requested the use of traditional healing rituals, it was unknown whether this was a preferred mechanism for intervention among child soldiers.

Therefore, the first goal was develop a therapeutic alliance with former child soldiers and set a mutual agenda for outcomes and mechanisms for achieving such outcomes.

TPO-Nepal adopted a procedure identified as Child Led Indicators (CLI), which at the time was being evaluated by Save the Children Sweden in South Asia (Karki, Kohrt, & Jordans, 2009). CLI is a participatory action research process, in which children and adolescents identify challenges in their lives and community, as well as avenues to address these challenges. They then select indicators that they could observe and measure to determine a program's success. CLI's goal is to make children a part of the development process, including monitoring and evaluation, by selecting outcomes that would be meaningful to them.

The CLI process was adopted for psychosocial well-being and mental health outcomes and tailored to the experience of child soldiers (Karki et al., 2009). The CLI process revealed that for many child soldiers, the return home and the experience of stigma in the community was more distressing than the experience of war. Child soldiers, especially girls, reported discrimination from family members, teachers, and other community members. For the child soldiers, the discontinuity of self was more salient in the community discrimination than in their experiences of war. Child soldiers, especially girls, reported that they felt more like the person they wanted to be as soldiers than they did in subservient roles in the community. The return home, especially the discrimination, disrupted how they wanted to see themselves.

Child soldiers stated that community acceptance was a goal for positive mental health outcomes. However, they did not want traditional rituals because those activities were seen as forcing them into a role which they had rebelled against in becoming soldiers: Community acceptance via rituals came at the expense of how they wanted to see themselves (Kohrt, 2015). Girl soldiers explained that the ritual made them more palatable to the community by placing them in a subservient position to men. They saw the ritual as symbolic submission to patriarchy (Bennett, 1983; Denov, 2007; Dyregrov, Gupta, Gjestad, & Raundalen, 2002). Instead, the girls wanted to participate in school and secular activities, such as clubs and drama teams. Returning to school did not challenge their concept of self, but fulfilled their expectations of how they wanted to see themselves. Although the community had identified ritual pathways to reintegration that would reduce discrimination, for the girl soldiers this step came at the cost of their identity as independent women. They stated that they would prefer to be mistreated as rebel girls than to be accepted as submissive women. Instead, former child soldiers wanted to participate in nonreligious activities, and especially to return to school, as a way to foster positive psychosocial well-being (Kohrt, 2015; Kohrt, Tol, Pettigrew, & Karki, 2010; Morley & Kohrt, 2013).

In both the Nepal and Kosovo examples, initial expectations for programs were altered in dialogue with different levels of beneficiaries. In Nepal, where the key risks were assumed to derive from war trauma, and the expected intervention involved reintegration rituals, the beneficiaries revealed that discrimination at home and in the community was the primary stressor, and that secular activities rather than religious rituals were preferred. In Kosovo, families revealed that support for relatives with severe mental illness, rather than trauma-related disorders, was the primary need. The dialogical practices were utilized to develop shared goals with health professionals and families in Kosovo and with former child soldiers in Nepal.

The CLI process revealed that child soldiers were most distressed by family and community responses during their reintegration. Although the staff of TPO-Nepal had established therapeutic relationships with the child soldiers, the next question was how to develop therapeutic alliances with different members of the child soldiers' social ecology, and, ultimately, how to facilitate a therapeutic relationship between child soldiers and members of their communities. A community-based, rather than clinical, approach was employed. Members of local nongovernmental organizations (NGOs), working in communities with child soldiers, were empowered through twenty-eight-day trainings to become community psychosocial workers (CPSWs) (Kohrt, Perera et al., 2010). The training was divided into five sessions over three months to make the process iterative, with CPSWs bringing successes and challenges into the conversation at each phase to enable ongoing modifications. This arrangement followed Bateson's principle of shortening the duration for information to move fully through the system.

Central to CPSW training were elements of dialogical practices and other communication skills to facilitate therapeutic alliance. The intervention was then conducted largely through meetings between CPSWs and community members, with individualized work with child soldiers as needed. This pattern is the converse of many HICs' clinical approaches to child mental health problems, where individualized treatment dominates the care plan and community interventions are supplemental. CPSWs would meet with teachers, health workers, religious leaders, women's groups, youth clubs, and other community stakeholders to discuss their concerns and experiences related to the war, including experiences with war-affected children, and experiences with former child soldiers. These discussions revealed that fear of former child soldiers underlay the discriminatory practices. Teachers did not want child soldiers in their classrooms for two reasons: They felt unsafe, and they felt that the child soldiers' educational gap would be disruptive and slow down the class. These revelations opened up an opportunity to discuss with teachers the fact that most child soldiers reported that returning to school was their top priority and that they often regretted becoming child soldiers because of the impact on their education. After developing a relationship with teachers and hearing their emotional and professional concerns, the CPSW facilitated conversations between child soldiers and teachers so that each could be heard regarding their concerns and goals.

Thus, the CPSW fostered an environment for dialogical practices to occur between child soldiers and teachers. In addition to dialogue, teachers' concerns about academic delays were addressed by identifying individuals in the community who were willing to tutor former child soldiers so that they could keep pace with classmates. In the majority of cases, these components fostered child soldiers' return to school, which contributed to reduced psychiatric symptoms. Moreover, because teachers were leaders in the community, their acceptance of former child soldiers fostered acceptance by other students and community groups. Ultimately, a cascade of dialogical practices across groups in the community ecology supported community support and positive mental health outcomes.

Concept 3. Spaces, Places, Technologies, and Discourse for Dialogical Processes

Avoiding either capitulating to or dominating the perspective of the other necessitates dialogue. For the clinician [or public health worker], this means building conditions for dialogue where dialogue does not already exist. ... Finding a position from which to initiate conversation is key. It must be close enough to make contact but not so close as to threaten. (Griffith, 2010, pp. 247–8)

Based on our interpretation of Levinas and scholars of development, for example, Paulo Freire (1998), success in GMH should be measured not in production of sameness or subjugation, but in relational dialogue and creating spaces for learning. This raises questions about what kind of physical spaces, virtual meeting places, and cultural institutions, including policies, guidelines, and formulations, can contribute to relational dialogue. In anthropology and fields such as health geography, social configurations and physical structures with specific histories and meanings create spaces where dialogue can occur. In Western psychotherapy, the clinic creates a social space with a set of boundaries that the therapist establishes for the client. These boundaries include a shared agreement between psychotherapist and patient regarding session confidentiality and specified length, and the patient's expectations to express freely whatever thoughts or feelings he or she wishes without shame or punishment.

In GMH, what physical spaces are available for therapeutic exchanges to occur at different ecological levels? Community counselors in Africa and Asia have explained that one of the most important issues is space for therapy to occur. Whereas home-based counseling is convenient for clients, it often lacks space for confidentiality. The open-air structure of many homes in sub-Saharan Africa does not allow for individual physical spaces. Even in places where appropriate structures may be available, a lack of precedent for individual conversations makes requesting privacy difficult, uncomfortable, and potentially threatening. In India, a trial by the Community Care for People with Schizophrenia in India (COPSI) involving home-based care for persons with severe mental illnesses was seen as a threat because it could lead to disclosure to others in the community that a family member had a severe mental illness; therefore, some families refused to participate in services, and some requested other areas to meet (Chatterjee et al., 2011). The tension related to confidentiality and space in intervention adaptations in GMH programs reflects a broader distinction between Western psychiatric treatment (with locked wards and private consultation offices) and most non-Western cultural settings, where forms of healing ritual are often characterized by large public gatherings, even for individual treatments.

In Kosovo, fostering community-wide relationships was the basis for creating a broad alliance of advocates for community mental health services. In Gjakova, for example, KFPEC organized the first community meeting of police, school teachers, Catholic and Muslim religious leaders, social workers, and local counselors to discuss plans for community mental health services (Pulleyblank-Coffey et al., 2006). Gjakova, a regional capital city, had been at the epicenter of violence against Kosovar Albanians during the war. Such community-wide gatherings had never been permitted under the old Communist government. Out of this meeting came a decision to build residential housing near the downtown shopping mall for persons without families who were living with a chronic mental illness, rather than in a marginalized location outside the city. The thinking of the community leaders was that citizens of Gjakova could drop by after shopping for friendly visits with the residents. The community, thus, played a key role in choosing a physical space and site that would facilitate ongoing dialogue with mentally ill persons who did not have families.

Mental health practitioners in both HICs and LMICs may prefer having a private counseling space or center, associated with a clinic or health facility. However, most spaces in clinic settings are communal, and it is rare to have a separate room with a door on it to provide a confidential space. In Uganda, a nongovernmental organization, Transcultural Psychosocial Organization (TPO-Uganda), found a creative solution to both the space issue and the personnel issue for mental health services. TPO-Uganda obtained governmental permission to build a two-room addition onto health centers: one room as a waiting room and the other as a private room with a door for mental health consultations. Signs saying "mental health services" were hung above the rooms and in various places within the rooms to mark clearly the intended purpose of the space.

This occurred during a period of dialogue in the health ministry to provide mental health services. Initially, reported demand from regional health facilities was infrequent, but once the rooms were built, potential clients, health workers, and local government leaders saw the spaces and signs and began asking national health officials about when those spaces would be staffed. The work of TPO-Uganda demonstrated that first providing the space ultimately fostered provision of the services, in contrast to some LMICs that make trained community counselors available but provide limited services because they lack acceptable physical infrastructure.

Uganda has been a model in other ways for thinking creatively about the use of space to foster improved mental health care. By 2008, the African Development Bank had completed support for major renovation of Butabika Hospital, the country's major psychiatric hospital, which has capacity for over five hundred patients. During the renovation, a large outpatient facility for nonpsychiatric conditions was added, including highly desired dental facilities. This addition led to a large influx of nonpsychiatric patients and helped reduce felt stigma among hospital staff and visiting family members.

Spaces are also important for facilitating therapeutic alliance at other ecological levels. Vincent Mujune, a Ugandan public health researcher, refers to "software-only" training, which he characterizes as a didactic approach with limited exposure to patients and health care facilities. He critiques such training as the equivalent of trying to teach someone a computer program without using a computer. For the preferred "hardware-based" training, mid-level health professionals spend a significant part of their time in a psychiatric facility working with psychiatrists and interacting with patients. This leads to improved communication with instructors and continued communication after training about cases that these mid-level professionals encounter in their own communities. This also improves knowledge acquisition and referrals because mid-level professionals have greater experience in the psychiatric facility, and thus are better able to decide whom to refer, how to refer smoothly, and how to minimize anxiety among families of persons being referred. This likely also contributes acculturation to hierarchical processes in formal medical systems with expectations of who can speak to whom and rigid expectations of what is considered an acceptable referral.

International networks can also foster dialogue between mental health experts in HICs and LMICs. For researchers, there are increasing efforts to create spaces for exchange, where mental health researchers from LMICs are empowered with resources to conduct studies.[1] In addition to places and spaces, cultural documents, such as diagnostic manuals, shape dialogue and discourse. Psychiatry is developing tools that can structure and promote dialogical practices. For example, the Cultural Formulation Interview (CFI) included in the fifth edition of the *DSM* (*DSM-5*; APA, 2013) operationalizes the process of eliciting elements of culture in psychiatric care planning. The cultural formulation grew out of recognition that individuals' explanatory models influence relationships with care providers, care-seeking pathways, and perceptions of distress and health (Lewis-Fernández, 1996, 2009). The CFI uses narrative as a data collection approach to improving psychiatric care: "Narrative creates a humanized account of suffering fundamentally embedded in a particular setting through the assembling of telling contextual details as signs of truth" (Lewis-Fernández, 1996, p. 136). In clinical work, eliciting patients' narratives can improve engagement and alliance through greater awareness of cultural influences on behavior, distress, and healing, promoting a person-centered approach to mental health care (Lewis-Fernández & Aggarwal, Chapter 17, *this volume*).

At a global systems level, the World Health Organization Assessment Instrument for Mental Health Systems (WHO-AIMS), which produced

---

[1] Activities of the Wellcome Trust and Department for International Development (DfID) in the United Kingdom, Grand Challenges Canada, and the U.S. National Institutes of Health are supporting researchers from LMICs, as well as conducting meetings that bring together researchers representing high-, middle-, and low-income countries from around the world. Skype and other technologies increasingly facilitate exchange and clinical consultation between HICs and LMICs, and within LMICs. Mount Sinai's GMH program in New York uses teleconferencing for weekly case discussion with the maternal and child mental health department of Liberia's John F. Kennedy Hospital. Also in Liberia, the Carter Center Mental Health Initiative has started virtual discussion boards for psychiatric nurses and physicians' assistants to discuss difficult cases and foster quality improvement.

the WHO Mental Health Atlas in 2005 and 2011, has been key to facilitating dialogue among health policy makers and funders for services in LMICs (WHO, 2005a, 2005b, 2011). A major limitation in advocacy can be a lack of information about the severity of treatment gaps or specific resource needs. Being armed with such information, as well as having regional and international comparisons, facilitates dialogue. WHO-AIMS records information on health workforce, spending, and facilities to highlight any gaps in services (see Figures 22.3 and 22.4). This information can be used to make regional comparisons and to highlight disparities in workforce or funding. WHO-AIMS also records information on service-user, family, and advocacy groups to raise awareness about the need for these endeavors in LMICs.

Within countries, Health Management Information Systems (HMIS) are crucial to provide data about gaps in service. Adding mental health diagnoses and treatment indicators to HMIS is an advocacy success because it empowers dialogue. In Liberia, the Clinton Health Access Initiative supported a nationwide accreditation program for clinical facilities. In 2010, new mental health indicators were added to the documentation process, thus illustrating, for the first time, the gross absence of psychiatric medications in most facilities. Fewer than 8 percent of clinical facilities in Liberia carried medications to address epilepsy, psychotic disorders, or depression. Mental health advocates and health workers have used this information to push for greater availability of psychotropic medication.

An effective way to produce cultural documents and include mental health researchers and practitioners from LMICs has been through Delphi exercises, which can bring together diverse voices to identify research priorities. Recent Delphi activities involving LMICs practitioners and researchers have addressed *Grand Challenges in GMH* (Collins et al., 2011) and research priorities in humanitarian settings (Tol et al., 2011). Delphi exercises in LMICs regions (Ferri, Chisholm, Van Ommeren, & Prince, 2004) have included a suicide prevention exercise in India (Colucci, Kelly, Minas, Jorm, & Chatterjee, 2010). In the Programme for Improving Mental Health CarE (PRIME) sponsored by Department for International Development (U.K.; DFID), Delphi exercises were used to identify key conditions for intervention, based on priorities of local mental health practitioners in Uganda, Ethiopia, South Africa, India, and Nepal. Of note, Delphi exercises have been critiqued for reifying conceptions of those in power into policy, and their value is ultimately dependent on who participates in the exercise (Watson & Wakefield, 2014).

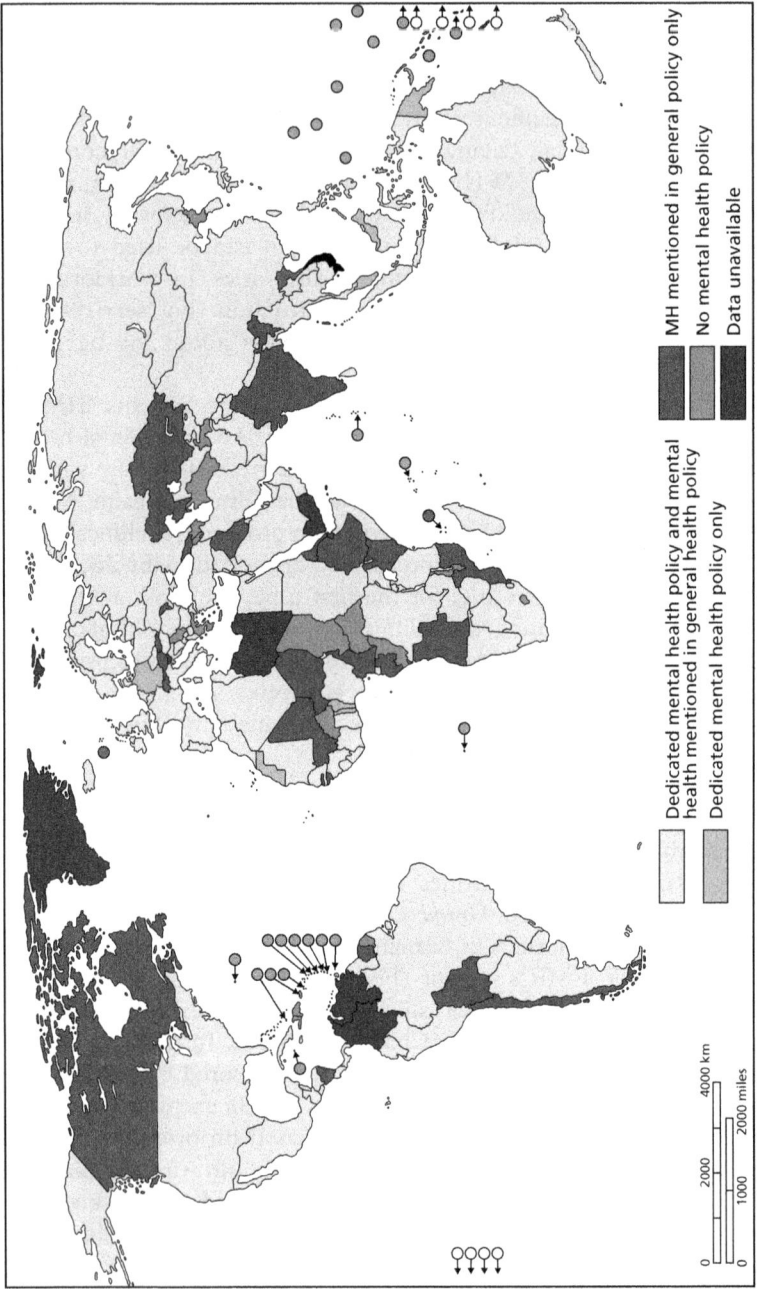

Figure 22.3. Mental health policy coverage by country. Reproduced, with the permission of the publisher, from *Mental Health Atlas 2011*. Geneva, World Health Organization, 2011 (Fig. 1.1.1, Page 19, http://www.who.int/mental_health/publications/mental_health_atlas_2011/en/, accessed 02 June 2015; see Color Plate).

Legend:
Dedicated mental health policy and mental health mentioned in general health policy
Dedicated mental health policy only
MH mentioned in general policy only
No mental health policy
Data unavailable

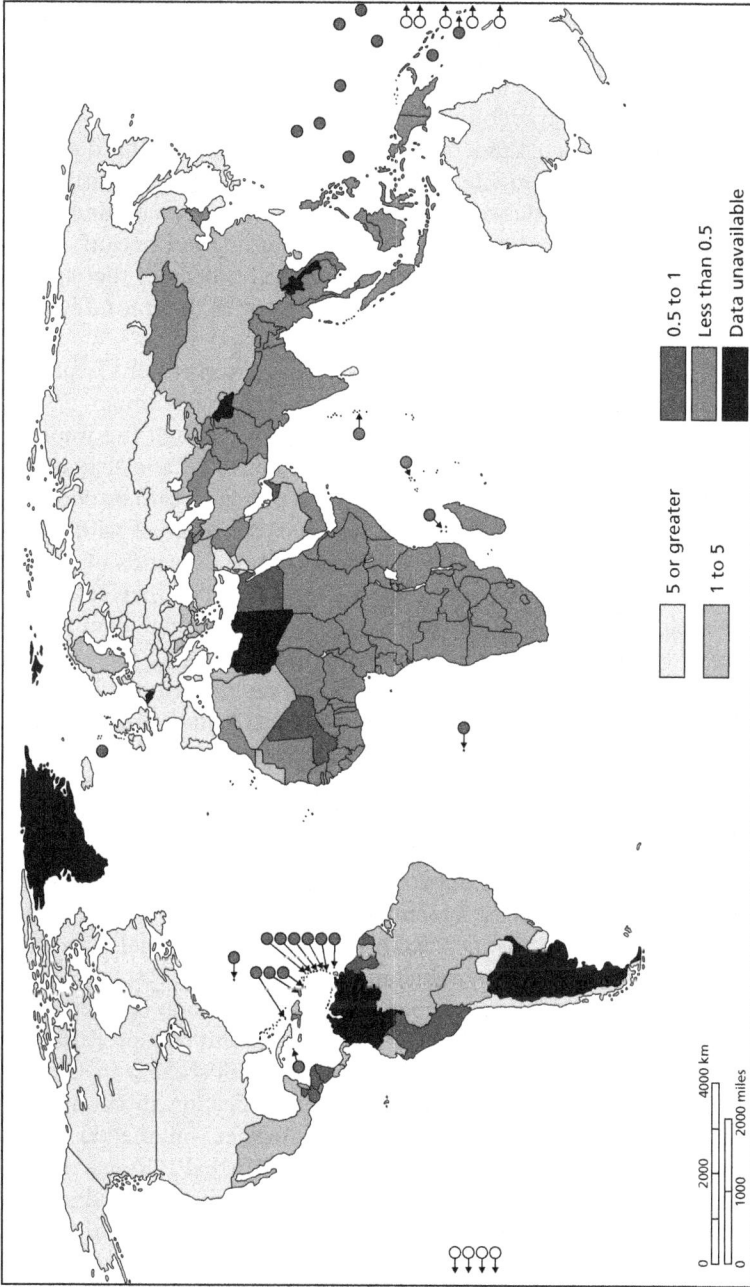

Figure 22.4. Psychiatrists per hundred thousand population by country. Reproduced, with the permission of the publisher, from *Mental Health Atlas 2011*. Geneva, World Health Organization, 2011 (Fig. 4.2.1, Page 57, http://www.who.int/mental_health/publications/mental_health_atlas_2011/en/, accessed 02 June 2015; see Color Plate).

Concept 4. Tradeoffs and Unintended Consequences

Tradeoffs and unintended consequences are crucial factors to keep in mind with global health initiatives, and an ecological framework helps conceptualize where tradeoffs happen and what unintended consequences might occur. Tradeoffs have been developed in detail in biocultural approaches to life history (Worthman, 2009; Worthman, & Kuzara, 2005). Theories of tradeoff help illustrate why certain behaviors viewed as maladaptive arise during developmental periods when they may be adaptive, and how certain biological processes that appear maladaptive may be adaptive in other domains or at different developmental periods.

The unintended consequences of policies and interventions is an area receiving increasing attention in global health work (Kleinman, 2010). Identifying such consequences requires thinking through the implications of a policy or intervention for the dynamics of social systems. This type of systems thinking is also pertinent to health care ecology. As new types of activities are introduced, what is the tradeoff within and across ecological levels? Within levels, how do new demands of mental health care impact on time, funding, and training to other activities? For example, in Nepal, a qualitative study of potential community volunteers (women from the community pharmacists, teachers) to engage in identification and referral found an "anyone but me" attitude toward adding this activity to other tasks (Jordans, Luitel, Tomlinson, & Komproe, 2013). Although all of the groups interviewed felt that increased identification and referral were important, they thought that any group but their own should actually take on these responsibilities. Each group already felt too burdened to take on additional responsibilities.

Task-shifting can also have impacts throughout the health care system. A desired outcome is increased identification of and referrals for persons in the community with mental health problems. These goals can have undesired impacts, such as overwhelming existing human resources (e.g., through increasing the need for supervision and evaluation of referrals by the overextended and limited number of mental health care professionals in low resource settings). A qualitative study of task-shifting in Uganda found that although allocating referral and identification to community health workers was intended to reduce the burden on mental health specialists (Petersen, Ssebunnya, Bhana, Baillie, & MhaPP Research Programme Consortium, 2011), it actually increased their time demands because of the greater number of referrals. One consequence was demoralization of those specialists, who felt they could not adequately address all needs. The issue of task-shifting leading to increased burden, either within or across levels, is crucial to consider because increased burden is a major ingredient in creating stigma. If individuals feel that their workload has been unfairly increased, the most vulnerable groups – those without a voice to reply – may become the target of animosity, stigma, and discrimination. In the area of mental health care, the persons with mental illness and their families end up with additional stigma placed on them by those who are expected to care for them.

Conclusion

GMH seeks to reduce human suffering from both social causes and mental illnesses. The challenge is that the impetus, targets, and resources for change typically originate in high-income, high-resource countries, whereas members of low-income, low-resource societies are the target populations for change. Furthermore, within both high and low-income settings, economically and educationally privileged groups tend to create policy and shape infrastructure for mental health care of more vulnerable groups. Regardless of how GMH professionals attempt to partner with members of the target population, the relationship remains an asymmetrical one in terms of power, scientific knowledge, and material resources.

The concepts of therapeutic alliance and dialogical practice can help us understand and address these issues of power by creating spaces and opportunities for dialogue and exchange. For GMH practitioners, we advocate a four-step approach: (1) use dialogical processes to develop therapeutic alliances; (2) contextualize therapeutic alliances within and across ecological levels; (3) develop and adapt spaces, places, technologies, and discourses that facilitate alliances within and across levels; and (4) be aware of potential tradeoffs and unintended consequences that may ripple through the health care and community ecologies. This approach is a process, rather than a claim for any universal type of content in diagnosis and treatment. Attending to process and incorporating these concepts holds promise for critical and engaged GMH praxis.

REFERENCES

Aggarwal, N. K., & Kohrt, B. A. (2013). Medical diplomacy and global mental health: From community and national institutions to regional centers of excellence. *Community Mental Health Journal, 49*(6), 805–14. http://dx.doi.org/10.1007/s10597-013-9644-0

American Psychiatric Association. (2013). *Diagnostic and statistical manual of mental disorders* (5th ed.). Washington, DC: Author.

Anderson, C. M., Reiss, D. J., & Hogarty, G. E. (1986). *Schizophrenia and the family: A practitioner's guide to psychoeducation and management.* New York, NY: Guilford Press.

Applbaum, K. (2009). Getting to yes: Corporate power and the creation of a psychopharmaceutical blockbuster. *Culture Medicine and Psychiatry, 33*(2), 185–215. http://dx.doi.org/10.1007/s11013-009-9129-3

Applbaum, K. (2010). Shadow science: Zyprexa, Eli Lilly and the globalization of pharmaceutical damage control. *Biosocieties, 5*(2), 236–55. http://dx.doi.org/10.1057/biosoc.2010.5

Applbaum, K. (2015). Solving global mental health as a delivery problem: Toward a critical epistemology of the solution. In L. J. Kirmayer, R. Lemelson, & C. A. Cummings (Eds.), *Re-visioning psychiatry: Cultural phenomenology, critical neuroscience, and global mental health* (pp. 544–74). New York, NY: Cambridge University Press.

Baer, H. A., Singer, M., & Susser, I. (2003). *Medical anthropology and the world system* (2nd ed.). Westport, CT: Praeger.

Baldwin, S. A., Wampold, B. E., & Imel, Z. E. (2007). Untangling the alliance-outcome correlation: Exploring the relative importance of therapist and patient variability in the alliance. *Journal of Consulting & Clinical Psychology, 75*(6), 842–52. http://dx.doi.org/10.1037/0022-006X.75.6.842

Barth, J., Munder, T., Gerger, H., Nüesch, E., Trelle, S., Znoj, H., … Cuijpers, P. (2013). Comparative efficacy of seven psychotherapeutic interventions for patients with depression: A network meta-analysis. *PLOS Medicine, 10*(5), e1001454. http://dx.doi.org/10.1371/journal.pmed.1001454

Bateson, G. (1971). The cybernetics of "self": A theory of alcoholism. *Psychiatry, 34*(1), 1–18.

Bennett, L. (1983). *Dangerous wives and sacred sisters: Social and symbolic roles of high-caste women in Nepal.* New York, NY: Columbia University Press.

Betancourt, T. S. (2005). Stressors, supports and the social ecology of displacement: Psychosocial dimensions of an emergency education program for Chechen adolescents displaced in Ingushetia, Russia. *Culture, Medicine, and Psychiatry, 29*(3), 309–40. http://dx.doi.org/10.1007/s11013-005-9170-9

Biehl, J. (2004). Life of the mind: The interface of psychopharmaceuticals, domestic economies, and social abandonment. *American Ethnologist, 31*(4), 475–96. http://dx.doi.org/10.1525/ae.2004.31.4.475

Biehl, J., & Petryna, A. (2013). *When people come first: Critical studies in global health.* Princeton, NJ: Princeton University Press.

Bracken, P., Thomas, P., Timimi, S., Asen, E., Behr, G., Beuster, C., … Double, D. (2012). Psychiatry beyond the current paradigm. *The British Journal of Psychiatry, 201*(6), 430–4. http://dx.doi.org/10.1192/bjp.bp.112.109447

Bracken, P. J. (2003). Postmodernism and psychiatry. *Current Opinion in Psychiatry, 16*(6), 673–7. http://dx.doi.org/10.1097/00001504-200311000-00012

Bronfenbrenner, U. (1979). *The ecology of human development: Experiments by nature and design.* Cambridge, MA: Harvard University Press.

Brown, R. A., Adler, N. E., Worthman, C. M., Copeland, W. E., Costello, E. J., & Angold, A. (2008). Cultural and community determinants of subjective social status among Cherokee and white youth. *Ethnicity & Health, 13*(4), 289–303. http://dx.doi.org/10.1080/13557850701837302

Chatterjee, S., Leese, M., Koschorke, M., McCrone, P., Naik, S., John, S., . . . Community care for people with schizophrenia in India group. (2011). Collaborative community based care for people and their families living with schizophrenia in India: Protocol for a randomised controlled trial. *Trials, 12,* 12.

Chisholm, D., Flisher, A. J., Lund, C., Patel, V., Saxena, S., Thornicroft, G., . . . Lancet Global Mental Health. (2007). Scale up services for mental disorders: A call for action. *Lancet, 370*(9594), 1241–52. http://dx.doi.org/10.1016/S0140-6736(07)61242-2

Choudhury, S., & Kirmayer, L. J. (2009). Cultural neuroscience and psychopathology: Prospects for cultural psychiatry. *Progress in Brain Research, 178,* 263–83. http://dx.doi.org/10.1016/S0079-6123(09)17820-2

Collins, P. Y., Patel, V., Joestl, S. S., March, D., Insel, T. R., Daar, A. S., . . . Stein, D. J. (2011). Grand challenges in global mental health. *Nature, 475*(7354), 27–30. http://dx.doi.org/http://dx.doi.org/10.1038/475027a

Colucci, E., Kelly, C. M., Minas, H., Jorm, A. F., & Chatterjee, S. (2010). Mental health first aid guidelines for helping a suicidal person: A Delphi consensus study in India. *International Journal of Mental Health Systems, 4*(1), 4. http://dx.doi.org/10.1186/1752-4458-4-4

Csordas, T. J., & Kleinman, A. (1996). The therapeutic process. In C. F. Sargent & T. M. Johnson (Eds.), *Handbook of medical anthropology: Contemporary theory and method* (rev. ed., pp. 3–20). Westport, CT: Greenwood Press.

de Jesus, M. J., Razzouk, D., Thara, R., Eaton, J., & Thornicroft, G. (2009). Packages of care for schizophrenia in low- and middle-income countries. *PLOS Medicine, 6*(10), e1000165. http://dx.doi.org/10.1371/journal.pmed.1000165

Del Re, A. C., Fluckiger, C., Horvath, A. O., Symonds, D., & Wampold, B. E. (2012). Therapist effects in the therapeutic alliance-outcome relationship: A restricted-maximum likelihood meta-analysis. *Clinical Psychology Review, 32*(7), 642–9. http://dx.doi.org/http://dx.doi.org/10.1016/j.cpr.2012.07.002

Denov, M. (2007). Is culture always right? The dangers of reproducing gender stereotypes and inequalities in psychosocial interventions for war-affected children. In L. Dowdney (Ed.), *Psychosocial web page.* London, England: Coalition to Stop the Use of Child Soldiers.

Dixon, L., McFarlane, W. R., Lefley, H., Lucksted, A., Cohen, M., Falloon, I., . . . Sondheimer, D. (2001). Evidence-based practices for services to families of people with psychiatric disabilities. *Psychiatric Services, 52*(7), 903–10. http://dx.doi.org/10.1176/appi.ps.52.7.903

Dow, J. (1986). Universal aspects of symbolic healing: A theoretical synthesis. *American Anthropologist, 88*(1), 56–69. http://dx.doi.org/10.1525/aa.1986.88.1.02a00040

Drew, N., Funk, M., Tang, S., Lamichhane, J., Chavez, E., Katontoka, S., . . . Saraceno, B. (2011). Human rights violations of people with mental and psychosocial disabilities: an unresolved global crisis. *Lancet, 378*(9803), 1664–75. http://dx.doi.org/10.1016/S0140-6736(11)61458-X

Duncan, B. L., Miller, S. D., Wampold, B. E., & Hubble, M. A. (Eds.). (2010). *The heart and soul of change: Delivering what works in therapy* (2nd ed.). Washington, DC: American Psychological Association.

Dyregrov, A., Gupta, L., Gjestad, R., & Raundalen, M. (2002). Is the culture always right? *Traumatology, 8*(3), 135–45. http://dx.doi.org/10.1177/153476560200800302

Earls, F., & Carlson, M. (2001). The social-ecology of child health and wellbeing. *Annual Review of Public Health, 22,* 143–66.

Ensink, K., & Robertson, B. (1999). Patient and family experiences of psychiatric services and African indigenous healers. *Transcultural Psychiatry, 36*(1), 23–43.

Farmer, P., Kim, J. Y., Kleinman, A., & Basilico, M. (2013). *Reimagining global health: An introduction.* Berkeley: University of California Press.

Fernando, S. (2011, September & October). A "global" mental health program or markets for big pharma? *Open Mind, 168.* See http://www.sumanfernando.com/openmind.htm

Ferri, C., Chisholm, D., Van Ommeren, M., & Prince, M. (2004). Resource utilisation for neuropsychiatric disorders in developing countries: A multinational Delphi consensus study. *Social Psychiatry & Psychiatric Epidemiology, 39*(3), 218–27.

Fluckiger, C., Del Re, A. C., Wampold, B. E., Symonds, D., & Horvath, A. O. (2012). How central is the alliance in psychotherapy? A multilevel longitudinal meta-analysis. *Journal of Counseling Psychology, 59*(1), 10–17.

Foucault, M. (1965). *Madness and civilization: A history of insanity in the Age of Reason.* New York, NY: Pantheon Books.

Frank, J. (1974). *Persuasions and healing.* New York, NY: Schocken. (Original work published 1961)

Frank, J. D., & Frank, J. B. (1991). *Persuasion and healing: A comparative study of psychotherapy* (3rd ed.). Baltimore, MD: Johns Hopkins University Press.

Freire, P. (1998). *Pedagogy of the oppressed* (3rd ed.). New York, NY: The Continuum Publishing Company.

Gaines, A. D. (1992). Ethnopsychiatry: The cultural construction of psychiatries. In A. D. Gaines (Ed.), *Ethnopsychiatry: The cultural construction of professional and folk psychiatries* (pp. 3–50). Albany: State University of New York Press.

Griffith, J. L. (2010). *Religion that heals, religion that harms: A guide for clinical practice.* New York, NY: Guilford Press.

Griffith, J. L., Agani, F., Weine, S., Ukshini, S., Pulleyblank-Coffey, E., Ulaj, J., … Kallaba, M. (2005). A family-based mental health program of recovery from state terror in Kosova. *Behavioral Sciences & the Law, 23*(4), 547–58.

Griffith, J. L., & Griffith, M. E. (1987). Structural family therapy in chronic illness: Intervention can help produce a more adaptive family structure. *Psychosomatics, 28*(4), 202–5.

(1994). *The body speaks: Therapeutic dialogues for mind–body problems.* New York, NY: Basic Books.

Gutlove, P., & Thompson, G. (2004). Psychosocial healing and post-conflict social reconstruction in the former Yugoslavia. *Medicine, Conflict & Survival, 20*(2), 136–50.

Habermas, J. (1987). *The theory of communicative action (Vol. 2). Lifeworld and system: A critique of functionalist reason* (T. McCarthy, Trans.). Boston, MA: Beacon Press.

Han, C. (2013). Labor instability and community mental health: the work of pharmaceuticals in Santiago, Chile. In J. Biehl & A. Petryna (Eds.), *When people come first: Critical studies in global health* (pp. 276–301). Princeton, NJ: Princeton University Press.

Hollan, D. (1997). The relevance of person-centered ethnography to cross-cultural psychiatry. *Transcultural Psychiatry, 34*(2), 219–34.

Jordans, M., Luitel, N., Tomlinson, M., & Komproe, I. (2013). Setting priorities for mental health care in Nepal: A formative study. *BMC Psychiatry, 13*(1), 332. http://dx.doi.org/10.1186/1471-244X-13-332

Kakuma, R., Minas, H., van Ginneken, N., Dal Poz, M. R., Desiraju, K., Morris, J. E., . . . Scheffler, R. M. (2011). Human resources for mental health care: Current situation and strategies for action. *The Lancet, 378* (9803), 1654–63.

Kane, S. S., Gerretsen, B., Scherpbier, R., Dal Poz, M., & Dieleman, M. (2010). A realist synthesis of randomised control trials involving use of community health workers for delivering child health interventions in low and middle income countries. *BMC Health Services Research, 10*, 286. http://dx.doi.org/ 10.1186/1472-6963-10-286

Karki, R., Kohrt, B. A., & Jordans, M. J. D. (2009). Child Led Indicators: Pilot testing a child participation tool for psychosocial support programmes for former child soldiers in Nepal. *Intervention: International Journal of Mental Health, Psychosocial Work & Counselling in Areas of Armed Conflict, 7*(2), 92–109.

Kirmayer, L. J. (1989). Psychotherapy and the cultural concept of the person. *Sante, Culture, Health, 6*(3), 241–70.

Kirmayer, L. J. (2004). The cultural diversity of healing: Meaning, metaphor and mechanism. *British Medical Bulletin, 69*, 33–48.

Kirmayer, L. J. (2006). Beyond the new cross-cultural psychiatry: Cultural biology, discursive psychology and the ironies of globalization. *Transcultural Psychiatry, 43*(1), 126–44.

Kirmayer, L. J., & Jarvis, E. (1998). Cultural psychiatry: From museums of exotica to the global agora. *Current Opinion in Psychiatry, 11*(2), 183–9.

Kleinman, A. (1980). *Patients and healers in the context of culture: An exploration of the borderland between anthropology, medicine, and psychiatry.* Berkeley: University of California Press.

Kleinman, A. (1987). Anthropology and psychiatry: The role of culture in cross-cultural research on illness. *British Journal of Psychiatry, 151*, 447–54.

Kleinman, A. (1988). *Rethinking psychiatry: From cultural category to personal experience.* New York, NY: Free Press.

Kleinman, A. (2010). Four social theories for global health. *The Lancet, 375*(9725), 1518–19.

Kleinman, A. (2012a). Medical anthropology and mental health: Five questions for the next fifty years. In M. C. Inhorn, *Medical anthropology at the intersections: Histories, activisms, and futures* (pp. 116–28). Durham, NC: Duke University Press.

Kleinman, A. (2012b). Rebalancing academic psychiatry: Why it needs to happen–and soon. *The British Journal of Psychiatry, 201*(6), 421–2.

Kleinman, A., & Desjarlais, R. R. (1995). Violence, culture, and the politics of trauma. In A. Kleinman (Ed.), *Writing at the margin: Discourse between anthropology and medicine* (pp. 173–92). Berkeley: University of California Press.

Kleinman, A., & Good, B. (1985). *Culture and depression: Studies in the anthropology and cross-cultural psychiatry of affect and disorder*. Berkeley, CA: University of California Press.

Kohrt, B. A. (2015). The role of traditional rituals for reintegration and psychosocial well-being of child soldiers in Nepal. In A. L. Hinton & D. E. Hinton (Eds.), *Gender and mass violence: Memory, symptom, and recovery*. (pp. 369–87). New York, NY: Cambridge University Press.

Kohrt, B. A., Hruschka, D. J., Kohrt, H. E., Panebianco, N. L., & Tsagaankhuu, G. (2004). Distribution of distress in post-socialist Mongolia: A cultural epidemiology of yadargaa. *Social Science & Medicine, 58*(3), 471–85.

Kohrt, B. A., Jordans, M. J. D., Tol, W. A., Perera, E., Karki, R., Koirala, S., & Upadhaya, N. (2010). Social ecology of child soldiers: child, family, and community determinants of mental health, psychosocial well-being, and reintegration in Nepal. *Transcultural Psychiatry, 47*(5), 727–53.

Kohrt, B. A., Perera, E., Jordans, M. J. D., Koirala, S., Karki, R., Karki, R., ... Upadhaya, N. (2010). *Psychosocial support model for children associated with armed forces and armed groups in Nepal*. Kathmandu, Nepal: Transcultural Psychosocial Organization-Nepal/ UNICEF.

Kohrt, B. A., Tol, W. A., Pettigrew, J., & Karki, R. (2010). Children and revolution: The mental health and psychosocial wellbeing of child soldiers in Nepal's Maoist army. In M. Singer & G. D. Hodge (Eds.), *The war machine and global health* (pp. 89–116). Lanham, MD: Altamira Press.

Lambert, M. J., & Bergin, A. E. (1994). The effectiveness of psychotherapy. In A. E. Bergin & S. L. Garfield (Eds.), *Handbook of psychotherapy and behavior change* (4th ed.; pp. 143–89). New York, NY: John Wiley.

Levi Strauss, C. (2000). The effectiveness of symbols. In R. Littlewood & S. Dein (Eds.), *Cultural psychiatry and medical anthropology: An introduction and reader* (pp. 162–78). New Brunswick, NJ: Athlone Press. (Original work published 1949)

Levinas, E. (1961). *Totality and infinity: An essay on exteriority*. Pittsburgh, PA: Duquesne University Press.

Lewis-Fernández, R. (1996). Cultural formulation of psychiatric diagnosis. *Culture, Medicine, and Psychiatry, 20*(2), 133–44.

Lewis-Fernández, R. (2009). The cultural formulation. *Transcultural Psychiatry, 46*(3), 379–82. http://dx.doi.org/http://dx.doi.org/10.1177/1363461509342519

Lewis-Fernández, R., & Kleinman, A. (1995). Cultural psychiatry: Theoretical, clinical, and research issues. *Psychiatric Clinics of North America, 18*(3), 433–48.

Littlewood, R. (1990). From categories to contexts: A decade of the "new cross-cultural psychiatry". *British Journal of Psychiatry, 159*, 308–27.

Littlewood, R., & Dein, S. (2000). Introduction. In R. Littlewood & S. Dein (Eds.), *Cultural psychiatry and medical anthropology: An introduction and reader* (pp. 1–34). New Brunswick, NJ: The Athlone Press.

Lopes Cardozo, B., Vergara, A., Agani, F., & Gotway, C. A. (2000). Mental health, social functioning, and attitudes of Kosovar Albanians following the war in Kosovo. *Journal of the American Medical Association, 284*(5), 569–77.

Luhrmann, T. M. (2000). *Of two minds: The growing disorder in American psychiatry* (1st ed.). New York, NY: Knopf.

Luty, J. (2014). Psychiatry and the dark side: Eugenics, Nazi and Soviet psychiatry. *Advances in Psychiatric Treatment, 20*(1), 52–60.

Maes, K. (2012). Volunteerism or labor exploitation? Harnessing the volunteer spirit to sustain AIDS treatment programs in urban Ethiopia. *Human Organization, 71*(1), 54–64.

Maes, K., Closser, S., & Kalofonos, I. (2014). Listening to community health workers: How ethnographic research can inform positive relationships among community health workers, health institutions, and communities. *American Journal of Public Health, 104*(5), e5–9.

Maes, K., & Kalofonos, I. (2013). Becoming and remaining community health workers: Perspectives from Ethiopia and Mozambique. *Social Science & Medicine, 87*, 52–9. http://dx.doi.org/10.1016/j.socscimed.2013.03.026

Maes, K. C., Kohrt, B. A., & Closser, S. (2010). Culture, status and context in community health worker pay: Pitfalls and opportunities for policy research. A commentary on Glenton et al. (2010). *Social Science & Medicine, 71*(8), 1375–18; discussion 1379–80.

Martino, S., Canning-Ball, M., Carroll, K. M., & Rounsaville, B. J. (2011). A criterion-based stepwise approach for training counselors in motivational interviewing. *Journal of Substance Abuse Treatment, 40*(4), 357–65.

McFarlane, W. R. (2002). *Multifamily groups in the treatment of severe psychiatric disorders.* New York, NY: Guilford Press.

McFarlane, W. R., Link, B., Dushay, R., Marchal, J., & Crilly, J. (1995). Psychoeducational multiple family groups: Four-year relapse outcome in schizophrenia. *Family Process, 34*(2), 127–44. http://dx.doi.org/10.1111/j.1545-5300.1995.00127.x

Miklowitz, D. J., Otto, M. W., Frank, E., Reilly-Harrington, N. A., Wisniewski, S. R., Kogan, J. N., … Sachs, G. S. (2007). Psychosocial treatments for bipolar depression: A 1-year randomized trial from the Systematic Treatment Enhancement Program. *Archives of General Psychiatry, 64*(4), 419–26.

Morley, C. A., & Kohrt, B. A. (2013). Impact of peer support on PTSD, hope, and functional impairment: A mixed-methods study of child soldiers in Nepal. *Journal of Aggression, Maltreatment & Trauma, 22*(7), 714–34. http://dx.doi.org/10.1080/10926771.2013.813882

Parsons, C. D. (1984). Idioms of distress: Kinship and sickness among the people of the Kingdom of Tonga. *Culture, Medicine, and Psychiatry, 8*(1), 71–93.

Patel, V. (2014). Why mental health matters to global health. *Transcultural Psychiatry, 51*(6), 777–89. http://dx.doi.org/10.1177/1363461514524473

Patel, V., Chowdhary, N., Rahman, A., & Verdeli, H. (2011). Improving access to psychological treatments: Lessons from developing countries.

Behaviour Research & Therapy, 49(9), 523–8. http://dx.doi.org/10.1016/j.
brat.2011.06.012

Patel, V., Collins, P. Y., Copeland, J., Kakuma, R., Katontoka, S., Lamichhane,
J., . . . Skeen, S. (2011). The movement for global mental health. *British
Journal of Psychiatry, 198*, 88–90.

Petersen, I., Ssebunnya, J., Bhana, A., Baillie, K., & MhaPP Research
Programme Consortium. (2011). Lessons from case studies of integrating
mental health into primary health care in South Africa and Uganda.
International Journal of Mental Health Systems, 5, 8. http://dx.doi.org/
10.1186/1752-4458-5-8

Petryna, A., Lakoff, A., & Kleinman, A. (2006). *Global pharmaceuticals: Ethics,
markets, practices.* Durham, NC: Duke University Press.

Prince, M., Patel, V., Saxena, S., Maj, M., Maselko, J., Phillips, M. R., & Rahman,
A. (2007). No health without mental health. *Lancet, 370*(9590), 859–77.

Pulleyblank-Coffey, E., Griffith, J. L., & Ulaj, J. (2006). Gjakova: The first
community mental health center in Kosova. In A. Lightburn & P. Sessions
(Eds.), *Community-based clinical practice.* New York, NY: Oxford University
Press.

Raviola, G., Becker, A. E., & Farmer, P. (2011). A global scope for global health–
including mental health. *Lancet, 378*(9803), 1613–15.

Rivers, W. H. R. (1924). *Medicine, magic, and religion: The Fitz Patrick lectures.*
New York, NY: Harcourt Brace.

Rutter, M. (1999). Resilience concepts and findings: Implications for family
therapy. *Journal of Family Therapy, 21*, 119–44.

Sapir, E. (1932). Cultural anthropology and psychiatry. *Journal of Abnormal
and Social Psychology, 27*, 229–42.

Selvini-Palazzoli, M. Boscolo, L., Prata, G., & Cecchin, G. (1978). *Paradox and
counterparadox.* New York, NY: Jason Aronson.

Shotter, J. (1993a). *Conversational realities: Constructing life through language.*
Thousand Oaks, CA: Sage.

Shotter, J. (1993b). *Cultural politics of everyday life: Social constructionism,
rhetoric and knowing of the third kind.* Toronto, Canada: University of
Toronto Press.

Singer, M. (1989). The coming of age of critical medical anthropology.
Social Science & Medicine, 28(11), 1193–1203.

Singer, M. C. (1995). Beyond the ivory tower: Critical praxis in medical
anthropology. *Medical Anthropology Quarterly, 9*, 80–106.

Summerfield, D. (1999). A critique of seven assumptions behind psychological
trauma programmes in war-affected areas. *Social Science & Medicine, 48*(10),
1449–62.

Summerfield, D. (2008). How scientifically valid is the knowledge base of
global mental health? *BMJ, 336*(7651), 992–4.

Summerfield, D. (2012). Afterword: Against global mental health. *Transcultural
Psychiatry, 49*(3), 519–30. http://dx.doi.org/10.1177/1363461512454701

Swartz, L. (2012). An unruly coming of age: The benefits of discomfort for
GMH. *Transcultural Psychiatry, 49*(3–4), 531–8. http://dx.doi.org/10.1177/
1363461512454810

Szasz, T. S. (1961). *The myth of mental illness: Foundations of a theory of personal conduct*. New York, NY: Dell.

Tol, W. A., Patel, V., Tomlinson, M., Baingana, F., Galappatti, A., Panter-Brick, C., ... van Ommeren, M. (2011). Research priorities for mental health and psychosocial support in humanitarian settings. *PLOS Medicine, 8*(9), e1001096.

Turner, V. W. (1967). *The forest of symbols: Aspects of Ndembu ritual*. Ithaca, NY: Cornell University Press.

van Voren, R. (2010). Political abuse of psychiatry: An historical overview. *Schizophrenia Bulletin, 36*(1), 33–5.

Wampold, B. E. (2011). The research evidence for common factors models: a historically situated perspective. In B. L. Duncan, S. D. Miller, B. E. Wampold & M. A. Hubble (Eds.), *The heart and soul of change: Delivering what works in therapy* (2nd ed., pp. 49–82). Washington, DC: American Psychological Association.

Wampold, B. E. (2012). Humanism as a common factor in psychotherapy. *Psychotherapy: Theory, Research, Practice, Training, 49*(4), 445–9. http://dx.doi.org/http://dx.doi.org/10.1037/a0027113

Watson, T., & Wakefield, R. (2014). Delphi 2.0: A reappraisal of Delphi method for public relations research. *Public Relations Review, 40*, 577–84. http://dx.doi.org/10.1016/j.pubrev.2013.12.004

Weine, S., Ukshini, S., Griffith, J., Agani, F., Pulleyblank-Coffey, E., Ulaj, J., ... Weingarten, K. (2005). A family approach to severe mental illness in post-war Kosovo. *Psychiatry, 68*(1), 17–27.

Wittkower, E. D. (1970). Transcultural psychiatry in the Caribbean: Past, present, and future. *American Journal of Psychiatry, 127*(2), 162–6.

World Health Organization. (2001). *The world health report 2001 – Mental health: New understanding, new hope*. Retrieved from http://www.who.int/whr/2001/en/

World Health Organization. (2005a). *Mental health atlas 2005*. Retrieved from http://www.who.int/mental_health/evidence/mhatlas05/en/

World Health Organization. (2005b). World Health Organization Assessment Instrument for Mental Health Systems (WHO-AIMS). Retrieved from http://www.who.int/mental_health/publications/who_aims_instrument/en/

World Health Organization. (2008). Task-shifting: Rational redistribution of tasks among health workforce teams: Global recommendations and guidelines. Retrieved from http://apps.who.int/iris/handle/10665/43821

World Health Organization. (2010). mhGAP Intervention Guide for mental, neurological and substance-use disorders in non-specialized health setting. Mental health Gap Action Programme (mhGAP). Retrieved from http://www.who.int/mental_health/publications/mhGAP_intervention_guide/en/

World Health Organization. (2011). *Mental health atlas 2011*. Retrieved from http://www.who.int/mental_health/publications/mental_health_atlas_2011/en/

Worthman, C. M. (2009). Habits of the heart: life history and the developmental neuroendocrinology of emotion. *American Journal of Human Biology, 21*(6), 772–81.

Worthman, C. M., & Kuzara, J. (2005). Life history and the early origins of health differentials. *American Journal of Human Biology, 17*(1), 95–112.

Yang, L. H., Thornicroft, G., Alvarado, R., Vega, E., & Link, B. G. (2014). Recent advances in cross-cultural measurement in psychiatric epidemiology: Utilizing "what matters most" to identify culture-specific aspects of stigma. *International Journal of Epidemiology, 43*(2), 494–510. http://dx.doi.org/10.1093/ije/dyu039

Yap, P.-M. (2000). Mental diseases peculiar to certain cultures: a survey of comparative psychiatry. In R. Littlewood & S. Dein (Eds.), *Cultural psychiatry and medical anthropology: An introduction and reader* (pp. 179–98). New Brunswick, NJ: Athlone Press. (Original work published 1951)

Young, A. (1995). *The harmony of illusions: Inventing post-traumatic stress disorder.* Princeton, NJ: Princeton University Press.

23 *Reflections*
Social Inequalities and Mental Health Outcomes
Toward a New Architecture for Global Mental Health

Duncan Pedersen

Global Mental Health (GMH) is an emerging and relatively new field of enquiry and practice, where policies, research, and action initiatives are driven by a heterogeneous group of actors and agencies, who have convergent, at times overlapping, but often also divergent views and incommensurate aims (McGoey, Reiss, & Wahlberg, 2011). The preceding chapters in this section reflect this diversity.

Globalization is a dominant force, exerting major influences in the configuration of vast social sectors, as well as realigning political fronts and generating alliances and antagonistic tensions and conflict in various forms, all of which give rise to a range of consequences in the quality of life, health status, and life expectancy of the world's populations. Several related factors – both positive and negative – contribute to global health, including: growing concerns with national security and the emergence of devastating epidemics in African countries (e.g., Ebola, HIV/AIDS); increasing interdependence and competition for world markets; the expansion of transnational corporations; WTO trade agreements (e.g., Trade-Related Aspects of International Property Rights [TRIPS]) that regulate the transnational flow of financial resources, goods, and services; and increased transfer of medical technologies, drugs and pharmaceuticals (Kim, Millen, Irwin, & Gershman, 2001; Labonté, Mohindra & Schrecker, 2011; Pedersen, 2012).

GMH has evolved at a faster pace in the last decade or so, shaping the discourse of policy makers, service providers, and the public at large, involving public and private sectors, multi- and bilateral agencies and private foundations, and more recently attracting donors and new funding sources, as well as increasing interest in academic circles and younger generations of medical and social scientists.

In the chapters encompassed in this section, the authors approach the GMH field in different ways and from different perspectives. In Chapter 20, Anne E. Becker and Jennifer J. Thomas's analysis tackles a central concern in GMH: the cross-cultural variation of mental illness in clinical presentations, which has received little attention in constructing Western nosologies of mental disorders. The cross-cultural heterogeneity and phenomenological diversity of mental health problems like eating disorders contribute to their relative invisibility among patients and populations, despite their significant health burden and potential lethality, resulting in lack of attention and neglect in public health programs and clinical settings. Eating disorders represent a special challenge but remain virtually nonexistent in today's GMH agenda and, for structural reasons, the voices of the most vulnerable still remain unheard.

In Chapter 19, Lemelson and Tucker remind us of the crucial importance of ethnography in the cross-cultural study of mental illness. Film images and narratives allow us to engage the lifeworld of patients and capture both the context and the particularities of the "local," revealing how globalized models of mental health care and access to psychopharmacological treatments penetrate deeply into subjects' lives and illness experience. In this regard, perhaps the most important contribution of ethnography, as a methodology applied to the study of GMH in contemporary Indonesia, consists in allowing thick description and interpretation of the social and cultural context and its linkages with specific mental health outcomes allowing for a more humane and comprehensive view than either neurobiological or clinical-phenomenological approaches alone can achieve. The two case studies that Lemelson and Becker present are connected by analogous diagnoses, and, although they belong to different generations, they share similar histories of colonialism, exposure to sweeping social and economic changes, including political violence, and an emerging context of globalized mental health economies of care and recovery.

In Chapter 21, Kalman Applbaum adopts a critical view of the GMH movement, in particular, its "packages of care" (Patel & Thornicroft, 2009). In doing so, Applbaum identifies subjacent tensions in the models of GMH, including those between a "public health approach" and a "social and culturally based approach." The former is grounded in biology and current evidence-based practices (which are still largely produced in high-income countries), with Western-driven taxonomies and classifications for mental disorders, and most often exogenous, vertically organized (or "top-down") interventions. The latter approach emphasizes the social origins of mental illness and the imperatives to listen to culture and its local discourses, starting with local taxonomies and priorities, and empowerment of endogenous resources, in order to build horizontal, community-based, and more sustainable solutions.

Another tension is created by discrepancies between the professionally claimed global epidemic of mental disorders and the popular perceptions of mental illness. Government statistics about prevalence and incidence rates of mental illness are often rough estimates based on weighted averages but are presented by international agencies such as WHO as global probabilities, often comparing the North to the South, with the North tacitly accepted as the "gold standard."

For instance, according to WHO estimates, in 2001 more than 25 percent of the world's population were affected by mental health disorders at some point in their lives, and depression affected over 340 million people worldwide. Extrapolating these trends, WHO predicted that by the year 2020, depression would be second only to ischemic heart disease for DALYs[1] worldwide, and first in the burden of disease ranking in developed countries, mostly in North America and Europe (World Health Organization, 2001). In 2005, Kessler and colleagues published the results of a household survey using a diagnostic interview, in which in any one year, about 26.2 percent of Americans reported symptoms compatible with a *DSM-IV* diagnosis of mental disorder (Kessler et al., 2005).

This rather alarming figures for the United States and northern European countries lends credence to the claim made by some GMH advocates – namely WHO and the "GMH movement" (http://www.global mentalhealth.org) – of a worldwide "crisis of epidemic proportions" with global figures of 25, 50, and 75 percent for annual, lifetime, and untreated incidence of neuropsychiatric disorders respectively, which Applbaum points out are not "... just epidemiological estimates, but large, rounded numbers intended to spur action." Much of this action implies the dispensing of Western psychiatric solutions, including the marketing and delivery of psychotropic drugs to "on the massive scale implied: 25 percent or half of 75 percent of the world's population." The problem with these global estimates is not so much the questionable validity of the categories used, but the totally arbitrary way in which the numbers are juggled. To estimate DALYs for a particular health condition or group of disorders you need to know the incidence rate, the level of disability caused, the average length of episodes, and the life expectancy. Of course, these variables are simply not available in most poverty-stricken countries; usually, they are just educated "guesstimates" which are later published as DALYs and used as justification for conducting massive interventions. Then there is the problem of comorbidity, which we know is high for common mental disorders such as depression. It is known that people tend

---

[1] DALYs, or disability adjusted life years, provide an estimate of the burden of illness that factors in both mortality and morbidity (disability or functional impairment; Murray, 1994).

to feel low when they are sick, and at the same time they are not up to doing much. How much of the disability resulting from physical illness gets attributed to depression? (Ingleby, 2013).

The final chapter of this section by Brandon A. Kohrt and James L. Griffith, presents four sets of concepts which they find useful for thinking about GMH praxis, based on their own experiences working with the Kosova American Family Therapy Academy in Kosovo, the Clinton Health Access Initiative in Liberia, and the Transcultural Psychosocial Organization (TPO) in Uganda and Nepal. These sets are presented under the following titles: (1) dialogical practices and the therapeutic alliance; (2) ecological systems; (3) spaces, places, technology, and discourse; and (4) tradeoffs and unintended consequences. Despite the fact that these interventions share important features with many other initiatives in post-conflict humanitarian assistance, little information is provided regarding the criteria used to assess these interventions and how mental health outcomes were measured. Given that such interventions are typically of brief duration, the concern is that they may, in fact, have limited impact, and even when effectiveness can be shown, it is usually unclear if any positive results can be attributed to the intervention itself. Indeed, the fact that these examples involve interventions mostly conducted by foreign agencies exporting Western approaches in low-income country settings may be viewed with scepticism by scholars critical of neocolonial approaches in GMH, with its medicalized models of care (Fernando, 2014; Mills, 2014).

One of the crucial questions that remains unexplored in these chapters concerns what are the main pathways that link social inequities with mental health outcomes. Poverty, racism, and social exclusion can have powerful influences in mental and physical health, both in terms of morbidity and mortality (Lund et al., 2010). Material insecurity, which comes along with poverty, is itself a source of distress, worry and a constant threat, which should not be underestimated. It is fairly well established that people exposed to stressful life events (i.e., marriage dissolution, job insecurity, death of family member, legal prosecution, eviction, serious financial trouble, etc.) have higher mortality rates (Link & Phelan, 1995; Robinson, McBeth & Macfarlane, 2004; Wilkinson, 1996).

There are several possible psychosocial pathways linking stressful life events with higher morbidity and mortality, some involve biological factors such as immune and neuroendocrine systems, while others are related to psychosocial and cultural dimensions. A research program centered on social inequity, disease and poor mental health outcomes offers an opportunity to explore pressing health and social issues while forging links among different disciplines and research topics. Societies where social inequality tends to increase, experience higher death rates from most causes and higher rates of alcohol-related deaths, drug abuse, self-inflicted injuries and suicide, crime, homicide and both, interpersonal and collective violence (Wilkinson & Picket, 2006). Violent death in urban settings in both industrial and less developed nations has become one of the main causes of mortality among young men in low-income sectors of cities such as Cape Town, Kingston, and El Salvador (Geneva Declaration Secretariat, 2008).

While diseases resulting from poverty and poor environmental conditions, such as diarrhoea or tuberculosis, have often been medicalized (transforming largely social and political problems into narrow biomedical concerns) and subject to massive technological interventions, mental disorders and the newly emerging behavior-related problems in GMH challenge conventional biomedical solutions and demand a different approach. As implied by the work in some of the chapters in this volume, the course and outcome of severe mental disorders depend not solely on access to services, medication, skills and the availability of professional care, but also on the reactions, care, and support provided by family members and the immediate social network of community resources (Bracken et al., 2012; Campbell & Burgess, 2012). Likewise, many behavior-related disorders have no simple, effective, and readily available biotechnological solution, but will require changes in individual *and* collective behaviours as well as interventions directed to both "microsocial processes" and the broader social context (Pedersen, 2012).

There is increasing awareness of the risks and potential harm that can be caused by exporting evidence-based Western biomedical psychiatry to non-Western cultures. For example, flaws in the published data on results of psychopharmaceutical therapies and the dangers arising from excessive use of psychotropic drugs in Europe and North America have been widely documented (Angell, 2011; Moncrieff, 2009; Whitaker, 2010). Moreover, the damage caused to people with mental illness by current custodial systems of care is now evident (Coles, Keenan, & Diamond, 2013; Davar, 2012). Given these limitations of contemporary psychiatric knowledge and practice, there may be a great deal to learn from non-Western societies in low- and middle-income countries (LMICs), where psychiatry has had relatively little or peripheral influence.

A final issue pertinent to this review relates to current calls to increase the value and reduce the waste of research in GMH. The increase in annual global investment in biomedical research – reaching $240 billion in 2010 – has resulted in important health dividends for patients and the public (Chalmers et al., 2014). However, most of the research undertaken does not lead to worthwhile achievements, partly because studies either do not have direct relevance to human health or because potential users' needs and perspectives are ignored. Much wasteful research is now being funded and it can be argued that what we need is not simply more research, but more relevant research that addresses key GMH issues. In particular, we need to improve the yield of basic research on social determinants of mental health, as well as applied research addressing practical questions of governance, policy, service delivery, and implementation (Chalmers et al., 2014).

This points to the need for a new architecture for global mental health (Kirmayer & Pedersen, 2014). A first step in this direction would be to acknowledge the fact that unless cultural, social and economic realities are incorporated into our research and action programs, and we begin to address existing social inequalities in the global North (and the global South), the gap between the rich and the poor will continue widening, with impoverishment of large segments of the population, devastation of the natural environment, and poor health outcomes, including mental health, for increasing numbers of people (Pedersen, 2013).

The quest in wealthy nations for perpetual development utopias and endless economic growth has come to a sudden end in the current global financial meltdown. But if we continue our current pattern of funding global mental health, investing primarily in the North-South transfer of pharmaceuticals and psychotropic drugs in "silos" narrowly constrained approaches to improve global mental health, we are likely to repeat only to perpetuate our current "failure of humanity" (Kleinman, 2009). To continue relying on the philanthropy of a few donors, the private industry, or the pharmaceutical corporations is not a long-term solution to global health problems (Benatar, 2009).

A balanced global mental health research agenda for the future must focus not only on the biological (i.e., molecular) bases and global burden of mental disorders but also on the social, environmental, and economic (i.e., molar) determinants within which these diseases occur. To maximize the research capacity for innovation in LMICs and knowledge transfer for GMH, we need to travel on at least two distinct directions of the innovation process: *downstream*, continuing the search for biotechnological and psychosocial solutions exemplified by global population-based development partnerships to build more efficacious screening, diagnostic, and therapeutic interventions in the secondary prevention and clinical management domains; and *upstream*, in exploring more actively the more distal causes: that is, the social and environmental origins of health and disease or the "causes of the causes," in search of systemic social solutions and collective interventions, exemplified by health policy and health systems research from a multisectoral, cross-cultural and transdisciplinary perspective. A unifying new paradigm for global mental health needs to be driven by both biotechnological and social innovations (Gardner, Acharya, & Yach, 2007).

REFERENCES

Angell, M. (2011, June 23). The epidemic of mental illness: Why? *The New York Review of Books*.

Applbaum, K. (2015). Solving global mental health as a delivery problem: Toward a critical epistemology of the solution. In L. J. Kirmayer, R. Lemelson, & C. A. Cummings (Eds.), *Re-visioning psychiatry: Cultural phenomenology, critical neuroscience, and global mental health* (pp. 544–74). New York, NY: Cambridge University Press.

Becker, A. E., & Thomas, J. J. (2015). Eating pathology in Fiji: Phenomenologic diversity, visibility, and vulnerability. In L. J. Kirmayer, R. Lemelson, & C. A. Cummings (Eds.), *Re-visioning psychiatry: Cultural phenomenology, critical neuroscience, and global mental health* (pp. 515–43). New York, NY: Cambridge University Press.

Benatar, S. R. (2009). Global health: Where to now? *Global Health Governance*, 2(2), 1–11.

Bracken, P., Thomas, P., Timimi, S., Asen, E., Behr, G., Beuster, C., . . . Yeomans, D. (2012). Psychiatry beyond the current paradigm. *British Journal of Psychiatry*, 201, 430–4. http://dx.doi.org/10.1192/bjp.bp.112.109447

Campbell, C., & Burgess, R. (2012). The role of communities in advancing the goals of the Movement for Global Mental Health. *Transcultural Psychiatry*, 49(3–4), 379–95. http://dx.doi.org/10.1177/1363461512454643

Coles, S., Keenan, S., & Diamond, B. (Eds.). (2013). *Madness contested: Power and practice*. Ross-on-Wye, England: PCCS Books.

Chalmers, I., Bracken, M. B., Djulbegovic, B., Garattini, S., Grant, J., Gülmezoglu, A. M., . . . Oliver, S. (2014). How to increase value and reduce waste when research priorities are set. *Lancet*, 383, 156–65. http://dx.doi.org/10.1016/S0140-6736(13)62229-1

Davar, B. V. (2012). Legal frameworks for and against persons with psychosocial disabilities. *Economic and Political Weekly*, XLVI(52), 123–31.

Fernando, S. (2014). *Mental health worldwide: Culture, globalization and development*. London, England: Palgrave-Macmillan. http://dx.doi.org/10.1057/9781137329608

Gardner, C. A., Acharya, T., & Yach, D. (2007). Technological and social innovation: A unifying new paradigm for global health. *Health Affairs*, 26(4), 1052–61. http://dx.doi.org/10.1377/hlthaff.26.4.1052

Geneva Declaration Secretariat (2008). *Global burden of armed violence*. London, England: Paul Green.

Ingleby, D. (2013). Personal communication. *January* 14, 2013.

Kessler, R. C., Berglund, P., Demler, O., Jin, R., Merikangas, K. R., & Walters, E. E. (2005). Lifetime prevalence and the age of onsetdistributions of *DSM-IV* disorders in the National Comorbidity Survey Replication. *Archives of General Psychiatry, 62*(6), 593–60. http://dx.doi.org/10.1001/archpsyc.62.6.593

Kim, J. Y., Millen, J. V., Irwin, A., & Gershman, J. (2001). *Dying for growth: Global inequality and the health of the poor.* Monroe, ME: Common Courage Press.

Kirmayer, L. J., & Pedersen, D. (2014). Toward a new architecture for global mental health. *Transcultural Psychiatry, 51*(6): 759–76.

Kleinman, A. (2009). Global mental health: A failure of humanity. *Lancet, 374* (9690), 603–4.

Kohrt, B. A., & Griffith, J. L. (2015). Global mental health praxis: Perspectives from cultural psychiatry on research and intervention. In L. J. Kirmayer, R. Lemelson, & C. A. Cummings (Eds.), *Re-visioning psychiatry: Cultural phenomenology, critical neuroscience, and global mental health* (pp. 575–612). New York, NY: Cambridge University Press.

Labonté, R., Mohindra, K., & Schrecker, T. (2011). The growing impact of globalization for health and public health practice, *Annual Review of Public Health, 32*, 263–83. http://dx.doi.org/10.1146/annurev-publhealth-031210-101225

Lemelson, R., & Tucker, A. (2015). Afflictions: Psychopathology and recovery in cultural context. In L. J. Kirmayer, R. Lemelson, & C. A. Cummings (Eds.), *Re-visioning psychiatry: Cultural phenomenology, critical neuroscience, and global mental health* (pp. 483–514). New York, NY: Cambridge University Press.

Link, B. G., & Phelan, J. (1995). Social conditions as fundamental causes of disease. *Journal of Health and Social Behavior, 35*(extra issue), 80–94. http://dx.doi.org/10.2307/2626958

Lund, C., Breen, A., Flisher, A. J., Kakuma, R., Corrigall, J., Joska, J. A., . . . Patel, V. (2010). Poverty and common mental disorders in low and middle income countries: A systematic review. *Social Science & Medicine, 71*(3), 517–28. http://dx.doi.org/10.1016/j.socscimed.2010.04.027

McGoey, L., Reiss, J., & Wahlberg, A. (2011). The global health complex. *BioSocieties, 6*(1), 1–9. http://dx.doi.org/10.1057/biosoc.2010.45

Mills, C. (2014). *Decolonizing global mental health: The psychiatrization of the majority world.* London, England: Routledge.

Moncrieff, J. (2009). *The myth of the chemical cure: A critique of psychiatric drug treatment.* Basingstoke, England: Palgrave Macmillan.

Murray, C. J. L. (1994). Quantifying the burden of disease: The technical basis for disability-adjusted life years. *WHO Bulletin, 72*(3), 429–45.

Patel, V., & Thornicroft, G. (2009). Packages of care for mental, neurological and substance abuse disorders in low- and middle-income countries. *PLOS Medicine, 6*, 1–2.

Pedersen, D. (2012). Vers un paradigme unificateur en santé mondiale. In J. C. Suárez-Herrera & M. J. Blain (Eds.), *La recherche en santé mondiale: Perspectives socio-anthropologiques – Actes du colloque # 652* (pp. 45–62). Sherbrooke, Canada: ACFAS 2011.

Pedersen, D. (2013). A step in the right direction. Canadian Coalition of Global Health Research (CCGHR). Retrieved from http://www.ccghr.ca/coalition-connect-your-global-health-news-blog/page/4

Robinson, K.L., McBeth, J., & Macfarlane, G.J. (2004). Psychological distress and premature mortality in the general population: A prospective study. *Annals of Epidemiology, 14*(7), 467–72.

World Health Organization. (2001). *The world health report 2001: Mental health – New understanding, new hope.* Retrieved from http://www.who.int/whr/2001/en/

Wilkinson, R. (1996). *Unhealthy societies: The afflictions of inequality.* London, England: Routledge. http://dx.doi.org/10.4324/9780203421680

Wilkinson, R. G., & Pickett, K. E. (2006). Income inequality and population health: A review and explanation of the evidence. *Social Science & Medicine, 62*(7), 1768–84. http://dx.doi.org/10.1016/j.socscimed.2005.08.036

Whitaker, R. (2010). *Anatomy of an epidemic: Magic bullets, psychiatric drugs, and the astonishing rise of mental illness in America.* New York, NY: Broadway.

24 Re-Visioning Psychiatry
Toward an Ecology of Mind in Health and Illness

Laurence J. Kirmayer

Introduction

Although mental afflictions are probably as old as humanity, psychiatry is a young discipline that has undergone dramatic changes in theory and practice over the last 150 years. With the rise of biological approaches to the mind, the mandate of psychiatry is being rethought. Will psychiatry disappear in the years to come, as the centuries-old mind/body dualism is resolved in favor of a reductive materialism, with the study of the mind's afflictions absorbed by neuroscience? Will psychiatry become "clinically applied neuroscience" with its broader concerns taken over by other professions that are more explicitly focused on the psychological and social dimensions of suffering? Or will the field find a way forward that realizes its promise of an integrative view and response to human suffering? The answers to these questions depend not only on scientific advances but on the social, cultural, political, and economic contexts of psychiatry as an evolving field of inquiry, profession, and social institution.

Over the last century, psychiatry embraced three broad views of psychopathology and corresponding notions of human personhood. One view, present from the start of modern psychiatry and currently in ascendance, sees the person as a biological organism, shaped by constitution and experience and vulnerable to specific kinds of disease related to the effects of adverse genes, environments, toxins, infections, and injuries to the brain. A second view of personhood, advanced by psychoanalysis, centers on the psychological self, with its inner theater of conflict, fantasies, and self-deceptions driven by largely unconscious projects of managing anxiety, avoiding death, pursuing pleasure, and achieving coherence and stability. A third view, favored in the social sciences, emphasizes the ways in which individual agency and capabilities are shaped and constrained by social contexts and the environment. In this view, individuals' plans and aspirations are structured by society, which affords some people advantages and confronts others with endless obstacles and structural violence.

Each of these views of the person corresponds to modes of explanation in psychiatry: biological, psychodynamic, and psychosocial.

Of course, these concepts of personhood are not mutually exclusive, and each offers only a partial truth; but at certain historical moments, particular models or modes of explanation have tended to dominate discourse, both within psychiatry and in the popular imagination. Indeed, the relative emphasis placed on one or another model in accounts of mental health problems or recovery has varied, not so much with advances in scientific knowledge, but with larger forces in society. Dominant social values have also figured in the evolution of psychiatry. For example, in its transplantation from fin-de-siècle Vienna to mid-century North America, psychoanalysis was transformed from an exploration of the inevitable conflicts of psyche and society that leads to a tragic view of life, to a method to promote better functioning by realizing the person's individuality, authentic feelings, and desires (Zaretsky, 2004). Although it served to support cultural critique and changes in gender roles and family life, this valorization of the individual culminated in what Bellah (1985) called "expressive" and "utilitarian" forms of individualism, which define well-being in terms of individuals' capacities to articulate and advance their personal agendas. This configuration of personhood has its own forms of pathology related to narcissism, social fragmentation, and the hedonic treadmill of competition and consumption (Cushman, 1995; Kasser, 2002). This cultural history is essential to understand the broad range of "neurotic" problems gathered under the umbrella of psychiatry.

In the last few decades, neuroscience has displaced psychodynamics as the conceptual language of psychiatry, and the focus has shifted toward working with a neurological notion of personhood in which "I am my brain" and my suffering reflects "bad chemicals" or structural changes due to stress and trauma more than "bad learning," social disadvantage, or miserable life circumstances (Rose & Abi-Rached, 2013; Vidal, 2009). This kind of neurological personhood allows the person to look for practical biological solutions as part of the care of the self, aimed at restoring good functioning. This concept has been supported by a refashioning of personhood in popular psychology in terms of a neurochemical self that must be kept in balance to optimize efficiency and flexibility (Malabou, 2008). But this view of the person as a well-tempered brain fails to capture the embodied, experiential, social, environmental, and ethical dimensions of well-being and affliction. Hence, it seems woefully inadequate for psychiatry as a clinical discipline and helping profession.

The work collected in this volume encourages the hope that psychiatric theory is on the threshold of a renaissance, in which complex-systems thinking will allow us to integrate neuroscience, psychology, and the social sciences in modes of practice that are more self-aware and self-critical – and therefore better able to recognize and respond to others in all their diversity. In this concluding chapter, I draw together some of these strands to articulate a vision of how psychiatry might move forward in ways that respect the complexity of its subject, clinical mandate, and ethical commitments. The discussion is organized in terms of the four overarching themes of this volume: (1) the nature of psychiatric knowledge and the place of phenomenology in research and clinical practice; (2) the significance of recent advances in cognitive and social neuroscience; (3) the development of social-ecological and cultural models of mental disorders; and (4) the challenges of responding to global disparities in mental health.

The Place of Phenomenology in Psychiatry

Phenomenology, the systematic study of the structure of experience, has been central to psychiatric theory from its inception because of the need to clearly characterize the strange ("alien") experiences that are the hallmark of psychopathology (Stanghellini & Fuchs, 2013). Phenomenology can also contribute in essential ways to the process of empathic understanding – the ability to recognize others and meet them at the level of their most intimate subjectivity and concerns. A phenomenological appreciation of illness experience is therefore basic to psychiatric theory and practice.

Unfortunately, the move to operationalize diagnostic criteria in *DSM-III* evacuated much of the content of clinical phenomenology (Andreasen, 2007). Patients' illness experiences were taken out of context and reduced to checklists of symptoms and signs that were tallied up to make a diagnosis. Psychiatric training followed suit, so that practitioners had less interest in the intricacies or details of patients' experiences. Complex experiences like hallucinations or delusions were treated as simply one more indicator of psychosis, relevant mainly for differential diagnosis. The details of content, quality, and relationship to other symptoms were treated as secondary or peripheral to treatment. Much recent work, including the contributions to this volume, shows how renewed attention to phenomenology and the grounding of subjectivity and illness experience in personal and social context has epistemological, ethical, and pragmatic implications for psychiatry (Parnas, Sass, & Zahavi, 2012).

The continued relevance of phenomenology for psychiatry is not accepted in every quarter. In North American psychiatry, the claim has been made that the descriptive task of clinical phenomenology has been largely completed and has proven to be of little value in identifying underling mechanisms of disease. The failure to find simple, unique, and reliable biological correlates of existing psychiatric disorders has led to suggestions to abandon clinical phenomenology as a way to distinguish between different types of problems. The proposed alternative is to work from the bottom up, studying the brain to identify the organization of behavior in health and illness. The hope is that this focus on the brain will yield a new classification of problems that more accurately reflects the nature of mental health problems and that can guide more effective interventions. However, abandoning the phenomenological analysis of first-person experience is misguided for many reasons.

First, whatever its merits or limitations for identifying underlying mechanisms, phenomenology can help us recognize, understand, and empathize with the lived experience of mental illness (Ratcliffe, 2012). Without attention to phenomenology there is little basis for mutual understanding and negotiation of effective treatment. An account of psychiatric disorders purely in terms of biological mechanisms ignores the experiential reality of suffering, which motivates help-seeking, and the experience of wellness that is the measure of successful outcome (Stanghellini, Bolton & Fulford, 2013). Understanding the patient's perspective is essential for clinical communication, rapport, and a working alliance. Moreover, viable definitions of illness and wellness depend on values that are articulated at the level of experience. Indeed, there are many kinds of problems central to psychiatry that are not only expressed through symptom experience but that reflect specific alterations in the structure of and capacity for experience itself.

Without attention to patients' experience, we might end up with a kind of psychiatry that identifies and treats underlying mechanisms, but that fails to address patients' fundamental concerns. For example, in a landmark study in Hunan, China, Arthur Kleinman (1986) found that although diagnosing depression and treating patients with antidepressants provided symptomatic improvement, many patients did not see themselves as well because their illnesses were linked to the losses and dislocations created by the Cultural Revolution, and the biomedical treatments they received failed to address the personal, social, and existential dimensions of their suffering. This speaks to a larger critique of forms of psychiatric theory and practice that frame mental health problems and solutions in terms of discrete biological disorders and drug interventions, rather than human predicaments and concerns that require mobilizing the full range of adaptive strategies, meaning-making processes, and social resources (Bracken et al., 2012).

A second set of arguments concerns the continued relevance of phenomenology for psychiatric research. Although the history of phenomenological studies of psychopathology can be traced back to the beginnings of modern psychiatry in the work of Karl Jaspers (Stanghellini & Fuchs, 2013), many common phenomena remain poorly described and understood in phenomenological terms. Indeed, phenomenological analyses of symptoms change with available interpretive frameworks. For example, recent work on the phenomenology of hallucinations in people with schizophrenia, as well as the much larger group of people who hear voices, is contributing to more refined understanding of the phenomena than biological theory alone can offer (Woods et al., 2014). This work is also clarifying the range and significance of cultural variation in hallucinations (Larøi et al., 2014). Similar work is refining our understanding of mood and anxiety disorders, as well as the more basic qualities of bodily experiences of distress (and well-being), which have been at the core of phenomenological reflections (Fuchs, Breyer, & Mundt, 2014; Ratcliffe, 2014).

Whether and to what extent phenomenology can shed light on under- lying mechanisms of psychopathology raises complex methodological issues. Layered over the physiological, psychological, and social processes that contribute to symptoms and suffering are individuals' ongoing efforts to make sense of and adapt to their condition. As a result, it is often not clear what constitutes an early and intrinsic part of a problem and what reflects a secondary response – whether biological, cognitive, or social elaboration – that has emerged over time. Of course, these "secondary" characteristics may be just as important (often more important) for the individual because of their experiential salience and personal conse- quences. Hence, they are valid – indeed, essential – objects of clinical attention and intervention. But these psychological and social responses may involve quite different processes than the mechanisms that initially set the problem in motion. For many conditions, therefore, simple biological correlates may not exist or may be incidental to the clinician's task; the failure of phenomenology to point to discrete underlying mechanisms, therefore, is not an indictment of its methods but a direct consequence of the complex, hierarchical, and interactional processes that give rise to psychopathology. Diagnostic assessment and effective interventions will need to focus on these aggravating or maintaining factors.

Various approaches to neurophenomenology attempt to link the struc- ture and quality of first-person experience and underlying brain processes (Thompson, 2007; Varela, 1996). In his contribution to this volume, Georg Northoff (Chapter 4) proposes what he terms a *neurophenomenal* approach, which links aspects of self-experience, such as self-focus, to the brain's intrinsic ("resting-state") activity. This allows him to consider the ways in which differences in neural processing, including those that are "more basic and prior" to consciousness, may give rise to different struc- tures of experience. Although this approach may ultimately help us understand how complex experiential phenomena are shaped by neuro-pathology, patterns and processes in the brain are even more dynamic and open-ended in the sense that they reflect not only the individual's history of experience but also aspects of shared or collective history (Northoff, 2013; Seligman, Choudhury, & Kirmayer, in press). The interplay of neurobiology, personal history, and collective systems of knowledge and practice occurs throughout the lifespan so that, in effect, all phenomenology reflects both neurobiological and cultural processes (Figure 24.1). Neurobiological processes may give rise to experiences directly, but these are immediately interpreted, elaborated, and transformed through cognitive, attentional, and interpersonal processes that interact with the underlying neurobiology. As a result, the neurophenomenological processes (represented as the bidirectional arrow between neurobiological process and experience) are embedded in cognitive and social processes that give rise to cultural phenomenology. The same kinds of interaction occur over the course of any mental health problem from inception to recovery, as well as in the moment-to-moment experience of affliction (Kirmayer, 2009). Hence, psychiatry needs a cultural neurophenomenology that examines how cultural knowledge, social roles, and contexts interact with an individual's neurobiological and psychological processes to give rise to experiences of affliction as well as to healing, resilience, and recovery.

Clearly, then, the project of a comprehensive phenomenology of mental disorders is unfinished; in fact, to the extent that phenomenology emerges from cultural-interpretive processes, it will never be complete. As culture changes, so too will the ways in which people experience mental disorders, requiring new phenomenological research. Clinically, this points to the need to understand patients' experience as embedded in and emerging from multiple levels of meaning based on both cognitive and social inter-pretative processes, as illustrated in Figure 24.2. The semiotics of psychiatry assumes that reliable symptom reports are based on underlying physiology. However, illness experience is embedded in cognitive and social processes that mediate and modify the translation of physiological or psychological disturbance into symptoms and behaviors. The interpretation of sensations, behaviors, and events is guided by symptom schemas, interpersonal interactions involving narrative conventions and social positioning, the exigencies of the health care system, and both local and global social and political processes. Each of these levels requires its own methods of research and clinical assessment. As the bi-directional arrows in Figure 24.2 indicate, these processes reach down from global social and political processes to the very earliest experiences of distress to shape illness experience. Clinical assessment must, therefore, consider symptoms not simply as indicators of underlying physiological problems or as

Personal history, attentional strategies
& interpretive frameworks

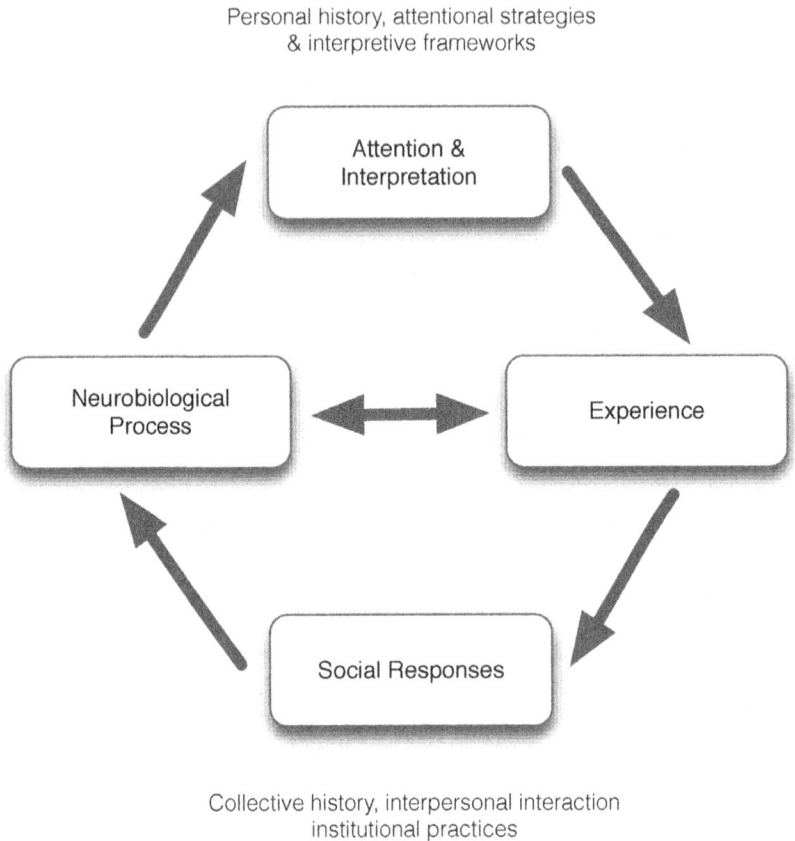

Collective history, interpersonal interaction
institutional practices

Figure 24.1. Cultural neurophenomenology. (See text; Kirmayer, 2009; Seligman, Choudhury & Kirmayer, in press.)

criteria of disorder but as part of modes of self-understanding that are socially configured and that have psychological, interpersonal, and socio-political consequences.

What Kind of Neuroscience for Psychiatry?

Our second theme concerns the kinds of neuroscientific theory and research that psychiatry needs in order to meet its mandate. Thomas Insel and other influential advocates of biological psychiatry contend that "psychiatric disorders are brain disorders" (Insel & Quirion, 2005). This statement is an expression of faith, not a judgment grounded in evidence;

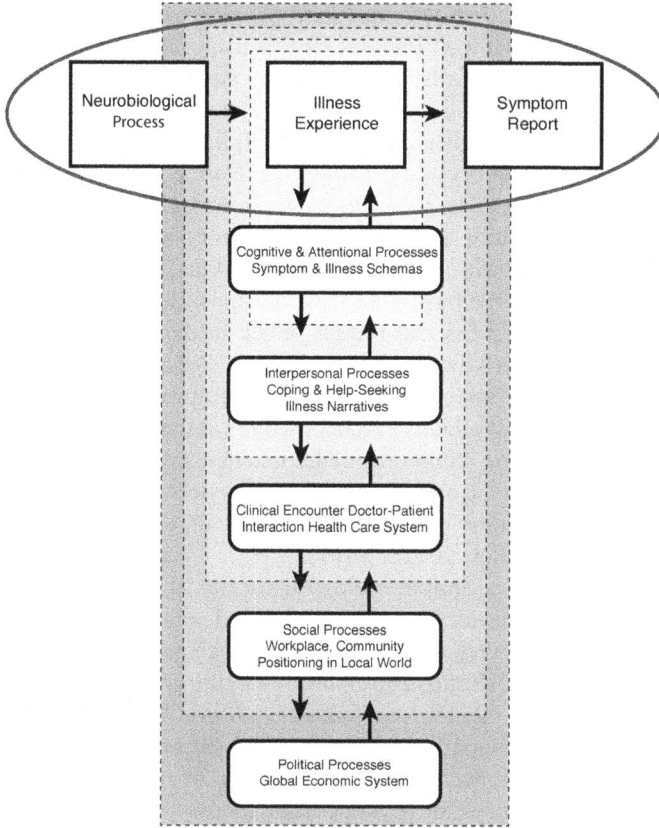

Figure 24.2. Clinical epistemology and the context of illness experience. Adapted from "Culture and the Metaphoric Mediation of Pain," by L. J. Kirmayer, 2008, *Transcultural Psychiatry, 45*(2), p. 321.

it is belied by the many ways in which psychiatric problems depend for their causes, course, and outcomes on social and psychological processes that, while they certainly are reflected in – and partially mediated by – neurobiology, are not located in the brain but in transactions between person and environment (Kirmayer & Gold, 2012). Psychiatric disorders are as much psychological and social disorders as they are brain disorders, and there is simply no way to dispense with the need for multiple levels of explanation in research and clinical practice (Kendler, 2012a, 2014).

However, this critique of the limits of reductionistic neuroscience should not be taken as a negative or nihilistic position. There is no doubt that much has been learned, and many new insights about psychopathology and healing will continue to emerge from neuroscience. Moreover, methodological reductionism is a necessary strategy in scientific research. The aim is to find simple systems that can be studied rigorously, and this has led to remarkable advances in understanding the molecular biology of various forms of memory and learning (e.g. Kandel, 2001; Kandel, Dudai, & Mayford, 2014). Yet, there is a great distance between the animal models used to study the biology of memory and the origins of the suffering of people with mental disorders. Many levels of structure and process lie between the molecular mechanisms of learning and the ways in which narrative practices and modes of self-understanding shape experience. Still more levels lie between individual behavior and the emergent dynamics of family systems, groups, or communities – all of which are relevant to clinical psychiatry. Hence, while we need reductive models to advance the scientific study of specific mechanisms, we need more complex, hierarchically structured, systems models to understand many aspects of psychopathology and make clinically useful predictions and interventions (Kendler, 2012a, 2014).

In some instances, simple biological mechanisms may be found that lead to complex behavioral manifestations. Indeed, one lesson of automata theory is that even very simple recursive processes can yield patterns of great complexity (Wolfram, 2002). However, the systems view implies that it may be unreasonable to expect clinically useful biological correlates for most forms of psychopathology because the causal pathways and underlying mechanisms may not be simple, unique, or reliable.

The causal pathways for psychopathology may not be simple, because they do not involve linear relationships between single factors or elements. Most causal pathways are part of dynamical systems with feedback loops in which multiple factors interact over time, both along developmental trajectories and over the course of the illness itself. Under certain circumstances, some systems can be decomposed into subsystems or component processes (Bechtel, 2013; Bechtel & Richardson, 2010). These can be studied in isolation, and, once their dynamics are understood, they can be resituated in the larger systems to which they belong in order to identify the emergent dynamics. However, many biological systems with emergent properties cannot be decomposed into discrete subsystems without losing essential features of their dynamics (Bechtel & Richardson, 2010; Bedau & Humphreys, 2008). The crucial question for psychiatry, then, is, what are the minimum components and levels of explanation that must be included in a useful model of the real-world systems of psychopathology. The NIMH RDoC program wagers that analyzing neurobiological systems at the level of circuits will be sufficient to explain mental disorders (Cuthbert, 2014). For most mental health problems, however, the pertinent systems likely include not just individual neural circuits, but whole brains, bodies, persons, and interpersonal networks that are irreducibly social (Kendler, 2014; Kirmayer & Gold, 2012).

The links between genetic, molecular, or neurophysiological mechanisms and psychopathology may not be unique because any given biological process interacts with many others to give rise to a wide variety of different manifestations. The causal path from one type of genetic or neural variation or abnormality to behavioral vulnerability, symptoms, and pathology is long and may have both branching and converging trajectories; that is to say, for different people at different times, the same causal factors may lead to several different outcomes (depending on small variations in initial conditions), and the same outcome might be caused by many different configurations of underlying processes converging on a final common pathway or attractor (Pavão, Tort, & Amaral, 2014). In formal terms, the mapping from neurobiology to psychopathology is not one-to-one, but many-to-many. A corollary is that, in general, no reversible mapping will unambiguously link each form of psychopathology to distinct underlying neurobiology. Hence, we cannot dispense with the descriptive language of psychopathology by replacing it with descriptions of neuropathology.

In recent years, the search for fundamental causes of mental disorders has emphasized genetic mechanisms. The recent discovery of multiple genes that contribute to the risk for schizophrenia, for example, has been touted as opening up new avenues for drug development and for understanding the underlying mechanisms (Schizophrenia Working Group of the Psychiatric Genomics Consortium, 2014). However, the implications of these findings are complex for several reasons. Some of these genes may code for proteins, but many likely play a role in poorly understood regulatory systems that may have different effects at particular stages of development: shaping basic neural architecture, influencing later developmental transitions, modulating mechanisms of stress response, or altering neuroplasticity and learning. Hence, the effects of any given gene will depend on other genes, as well as on specific developmental and environmental contexts that remain unclear (Duncan, Pollastri & Smoller, 2014; Keller, 2010; Maheu & Macdonald, 2011). Very likely, the effects of many of these genes will turn out to be nonspecific, affecting the risk for many other disorders as well. The implications for treatment are particularly challenging. Given that the same genes may have many different roles at different points in time or in relation to specific biological and environmental contexts, influencing a specific gene or its related system at the right developmental time might decrease risk for schizophrenia, but have other unexpected and unwanted effects.

The genome is now understood to be a set of complex regulatory systems rather than a "blueprint" for the final organism (Davidson, 2010; Griffiths & Stotz, 2013). Moreover, the genome represents only one level of organization of information in developmental systems, which include epigenetic mechanisms and ongoing interactions with the environment that give rise to their final phenotypic expressions in brain, body, and behavior (Oyama, Griffiths, & Gray, 2003). Moreover, the social environment is salient in many distinctive ways in the regulation of the genome across the lifespan (Meloni, 2014). Researchers have searched for *endophenotypes* – structural or functional characteristics that might underlie the variable manifestations of psychopathology (Gottesman & Gould, 2003; Kendler & Neale, 2010). But there are many steps from genes through endophenotypes to clinical symptoms, and there are additional sources of variation at each point along the causal paths from genetic, epigenetic, or developmental events to derangement of physiological or psychological processes. Again, the relationships across these levels of biological organization and over time are not one-to-one but many-to-many. Numerous genes contribute to neurodevelopment and to the ongoing regulation of multiple neural circuits, which in turn interact with many features of the environment, leading to changes in multiple behaviors that feed back to circuits and to gene expression. Hence, the same genome, circuitry, behavior, or environmental situation may have different consequences, depending on the history and current context of activity at each systemic level.

Even when correlations or causal links are found between neurobiology and behavioral manifestations of psychopathology in particular clinical or laboratory settings, they may not be reliable or generalizable. That is, the same underlying process may or may not give rise to psychopathology depending on a host of external or extrinsic factors that can mitigate its effects. Even the most heritable psychiatric conditions have great variability in expression based on developmental experiences and environmental conditions (Kendler, 2012a; Maheu & Macdonald, 2011). Most psychiatric problems arise from interactions between multiple genes, neural circuits, and environments over the course of development (Karmiloff-Smith, 2009; Kendler, 2014; see also Labonté, Farah, & Turecki, Chapter 9, and McKenzie & Shah, Chapter 13, *this volume*). Moreover, the same processes may be instantiated in different ways in people with different learning histories, developmental trajectories, and (hence) different premorbid brain architecture.

Although research requires simple models that can be rigorously controlled, predicting real-world outcomes may require reconstituting crucial structures of the larger system (Bechtel, 2013; Bechtel & Richardson, 2010). As a result, clinical or public health interventions may have unexpected effects when based on a simplified view that does not consider the dynamics of systems (Mitchell, 2009). This is true even for the dynamics of neural circuitry itself, which may have self-regulating organization that resists or compensates for changes brought about by clinical interventions. For example, there is evidence that blocking of dopamine D_2 receptors, which is part of the mechanism of action of most antipsychotic medications, may lead to an increase in sensitivity of related pathways, which can cause a rebound "supersensitivity" psychosis if the medication is stopped (Chouinard & Jones, 1980; Moncrieff, 2006; Seeman & Seeman, 2014). The same process may account for the symptoms of tardive dyskinesia, a movement disorder caused by long-term use of these medications. A similar process of habituation may occur with the use of antidepressant medication, resulting in loss of its effectiveness, relapse, and treatment-resistant depression (Fava & Offidani, 2011). It is not clear how frequently these problems occur, nor indeed, their precise mechanisms, but there is an urgent need to study such medication effects from a systems perspective that looks at a broad range of outcomes at multiple levels from synapse, to circuit and behavior (Remington et al., 2014).

To better understand the complexity of neural dynamics, including feedback and feedforward effects and multilevel interactions, neuroscience research is increasingly focusing on *connectomics* – the systems-level study of the brain's networks, which orchestrate the activity within and between brain regions (Byrge, Sporns & Smith, 2014; Sporns, Honey, & Kotter, 2005; Sporns, 2012). Recent work has focused on various "hub nodes," which mediate connectivity between regions and may be important for integrative information processing and adaptive behavior (Crossley et al., 2013; van den Heuvel, Kahn, Goni, & Sporns, 2012). Disruptions to these hubs may contribute to some psychiatric disorders (Crossley et al., 2014; Fornito & Bullmore, 2014).

Network science can be applied to a broad range of systems with interacting elements, including transportation, telecommunication, and social systems (Newman, 2010). Although such systems-level approaches in neuroscience hold promise for explaining many aspects of psychopathology, it is worth reemphasizing that the underlying mechanisms of psychiatric disorder need not be biological – at least in the narrow sense of neurobiology – because psychological and social processes may play a crucial role in their origins, manifestations, and evolution. Hence, the kind of neuroscience we need to understand complex human behavior in health and illness must take into account all that is distinctive about us as human beings. Most of the forms of psychopathology human beings experience have only rough analogues in other animals. There are distinctive features of the human brain that reflect our evolutionary history.

Human beings have been selected to be intensely social with unique capacities for learning, communication, and cooperative action (Tomasello, 2014). Spinoffs from this evolutionary history include our immense capacity for imagination and creativity, which is manifest everywhere in the complexity of our social worlds – both outwardly in terms of institutions and practices, and inwardly in terms of our own psychological constructions, aspirations, and conflicts. As social animals we have evolved to function in groups capable of extremely elaborate coordinated activity (Adolphs, 2009; Frith, 2007). Human thinking involves imaginative and linguistic capacities not found in even our closest primate relatives (Tomasello, 2014). This can be directly related to our ability to work together by tracking and anticipating each other's desires, intentions, and plans. The human brain is a social brain, and the social world is a cultural world. Our brains remain highly plastic for two decades after birth as we continue to acquire all the knowledge, skills, and capabilities needed to embody and enact culture (Wexler, 2006).

The kind of neuroscience that is most directly relevant to psychiatry, therefore, is social and cultural neuroscience, which models those functions of the brain involved in navigating social relationships, knowledge, positions, and actions (J. T. Cacioppo, Cacioppo, Dulawa, & Palmer, 2014; Kennedy & Adolphs, 2012). A thoroughgoing social neuroscience will not simply map the social world onto the brain, or explain social processes in terms of neural circuitry, but will seek to understand how social processes, contexts, histories, and exigencies lead us to engage the world in ways that reorganize the brain's functional architecture.

From Neural Systems to Situated Cognition: Thinking About the Brain in Context

An important insight from evolutionary biology is that the brain is not simply a general purpose computer equally capable of any arbitrary computation but an organ of adaptation designed for specific tasks. This view suggests that the brain can be understood as a collection of more or less specialized modules, cobbled together by evolution to meet new and increasingly diverse tasks (Barrett & Kurzban, 2006). This modularity may include functional systems for recognizing faces and facial expressions, for tracking the gaze of others and figuring out their probable focus of attention, for constructing models of others' perspectives, and for translating sequences of sound into words and language (Baron-Cohen, 1995). These specialized circuits organize bodily, emotional, and motivational processes that allow specific types of adaptive learning (Adolphs, 2009; Panksepp & Biven, 2012). Indeed, human beings are capable of many forms of learning and, correspondingly, many kinds of memory (Squire, 2004).

Modularity theories probably misrepresent the nature of the intrinsic structure of the brain. Although specific brain regions and circuits may subserve particular functions, they are highly interconnected and modified over time to serve new functions. The brain has many plastic neural systems that are pruned and shaped over the course of development and enculturation to fit the adaptive demands of particular social-ecological and cultural niches (Lende & Downey, 2012; Wexler, 2006). This points to the need for a "neuroconstructivist" approach that examines the co-construction of brain and world (Karmiloff-Smith, 2009).

The brain does not simply react to the environment but has ongoing intrinsic activity; both globally and through various subsystems, the brain modifies its processing to anticipate the demands of local environments. The role of intrinsic activity was recognized by D. O. Hebb (1949) long ago, and involves not simply the "resting state" but the constant process of anticipating and predicting both action and perception. In a sense, the brain is a "prediction machine," designed to generate expectations and to respond to discrepancies between its evolving models of the world and actual events (Clark, 2013; Friston, Stephan, Montague, & Dolan, 2014; Hohwy, 2013). The networks of the brain are modified or tuned to reduce discrepancies between expectation and outcome, both at the level of basic sensory and motor functions, which are more or less automatic, and in relation to larger goals that involve conscious planning and action (Miller, Galanter, & Pribram, 1960).

Although models of the predictive brain involve processes that occur at the subpersonal levels of neural networks, there are parallels at the levels of personal agency and awareness. When these processes work well, we find our environment predictable (with just enough novelty and surprise to be engaging and motivate learning), and we can navigate our world confidently and adapt to new circumstances on the basis of what we already know. When predictions break down, we experience distress, feeling overloaded and cognitively exhausted. Depending on the type of predictions that are failing, we may feel anxious (too much threat), depressed (too little reward), or disorganized (too little coherence). We can try to reestablish predictability with many strategies, including: instrumentally acting on the world to bring it into line with our expectations; cognitively adjusting our models of the world; or through attention, by ignoring those aspects that do not fit our preconceptions. These compensatory processes may give rise to their own symptomatology.

In addition to common instances where the environment violates our predictions and challenges us to modify our stance, the machinery of prediction itself can go awry in various ways (Friston et al., 2014). Specific kinds of psychopathology may be associated with these forms of dysfunction: entirely replacing or occluding the perception of external events with our predictions (e.g., hallucinations, delusions), generating excessively negative or terrifying predications (e.g. catastrophizing thoughts in anxiety), or failing to anticipate avoidable dangers.

The view of the brain as a prediction system fits with approaches to embodied cognition in terms of sensorimotor loops that relate organism and environment. A wealth of work on body perception, for example, shows how our sense of self is constantly constructed and reconstructed through sensorimotor or perception-action loops. Our sense of the location of body and self can be altered simply by altering visual, tactile, or other sensory feedback. For example, phantom limb pain can be treated by presenting the patient with a mirror image of the healthy limb that corresponds to the phantom limb (Ramachandran & Hirstein, 1998). Presumably, this alters the loop between action, perception, and sensation. In effect, specific kinds of action and response from the environment can "reprogram" the brain (or modify neural networks) to change basic experiences of embodiment. Thus, whatever "hard wiring" we inherit, learning and experience are constantly reshaping and reprograming our brains – for better and for worse.

This metaphor of learning or experience as "programing" is based on an analogy between the brain and the digital computer (von Neumann, 1958), which contrasts hardware (i.e., the wetware of the brain) and software (the structured, rule-governed, or self-regulating sequences of computations that are acquired by learning). Because software can be self-referencing, it can create its own hierarchical structures and processes. For example, we have many kinds of memory systems (e.g., cognitive, habitual); some of these involve completely different neural circuitry and neurochemistry; others are based on modes of recoding or interpreting experience that are themselves software strategies (e.g., learning mnemonic tricks or strategies). Hence, learning new strategies (or self-programming) can create new kinds of memory. Indeed, the idea of extended mind is based on the recognition that we often instantiate these mnemonic strategies outside of the person: in interactions with others, social institutions, routines, and practices (Clark & Chalmers, 1998; Gallagher, 2013; Menary, 2010). In the Renaissance, the art of memory allowed great feats of recollection by using mental imagery based on internalized architectural spaces (Sutton, 2010; Yates, 1992). Today, the Internet and search engines such as Google present us with new kinds of extended memory that let us locate and store information, learn how to do things, and even find and connect with other people to ratify our self-understanding and carry out collective tasks. These abilities, in turn, lead to new forms of pathology, as well as new possibilities for help and healing (Kirmayer, Raikhel, & Rahimi, 2013).

The hardware/software distinction is compelling, but it is not a precise analogy for the relationship between mind and brain because the software of the mind is acquired through structural changes to its hardware. Moreover, problems in software can result in hardware problems and vice versa, and these effects unfold over time, so that no sharp distinction between the two is usually possible (Kendler, 2012b). Then, too, if experience changes the brain by tuning neural networks, there may be nothing in this process that corresponds to discrete programs, rules, or instructions. Despite these limitations, the conceptual distinction between hardware and software provides a useful analogy that can enlarge our understanding of the variety of mental mechanisms.

If the hardware of the mind is the brain, the software is provided by culture (Rorty, 2004). Culture is not just a set of discrete variables that can be identified from the perspective of the biology of the organism, but constitutes a larger system with its own emergent structures and dynamics. Culture provides systems of meaning and communication through which the world is conceived, perceived, and interpreted. But culture involves both explicit knowledge, rules, and institutions and implicit or procedural knowledge, skills, and dispositions to respond. Each kind of cultural knowledge has its place in causal explanations of behavior and pathology. Psychiatric conditions, therefore, can involve problems that reside in the tuning of neural networks or in the content and execution of cognitive plans or programs. Clinicians must be able to think in terms of both kinds of process. Although rule-governed processes may be approached through explicit cognitive interventions, those that involve embodied procedural learning require changing contexts or contingencies in ways that allow new behavioral enactments.

Toward An Ecology of Mind

The subtitle of this chapter pays homage to Gregory Bateson's seminal collection of papers "Steps to an Ecology of Mind" (Bateson, 1972). A key notion in Bateson's theoretical work was that mind could not be understood as a purely psychological phenomenon confined to the brain of one individual. Bateson saw mind as embodied and enacted through brain-body-environment loops (Bateson, 1979; Harries-Jones, 1995). Bateson was a key participant in the Macy conferences, which advanced systems theory and cybernetics as conceptual tools for understanding human behavior and experience (Pickering, 2010; Wiener, 1961). These early versions of systems theory were criticized as too general and vague to address key questions in neuroscience and psychiatry and make useful predictions. Most of human biology and behavior is historically contingent, and general systems models did not seem to grasp enough of the particulars relevant to specific problems. Nevertheless, cybernetics had wide influence on work in neural systems theory and cognitive psychology (Dawson, 2013; McCulloch, 1965/1988). In psychiatry, Bateson's ideas inspired work on communication and interaction as the basis of mental disorders (Watzlawick, Beavin & Jackson, 1967), as well as the field of family therapy, which found ways to apply systems thinking to develop innovative interventions (Beels, 2002).

The ensuing years have brought advances in systems science, both mathematically, under the rubric of dynamical systems theory and complexity theory (Mainzer, 2004; Miller & Page, 2009; Scott, 2007), and empirically in the biological sciences as systems biology (Bechtel & Richardson, 2010; Boogerd, Bruggeman, Hofmeyer, & Westerhoff, 2007; Kitano, 2002). We now know that some of the complexity seen in biological systems is inherent in the dynamics of even simple model systems, which may have trajectories that show great sensitivity to initial conditions (Kellert, 1993; Mainzer, 2004; Scott, 2007). Thus, the critique concerning the limits of predictability of systems models may reflect something intrinsic to the dynamics of the real-world systems they try to capture, rather than any limitation of theory. These new ways of thinking about complexity have important implications for psychiatric theory and practice, as well as for public health policy and prevention (Mitchell, 2009).

Systems are networks or other ensembles in which the parts are interrelated and interact in ways that give rise to new structures and dynamics; in that sense, it is meaningful to speak of various kinds of emergent properties of systems which occur by virtue of their organization (Bedau & Humphreys, 2008; Silberstein, 2012). Mental processes are examples of just such emergence. Mind, in this view, resides in systems that include brains, bodies, and the environment in interacting relationships (Juarrero, 1999; Maturana & Varela, 1987; Thompson, 2007). The environment, including the social world of persons and institutions has its own dynamics that supervene on the lower levels of organization (individual minds, brains, and bodies). In effect, we live within and are inextricably part of social "ecosystems" or environments, hence the system of body-mind and person is an ecosocial system.

This way of looking at mental phenomena as emergent from inter-actions between brains, bodies, persons and environment has important implications for psychiatry (Henningsen & Kirmayer, 2000). This con-cept can be elaborated through recent work in cognitive science that emphasizes the embodied, situated, and enacted nature of human thought and experience (Chemero, 2011; Clark & Hansen, 2009; Galla-gher, 2005; Gibbs, 2006; Menary, 2010; Rowlands, 2010; Semin & Smith, 2008; Shapiro, 2011; Hutto & Myin, 2013; Stewart, Gapenne, & Di Paolo, 2010; Varela, Thompson, & Rosch, 1991). Cognition is embodied in that it depends on the physiological and experiential conse-quences of the body's structure, functions, and development. Cognition is situated in that it not only responds to the stimuli or exigencies of specific contexts, but also depends on contexts to organize thought and action. Cognition is enacted in that much thinking occurs not only or primarily through manipulating mental representations or symbols, but by taking action in the world and responding to the consequences of previous actions. Consequently, psychological processes like cognition, emotion, perception, and action must be understood as part of ongoing streams of behavior that emerge from interactions that occur in specific social-environmental contexts. Together, the many people who interact with each other, along with their histories, communities, and institutions, constitute larger social systems in what we might call, following Bateson, "an ecology of mind."

To the extent that mental phenomena involve embodied, situated, and enacted cognitive processes, what goes wrong in psychopathology may involve problems that are not just in the brain, but in the loops that mutually constitute self and other, person, and environment. Thus, we need ways of categorizing mental health problems in terms of systemic processes: for example, a typology of looping effects that would identify the multiple levels and paths through which problems can be amplified and become self-sustaining (Table 24.1; Kirmayer & Sartorius, 2009). Hierarchical systems models suggest that psychopathology can emerge from problems at different levels and, whatever the primary or initial level of disturbance, problems will tend to propagate up and down the hierarchy to affect other levels. A corollary is that interventions applied at one level may also have effects at many other levels, either directly or through their propagation up and down the hierarchy. However, the existence of emergent structures and processes also implies that causal

Table 24.1 *A Typology of Looping Effects*

Level	Example
1. Attentional	Attention to bodily sensations increases their salience and intensity leading to more sensations and still greater bodily-focussed attention
2. Emotional exacerbation (arousal-performance)	Emotional arousal interferes with motor, cognitive and social functioning leading to performance decrements, negative self-appraisal and greater emotional arousal
3. Attributional	Attributing sensations to bodily, psychological or some other form of pathology leads to conviction that one is ill, increasing the tendency to attribute new sensations to pathology
4. Family system and interpersonal interaction	Reactions of others to distress reinforces illness experience and expressions of distress, which leads to further response from others
5. Help-seeking, health care services, iatrogenic	Availability of health care services, diagnostic labels, and interventions increases tendency to seek care for specific types of problems
6. Disability/avoidance	Disability allows individual to obtain support and avoid unpleasant work, family or other situations and so reinforces disability
7. Political economic	Marketing of pharmaceuticals for specific diagnostic entities increases professional use of the diagnostic label and consumer demand leading to greater profits which are then invested in further marketing.

Adapted from L. J. Kirmayer & N. Sartorius, "Cultural Models and Somatic Symptoms," *Psychosomatic Medicine*, 69(9), p. 836. Copyright 2007 by Wolters Kluwer.

influences across levels have their own dynamics; hence, simply using an analogy or metaphor to predict an effect across levels will not likely provide a reliable guidelines for intervention. Instead, we need an adequate understanding of the dynamics at each level as well as of the processes that link the levels. These causal chains run not only within the neural circuits of the brain, but also between brain/body and environment. Hence, an adequate model of problems treated by psychiatry cannot be limited to molecular or neurocentric diagnoses and interventions.

Human systems – persons, families, societies – are complex adaptive systems; that is, they are self-organized and evolve under selective forces that favor configurations that are flexible and adaptable to changing circumstances. One way to approach this complexity is through models of system dynamics that include both individual and collective processes of meaning-making which involve social processes of participation, legitimation, and resistance. These loops can be separated into subsystems, involving psychophysiological and sociopolitical processes, and studied independently. But they are linked through social psychology (in which mental processes interact with social structure and process) and sociophysiology (in which social structure has effects on physiology, not all of which are mediated by psychology). Psychophysiological looping processes like those described by Hinton and Simon (Chapter 14) and Ryder and Chentsova-Dutton (Chapter 16) can explain symptom amplification and persistence for many types of problems. Transient alterations in mental state or functioning that are amplified by patterns of internal or external interaction can result in major pathology (van Os, Lataster, Delespaul, Wichers, & Myin-Germeys, 2014). Recognizing these loops means that theoretical efforts to define distal and proximal (or primary and secondary) causes break down, since the outcomes of one process become inputs to the next in cycles of symptom amplification, maintenance, and social reification (Figure 24.3; Kirmayer & Bhugra, 2009). Although posing challenges for scientific research, this perspective fits well with the orientation of much clinical work, which often focuses not on causality but on how to interrupt or change the vicious cycles that amplify and maintain symptomatology, disability, and distress (Hofmann, 2014). To identify the vicious cycles that result in psychopathology, we need to look not only at the network structure of the brain's connectome, but at the cognitive and social "interactome" (van Os et al., 2014).

At the sociopolitical level (the interface between individual illness experience and collective processes), looping effects can help explain how psychiatric modes of explanation and intervention become part of popular knowledge and reconfigure the ways that people understand themselves. To understand this process, we need both a macro-level sociology of knowledge and power (following Foucault) and a microsociology of interpersonal interaction in everyday life and in crucial social settings like psychiatric clinics, hospitals, and families (following Goffman) (Hacking, 2004).

Cultural Psychiatry and Critical Neuroscience

Explicit attention to culture means not simply looking at variation across different geographic or ethnocultural regions, but also considering the ways in which our own concepts and practices are shaped by historical traditions, current commitments, and political and economic forces. Critical perspectives are needed to expose the tangle of interests involved in an enterprise like psychiatry. We need to understand psychiatry as part of ecosocial system dynamics in real-world contexts. Science can capture

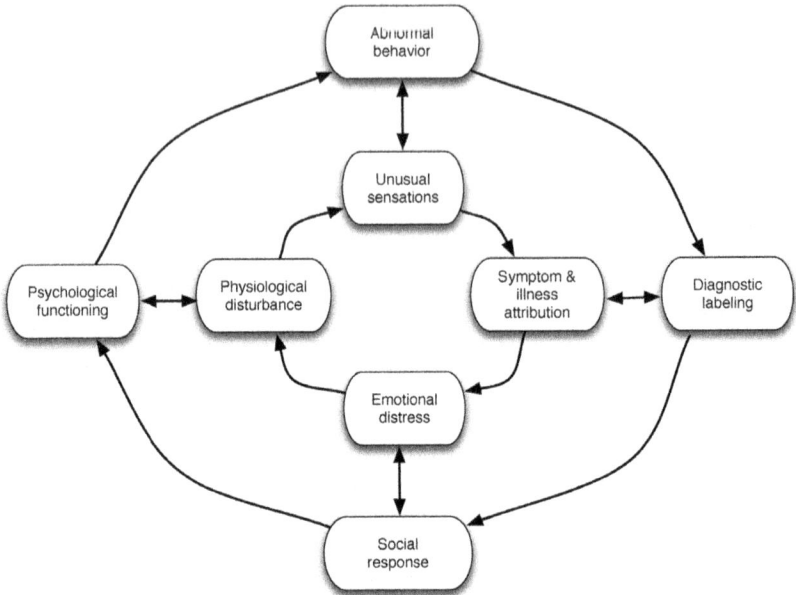

Figure 24.3. Looping processes that amplify or maintain mental disorders. The inner loop represents the cognitive-emotional processes within the person that amplify and maintain symptoms or maladaptive behavior: Physiological disturbances give rise to sensations, which become symptoms when they are attributed to specific types of illness. This attribution may then cause emotional distress, leading to more physiological disturbance and a vicious cycle of symptom amplification, resulting in more severe and persistent symptoms. Attention and other processes play important roles in this cycle. The outer loop stands for some of the social processes that reify, amplify, and stabilize diagnostic entities. Symptom reports and behaviors are interpreted as evidence of particular types of problems and given diagnostic labels. These labels result in social responses, for example, creating new kinds illness identities, treatments, forms of disability, or stigmatization. These social responses have effects on psychological functioning, for example, diminished self-esteem, increased self-consciousness, and demoralization, which then result in more symptomatic behaviors. These two vicious cycles can influence each other at many points: for example, impaired psychological functioning can result physiological disturbance; available diagnostic labels influence the process of attribution and interpretation of sensations. Patients may then return to the clinic with new symptoms that confirm the diagnosis. Adapted from "Culture and Mental Illness: Social Context and Explanatory Models," by L. J. Kirmayer & D. Bhugra, 2009, *Psychiatric diagnosis: Patterns and prospects*, pp. 29–37.

part of these dynamics, but we are hampered by the fact that we also live and participate in the politics of knowledge production at the ecosocial level. Hence, we need not only scientific research but also critical theory – that is, philosophical and social science methods of exposing the tacit, taken for grant, or hidden underpinnings of our assumptive worlds (Choudhury & Slaby, 2011; Whitley, 2014)

As a body of knowledge, social institution, and form of clinical practice, psychiatry is both a product of cultural history and a significant influence on contemporary culture. How we think about normal human functioning and pathology is rooted in our ideas about human personhood. Psychiatry both reflects central cultural preoccupations and has contributed in many ways to changing our understanding of ourselves. This cycle of influence – from everyday concepts of the person to psychiatric notions of affliction and back – is an example of what the philosopher Ian Hacking has called "the looping effect of human kinds" (Hacking, 1995, 1999, 2002). That is, the ways in which we understand ourselves in health and illness and the corresponding modes of suffering are both cause and consequence of institutionalized theories and practices in mental health. Indeed, there are two nested loops here: one between modes of suffering and self-understanding and a second larger loop between experiences of suffering and self-understanding and institutional knowledge and practice (Figure 24.3). The insights into the human condition offered by psychiatry, therefore, do not simply describe "human nature" or psychopathology, but are interventions that contribute to the social construction of personhood, reshaping our notions of self and ways of being.

Psychiatric diagnoses have a social life of their own, and diagnostic systems are part of institutions with powerful impacts on the health and well-being of individuals and communities. Although psychiatric disorders are formally defined by diagnostic criteria that are presented as based on scientific evidence, our current diagnostic systems actually result from highly contentious debates and struggle among various competing interests. The formal definitions enshrined in nosology, moreover, are only part of larger systems of knowledge, institutions, and practices that create, disseminate, and apply psychiatric labels. The official publication of a nosology punctuates this ongoing development, setting standards and authorizing specific diagnostic practices. However, labels have meanings and effects beyond their implications for medical care through popular illness representations. Consideration of the impact of definitions of psychiatric disorders must therefore consider their different uses in a range of specific social contexts and institutions.

The economic factors shaping nosology are enormously important because of the power of the pharmaceutical industry and also the ways in which popular representations – influenced by cultural changes, marketing, and global information flows – can change local health behavior and illness experience (Ecks, 2013). The recent growth in popularity of the diagnosis of depression in Japan is a striking example of this kind of change (Applbaum, Chapter 22, *this volume*; Kitanaka, 2012). This whole area is difficult to address because the generation of "evidence" in psychiatry is largely determined by economic interests (Lexchin, 2012).

To explain why the promise of neuroscientific explanations and solutions for psychiatric problems has gained such popularity, however, we need to understand not only economic interests, and the influence of technology (e.g., brain imaging and genomics) in the remaking of our identities as biological beings, but also the resistance to addressing the social-structural, political, and economic determinants of mental health. The shrinking of psychiatry to a discipline focused on diagnosis and medication prescription has occurred in conjunction with the corporatization and globalization of health care. The consequences include the dehumanization of patients, the overuse of medication, the overselling of biological solutions, and ruling out as impractical any consideration of changes in social structure and values that could promote healthier and more sustainable environments and communities.

Global Mental Health

The fourth theme in this volume invites us to step back from the intricacies of individual psychopathology and local cultural histories to take in the big picture. On a global scale, we can understand mental health problems not just as humanity's shared vulnerability to certain kinds of neuropsychiatric problems, but as a reflection of the structural processes, driven by power and interests, that generate, amplify, and maintain inequality. The geographic distribution and variations of mental disorders show enormous inequities that result from both local and global forces that reflect economic, political, and ecological dynamics (Bourque & Consulo Willox, 2014; Labonté, Mohindra, & Schrecker, 2011; Ruckert & Labonté, 2014). These forces affect the prevalence, form, course, and outcome of mental disorders in several ways: (1) by determining the distribution of social determinants of health (e.g., exposure to violence, poverty, malnutrition, education, economic opportunity); (2) by creating new types of stressors related precisely to the tensions between the local and the global (e.g., awareness of global disparities, feelings of threat or vulnerability associated with particular kinds of identity or social status); (3) by disseminating new models and ways of thinking about the self, new structures of social life, and new sets of aspirations and expectations with health consequences; and (4) by setting up new contingencies between the local and the global that create looping effects, which stabilize new forms of self, affliction, and healing.

These processes occur at many levels, including families, communities, and transnational networks, each of which makes use of psychiatric models and services and, in doing so, reinforce particular ways of thinking about suffering. The largest circle stabilizing our constructions of mental health and illness involve our global institutions. Psychiatric knowledge circulates internationally, motivated by humanitarian, political, and clinical concerns to respond to suffering, as well as by economic interests, especially, those of pharmaceutical corporations. In the process, psychiatry changes the way we think about problems and the sorts of solutions that seem feasible and appropriate.

Global mental health is the latest incarnation of international efforts to address inequities. Efforts to quantify the impact of health problems in terms of disability and quality of life have served to raise the profile of mental health and increase its priority in health policy and planning. Much of this work has gone forward on the assumption that we have good models for assessment and intervention in the wealthy, urbanized countries of the global North and West, so that the major challenge for health equity is how to implement and scale-up existing approaches for the majority of the world's population who reside in low-income countries. However, given the limited evidence-base of existing knowledge, the substantial critique of the limitations of current psychiatric practice, and the conflicts of interest evident in research, clinical, and policy domains, the global export of existing practices in the urbanized West requires careful consideration.

How can psychiatry address these wider contexts of mental health, balancing the local and the global in its theory and practice? This question has economic and political dimensions and leads us toward an engaged psychiatry in which our concern to address human suffering is guided by critical analysis of the overarching agendas that frame problems and their solutions. Without this critical perspective, there is the very real possibility we will be subverted by powerful forces that aim to maintain the status quo, advancing the interests of international institutions, corporations, and professions at the cost of any real liberation for those most grievously afflicted. To trace these influences, we need an analysis of economic and political power, but also an understanding of global system dynamics that transcend individual plans and intentions. We can use some of the same tools identified in our analysis of neural and social systems to consider these larger political and economic frames. Indeed, much of our understanding of system dynamics has come from considering the large-scale systems in which we are embedded.

Psychopharmaceuticals have become big business and there are now many examples of exploitation, dissimulation, and criminal activity by corporations in the promotion of these medications (Angel, 2011; Sadler, 2013). Ironically, the growing evidence of malfeasance has been accompanied by increases in the social acceptability of medications and by marketing forces that have sought to steer and exploit these cultural changes. Psychiatrists represent middle- or low-level players in this economic system: they are closer to patients than are administrators or planners, and they ought to be able to consider the ways in which particular styles of practice and technologies will affect everyday care and concern. But clinicians are strongly influenced by both direct and indirect marketing forces, and this influences the extent to which they resist profit-generation considerations in reflecting on the implications of the diagnostic practices, treatment recommendations, or any other aspect of health care.

These are not just issues in wealthy countries, but increasingly part of a larger global economy that struggles to find solutions to problems that involve sociopolitical conflict and economic disparities that amplify and maintain mental health problems (Mills, 2014). Despite our understanding of the socially contingent nature of psychiatric illness, the global mental health movement has moved to expand and promote a universalized picture of mental disorders; although leaders in the field are well aware of cultural variation, they see the urgency of responding to reduce suffering, and so aim for the lowest common denominator in mental health care. The questions that remain are whether and when these efforts are adequate and what the tradeoffs may be in terms of unintended harms

The current critique of global mental health emphasizes the importance of social structural processes in determining health and illness (Kirmayer & Pedersen, 2014). This emphasis requires rethinking the nature of mental health problems in terms of the environments in which we live, and points toward the need for political and economic change to directly reduce inequality. Psychiatry can contribute by identifying the impacts of inequality on mental health and the beneficial effects of more equitable social arrangements on both local and global scales. The movements for recovery and for person-centered medicine represent potential organized resistance to the market-driven, neoliberal logic that pervades mental health research, policy, and service delivery (Slade et al., 2014). Even global public health interventions that aim to address the larger social determinants of health affecting groups, communities, or whole populations can benefit from adopting an ethic that is people- and person-centered (Cloninger et al., 2014).

Conclusion: An Ecosocial View for Psychiatry

Taken together, the contributions to this volume and the work touched on in this conclusion point toward the importance of elaborating a dynamic ecosocial view of mental health and illness. This approach would be ecological in that it understands humans as deeply embedded in and interdependent with their environment, occupying specific niches in local worlds. The approach is social in that the local world is both constructed by and constituted of other human beings and cooperative institutions. On analogy to the study of ecosystems, this social context has its own dynamics, which can be self-sustaining and adapt to perturbations, but can also develop its own pathologies.

A key lesson of dynamical systems theory is that even simple systems can show exquisite sensitivity to initial conditions or boundary values, limiting the ability of any model to predict outcomes (Mitchell, 2009). In the case of the complex systems that underlie human behavior and psychopathology – which occur at the levels of genome, brain, and social world – these initial conditions include the individual's developmental history. In general, this means that we cannot understand the causes and course of psychopathology with any specificity without knowing a great deal about the developmental trajectory and contexts of behavior. Of course, some forms of pathology may turn out to be more predictable precisely because they are constrained in particular ways. For example, they may represent a final common pathway constrained by the structures of a limited behavioral repertoire; they might reflect environmental constraints that allow, select for, or support only certain modes of adaptation; or they may be imposed from the "top down" to the extent that behavior is governed by particular cognitive schemas, templates, goals, or plans that we strive to adhere to.

This imposition of top-down control by an individual's plans and intentions or by social norms and expectations is crucial to understanding human behavior. Human systems have both dynamical and linguistic modes (Pattee, 1977). We are self-describing beings who are partly governed by our own self-descriptions expressed in images, metaphors, narratives, and scripts which are partly self-descriptions but largely produced by others and transmitted through social institutions and practices that are ready-to-hand and that shape our experience, self-understanding, and opportunities for action. In the end, complex systems theory points to the importance of understanding human behavior in terms of individual biography and social context – ways of knowing central to literature, the arts, and humanities. If we want a more precise understanding of an individual's behavior, pathology, illness trajectory, or treatment outcomes, therefore, we will usually need much information about personal history and social context. Because we are narrative beings – constituted in essential ways by the stories we enact, which draw their meaning from the social contexts we inhabit – psychiatry must remain a practice that bridges understandings of behavior in terms of both biosocial mechanisms and the cultural-historical narratives that frame human action and experience (Glover, 2014; Hamkins, 2013; Kleinman, 1988; Lewis, 2011). Further, psychiatrists must also engage the larger social and cultural meanings of patients' narratives – and of psychiatric models of illness and healing – to appreciate their power, consequences, and constraints.

The ecosocial systems view has implications for psychiatric theory, research, policy, and practice. Theoretically, the person is seen as part of larger networks and looping processes, so that understanding mental health problems requires considering multiple levels. Research must also address these multiple levels and must consider how different components, isolated for study, interact to give rise to the complex phenomena of psychiatric conditions. No single level of analysis for studying brain and behavior can be privileged a priori since problems can potentially occur at any level in the hierarchy from molecular biology to society. Similarly, interventions may operate at many levels (Figure 24.4). Even when an intervention is designed to work at one level, it will usually have effects at many levels, which may reinforce or undermine the benefit or have other unintended consequences. Hence, an analysis of the impact of an intervention and its potential tradeoffs at multiple levels is essential.

Phenomenology remains important for psychiatric practice because it focuses on how people experience, understand, and describe their suffering. The configuration of experience, which inevitably includes elements of self-understanding, structures individuals' responses to illness, including coping and help-seeking. Close attention to the quality and structure of illness experience therefore constitutes an essential bridge between sufferer and helper – a platform for mutual understanding and for organizing meaningful interventions.

Clinically applied neuroscience provides a set of models and metaphors for explaining aspects of illness experience and a rough guide for the use of pharmacological treatments (Griffith, 2014; Zorumski & Rubin, 2011). At present, these models provide only crude rules of thumb for clinical decisions, which remain largely matters of trial and error. No matter how refined it becomes in the years to come, though, it is likely that neuroscience will always yield only a partial guide to

MODE OF HEALING	LEVEL OF ORGANIZATION	MEDIATING PROCESS
Social or political activism, religious or spiritual engagement	**Society**	Changing relationship to environment, political system & spiritual order
Communal & religious ritual Social network interventions	**Community** Meaning & Morale	Creating & restoring order of community & collective identity
Family ritual or therapy	**Family System**	Change in structure or rules of interaction
Cognitive-behavior therapy, Insight-oriented (psychodynamic or existential) psychotherapy	**Cortical Networks** Cognition	Insight, cognitive restructuring, metaphoric transformation, dissociation Catharsis
Relationship ("supportive") psychotherapy	**Limbic System** Motivation & emotion	Attachment, bonding, soothing & social support
Touch, massage, sensory reduction, environmental manipulation	**Brainstem** Regulation of autonomic function, arousal, & pain systems	Endogenous pain control mechanisms, habituation, conditioning

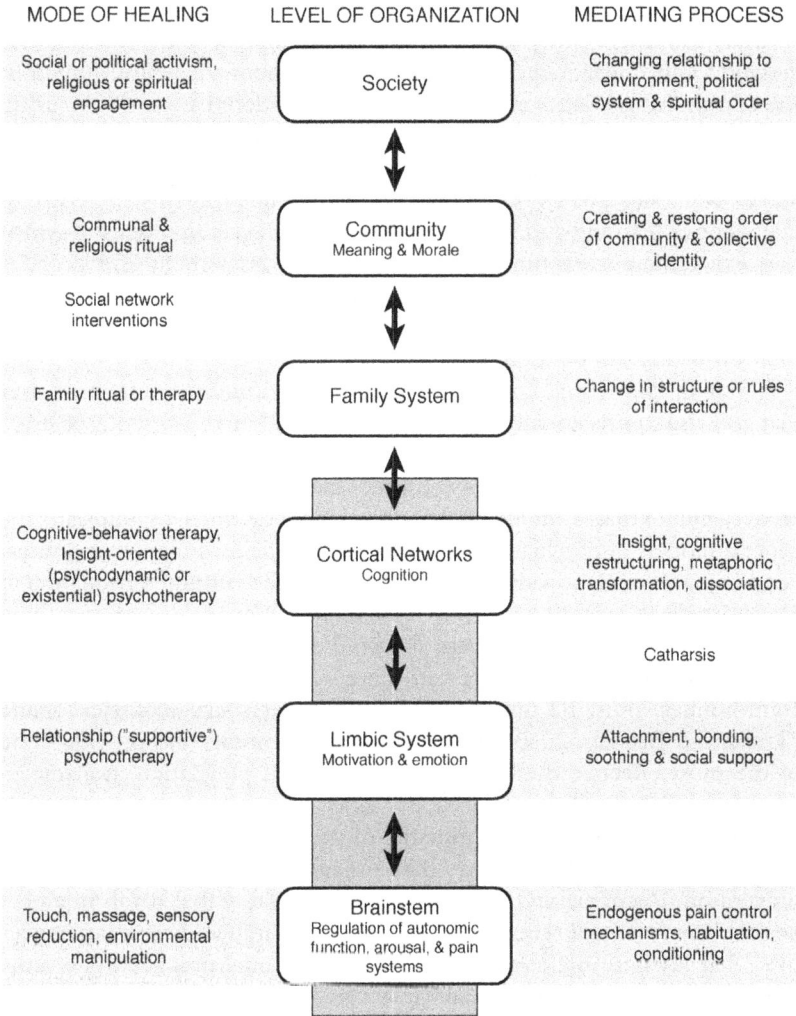

Figure 24.4. Levels of intervention in mental health problems. Treatment interventions and mental health promotion can occur at many levels, represented schematically here as levels of organization within the brain, and in the social world. Although particular kinds of intervention may target specific levels, any intervention will have effects at multiple levels. Hence, conceptualizing any treatment as a multilevel, systemic intervention will allow the clinician to identify complementary strategies to reinforce its effect and anticipate potential wider ramifications. This requires knowledge of the dynamics at each level and how they may work together synergistically or in ways that conflict and require thinking through potential tradeoffs between psychological and social benefits and costs. Adapted from L. J. Kirmayer, "The Cultural Diversity of Healing: Meaning, Metaphor and Mechanism," *British Medical Journal*, 2004, *69*(1), 33–48, by permission of Oxford University Press.

assessment and treatment. Other contextual factors at the level of individuals' learning history and current social context will influence the meaning and consequences of any given alteration in neural function. All of this history and context must be considered even when using medication to ameliorate symptoms. Moreover, the neural level of explanation and intervention cannot cover the whole of psychiatry (Kirmayer & Crafa, 2014). Ways of understanding problems in terms of maladaptive learning and social contingencies that set up cycles of symptom exacerbation are fundamental to clinical assessment and broader intervention planning (Hofmann, 2014). These are relevant to all patients, regardless of whether any specific neurobiological aspect to their problems can be identified.

Although the neural, cognitive-emotional, and interpersonal processes that give rise to psychopathology can be described in a sufficiently abstract way to be applied across cultures, in any given instance they reflect specific details of the person's life history, cultural background, and social context. Hence, contextual framing of the problem is essential to translate the general models of psychiatric theory into a specific formulation and intervention plan for an individual. Frameworks like the cultural formulation in *DSM-5* reflect current efforts to systematize the process of including context in psychiatric assessment (Lewis-Fernández et al., 2014). Interventions, too, whether delivered in the clinic to individuals or to whole communities, must be understood in a broader social-ecological frame (Trickett, & Beehler, 2013). Psychosocial interventions may provide some of the most effective methods of treatment and prevention available to psychiatry (Priebe, Omar, Giacco, & Slade, 2014).

Identifying the social determinants of mental health is a central concern for any vision of psychiatry that aims to move beyond treatment to prevention. Recognizing the structures of inequality that result in global health disparities will require social science research and critical perspectives that lay bare the assumptions of conventional practice. The same broad systemic and contextual view can also inform psychiatry as a clinical practice that aims to meet individuals on their own terms and work with them to find effective ways to help and heal.

REFERENCES

Adolphs, R. (2009). The social brain: Neural basis of social knowledge. *Annual Review of Psychology, 60*, 693–716. http://dx.doi.org/10.1146/annurev.psych.60.110707.163514

Alivisatos, A. P., Chun, M., Church, G. M., Greenspan, R. J., Roukes, M. L., & Yuste, R. (2012). The brain activity map project and the challenge of

functional connectomics. *Neuron, 74*(6), 970–4. http://dx.doi.org/10.1016/j.
neuron.2012.06.006

Andreasen, N. C. (2007). *DSM* and the death of phenomenology in America:
An example of unintended consequences. *Schizophrenia Bulletin, 33*(1),
108–12. http://dx.doi.org/10.1093/schbul/sbl054

Angell, M. (2011, July 14). The illusions of psychiatry. *The New York Review of
Books, 58*, 12. Retrieved from http://www.nybooks.com/articles/archives/
2011/jul/14/illusions-of-psychiatry/

Applbaum, K. (2015). Solving global mental health as a delivery problem:
Toward a critical epistemology of the solution. In L. J. Kirmayer,
R. Lemelson, & C. A. Cummings (Eds.), *Re-visioning psychiatry: Cultural
phenomenology, critical neuroscience, and global mental health* (pp. 544–74).
New York, NY: Cambridge University Press.

Baron-Cohen, S. (1995). *Mindblindness*. Cambridge, MA: MIT Press.

Barrett, H. C., & Kurzban, R. (2006). Modularity in cognition: Framing the
debate. *Psychological Review, 113*(3), 628–47. http://dx.doi.org/10.1037/
0033-295X.113.3.628

Bateson, G. (1972). *Steps to an ecology of mind: Collected essays in anthropology,
psychiatry, evolution, and epistemology.* New York, NY: Ballantine.

Bateson, G. (1979). *Mind and nature: A necessary unity.* New York, NY: Dutton.

Bateson, M.C. (1972). *Our own metaphor: A personal account of a conference on the
effects of conscious purpose on human adaptation.* New York, NY: Knopf.

Bechtel, W. (2013). Network organization in health and disease: On being a
reductionist and a systems biologist too. *Pharmacopsychiatry, 46*(Suppl. 01),
S10–21. http://dx.doi.org/ 10.1055/s-0033-1337922

Bechtel, W., & Richardson, R. C. (2010). *Discovering complexity: Decomposition
and localization as strategies in scientific research.* Cambridge, MA: MIT Press.

Bedau, M. A., & Humphreys, P. (Eds.). (2008). *Emergence: Contemporary readings
in philosophy and science.* Cambridge, MA: MIT Press. http://dx.doi.org/
10.7551/mitpress/9780262026215.001.0001

Beels, C. C. (2002). Notes for a cultural history of family therapy. *Family Process,
41*(1), 67–82. http://dx.doi.org/10.1111/j.1545-5300.2002.40102000067.x

Bellah, R. N. (1985). *Habits of the heart: Individualism and commitment in
American life.* Berkeley: University of California Press.

Boogerd, F., Bruggeman, F. J., Hofmeyr, J. H. S., & Westerhoff, H. V. (Eds.).
(2007). *Systems biology: Philosophical foundations.* Amsterdam, The
Netherlands: Elsevier.

Bourque, F., & Cunsolo Willox, A. (2014). Climate change: The next challenge
for public mental health? *International Review of Psychiatry, 26*(4), 415–22.
http://dx.doi.org/10.3109/09540261.2014.925851

Bracken, P., Thomas, P., Timimi, S., Asen, E., Behr, G., Beuster, C., ... &
Yeomans, D. (2012). Psychiatry beyond the current paradigm. *The British
Journal of Psychiatry, 201*(6), 430–4. http://dx.doi.org/10.1192/bjp.
bp.112.109447

Byrge, L., Sporns, O., & Smith, L. B. (2014). Developmental process emerges
from extended brain–body–behavior networks. *Trends in Cognitive Sciences,
18*(8), 395–403. http://dx.doi.org/10.1016/j.tics.2014.04.010

Cacioppo, J. T., Cacioppo, S., Dulawa, S., & Palmer, A. A. (2014). Social neuroscience and its potential contribution to psychiatry. *World Psychiatry, 13*, 131–9. http://dx.doi.org/10.1002/wps.20118

Chemero, A. (2011). *Radical embodied cognitive science.* Cambridge, MA: MIT press.

Choudhury, S., & Slaby, J. (Eds.). (2011). *Critical neuroscience: A handbook of the social and cultural contexts of neuroscience.* Chichester, England: Wiley-Blackwell. http://dx.doi.org/10.1002/9781444343359

Chouinard, G., & Jones, B. D. (1980). Neuroleptic-induced supersensitivity psychosis: Clinical and pharmacologic characteristics. *American Journal of Psychiatry, 137*(1), 16–21. http://dx.doi.org/10.1176/ajp.137.1.16

Clark, A. (2013). Whatever next? Predictive brains, situated agents, and the future of cognitive science. *Behavioral and Brain Sciences, 36*(3), 181–204. http://dx.doi.org/10.1017/S0140525X12000477

Clark, A., & Chalmers, D. (1998). The extended mind. *Analysis, 58*(1), 7–19. http://dx.doi.org/10.1093/analys/58.1.7

Clarke, B., & Hansen, M. B. N. (2009). *Emergence and embodiment: New essays on second-order systems theory.* Durham, NC: Duke University Press. http://dx.doi.org/10.1215/9780822391388

Cloninger, C. R., Salvador-Carulla, L., Kirmayer, L. J., Schwartz, M. A., Appleyard, J., Goodwin, N., . . . Rawaf, S. & (2015). A time for action on health inequities: Foundations of the 2014 Geneva Declaration on Person- and People-centered Integrated Health Care for All. *International Journal of Person Centered Medicine, 4(2)*, 69–89.

Crossley, N. A., Mechelli, A., Vértes, P. E., Winton-Brown, T. T., Patel, A. X. Ginestet, C. E., . . . Bullmore, E. T. (2013). Cognitive relevance of the community structure of the human brain functional coactivation network. *Proceedings of the National Academy of Sciences of the United States of America, 110*(28), 111583–88. http://dx.doi.org/ 10.1073/pnas.1220826110

Crossley, N. A., Mechelli, A., Scott, J., Carletti, F., Fox, P. T., McGuire, P., & Bullmore, E. T. (2014). The hubs of the human connectome are generally implicated in the anatomy of brain disorders. *Brain, 137*(8), 2382–95. http://dx.doi.org/10.1093/brain/awu132

Cushman, P. (1995). *Constructing the self, constructing America: A cultural history of psychotherapy.* Boston, MA: Addison-Wesley.

Cuthbert, B. N. (2014). The RDoC framework: Facilitating transition from *ICD/DSM* to dimensional approaches that integrate neuroscience and psychopathology. *World Psychiatry, 13*(1), 28–35. http://dx.doi.org/10.1002/wps.20087

Davidson, E. H. (2010). *The regulatory genome: Gene regulatory networks in development and evolution.* New York, NY: Academic Press.

Dawson, M. R. (2013). *Mind, body, world: Foundations of cognitive science.* Edmonton, Canada: Athabasca University Press.

Duncan, L. E., Pollastri, A. R., & Smoller, J. W. (2014). Mind the gap: Why many geneticists and psychological scientists have discrepant views about gene–environment interaction (G× E) research. *American Psychologist, 69*(3), 249–68. http://dx.doi.org/10.1037/a0036320

Ecks, S. (2013). *Eating drugs: Psychopharmaceutical pluralism in India.* New York, NY: New York University Press.

Fava, G. A., & Offidani, E. (2011). The mechanisms of tolerance in antidepressant action. *Progress in Neuro-Psychopharmacology and Biological Psychiatry, 35*(7), 1593–1602. http://dx.doi.org/10.1016/j.pnpbp.2010.07.026

Friston, K. J., Stephan, K. E., Montague, R., & Dolan, R. J. (2014). Computational psychiatry: The brain as a phantastic organ. *The Lancet Psychiatry, 1*(2), 148–58. http://dx.doi.org/10.1016/S2215-0366(14)70275-5

Frith, C. D. (2007). The social brain? *Philosophical Transactions of the Royal Society B: Biological Sciences, 362*(1480), 671–8. http://dx.doi.org/10.1098/rstb.2006.2003

Fornito, A. & Bullmore, E. T. (2015). Connectomics: A new paradigm for understanding brain disease. *European Neuropsychopharmacology, 25*(5), 733–48. http://dx.doi.org/10.1016/j.euroneuro.2014.02.011

Fuchs, T., Breyer, T., & Mundt, C. (2014). *Karl Jaspers' philosophy and psychopathology.* New York, NY: Springer. http://dx.doi.org/10.1007/978-1-4614-8878-1

Gallagher, S. (2005). *How the body shapes the mind.* New York, NY: Clarendon Press. http://dx.doi.org/10.1093/0199271941.001.0001

Gallagher, S. (2013). The socially extended mind. *Cognitive Systems Research, 25,* 4–12. http://dx.doi.org/10.1016/j.cogsys.2013.03.008

Gibbs, R. W. (2006). *Embodiment and cognitive science.* New York, NY: Cambridge University Press.

Gottesman, I.I., & Gould, T.D. (2003). The endophenotype concept in psychiatry: Etymology and strategic intentions. *American Journal of Psychiatry, 160*(4), 636–45. http://dx.doi.org/10.1176/appi.ajp.160.4.636

Glover, J. (2014). *Alien landscapes?: Interpreting disordered minds.* Cambridge, MA: Harvard University Press. http://dx.doi.org/10.4159/harvard.9780674735743

Griffith, J. L. (2014). Neuroscience and humanistic psychiatry: A residency curriculum. *Academic Psychiatry, 38*(2), 177–84. http://dx.doi.org/10.1007/s40596-014-0063-5

Griffiths, P., & Stotz, K. (2013). *Genetics and philosophy: An introduction.* Cambridge, England: Cambridge University Press. http://dx.doi.org/10.1017/CBO9780511744082

Hacking, I. (1995). The looping effect of human kinds. In D. Sperber, D. Premack, & A. J. Premack (Eds.), *Causal cognition: A multidisciplinary debate* (pp. 351–83). Oxford, England: Oxford University Press.

Hacking, I. (1999). *The social construction of what?* Cambridge, MA: Harvard University Press.

Hacking, I. (2002). *Historical ontology.* Cambridge, MA: Harvard University Press.

Hacking, I. (2004). Between Michel Foucault and Erving Goffman: Between discourse in the abstract and face-to-face interaction. *Economy and Society, 33,* 277–302. http://dx.doi.org/ 10.1080/0308514042000225671

Hamkins, S. (2013). *The art of narrative psychiatry: Stories of strength and meaning.* New York, NY: Oxford University Press.

Harries-Jones, P. (1995). *A recursive vision: Ecological understanding and Gregory Bateson.* Toronto, Canada: University of Toronto Press.

Hebb, D. O. (1949). *The organization of behavior.* New York, NY: John Wiley & Sons.

Henningsen, P., & Kirmayer, L. J. (2000). Mind beyond the net: Implications of cognitive neuroscience for cultural psychiatry. *Transcultural Psychiatry, 37*(4), 467–94. http://dx.doi.org/10.1177/136346150003700401

Hinton, D. E., & Simon, N. M. (2015). Toward a cultural neuroscience of anxiety disorders: The multiplex model. In L. J. Kirmayer, R. Lemelson, & C. A. Cummings (Eds.), *Re-visioning psychiatry: Cultural phenomenology, critical neuroscience, and global mental health* (pp. 343–74). New York, NY: Cambridge University Press.

Hofmann, S. G. (2014). Toward a cognitive-behavioral classification system for mental disorders. *Behavior Therapy, 45,* 576–87. http://dx.doi.org/10.1016/j.beth.2014.03.001

Hohwy, J. (2013). *The predictive mind.* New York, NY: Oxford University Press. http://dx.doi.org/10.1093/acprof:oso/9780199682737.001.0001

Hutto, D. D., & Myin, E. (2013). *Radicalizing enactivism: Basic minds without content.* Cambridge, MA: MIT Press.

Insel, T. R., & Quirion, R. (2005). Psychiatry as a clinical neuroscience discipline. *JAMA, 294*(17), 2221–4. http://dx.doi.org/10.1001/jama.294.17.2221

Juarrero, A. (1999). *Dynamics in action: Intentional behavior as a complex system.* Cambridge, MA: MIT Press.

Kandel, E. R. (2001). The molecular biology of memory storage: A dialogue between genes and synapses. *Science, 294*(5544), 1030–8. http://dx.doi.org/10.1126/science.1067020

Kandel, E. R., Dudai, Y., & Mayford, M. R. (2014). The molecular and systems biology of memory. *Cell, 157*(1), 163–86. http://dx.doi.org/10.1016/j.cell.2014.03.001

Karmiloff-Smith, A. (2009). Nativism versus neuroconstructivism: rethinking the study of developmental disorders. *Developmental Psychology, 45*(1), 56–63. http://dx.doi.org/10.1037/a0014506

Kasser, T. (2002). *The high price of materialism.* Cambridge, MA: MIT Press.

Keller, E. F. (2010). *The mirage of a space between nature and nurture.* Durham, NC: Duke University Press. http://dx.doi.org/10.1215/9780822392811

Kellert, S. H. (1993). *In the wake of chaos: unpredictable order in dynamical systems.* Chicago, IL: University of Chicago Press. http://dx.doi.org/10.7208/chicago/9780226429823.001.0001

Kendler, K. S. (2012a). Levels of explanation in psychiatric and substance use disorders: Implications for the development of an etiologically based nosology. *Molecular Psychiatry, 17*(1), 11–21. http://dx.doi.org/10.1038/mp.2011.70

Kendler, K. S. (2012b). The dappled nature of causes of psychiatric illness: Replacing the organic-functional/hardware-software dichotomy with empirically based pluralism. *Molecular Psychiatry, 17*(4), 377–88. http://dx.doi.org/10.1038/mp.2011.182

Kendler, K. S. (2014). The structure of psychiatric science. *American Journal of Psychiatry, 171*, 931–8. http://dx.doi.org/10.1176/appi.ajp.2014.13111539

Kendler, K. S., & Neale, M. C. (2010). Endophenotype: A conceptual analysis. *Molecular Psychiatry, 15*(8), 789–97. http://dx.doi.org/10.1038/mp.2010.8

Kennedy, D. P., & Adolphs, R. (2012). The social brain in psychiatric and neurological disorders. *Trends in Cognitive Sciences, 16*(11), 559–72. http://dx.doi.org/10.1016/j.tics.2012.09.006

Kirmayer, L. J. (2004). The cultural diversity of healing: Meaning, metaphor and mechanism. *British Medical Bulletin, 69*, 33–48. http://dx.doi.org/10.1093/bmb/ldh006

Kirmayer, L. J. (2008). Culture and the metaphoric mediation of pain. *Transcultural Psychiatry, 45*(2), 318–38. http://dx.doi.org/10.1177/1363461508089769

Kirmayer, L. J. (2009). Nightmares, neurophenomenology and the cultural logic of trauma. *Culture, Medicine, and Psychiatry, 33*(2), 323–31. http://dx.doi.org/10.1007/s11013-009-9136-4

Kirmayer, L. J. (2012). The future of critical neuroscience. In S. Choudhury & J. Slaby (Eds.), *Critical Neuroscience: A Handbook of the Social and Cultural Contexts of Neuroscience* (pp. 367–83). Chichester, England: Wiley-Blackwell.

Kirmayer, L. J., & Bhugra, D. (2009). Culture and mental illness: Social context and explanatory models. In I. M. Salloum & J. E. Mezzich (Eds.), *Psychiatric diagnosis: Patterns and prospects* (pp. 29–37). New York, NY: Wiley. http://dx.doi.org/10.1002/9780470743485.ch3

Kirmayer, L. J., & Crafa, D. (2014). What kind of science for psychiatry? *Frontiers in Human Neuroscience, 8*, 435. http://dx.doi.org/ 10.3389/fnhum.2014.00435

Kirmayer, L. J., & Gold, I. (2012). Re-socializing psychiatry: Critical neuroscience and the limits of reductionism. In S. Choudhury & J. Slaby (Eds.), *Critical neuroscience: A handbook of the social and cultural contexts of neuroscience* (pp. 307–30). Oxford, England: Blackwell.

Kirmayer, L. J., & Pedersen, D. (2014). Toward a new architecture for global mental health. *Transcultural Psychiatry, 51*(6), 759–76. http://dx.doi.org/10.1177/1363461514557202

Kirmayer, L.J., Raikhel, E., & Rahimi, S. (2013). Cultures of the Internet: Identity. Community, and mental health. *Transcultural Psychiatry, 50*(2), 165–91. http://dx.doi.org/10.1177/1363461513490626

Kirmayer, L. J., & Sartorius, N. (2009). Cultural models and somatic syndromes. In J. E. Dimsdale, V. Patel, Y. Xin, A. Kleinman, P. J. Sirovatka, & D. A. Regier (Eds.), *Somatic presentations of mental disorders: Refining the research agenda for "DSM-V"* (pp. 23–46). Washington, DC: American Psychiatric Press.

Kitanaka, J. (2012). *Depression in Japan: Psychiatric cures for a society in distress.* Princeton, NJ: Princeton University Press.

Kitano, H. (2002). Systems biology: a brief overview. *Science, 295*(5560), 1662–4. http://dx.doi.org/10.1126/science.1069492

Kleinman, A. (1986). *Social origins of distress and disease: Depression, neurasthenia, and pain in Modern China.* New Haven, CT: Yale University Press.

Kleinman, A. (1988). *The illness narratives*. New York, NY: Basic Books.

Labonté, B., Farah, A., & Turecki, G. (2015). Early-life adversity and epigenetic changes: Implications for understanding suicide. In L. J. Kirmayer, R. Lemelson, & C. A. Cummings (Eds.), *Re-visioning psychiatry: Cultural phenomenology, critical neuroscience, and global mental health* (pp. 206–35). New York, NY: Cambridge University Press.

Labonté, R., Mohindra, K., & Schrecker, T. (2011). The growing impact of globalization for health and public health practice. *Annual Review of Public Health, 32*, 263–83. http://dx.doi.org/10.1146/annurev-publhealth-031210-101225

Larøi, F., Luhrmann, T. M., Bell, V., Christian, W. A., Deshpande, S., Fernyhough, C...Woods, A. (2014). Culture and hallucinations: Overview and future directions. *Schizophrenia Bulletin, 40*(Suppl. 4), S213–20. http://dx.doi.org/10.1093/schbul/sbu012

Lende, D. H., & Downey, G. (Eds.). (2012). *The encultured brain: An introduction to neuroanthropology*. Cambridge, MA: MIT Press.

Lewis, B. (2011). *Narrative psychiatry: How stories can shape clinical practice*. Baltimore, MD: Johns Hopkins University Press.

Lewis-Fernández, R., Aggarwal, N. K., Bäärnhielm, S., Rohlof, H., Kirmayer, L. J., Weiss, M. G., ... & Lu, F. (2014). Culture and psychiatric evaluation: Operationalizing cultural formulation for *DSM-5*. *Psychiatry: Interpersonal and Biological Processes, 77*(2), 130–54. http://dx.doi.org/10.1521/psyc.2014.77.2.130

Lexchin, J. (2012). Those who have the gold make the evidence: How the pharmaceutical industry biases the outcomes of clinical trials of medications. *Science Engineering Ethics, 18*(2), 247–61. http://dx.doi.org/10.1007/s11948-011-9265-3

Maheu, L., & Macdonald, R. A. (Eds.). (2011). *Challenging genetic determinism: New perspectives on the gene in its multiple environments*. Montreal, Canada: McGill-Queen's Press.

Mainzer, K. (2004). *Thinking in complexity: The computational dynamics of matter, mind, and mankind*. New York, NY: Springer. http://dx.doi.org/10.1007/978-3-662-05364-5

Malabou, C. (2008). *What should we do with our brain?* (S. Rand, Trans.). New York, NY: Fordham.

Maturana, H. R., & Varela, F. J. (1987). *The tree of knowledge: The biological roots of human understanding*. Boston, MA: Shambhala Publications.

McCulloch, W. S. (1988). *Embodiments of mind*. Cambridge, MA: MIT Press. (Original work published 1965)

McKenzie, J., & Shah, J. (2015). Understanding the social etiology of psychosis. In L. J. Kirmayer, R. Lemelson, & C. A. Cummings (Eds.), *Re-visioning psychiatry: Cultural phenomenology, critical neuroscience, and global mental health* (pp. 317–42). New York, NY: Cambridge University Press.

Meloni, M. (2014). The social brain meets the reactive genome: Neuroscience, epigenetics and the new social biology. *Frontiers in Human Neuroscience, 8*, 309. http://dx.doi.org/10.3389/fnhum.2014.00309

Menary, R. (Ed.) (2010). *The extended mind*. Cambridge, MA: MIT Press. http://dx.doi.org/10.7551/mitpress/9780262014038.001.0001c

Mezzich, J. E., Salloum, I. M., Cloninger, C. R., Salvador-Carulla, L., Kirmayer, L. J., Banzato, C. E. M., . . . Botbol, M. (2010). Person-centered Integrative Diagnosis: Conceptual basis and structural model. *Canadian Journal of Psychiatry, 55*(11), 701–8.

Miller, G. A., Galanter, E., & Pribram, K. H. (1960). *Plans and the structure of behavior*. New York, NY: Holt, Rinehart and Winston. http://dx.doi.org/10.1037/10039-000

Miller, J. H., & Page, S. E. (2009). *Complex adaptive systems: An introduction to computational models of social life: An introduction to computational models of social life*. Princeton, NJ: Princeton University Press. http://dx.doi.org/10.1515/9781400835522

Mills, C. (2014). *Decolonizing global mental health: The psychiatrization of the majority world*. New York, NY: Routledge.

Mitchell, S. D. (2009). *Unsimple truths: Science, complexity, and policy*. Chicago, IL: University of Chicago Press. http://dx.doi.org/10.7208/chicago/9780226532653.001.0001

Moncrieff, J. (2006). Does antipsychotic withdrawal provoke psychosis? Review of the literature on rapid onset psychosis (supersensitivity psychosis) and withdrawal-related relapse. *Acta Psychiatrica Scandinavica, 114*(1), 3–13. http://dx.doi.org/10.1111/j.1600-0447.2006.00787.x

Newman, M. (2010). *Networks: An introduction*. New York, NY: Oxford University Press. http://dx.doi.org/10.1093/acprof:oso/9780199206650.001.0001

Northoff, G. (2013). What is culture? Culture is context-dependence! *Culture and Brain, 1*(2–4), 77–99. http://dx.doi.org/10.1007/s40167-013-0008-y

Northoff, G. (2015). How the self is altered in psychiatric disorders: A neurophenomenal approach. In L. J. Kirmayer, R. Lemelson, & C. A. Cummings (Eds.), *Re-visioning psychiatry: Cultural phenomenology, critical neuroscience, and global mental health* (pp. 81–116). New York, NY: Cambridge University Press.

Oyama, S., Griffiths, P. E., & Gray, R. D. (Eds.). (2003). *Cycles of contingency: Developmental systems and evolution*. Cambridge, MA: MIT Press.

Panksepp, J., & Biven, L. (2012). *The archaeology of mind: Neuroevolutionary origins of human emotions*. New York, NY: Norton.

Parnas, J., Sass, L. A., & Zahavi, D. (2012). Rediscovering psychopathology: The epistemology and phenomenology of the psychiatric object. *Schizophrenia Bulletin, 39*(2), 270–7. http://dx.doi.org/10.1093/schbul/sbs153

Pattee, H. H. (1977). Dynamic and linguistic modes of complex systems. *International Journal of General Systems, 3*(4), 259–66. http://dx.doi.org/10.1080/03081077708934771

Pavão, R., Tort, A. B. L., & Amaral, O. B. (2014). Multifactoriality in psychiatric disorders: A computational study of schizophrenia. *Schizophrenia Bulletin*. http://dx.doi.org/10.1093/schbul/sbu146

Pickering, A. (2010). *The cybernetic brain: Sketches of another future*. Chicago, IL: University of Chicago Press. http://dx.doi.org/10.7208/chicago/9780226667928.001.0001

Priebe, S., Omer, S., Giacco, D., & Slade, M. (2014). Resource-oriented therapeutic models in psychiatry: conceptual review. *British Journal of Psychiatry, 204*(4), 256–61. http://dx.doi.org/10.1192/bjp.bp.113.135038

Ramachandran, V. S., & Hirstein, W. (1998). The perception of phantom limbs. The DO Hebb lecture. *Brain, 121*(9), 1603–30. http://dx.doi.org/10.1093/brain/121.9.1603

Ratcliffe, M. (2012). Phenomenology as a form of empathy. *Inquiry, 55*(5), 473–95. http://dx.doi.org/10.1080/0020174X.2012.716196

Ratcliffe, M. (2014). *Experiences of depression: A study in phenomenology.* Oxford, England: Oxford University Press.

Remington, G., Foussias, G., Agid, O., Fervaha, G., Takeuchi, H., & Hahn, M. (2014). The neurobiology of relapse in schizophrenia. *Schizophrenia Research, 152*(2), 381–90. http://dx.doi.org/10.1016/j.schres.2013.10.009

Rorty, R. (2004). The brain as hardware, culture as software. *Inquiry, 47*(3), 219–35. http://dx.doi.org/10.1080/00201740410006348

Rose, N. S., & Abi-Rached, J. M. (2013). *Neuro: The new brain sciences and the management of the mind.* Princeton, NJ: Princeton University Press.

Rowlands, M. (2010). *The new science of the mind: From extended mind to embodied phenomenology.* Cambridge, MA: MIT Press. http://dx.doi.org/10.7551/mitpress/9780262014557.001.0001

Ruckert, A., & Labonté, R. (2014). The global financial crisis and health equity: Early experiences from Canada. *Globalization and Health, 10*(1), 2. http://dx.doi.org/10.1186/1744-8603-10-2

Ryder, A. G., & Chentsova-Dutton, Y. E. (2015). Cultural clinical psychology: From cultural scripts to contextualized treatments. In L. J. Kirmayer, R. Lemelson, & C. A. Cummings (Eds.), *Re-visioning psychiatry: Cultural phenomenology, critical neuroscience, and global mental health* (pp. 400–33). New York, NY: Cambridge University Press.

Sadler, J. Z. (2013). Considering the economy of *DSM* alternatives. In J. Paris & J. Phillips (Eds.), *Making the "DSM-5"* (pp. 21–38). New York, NY: Springer. http://dx.doi.org/10.1007/978-1-4614-6504-1_2

Schizophrenia Working Group of the Psychiatric Genomics Consortium. (2014). Biological insights from 108 schizophrenia-associated genetic loci. *Nature, 511*, 421–7. http://dx.doi.org/10.1038/nature13595

Scott, A. (2007). *The nonlinear universe: Chaos, emergence, life.* New York, NY: Springer.

Seeman, M. V., & Seeman, P. (2014). Is schizophrenia a dopamine supersensitivity psychotic reaction? *Progress in Neuro-Psychopharmacology and Biological Psychiatry, 48*, 155–60. http://dx.doi.org/10.1016/j.pnpbp.2013.10.003

Seligman, R., Choudhury, S. & Kirmayer, L. J. (forthcoming). Locating culture in the brain and in the world: From social categories to the ecology of mind. In J. Chiao, S.-C. Li, R. Seligman, & R. Turner (Eds.), *Handbook of cultural neuroscience,* New York, NY: Oxford University Press.

Semin, G. R., & Smith, E. R. (2008). *Embodied grounding: Social, cognitive, affective, and neuroscientific approaches.* New York, NY: Cambridge University Press. http://dx.doi.org/10.1017/CBO9780511805837

Shapiro, L. A. (2011). *Embodied cognition.* London, England: Routledge. http://dx.doi.org/10.1016/j.nlm.2004.06.005

Silberstein, M. (2012). Emergence and reduction in context: Philosophy of science and/or analytic metaphysics. *Metascience, 21*(3), 627–42. http://dx.doi.org/10.1007/s11016-012-9671-4

Slade, M., Amering, M., Farkas, M., Hamilton, B., O'Hagan, M., Panther, G., ... & Whitley, R. (2014). Uses and abuses of recovery: implementing recovery-oriented practices in mental health systems. *World Psychiatry*, *13*(1), 12–20. http://dx.doi.org/10.1002/wps.20084

Sporns, O. (2012). *Discovering the human connectome*. Cambridge, MA: MIT Press.

Sporns, O., Honey, C. J., & Kotter, R. (2005). The human connectome: A structural description of the human brain. *PLOS Computational Biology*, *1*, e42. http://dx.doi.org/10.1371/journal.pcbi.0010042

Squire, L. R. (2004). Memory systems of the brain: A brief history and current perspective. *Neurobiology of Learning and Memory*, *82*(3), 171–7. http://dx.doi.org/10.1016/j.nlm.2004.06.005

Stanghellini, G., Bolton, D., & Fulford, W. K. (2013). Person-centered psychopathology of schizophrenia: Building on Karl Jaspers' understanding of patient's attitude toward his illness. *Schizophrenia Bulletin*, *39*(2), 287–94. http://dx.doi.org/10.1093/schbul/sbs154

Stanghellini, G., & Fuchs, T. (Eds.). (2013). *One century of Karl Jaspers' general psychopathology*. New York, NY: Oxford University Press.

Stewart, J. R., Gapenne, O., & Di Paolo, E. A. (Eds.). (2010). *Enaction: Toward a new paradigm for cognitive science*. Cambridge, MA: MIT Press. http://dx.doi.org/10.7551/mitpress/9780262014601.001.0001

Sutton, J. (2010). Exograms and interdisciplinarity: History, the extended mind, and the civilizing process. In: Menary, R. (Ed.) *The extended mind* (pp. 189–225). Cambridge, MA: MIT Press. http://dx.doi.org/10.7551/mitpress/9780262014038.003.0009

Thompson, E. (2007). *Mind in life: Biology, phenomenology, and the sciences of mind*. Cambridge, MA: Harvard University Press.

Tomasello, M. (2014). *A natural history of human thinking*. Cambridge, MA: Harvard University Press.

Trickett, E. J., & Beehler, S. (2013). The ecology of multilevel interventions to reduce social inequalities in health. *American Behavioral Scientist*, *57*(8), 1227–46. http://dx.doi.org/10.1177/0002764213487342

van den Heuvel, M. P., Kahn, R. S., Goni, J., & Sporns, O. (2012). High-cost, high-capacity backbone for global brain communication. *Proceedings of the National Academy of Sciences of the United States of America*, *109*, 11372–7. http://dx.doi.org/ 10.1073/pnas.1203593109

van Os, J., Lataster, T., Delespaul, P., Wichers, M., & Myin-Germeys, I. (2014). Evidence that a psychopathology interactome has diagnostic value, predicting clinical needs: An experience sampling study. *PloS One*, *9*(1), e86652. http://dx.doi.org/10.1371/journal.pone.0086652

Varela, F. J. (1996). Neurophenomenology: A methodological remedy for the hard problem. *Journal of Consciousness Studies*, *3*(4), 330–49.

Varela, F. J., Thompson, E., & Rosch, E. (1991). *The embodied mind: Cognitive science and human experience*. Cambridge, MA: MIT Press.

Vidal, F. (2009). Brainhood, anthropological figure of modernity. *History of the Human Sciences*, *22*(1), 5–36. http://dx.doi.org/10.1177/0952695108099133

von Neumann, J. (1958). *The computer and the brain*. New Haven, CT: Yale University Press.

Watzlawick, P., Beavin, J., & Jackson, D. D. (1967). *Pragmatics of human communication*. New York, NY: Random House.

Wexler, B. E. (2006). *Brain and culture: Neurobiology, ideology, and social change*. Cambridge, MA: MIT Press.

Whitley, R. (2014). Beyond critique: Rethinking roles for the anthropology of mental health. *Culture, Medicine, and Psychiatry, 38*(3), 499–511. http://dx.doi.org/10.1007/s11013-014-9382-y

Wiener, N. (1961). *Cybernetics, or control and communication in the animal and the machine* (2nd ed.). Cambridge, MA: MIT Press. http://dx.doi.org/10.1037/13140-000

Wolfram, S. (2002). *A new kind of science*. Champaign, IL: Wolfram Media.

Woods, A., Jones, N., Bernini, M., Callard, F., Alderson-Day, B., Badcock, J. C., ... & Fernyhough, C. (2014). Interdisciplinary approaches to the phenomenology of auditory verbal hallucinations. *Schizophrenia Bulletin, 40* (Suppl. 4), s246–54. http://dx.doi.org/10.1093/schbul/sbu003

Yates, F. A. (1992). *The art of memory*. New York, NY: Random House.

Zaretsky, E. (2004). *Secrets of the soul: A social and cultural history of psychoanalysis*. New York, NY: Knopf.

Zorumski, C., & Rubin, E. (2011). *Psychiatry and clinical neuroscience*. New York, NY: Oxford University Press. http://dx.doi.org/10.1093/med/9780199768769.001.1

Index

prodromes, schizophrenia, 10
Programme for Improving of Mental Health
    Care (PRIME), 599
projection, empathy vs., 155
promoters, 209
proopiomelanocortin (POMC), 212–13,
    215, 221
propositional signals, 76
proteome, mechanistic links, 196
protocol-statements, 67
prototype-gestalt, 74–5
prototypes, 73, 77
prototypical mental disorders, 181
Prozac (fluoxetine), 547, 555–6, 562
pseudo-hallucinations, 452
pseudo-mutuality, 155
psychiatric categories, Western vs.
    non-Western, 583
psychiatric conditions, variability in
    expression, 632
psychiatric diagnoses, 643–4
psychiatric drugs, unregulated
    dissemination, 551
psychiatric objects, 65–6, 72
psychiatric syndromes, organic vs.
    functional, 188
psychiatrists by population, 601
psychiatry
    biological, 46
    critical, 1
    colonial, 161
    cultural, 576
    ecosocial approach, 3, 13, 638, 641,
        647–50
    future of, 3, 194–7, 260–1, 478
    history, 6–11, 44–6
    hybrid nature, 15, 43
    narrative, 41–2, 46, 60
    neurophenomenal approach, 15
    nosology, 4–7, 11–12, 24, 28, 382,
        434–8, 440, 444, 456–461, 495, 516,
        519, 522, 534, 553, 643, 644
    person-centered, 3, 15, 23–4, 68, 485,
        506, 598, 646
    phenomenological approach, 15
psychoactive substances, interpretation of
    sensation, 385, 387, 389
psychoanalysis, 119, 305, 623
psychodynamic theories, 154–5
psychoeducation, 584, 587
psychological safety valves, 352
psychological self, 622
psychometric approaches, bias, 187
psychopathology
    aCMS, 104

    cultural variation, 435–6
    developing interventions, 334–5
    dimensional approach, 181
    ecological-level social factors, 327
    empathy and, 152–5
    individual and social-level interaction,
        327–8
    individual-level social factors, 326–7
    integrative conceptual framework,
        326–9
    phenomenology, 434–5
    task-induced deactivation, 104
    taxonomies and research, 182–3
    time, 328–9
psychopharmaceuticals
    branding, 552, 560–5
    delivery, 546
    economics, 646
    globalization, 551
    LMIC trials, 550
    marketing, 503, 560–2, 562–3
    research funding, 66
    social exclusion, 558
psychopharmacological societies, 565
psychosis
    daily hassles, 322
    definition of, 152
    depression, 564
    experience, 152, 308–11
    fear of causing, 171
    not caused by culture, 493
    outside West, 310
    perceived discrimination and, 331–2
    RDoC approach, 311
    rebound, 633
    simulating, 153
    social factors, 318
    triggers, 494
    urban environment, 320, 324
    WHO incidence studies, 332
psychosocial looping processes, 641
psychosocial self, 622
psychostimulants, drug sales, 548
psychotherapy, 582, 584, 592
psychotic depression, 564
psychotic disorders, 189, 599
psychotropic medications, 172, 583, 615,
    617
PTSD (posttraumatic stress disorder),
    366–7
    Cambodian refugees, 344
    DNA methylation, 219
    dimensional, 186
    multiplex model, 343
    panic attacks, 346

Lightning Source UK Ltd.
Milton Keynes UK
UKOW01f0238020917
308446UK00010B/115/P